INSIGHTS IN GLOBAL HEALTH

A Compendium of Healthcare Facilities and Non-Profit Organizations

INSIGHTS IN GLOBAL HEALTH

A Compendium of Healthcare Facilities and Non-Profit Organizations

EDITED BY

Ebby Elahi, MD, MBA

CRC Press
Taylor & Francis Group
Boca Raton London New York

CRC Press is an imprint of the
Taylor & Francis Group, an **informa** business

First edition published 2021
by CRC Press
6000 Broken Sound Parkway NW, Suite 300, Boca Raton, FL 33487-2742

and by CRC Press
2 Park Square, Milton Park, Abingdon, Oxon, OX14 4RN

CRC Press is an imprint of Taylor & Francis Group, LLC

ISBN: 9780367693466(hbk)
ISBN: 9780367693190 (pbk)
ISBN: 9781003141440(ebk)

Contents

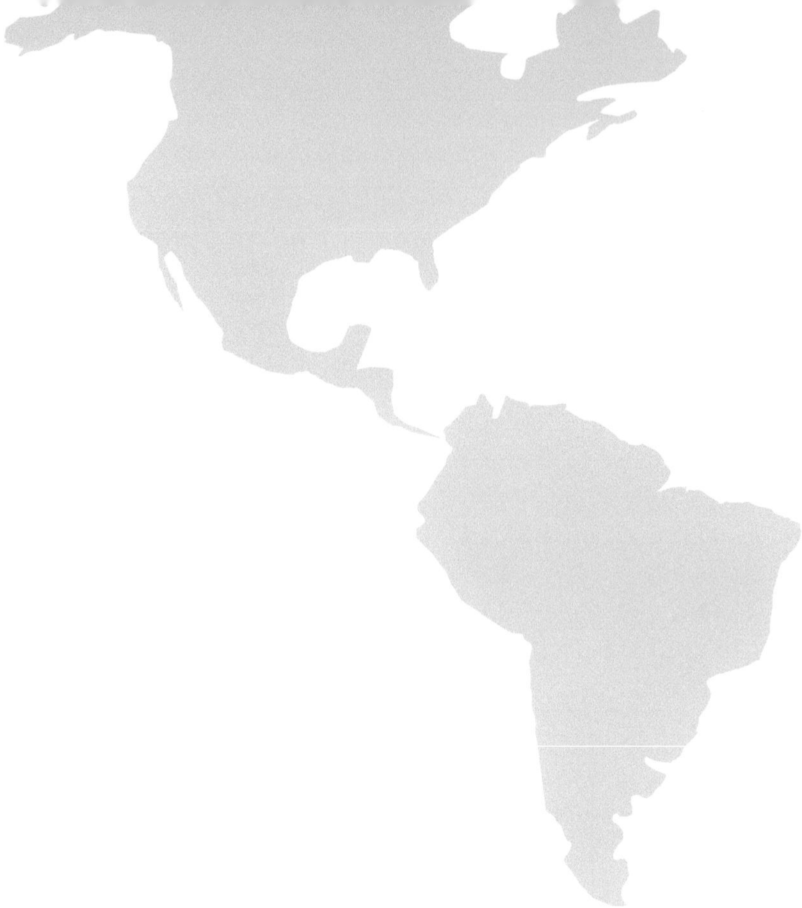

Preface

The journey that has led to this compendium began nearly two decades ago when a group of like-minded professionals came together to create the Virtue Foundation. Our idealism of wanting to serve those in need in resource-poor regions around the world was soon to be confronted with the challenging reality of making these interventions effective, ethical, and lasting. It was not long before I began questioning the long-term value of discrete missions and their potential harm on the communities they were intended to serve.

These concerns led me to reconsider the pursuit of short-term interventions in favor of complex but sustainable training programs overseas. Such efforts would require the cooperation of governments, international and national stakeholders, professionals, and philanthropists. Yet I was confronted time and again with seemingly insurmountable obstacles to effecting sustainable change in dynamic socio-political environments. As it soon became apparent, many long-term projects remained too heavily dependent on a complex set of factors to remain truly sustainable. Beyond the cacophony of well-intentioned voices calling for lasting change was an unsettling landscape dotted with graveyards of unfinished buildings and abandoned projects. Without such critical factors as a stable government, sustained economic support, personal security, protection from corruption, and community buy-in, even the most laudable philanthropic efforts would be destined to encounter insurmountable headwinds. Perhaps this explained the uneven presence of non-governmental organizations in well-known metropolitan centers despite rural and at times large population areas with greater need.

This concern was the core impetus behind the present compendium. Collaborating with a group of academics and professionals in fields ranging from healthcare and economics to data science and analytics, we thus sought ways to help optimize our interventions and engagements around the globe. To our great surprise, we found a dearth of practical resources to provide satisfactory answers to our questions. The search for solutions led us on a decade-long journey beginning with data mapping initiatives and culminating in the adoption of machine learning and artificial intelligence as a means to better define need and intervention opportunities worldwide. The ensuing outcome is the first-ever comprehensive compendium of healthcare facilities and nonprofits in low-income countries.

This book offers a fresh perspective on global health interventions. Philanthropic interventions need not conform to an all-or-nothing model whereby they are considered either *ineffective short-term neocolonial voluntourism*, or *complex, bureaucratic and inefficient undertakings marked by inertia and inflexibility*. By making data accessible, the information age promises customizable and targeted matching of needs and resources at the individual and organizational level, thereby reducing the inefficiencies that have historically plagued international healthcare philanthropy.

As a practicing physician for over two decades, I continue to believe that even a single life transformed reaffirms the inherent value of philanthropic medicine. Yet, by cooperating together and harnessing the power of data, we can exponentially expand our impact far beyond what any one individual can do alone. For me, this book is a testament to the power of collaboration in bringing about meaningful change.

Ebby Elahi

Editor Biography

Dr. Ebby Elahi is Clinical Professor of Ophthalmology, Otolaryngology and Public Health at the Icahn School of Medicine at Mount Sinai, and Director of Fifth Avenue Associates. An oculofacial surgeon, Dr. Elahi is a fellow of the American Academy of Ophthalmology, the American Society of Ophthalmic Plastic and Reconstructive Surgery, and past president of the New York Facial Plastic Surgery Society. Inducted into the Alpha Omega Alpha Medical Honor Society, he is actively involved in research and education, and holds several surgical device patents. He is the recipient of multiple awards for his academic teaching and contributions to the international community. Dr. Elahi completed his medical and postgraduate education at the Mount Sinai School of Medicine and earned his MBA from Columbia University.

For over twenty years, Dr. Elahi has been an advocate for issues surrounding global health and currently serves as Director of Global Affairs at the Virtue Foundation, an NGO in special consultative status to the United Nations Economic and Social Council.

Acknowledgments

Insights in Global Health is the product of a multi-year interdisciplinary collaboration. A deep debt of gratitude is owed to all those who have graciously given of their time, knowledge and wisdom in making this project become a reality, including, but not limited to: Dr. Joan LaRovere for sparing no effort and investing untold time on this compendium; Kim Azzarelli for her editorial leadership and unparalleled commitment to seeing this project to fruition; Anna Szczepanek for her selfless and tireless dedication to this project and exemplary work ethic; Nicolas Douard and Allen Nasseri for their thorough involvement and technical expertise; Dr. Omar Besbes for his enduring and sage role throughout as chief scientific advisor; Dr. Matthew Baker, Dr. Amine Allouah and Zidong Liu for their instrumental role in this project from its inception; and the litany of volunteers and physicians who provided invaluable input, especially Dr. Rosie Balfour-Lynn, Drs. Janak and Preeti Shah, Dr. Reza Yassari, Jared Dashevsky, Niki Elahi, Nysa Gandhi, and Hannah Oblak for going above and beyond in both time and effort. Of course, there is simply no way to individually acknowledge and thank the many selfless volunteers without whom this compendium would not become a reality. Lastly, the visionary leadership of Drs. Joseph Salim and Joan LaRovere at the Virtue Foundation merits special recognition.

Contributors

Eliza Abrams	Student/Researcher, Massachusetts General Hospital/Harvard Medical School	Volunteer
Ebrahim Afshinnekoo	Medical Student, New York Medical College	Volunteer
Amine Allouah, Ph.D.	Data Scientist, Columbia University	Volunteer
Adam Ammar, M.D.	Resident, Montefiore Medical Center/Albert Einstein College of Medicine, Department of Neurosurgery; Harvard Medical School, Program in Global Surgery and Social Change	Volunteer
Kimberly Ashayeri, M.D.	Resident, New York University, Department of Neurosurgery	Volunteer
Kim Azzarelli, J.D.	CEO, Seneca Women; Chair, Cornell Law School's Center for Women and Justice	Senior Advisor/Editor
Matthew Baker, Ph.D.	Associate Professor of Economics, CUNY Hunter	Advisor
Rosie Balfour-Lynn, MBBS BSc	Paediatric Trainee, North Thames Training Program, London, UK	Volunteer
Alexander Barash, M.D.	Ophthalmologist, New York Eye and Ear Infirmary of Mount Sinai	Volunteer
Joshua Benton	Medical Student, Albert Einstein College of Medicine	Volunteer
Omar Besbes, Ph.D.	Vikram S. Pandit Professor of Business, Columbia Business School	Advisor
Nitin Chopra, M.D., MBA	Resident, New York Eye and Ear Infirmary of Mount Sinai, Department of Ophthalmology	Volunteer
Jared Dashevsky	Medical Student, Icahn School of Medicine at Mount Sinai	Volunteer
Maria del Rio Sanin, M.S.	Service Designer and Project Manager, Barcelona, Spain	Volunteer
Nicolas Douard, M.S.	Data Scientist, Virtue Foundation	Virtue Foundation Staff

Murray Echt, M.D.	Resident, Montefiore Medical Center/Albert Einstein College of Medicine, Department of Neurosurgery	Volunteer
Niki Elahi, MPH	Student, Columbia University, School of Dental Medicine	Volunteer
Mattia Filiaci, Ph.D.	Director, Risk Management, Credit Suisse	Volunteer
Adison Fortunel, M.D.	Resident, Montefiore Medical Center/Albert Einstein College of Medicine, Department of Neurosurgery	Volunteer
Nysa Gandhi	Student, Roland Park Country School	Volunteer
Saadi Ghatan, M.D.	Associate Professor of Neurosurgery, Mount Sinai Health System	Volunteer
Yvonne Jones	Surgical Technician, Mount Sinai Medical Center	Volunteer
Ellen Kampinsky	Editorial Director, Seneca Women	Volunteer
Joan LaRovere, M.D., MSc, MBA	Assistant Professor of Pediatrics, Boston Children's Hospital/ Harvard Medical School	Contributor/Senior Editor
Michaela Leone	Data Scientist, Icahn School of Medicine	Volunteer
Zidong Liu	Data Scientist, University of Cambridge	Virtue Foundation Staff (former)
Michael Longo, M.D.	Resident, Vanderbilt University Medical Center, Department of Neurosurgery	Volunteer
Allen Nasseri, MBA	Product Manager, Virtue Foundation	Virtue Foundation Staff
Hannah Oblak	Research Intern, Yale University	Volunteer
Aleka Scoco, M.D.	Resident, Montefiore Medical Center/Albert Einstein College of Medicine, Department of Neurosurgery	Volunteer
Janak Shah, M.D.	Ophthalmologist, Netrapuja Research Centre/Netrapuja Eye Care	Volunteer
Preeti Shah, M.D.	Ophthalmologist, Netrapuja Research Centre/Netrapuja Eye Care	Volunteer
Noah Shohet	Office Administrator, Sea Surgery Center	Volunteer
Anna Szczepanek, M.S.	Program Director, Virtue Foundation	Virtue Foundation Staff/ Editor
Reza Yassari, M.D.	Professor of Neurosurgery, Montefiore Medical Center/Albert Einstein College of Medicine	Volunteer

Institutional Contributors

Columbia Business School

DataRobot

Dun & Bradstreet

Goldman Sachs Gives

Harvard University Center for Geographic Analysis

Icahn School of Medicine at Mount Sinai

Massachusetts Institute of Technology

Procter & Gamble

Wolfram Alpha

Specialty Abbreviations

Specialty	Abbreviation
Allergy and Immunology	All-Immu
Anesthesiology	Anesth
Cardiothoracic Surgery	CT Surg
Cardiovascular Medicine	CV Med
Critical Care Medicine	Crit-Care
Dentistry & Maxillofacial Surgery	Dent-OMFS
Dermatology	Derm
Emergency/Disaster Medicine	ER Med
Endocrinology	Endo
Family Medicine/General Practice	General
Gastroenterology	GI
Geriatric Medicine	Geri
Hematology & Oncology	Heme-Onc
Infectious & Tropical Diseases	Infect Dis
Internal Medicine	Medicine
Logistics and Operations	Logist-op
Maternal–Fetal Medicine	MF Med
Medical Genetics and Genomics	Genetics
Neonatology and Perinatology	Neonat
Nephrology	Nephro
Neurological Surgery	Neurosurg
Neurology	Neuro
Nutrition	Nutr
Ophthalmology/Optometry	Ophth-Opt
Orthopaedic Medicine & Surgery	Ortho
Otolaryngology	ENT
Palliative Medicine	Palliative
Pathology & Laboratory Medicine	Path
Pediatric Surgery	Ped Surg
Pediatrics	Peds
Physical Medicine and Rehabilitation	Rehab
Plastic Surgery	Plast
Podiatry	Pod
Psychiatry	Psych
Public Health	Pub Health
Pulmonology and Critical Care Medicine	Pulm-Critic
Radiation Oncology	Rad-Onc
Radiology & Nuclear Medicine	Radiol
Rheumatology	Rheum
Surgery	Surg
Urology	Urol
Vascular Surgery	Vasc Surg
Women's Health, Obstetrics and Gynecology	OB-GYN

Introduction

Today the global marketplace for delivery of targeted healthcare in resource-poor regions presents challenging barriers. That is to say, while human and capital resources available to care for underserved populations have increased, these resources remain unevenly distributed. The people and institutions that wish to deliver healthcare—volunteers, nonprofits, governments, the private sector—lack ready access to granular local data necessary to identify those most in need. **Insights in Global Health: A Compendium of Healthcare Facilities and Nonprofit Organizations** seeks to address this information asymmetry and thereby reduce the frictions that lead to inefficient delivery of services or disengagement.

Among the most comprehensive resources of its kind, *Insights in Global Health* presents a curated directory of nonprofits, non-governmental organizations (NGOs), hospitals, and healthcare facilities in 24 of the lowest-income countries as classified by the World Bank. Access to such data highlights areas that are underserved or in need of additional assistance. The content is classified by country and enhanced with custom maps and country overviews.

Insights in Global Health was born out of Virtue Foundation's considerable experience providing direct healthcare in resource-poor regions. For nearly 20 years, Virtue Foundation volunteers working in collaboration with local healthcare professionals have been providing surgical and medical services worldwide. During this time, much has been learned about the necessity for access to reliable targeted data as a means to provide efficient healthcare delivery.

Insights in Global Health is also an outgrowth of the *Virtue Foundation Actionable Data Initiative.* Harnessing advancements in technology and machine learning, the Foundation has created a first-of-its-kind mapping-and-matching global health platform for local nonprofits and healthcare organizations. This compendium represents the first product of this initiative, providing a curated view of demand-side data and enabling volunteer medical professionals, governments, and stakeholders to better identify where healthcare services are available and additional resources are needed. Each of the 24 chapters presents a brief country overview, a map depicting the locations of healthcare facilities, and a curated list of nonprofit organizations and healthcare facilities. QR codes associated with each listing link back to the web platform, providing access to further information about the organizations as well as the ability to interact with the data in a customizable manner.

Approach and Methodology

Nonprofit Data Collection and Curation

Using specific keywords and medical specialty descriptors, a pipeline for querying and identifying nonprofit websites was created for targeted regions. Forty-three separate medical specialties, 7 generic terms, and 4 nonprofit keywords were applied to produce a total of 5,076 unique query combinations and executed on various search engines and social media platforms. This resulted in 1,060,451 candidate nonprofit web pages that were subsequently indexed using custom crawlers built with open-source Python libraries as a distributed Spark application, running on parallel workers on Amazon Web Services. This list was complemented with known public resources, such as the United Nations database for NGOs.

A decision-tree script extracted the domains, deduplicated web pages, and created a recursive multilevel indexing tree, identifying 66,121 unique candidate nonprofit websites. Further data including contact information, donation links, and other metadata were captured using regular expressions and pattern matching techniques. To minimize the likelihood of collected websites not representing an actual healthcare nonprofit organization and to minimize noise, machine learning methods were employed to filter the data. A training set of 11,877 websites was thus manually labeled by the Virtue Foundation volunteer team. An auto-tuned word N-Gram text modeler using token occurrences, optimized for sensitivity over precision, achieved best performance on this training set. In addition to being able to predict whether or not a website represents a nonprofit, the classifier was also able to determine whether the organization's activities were concentrated on healthcare. The inference process applied to the 66,121 candidate websites returned 3,052 organizations as healthcare nonprofits. Predicting whether a nonprofit was involved in healthcare proved challenging as numerous healthcare-related websites belonging to educational organizations, publications, and for-profit entities have a high likelihood of being incorrectly classified as providing healthcare. Therefore, all 3,052 organizations underwent further manual review to establish legitimacy, identify healthcare services provided, confirm countries of activity, and find additional relevant information. At completion, the total number of nonprofit organizations was narrowed down to 1,610. Due to space constraints, only 1,070 nonprofit organizations were ultimately included in the book, based on their quality and relevance. The companion online platform provides a more comprehensive and regularly updated dataset.

Healthcare Facility Data Collection and Curation

Healthcare facility data was primarily sourced from the OpenStreetMap humanitarian data layer. Given the abundant, and at times outdated, hospital listings in the OpenStreetMap dataset, uniform filtering based on building footprint, facility name, and online presence was applied to limit the data to hospitals and facilities with the highest impact and capacity. Area-based filtering was employed to exclude buildings too small to be a hospital based on square footage. Keyword filtering was then used to exclude non-hospitals on name (e.g., "health post"), factoring for linguistic differences. Lastly, to establish activity, a scoring system was derived for each candidate facility by searching for related websites, local directories, government reports, social media posts, etc. Public APIs, including Bing Maps, OpenStreetMap Nominatim, and Geonames were called to capture and externally validate additional details. The purpose of these integrations was to (1) reverse-geocode hospital coordinates to return missing addresses, and (2) validate the location of the hospitals with close proximity to country borders. This approach was premised on the assumption that principal hospitals are more likely to be referenced online, whether by individuals, governments, or nonprofits. Filtering was complemented by several rounds of manual curation and review.

Future Directions

Data contained in this compendium presents only the first steps in improving the nonprofit and healthcare facility landscape in low-income countries. Much work remains to be done to better our understanding of the granularity specific to each region and healthcare system. The Foundations's development of a vulnerability index based upon macro-level health statistics, bed capacity, and population mobility in targeted regions is a step in this direction. Additionally, insights from social media activity can help identify acute medical conditions in real time and facilitate rapid assistance where needed. Information sources such as public satellite data and ground images obtained from online user activity can be further used in conjunction with machine-learning algorithms to validate the location of hospitals, estimate facility area, and even predict the number of beds needed. Together, these and other features will enhance the global marketplace for the exchange of healthcare services.

A Final Word

Insights in Global Health presents comprehensive healthcare data for 24 low-income countries, in an accessible single-source format. It is the result of countless hours of work by volunteers, data scientists, and healthcare professionals. Yet, it only marks the beginning of the journey. In due course, demand-side data—the healthcare facilities and NGOs that comprise the healthcare ecosystem—will be expanded to include more countries and regions. At the same time, machine-learning algorithms will provide the supply-side data—healthcare professionals and organizations delivering services. Ultimately, the combined data will be available to stakeholders on an optimized platform that best matches need to particular skill sets.

It should be noted that *Insights in Global Health* represents a snapshot of countries and organizations and is by no means exhaustive. The nature of the project has several limitations, including the lack of readily available information in certain resource-poor regions. In many instances, organizations do not have a digital presence, and up-to-date health data is often not available on a granular or regional level. Additionally, the query pipeline was constructed in English and, as a result, some candidate websites in non-English languages have not been included. Furthermore, the methodology applied here is subject to the technological limitations of capturing and processing large swaths of data, a limitation compounded by the unpredictable political, economic, and social changes that are often at play in low-income countries.

Today, advancements in technology and big data allow us to leverage information to improve decision-making and provide opportunities to effect change beyond isolated interventions. It is hoped that this compendium and its related platform will help to improve health outcomes for individuals, communities, and countries around the world.

About Virtue Foundation

The Virtue Foundation is a nonprofit organization with special consultative status to the United Nations Economic and Social Council. The Foundation's mission is to increase awareness, inspire action, and render assistance through healthcare, education, and empowerment initiatives. Virtue Foundation is guided by the principle that true global change must begin within each of us—one person at a time, one act at a time.

Country Directory

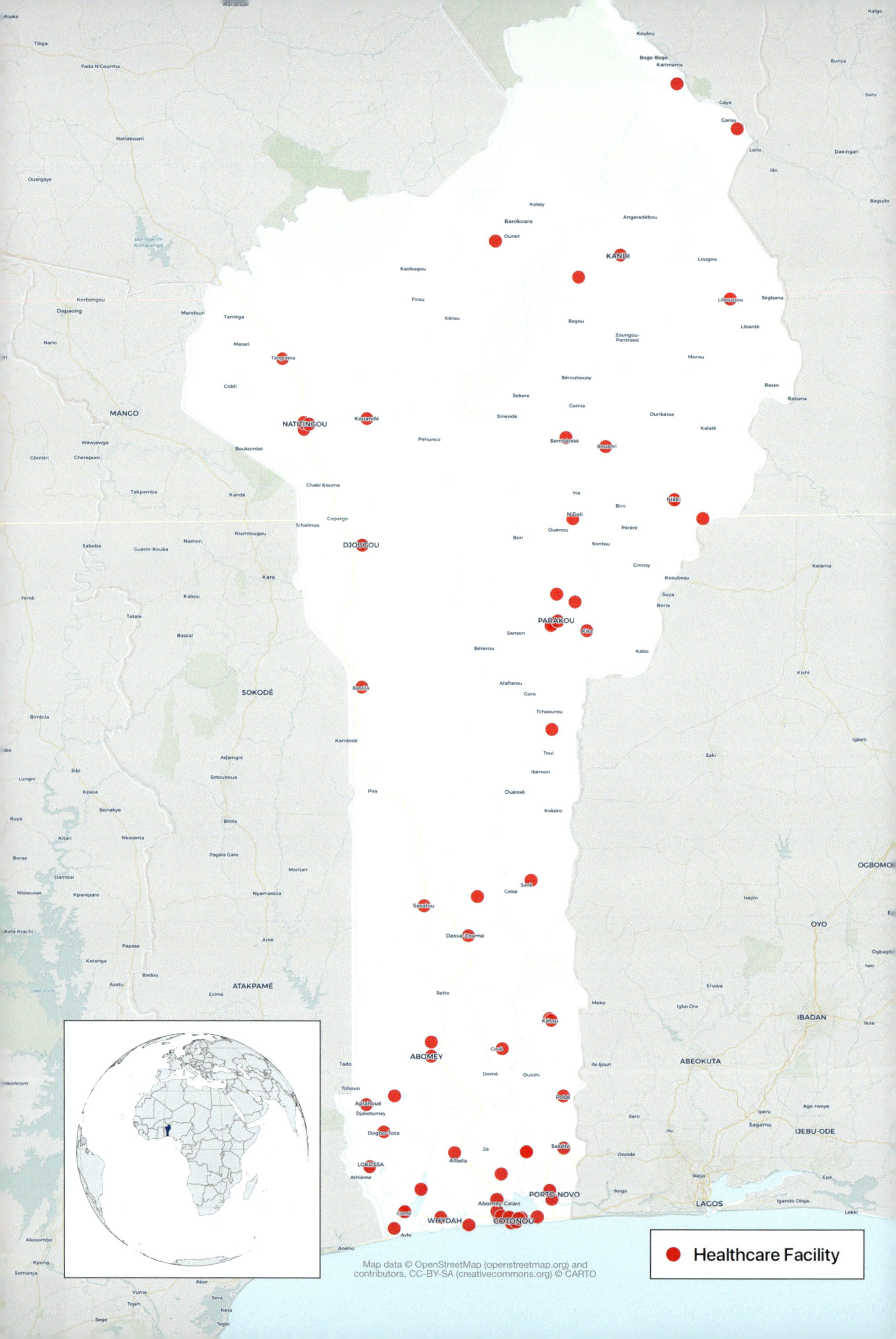
Healthcare Facility
Map data © OpenStreetMap (openstreetmap.org) and contributors, CC-BY-SA (creativecommons.org) © CARTO
KANDI
NATITINGOU
DJOUGOU
PARAKOU
ABOMEY
WHYDAH
COTONOU
PORTO NOVO
LOKOSSA
MANGO
SOKODÉ
ATAKPAMÉ
ABEOKUTA
IBADAN
OYO
LAGOS
IJEBU-ODE
OGBOMO
Koulou
Bogo-Bogo
Karimama
Gaya
Garou
Kokey
Banikoara
Ounet
Angaradébou
Lougou
Kaobagou
Firou
Kérou
Bagou
Libousou
Ségbana
Libanté
Zoungou-Pantrossi
Tantéga
Materi
Tanguiéta
Cobli
Morou
Béroubouay
Sekere
Gamia
Sinendé
Kouandé
Péhunco
Bembéréké
Bouanri
Dunkassa
Kalalé
Basso
Babana
Boukombé
Chabi Kouma
Ina
Biro
Nikki
N'Dali
Ouénou
Pèrèrè
Bori
Sontou
Copargo
Tchalinga
Gninsy
Kosubosu
Suya
Boria
Kika
Sanson
Bétérou
Kabo
Bassila
Alafiarou
Goro
Tchaourou
Kambolé
Toui
Ikèmon
Pira
Ouèssè
Kokoro
Savè
Cobè
Savalou
Dassa-Zoumé
Setto
Kétou
Covè
Tado
Domè
Ouinhi
Tohoun
Aplahoué
Djakotomey
Pobè
Dogbo-Tota
Zè
Sakété
Allada
Athiémé
Abomey-Calavi
Comè
Avlo
Aného
Tibga
Fada N'Gourma
Natiaboani
Ouargaye
Korbongou
Dapaong
Mandouri
Nano
Wawjawga
Gbintiri
Chereponi
Takpamba
Kandé
Namon
Niamtougou
Saboba
Guérin-Kouka
Kara
Yendi
Kabou
Tatale
Bassar
Bimbila
Adjengré
Sibi
Sotouboua
Lungni
Kpasa
Bonakye
Buya
Blitta
Kitari
Nkwanta
Borae
Pagala Gare
Moritan
Dambai
Ntewusae
Kparepare
Nyamassila
Kete Krachi
Anié
Papase
Katanga
Badou
Asatu
Ezimé
Lake Volta
Akosombo
Kpong
Somanya
Abor
Vume
Sogakope
Toje
Seva
Keta
Sege
Tegbi
Kalgo
Bunza
Suru
Dakingari
Lollo
Illo
Bagudo
Kalama
Kishi
Igbeti
Saki
Iseyin
Ogbagbi
Iwo
Eruwa
Meko
Igbo Ora
Ikire
Ile Ijoun
Ago-Iwoye
Iperu
Ilaro
Sagamu
Ifo
Owode
Ikeja
Epe
Ikoga
Igando Oloja
Lekki

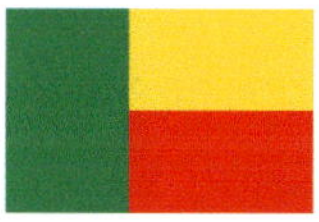

Benin

The Republic of Benin, in West Africa, lies between Togo, Nigeria, Burkina Faso, and Niger. Referred to as the birthplace of Vodou and home to centuries-old palaces in Abomey, Benin has a small, young population of 12.9 million. The country comprises several ethnic groups including the Fon, Adja, Yoruba, Bariba, and Fulani, who speak their namesake languages as well as the country's official language, French.

Benin gained independence from France in 1960. Since establishing its democratic system of government more than 20 years ago, Benin has become one of Africa's most stable democracies. Its farm-based economy, which employs about 70 percent of the country's population, has grown significantly from decade to decade. Benin has also invested in infrastructure, including renovating its port. Today, Benin has an economic growth rate of about 5 percent. Despite this growth, poverty remains a pressing issue faced by roughly 40 percent of the population. Benin is particularly vulnerable to climate hazards, as well as to the effect of economic and political changes in Nigeria, its largest trading partner.

Life expectancy continues to rise, nearing 61 years of age. Despite some improvements in health indicators, the health challenges that contribute most to death and disability in the country are communicable and non-communicable diseases. Significant causes of death include malaria, neonatal disorders, lower respiratory infections, diarrheal disease, stroke, ischemic heart disease, congenital defects, tuberculosis, HIV/AIDS, and measles. Stroke, ischemic heart disease and measles have significantly increased in recent years. Of note, trauma from road injuries is a major cause of disability.

12.9M
Population

$1,219
GDP Per Capita

61 years
Life Expectancy
↑ Improving

7.9
Doctors/100k
Physician Density

50
Beds/100k
Hospital Bed Density

397
Deaths/100k
Maternal Mortality

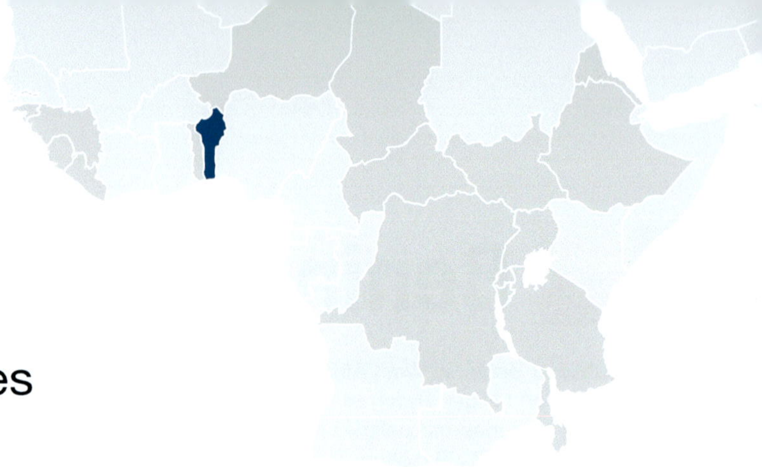

Benin

Healthcare Facilities

Centre de Santé de Tika
RN 4, Adjohoun, Ouémé, Benin
https://vfapp.org/acc9

Centre de Santé Oganla de Ketou
RNIE 4, Oke Ola, Plateau, Benin
https://vfapp.org/f66c

Centre Hospitalier Départemental de Borgou-Alibori
Parakou, Benin
https://vfapp.org/5921

Centre Hospitalier Départemental de Mono
RN 23, Possotomè, Mono, Benin
https://vfapp.org/a728

Centre Hospitalier Départemental de Natitingou (CHD)
RNIE 3;RN 7, Natitingou, Atakora, Benin
https://vfapp.org/832e

Centre Hospitalier Universitaire Départemental de l'Ouémé-Plateau
Rue l'Inspection, Porto-Novo, Benin
https://vfapp.org/a4f4

CHD Centre Hospitalier du Zou
Hospital, RNIE4, Abomey, Benin
https://vfapp.org/e916

CNHU Centre National Hospitalier Universitaire
Littoral, Cotonou, Benin
https://vfapp.org/c889

Enfant du Bénin
117 RNIE 1, Abomey-Calavi, Atlantique, Benin
https://vfapp.org/3665

Hospital Area Bembéréké-Sinendé
Bembéréké, Benin
https://vfapp.org/5dba

Hospital Dogbo
Dogbo, Benin
https://vfapp.org/7c74

Hospital Malanville Karimama
Malanville, Benin
https://vfapp.org/9d11

Hospital Zone de Kandi
RNIE2, Kandi, Benin
https://vfapp.org/e176

Hospital Zone de Tchaourou
Tchaourou, Benin
https://vfapp.org/ee9a

HZ Allada
Allada, Benin
https://vfapp.org/243c

HZ Saint-Jean de Dieu Parakou
Parakou, Benin
https://vfapp.org/3691

Hôpital Ahmadiyya
Parakou, Benin
https://vfapp.org/2bda

Hôpital Avlékété
Avlékété, Benin
https://vfapp.org/b81c

Hôpital Bethesda
Avenue du Renouveau, Sainte Rita, Littoral, Benin
https://vfapp.org/dc72

Hôpital Cent Lits
Boulevard de Comè, Akodéha Kpodji, Akodeha, Comé, Mono, Benin
https://vfapp.org/1ead

Hôpital d'Instructions des Armées de Cotonou
Rue 238, Cotonou, Benin
https://vfapp.org/1676

Hôpital de Grand Popo
Grand-Popo, Benin
https://vfapp.org/9d51

Hôpital de Karimama
Karimama, Benin
https://vfapp.org/c4b2

Hôpital de l'Enfant et de la Mère Lagune
Rue des Dako Donou, Cotonou, Benin
https://vfapp.org/e394

Hôpital de l'Ordre de Malte
RN 6, Djougou, Donga, Benin
https://vfapp.org/ee77

Hôpital de la Zone Sanitaire Djidja-Abomey-Agbangnizoun
Djidja, Benin
https://vfapp.org/fa92

Hôpital de Liboussou
RNIE 7, Liboussou, Alibori, Benin
https://vfapp.org/c788

Hôpital de Menontin
Rue 9.224, Kindonou, Littoral, Benin
https://vfapp.org/7568

Hôpital de Tchikandou
RNIE 6, Tchikandou, Borgou, Benin
https://vfapp.org/34d9

Hôpital de Zone Ayélawadjè
2ème Arrondissement, Cotonou, Benin
https://vfapp.org/7326

Hôpital de Zone Bassila
Rue 043, Bassila, Donga, Benin
https://vfapp.org/2ecd

Hôpital de Zone Comè
Comè, Benin
https://vfapp.org/d8cd

Hôpital de Zone d'Adjohoun
RN4, Akpro-Misserete, Benin
https://vfapp.org/1e4f

Hôpital de Zone d'Ekpè
Ekpè, Ouémé, Benin
https://vfapp.org/e66c

Hôpital de Zone de Aplahoué
RNIE 4, Aplahoué, Kouffo, Benin
https://vfapp.org/6213

Hôpital de Zone de Banikouara
RN 8, Banikoara, Benin
https://vfapp.org/c8df

Hôpital de Zone de Covè
RNIE 4, Flessa, Loko Alankpé, Zangnanado, Zou, Benin
https://vfapp.org/e4d6

Hôpital de Zone de Dassa-Zoumé
Dassa-Zoumé, Benin
https://vfapp.org/29b8

Hôpital de Zone de Glazoué
Glazoué, Benin
https://vfapp.org/49f7

Hôpital de Zone de Kouandé
Kouandé, Benin
https://vfapp.org/566e

Hôpital de Zone de Lokossa
Colodo, Lokossa, Mono, Benin
https://vfapp.org/1389

Hôpital de Zone de Natitingou
RNIE 3;RN 7, Natitingou, Atakora, Benin
https://vfapp.org/4152

Hôpital de Zone de Ouidah
Ouidah, Benin
https://vfapp.org/ca1c

Hôpital de Zone de Pobè
RN 3, Pobè, Plateau, Benin
https://vfapp.org/e74c

Hôpital de Zone de Sakété
Sakété, Benin
https://vfapp.org/9923

Hôpital de Zone de Savalou
Savalou, Benin
https://vfapp.org/c8a2

Hôpital de Zone de Suru Lere
Rue 1647, Cotonou, Benin
https://vfapp.org/5f13

Hôpital de Zone d'Abomey-Calavi
RNIE 2, Abomey-Calavi, Atlantique, Benin
https://vfapp.org/f92f

Hôpital de Zone KTL
Ayahohoué, Benin
https://vfapp.org/7988

Hôpital de Zone Savè
Savè, Benin
https://vfapp.org/b94c

Hôpital Djougou
Djougou, Benin
https://vfapp.org/8cc8

Hôpital du Militaire
RNIE 2, Parakou, Borgou, Benin
https://vfapp.org/8cd2

Hôpital Evangélique de Bembéréké
Bembéréké, Benin
https://vfapp.org/2393

Hôpital La Croix de Zinvié
RN 31, Zinvié, Atlantique, Benin
https://vfapp.org/8339

Hôpital Padre Pio N'Dali
N'Dali, Benin
https://vfapp.org/9b6f

Hôpital Saint Jean de Dieu Tanguiéta
RNIE 3, Tanguiéta, Atakora, Benin
https://vfapp.org/9362

Hôpital Saint Luc de Cotonou
Cotonou, Benin
https://vfapp.org/4c84

Hôpital Saint-Martin à Papané
Papané, Benin
https://vfapp.org/893d

Hôpital Sainte Bakhita
Natitingou, Benin
https://vfapp.org/ed13

Hôpital Sanitaire de N'Dali
RNIE 2, N'Dali, Borgou, Benin
🌐 https://vfapp.org/4594

Hôpital Sunon Séro
RN 10, TÈPA, Borgou, Benin
🌐 https://vfapp.org/edf1

Islamic Hospital
Porto-Novo, Benin
🌐 https://vfapp.org/b9f8

Médecins d'Afrique
RN 3, Idenan, Kétou, Plateau, Benin
🌐 https://vfapp.org/6fba

Nikki-Hospital
Nikki, Benin
🌐 https://vfapp.org/ca69

SAM Hospital
Sam, Benin
🌐 https://vfapp.org/8e62

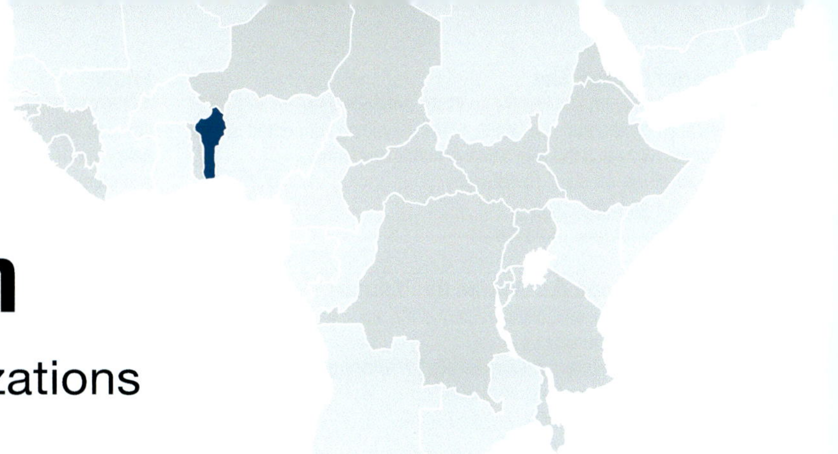

Benin

Nonprofit Organizations

Abt Associates
Seeks to improve the quality of life and economic well-being of people worldwide, while striving to meet and exceed the highest professional standards.

General, Logist-Op, MF Med, OB-GYN, Peds

+1 212-779-7700

https://vfapp.org/cec2

Advance Family Planning
Aims to achieve global expansion and access to quality contraceptive information, services, and supplies through financial investment and political commitment.

General, MF Med, Pub Health

+1 410-502-8715

https://vfapp.org/7478

Africa CDC
Aims to strengthen the capacity and capability of Africa's public health institutions as well as partnerships to detect and respond quickly and effectively to disease threats and outbreaks, based on data-driven interventions and programs.

Infect Dis, Logist-Op, Pub Health

+251 11 551 7700

https://vfapp.org/339c

African Health Now
Promotes and provides information and access to sustainable primary healthcare to women, children, and families living across Sub-Saharan Africa.

Dent-OMFS, Endo, General, Infect Dis, MF Med, OB-GYN

https://vfapp.org/c766

Africa Indoor Residual Spraying Project (AIRS)
Aims to protect millions of people in Africa from malaria by spraying insecticide on the walls, ceilings, and other indoor resting places of mosquitoes that transmit malaria.

Infect Dis

+1 301-347-5000

https://vfapp.org/9bd1

African Field Epidemiology Network (AFENET)
Strengthens field epidemiology and public health laboratory capacity to contribute effectively to addressing epidemics and other major public health problems in Africa.

All-Immu, Infect Dis, Path, Pub Health

https://vfapp.org/df2e

Amref Health Africa
Serves millions of people across thirty-five countries in Sub-Saharan Africa, strengthening health systems, and training African health workers to respond to the continent's most critical health issues.

All-Immu, General, Infect Dis, Logist-Op, MF Med, OB-GYN, Path, Pub Health, Surg

+254 20 6993000

https://vfapp.org/6985

AO Alliance
Builds solutions to lessen the burden of injuries in low- and middle-income countries, while enhancing the care of the injured to reduce human suffering, disability, and poverty.

Ortho, Surg

https://vfapp.org/8cd5

Asclepius Snakebite Foundation
Seeks to reverse the cycle of tragic snakebite outcomes through a combination of innovative research, clinical medicine, and education-based public health initiatives.

Infect Dis, Pub Health

https://vfapp.org/d37d

BroadReach
Collaborates with governments, multinational health organizations, donors, and private sector companies to affect healthcare reform and solve the world's biggest health challenges.

Logist-Op

+27 21 514 8300

https://vfapp.org/7812

Canada-Africa Community Health Alliance
Sends Canadian volunteer teams on two- to three-week missions to African communities to work hand-in-hand with local partners.

General, Infect Dis, MF Med, OB-GYN, Peds, Surg

+1 613-234-9992

https://vfapp.org/4c94

CARE
Works around the globe to save lives, defeat poverty, and achieve social justice.

ER Med, General

+1 800-422-7385

https://vfapp.org/7232

Carter Center, The
Seeks to prevent and resolve conflicts, enhance freedom and democracy, and improve health, while remaining committed to human rights and the alleviation of human suffering.

Infect Dis, MF Med, Ophth-Opt

📞 +1 800-550-3560

🌐 https://vfapp.org/6556

Chain of Hope (La Chaîne de l'Espoir)
Helps underprivileged children around the world by providing them with access to healthcare.

Anesth, CT Surg, Crit-Care, ER Med, Neurosurg, Ortho, Ped Surg, Surg, Vasc Surg

📞 +33 1 44 12 66 66

🌐 https://vfapp.org/e871

Challenge Initiative, The
Seeks to rapidly and sustainably scale up proven reproductive health solutions among the urban poor.

MF Med, OB-GYN, Peds

📞 +1 410-502-8715

🌐 https://vfapp.org/2f77

Christian Blind Mission (CBM)
Aims to improve the quality of life of persons with disabilities in the poorest countries, addressing poverty as a cause, and a consequence, of disability, and working in partnership to create a society for all.

ENT, General, Infect Dis, OB-GYN, Ophth-Opt, Ortho, Peds, Psych, Rehab, Surg

📞 +49 6251 131131

🌐 https://vfapp.org/3824

Christian Connections for International Health (CCIH)
Promotes global health and wholeness from a Christian perspective.

All-Immu, General, Infect Dis, MF Med, Neonat, OB-GYN, Psych

📞 +1 703-923-8960

🌐 https://vfapp.org/fa5d

Core Group
Aims to improve and expand community health practices for underserved populations, especially women and children, through collaborative action and learning.

General, Infect Dis, MF Med, Medicine, OB-GYN, Peds, Pub Health

📞 +1 202-380-3400

🌐 https://vfapp.org/9de3

Developing Country NGO Delegation: Global Fund to Fight AIDS, TB & Malaria
Works to strengthen the engagement of civil society actors and organizations in developing countries to contribute toward achieving a world in which AIDS, TB, and Malaria are no longer global, public health, and human rights threats.

Infect Dis, Pub Health

📞 +254 20 2515790

🌐 https://vfapp.org/3149

Direct Relief
Improves the health and lives of people affected by poverty or emergency situations by mobilizing and providing essential medical resources needed for their care.

ER Med, Logist-Op

📞 +1 805-964-4767

🌐 https://vfapp.org/58e5

Enabel
As the development agency of the Belgian federal government, charged with implementing Belgium's international development policy, carries out public service assignments in Belgium and abroad pursuant to the 2030 Agenda for Sustainable Development.

General, Infect Dis, Logist-Op, MF Med, OB-GYN, Peds, Pub Health

📞 +32 2 505 37 00

🌐 https://vfapp.org/5af7

EngenderHealth
Works to implement high-quality, gender-equitable programs that advance sexual and reproductive health and rights.

General, MF Med, OB-GYN, Peds

📞 +1 202-902-2000

🌐 https://vfapp.org/1cb2

Fistula Foundation
Aims to engage the support of people worldwide who are eager to see the day when no woman suffers from obstetric fistula. Raises and directs funds to doctors and hospitals providing life-transforming surgery to women in need.

OB-GYN

📞 +1 408-249-9596

🌐 https://vfapp.org/e958

Fondation Follereau
Promotes the quality of life of the most vulnerable African communities. Alongside trusted partners, the foundation supports local initiatives in healthcare and education.

General, Infect Dis, OB-GYN

📞 +352 44 66 06 34

🌐 https://vfapp.org/bcc7

Global Clubfoot Initiative (GCI)
Promotes and resources the treatment of children with clubfoot in developing countries using the Ponseti technique.

Ortho, Ped Surg

🌐 https://vfapp.org/f229

Global Oncology (GO)
Brings the best in cancer care to underserved patients around the world and collaborates across geographic, professional, and academic borders to improve cancer care, research, and education.

Heme-Onc, Path, Rad-Onc

🌐 https://vfapp.org/fcb8

Grace Dental and Medical (GDM) Missions
Sends and supports dental and medical missions, based in Christian ministry with the aim of church planting.

Dent-OMFS, ER Med, General

📞 +1 978-242-6724

🌐 https://vfapp.org/bdea

Grassroot Soccer
Leverages the power of soccer to educate, inspire, and mobilize at risk youth in developing countries to overcome their greatest health challenges, live healthier more productive lives, and be agents for change in their communities.

Infect Dis

📞 +1 603-277-9685

🌐 https://vfapp.org/3521

Health Equity Initiative
Aims to build and sustain a global community that engages across sectors and disciplines to advance health equity.
Pub Health
https://vfapp.org/e2e2

Health Volunteers Overseas (HVO)
Improves the availability and quality of healthcare through the education, training, and professional development of the health workforce in resource-scarce countries.
All-Immu, Anesth, CV Med, Dent-OMFS, Derm, ENT, ER Med, Endo, GI, Heme-Onc, Infect Dis, Medicine, Medicine, Nephro, Neuro, OB-GYN, Ophth-Opt, Ortho, Peds, Plast, Psych, Pulm-Critic, Rehab, Rheum, Surg
+1 202-296-0928
https://vfapp.org/42b2

Hernia Help
Provides free hernia surgery to underserved children and adults in the Western Hemisphere, practicing the preferential option for the poor. Trains, mentors, develops, and supports local general surgeons who will serve as trainers and future leaders to create self-sustaining teams.
Anesth, Surg
https://vfapp.org/6319

Hope Walks
Frees children, families, and communities from the burden of clubfoot, inspired by the Christian faith.
Ortho, Ped Surg, Peds, Rehab
+1 717-502-4400
https://vfapp.org/f6d4

Humanity & Inclusion
Works alongside people with disabilities and vulnerable populations, taking action and bearing witness in order to respond to their essential needs, improve their living conditions and health, and promote respect for their dignity and fundamental rights.
General, Infect Dis, MF Med, Medicine, Ortho, Peds, Psych, Pub Health, Rehab
+1 301-891-2138
https://vfapp.org/16b7

Humanity First
Provides aid and assistance to those in need, offering sustainable development solutions to society while providing and empowering local communities with the resources to help themselves.
ER Med, General, MF Med, Ophth-Opt
+44 20 8417 0082
https://vfapp.org/13cc

Hunger Project, The
Aims to end hunger and poverty by pioneering sustainable, grassroots, women-centered strategies and advocating for their widespread adoption in countries throughout the world.
Infect Dis, Nutr, OB-GYN, Pub Health
+1 212-251-9100
https://vfapp.org/3a49

International Agency for the Prevention of Blindness (IAPB), The
Leads international efforts in blindness-prevention activities, works toward a world where no one is needlessly visually impaired, and ensures that everyone has access to the best possible standard of eye health.
Infect Dis, Ophth-Opt, Pub Health
https://vfapp.org/87a2

International Council of Ophthalmology
Works with ophthalmologic societies and others to enhance ophthalmic education and improve access to the highest quality eye care in order to preserve and restore vision for the people of the world.
Ophth-Opt
https://vfapp.org/ffd2

International Federation of Gynecology and Obstetrics (FIGO)
Implements global projects on specific women's health issues.
MF Med, Medicine, Neonat, OB-GYN, Surg, Urol
+44 20 7928 1166
https://vfapp.org/c4b4

International Federation of Red Cross and Red Crescent Societies (IFRC)
Coordinates and directs international assistance following natural and man-made disasters in nonconflict situations through the world's largest humanitarian and development network. Provides disaster-preparedness programs, healthcare activities, and promotes humanitarian values.
ER Med, General, Infect Dis, Nutr
+1 212-338-0161
https://vfapp.org/b4ee

International Organization for Migration (IOM) – The UN Migration Agency
Promotes evidence-informed policies and holistic, preventive, and curative health programs that are beneficial, accessible, and equitable for vulnerable migrants.
General, Infect Dis, OB-GYN
+27 12 342 2789
https://vfapp.org/621a

International Pediatric Nephrology Association (IPNA)
Leads the global efforts to successfully address the care for all children with kidney disease through advocacy, education, and training.
Medicine, Nephro, Peds
https://vfapp.org/b59d

International Planned Parenthood Federation (IPPF)
Leads a locally owned, globally connected civil society movement that provides and enables services and champions sexual and reproductive health and rights for all, especially the underserved.
Infect Dis, MF Med, OB-GYN
+44 20 7939 8200
https://vfapp.org/dc97

International Trachoma Initiative (iTi)
Works toward a world free from trachoma, a preventable cause of blindness, and provides comprehensive support to national ministries of health and governmental and nongovernmental organizations to implement a comprehensive approach to fight trachoma.
Infect Dis, Ophth-Opt
+1 404-371-0466
https://vfapp.org/3278

International Union Against Tuberculosis and Lung Disease
Develops, implements, and assesses anti-tuberculosis, lung health, and noncommunicable disease programs.
Infect Dis, Pub Health, Pulm-Critic
+33 1 44 32 03 60
https://vfapp.org/3e82

IntraHealth International
Improves the performance of health workers and strengthens the systems in which they work.
CV Med, Endo, General, Infect Dis, MF Med, Neonat, Nutr, OB-GYN
+1 919-313-3554
https://vfapp.org/ddc8

Ipas
Focuses efforts on women and girls who want contraception or abortion, and builds programs around their needs and how best to support them.
OB-GYN
https://vfapp.org/8e39

Jhpiego
Creates and delivers transformative healthcare solutions that save lives in partnership with national governments, health experts, and local communities.
General, Infect Dis, OB-GYN, Surg
+1 410-537-1800
https://vfapp.org/45b8

John Snow, Inc. (JSI)
Aims to improve the health and well-being of underserved and vulnerable people and communities throughout the world.
General, Infect Dis, Logist-Op, MF Med, OB-GYN, Peds, Psych, Pub Health
+1 617-482-9485
https://vfapp.org/ba78

Johns Hopkins Center for Communication Programs
Believes in the power of communication to save lives, by empowering people to adopt healthy behaviors for themselves, their families, and their communities.
General, Infect Dis, Logist-Op, OB-GYN, Pub Health
+1 410-659-6300
https://vfapp.org/1bf9

Joint United Nations Programme on HIV/AIDS (UNAIDS)
Aims to place people living with HIV and people affected by the virus at the decision-making table and at the center of designing, delivering, and monitoring the AIDS response.
Infect Dis
+41 22 791 36 66
https://vfapp.org/464a

Lions Clubs International
Empowers volunteers to serve their communities, meet humanitarian needs, encourage peace, and promote international understanding through Lions clubs.
Heme-Onc, Medicine, Nutr, Ophth-Opt
+1 630-571-5466
https://vfapp.org/7b12

Management Sciences for Health (MSH)
Works with countries and communities to save lives and improve the health of the world's poorest and most vulnerable people by building strong, resilient, sustainable health systems.
Infect Dis, Logist-Op, Pub Health
+1 617-250-9500
https://vfapp.org/6aa2

MAP International
Provides medicines and health supplies to those in need around the world so they might experience life to the fullest.
Logist-Op
+1 800-225-8550
https://vfapp.org/deed

Maternity Foundation
Works to ensure safer childbirth for women and newborns everywhere through innovative mobile health solutions such as the Safe Delivery App, a mobile training tool for skilled birth attendants.
MF Med, OB-GYN, Pub Health
https://vfapp.org/ff4f

Médecins du Monde/Doctors of the World
Provides care, bears witness, and supports social change worldwide with innovative medical programs and evidence-based advocacy initiatives.
ER Med, General, Infect Dis, MF Med, Neonat, OB-GYN, Peds, Pub Health
+33 1 44 92 15 15
https://vfapp.org/a43d

Medical Care Development International (MCD International)
Works to strengthen health systems through innovative, sustainable interventions.
Infect Dis, Logist-Op, OB-GYN, Pub Health
+1 301-562-1920
https://vfapp.org/dc5c

MedShare
Aims to improve the quality of life of people, communities, and the planet by sourcing and directly delivering surplus medical supplies and equipment to communities in need around the world.
Logist-Op
+1 770-323-5858
https://vfapp.org/c8bc

Mercy Ships
Operates hospital ships staffed by volunteers to bring hope, healing, and healthcare to underserved communities worldwide.
Anesth, Dent-OMFS, Logist-Op, Neonat, OB-GYN, Ophth-Opt, Ortho, Palliative, Plast, Psych, Surg
+1 903-939-7000
https://vfapp.org/2e99

Mérieux Foundation
Committed to fighting infectious diseases that affect developing countries by capacity building, particularly in clinical laboratories, and focusing on diagnosis.
Logist-Op, Path
+33 4 72 40 79 79
https://vfapp.org/a23a

Mission Partners for Christ
Provides medication, treatment, screenings, and health education in underserved communities around the world, inspired by the Christian faith.
Dent-OMFS, General, Ophth-Opt
+1 312-307-5475
https://vfapp.org/eb25

Partners for Development (PfD)
Works to improve quality of life for vulnerable people in underserved communities through local and international partnerships.
Infect Dis, MF Med, Neonat, Peds
+1 301-608-0426
https://vfapp.org/d2f6

PINCC Preventing Cervical Cancer
Seeks to prevent female-specific diseases in developing countries by utilizing low-cost and low-technology methods to create sustainable programs through patient education, medical personnel training, and facility outfitting.
OB-GYN
+1 830-708-6009
https://vfapp.org/9666

PSI – Population Services International
Dedicates efforts to improving the health of people in the developing world by focusing on challenges such as a lack of family planning, HIV/AIDS, barriers to maternal health, and the greatest threats to children under the age of 5, including malaria, diarrhea, pneumonia, and malnutrition.
Infect Dis, MF Med, OB-GYN, Peds
+1 202-785-0072
https://vfapp.org/ffe3

RestoringVision
Empowers lives by restoring vision for millions of people in need.
Ophth-Opt
+1 209-980-7323
https://vfapp.org/e121

Rockefeller Foundation, The
Works to promote the well-being of humanity.
Logist-Op, Nutr, Pub Health
+1 212-869-8500
https://vfapp.org/5424

Rotary Action Group for Family Health & AIDS Prevention (RFHA)
Works to save and improve the lives of children and families who lack access to preventive healthcare and education.
Dent-OMFS, Infect Dis, OB-GYN, Ophth-Opt, Peds
+27 83 456 3923
https://vfapp.org/6563

Rotary International
Provides service to others, improves lives, and advances world understanding, goodwill, and peace through its fellowship of business, professional, and community leaders.
ER Med, General, Infect Dis, MF Med, OB-GYN
https://vfapp.org/8fb5

Sanofi Espoir Foundation
Contributes to reducing health inequalities among populations that need it most by applying a socially responsible approach focused on fighting childhood cancers in low-income countries, improving maternal and newborn health, and improving access to care.
ER Med, OB-GYN, Peds
+33 1 53 77 91 38
https://vfapp.org/943b

SATMED
Serves non-governmental organizations, hospitals, medical universities, and other healthcare providers active in resource-poor areas, by providing open-access e-health services for the health community.
Logist-Op
https://vfapp.org/b8d5

Shammesh – Vers un Monde Meilleur
Aims to transfer skills, knowledge, financial means, and resources to populations in distress or in situations of extreme poverty, in France and abroad.
Dent-OMFS, General, Peds, Pub Health
https://vfapp.org/9aed

Sightsavers
Prevents avoidable blindness in some of the poorest parts of the world by treating debilitating eye diseases.
Infect Dis, Ophth-Opt, Surg
+1 800-707-9746
https://vfapp.org/aa52

Smile Train
Seeks to give every child with a cleft the opportunity for a healthy, productive life by providing free cleft repair surgery and comprehensive cleft care in their own communities.
Dent-OMFS, ENT, Plast
+1 800-932-9541
https://vfapp.org/f21d

Solthis
Improves disease prevention and access to quality care by strengthening the health systems and services of the countries served.
General, Infect Dis, Logist-Op, MF Med, Neonat, Path
+33 1 81 70 17 90
https://vfapp.org/a71d

SOS Children's Villages International
Supports children through alternative care and family strengthening.
ER Med, Peds
+43 1 36824570
https://vfapp.org/aca1

Sustainable Kidney Care Foundation (SKCF)
Works to provide treatment for kidney injury where none exists, and aims to reduce mortality from treatable acute kidney injury (AKI).
Infect Dis, Medicine, Nephro
https://vfapp.org/1926

Swiss Tropical and Public Health Institute
Contributes to the improvement of the health of populations internationally, nationally, and locally through excellence in research, education, and services.
Infect Dis, Pub Health
+41 61 284 81 11
https://vfapp.org/2ee4

Task Force for Global Health, The
Consists of programs and focus areas that cover a range of global health issues including neglected tropical diseases, infectious diseases, vaccines, field epidemiology, public health informatics, health workforce development, and global health ethics.
Infect Dis, Logist-Op, Medicine, Ophth-Opt, Peds
☎ +1 404-371-0466
🌐 https://vfapp.org/714c

Terre Des Hommes
Works to improve the conditions of the most vulnerable children worldwide by improving the health of children under the age of 3, protecting migrant children, providing humanitarian aid to children and their families in times of crisis, and preventing child exploitation.
ER Med, MF Med, Neonat, OB-GYN, Ped Surg, Peds
☎ +41 58 611 06 66
🌐 https://vfapp.org/2689

Turing Foundation
Aims to contribute toward a better world and a better society by focusing on efforts such as health, art, education, and nature.
Infect Dis
☎ +31 20 520 0010
🌐 https://vfapp.org/6bcc

U.S. President's Malaria Initiative (PMI)
Supports low-income countries to help control and eliminate malaria through cost-effective, lifesaving malaria interventions.
Infect Dis, MF Med, OB-GYN
☎ +1 202-712-0000
🌐 https://vfapp.org/dc8b

Union for International Cancer Control (UICC)
Unites and supports the cancer community to reduce the global cancer burden, promote greater equity, and ensure that cancer control continues to be a priority in the world health and development agenda.
Heme-Onc, Pub Health
☎ +41 22 809 18 11
🌐 https://vfapp.org/88b1

United Nations Children's Fund (UNICEF)
Works in over 190 countries and territories to save children's lives, to defend their rights, and to help them fulfill their potential, from early childhood through adolescence.
All-Immu, Infect Dis, MF Med, Neonat, Nutr, OB-GYN, Ped Surg, Peds, Pub Health
🌐 https://vfapp.org/42d7

United Nations Development Programme (UNDP)
Helps countries achieve the simultaneous eradication of extreme poverty and significant reduction of inequalities and exclusion using a sustainable human development approach.
Infect Dis, Logist-Op, Pub Health
🌐 https://vfapp.org/935c

United Nations High Commissioner for Refugees (UNHCR)
Safeguards the rights and well-being of people who have been forced to flee, ensuring that everybody has the right to seek asylum and find safe refuge in another country, with the goal of seeking lasting solutions.
General, MF Med, Medicine, OB-GYN, Peds, Psych, Pub Health
🌐 https://vfapp.org/6636

United Nations Population Fund (UNFPA)
Supports reproductive healthcare for women and youth in more than 150 countries, focusing on delivering a world where every pregnancy is wanted, every childbirth is safe, and every young person's potential is fulfilled.
Infect Dis, MF Med, Neonat, OB-GYN, Peds, Pub Health
☎ +1 212-963-6008
🌐 https://vfapp.org/c969

United Surgeons for Children (USFC)
Pursues greater health and opportunity for children in the most neglected pockets of the world, with a specific focus and expertise in surgery.
Anesth, CT Surg, Neonat, Neurosurg, OB-GYN, Peds, Radiol, Surg
🌐 https://vfapp.org/3b4c

USAID: African Strategies for Health
Identifies and advocates for best practices, enhancing technical capacity of African regional institutions and engaging African stakeholders to address health issues in a sustainable manner.
All-Immu, Infect Dis, OB-GYN, Peds
🌐 https://vfapp.org/c272

USAID: Health Finance and Governance Project
Uses research to implement strategies to help countries develop robust governance systems, increase their domestic resources for health, manage those resources more effectively, and make wise purchasing decisions.
Logist-Op
☎ +1 202-712-0000
🌐 https://vfapp.org/8652

USAID: Leadership, Management and Governance Project
Improves leadership, management, and governance practices to strengthen health systems and improve health for all, including vulnerable populations worldwide.
Logist-Op
🌐 https://vfapp.org/d35e

World Blind Union (WBU)
Represents those experiencing blindness, speaking to governments and international bodies on issues concerning visual impairments.
Ophth-Opt
🌐 https://vfapp.org/2bd3

World Health Organization, The (WHO)
The United Nations' agency for health provides leadership on global health matters, shapes the health research agenda, setting norms and standards, articulates evidence-based policy options, provides technical support and monitoring to countries, and assesses health trends.
ER Med, General, Infect Dis, Logist-Op, MF Med, OB-GYN, Peds, Psych, Pub Health
☎ +41 22 791 21 11
🌐 https://vfapp.org/c476

World Medical Relief
Facilitates the distribution of surplus medical resources where they are needed.

Logist-Op

+1 313-866-5333

https://vfapp.org/72dc

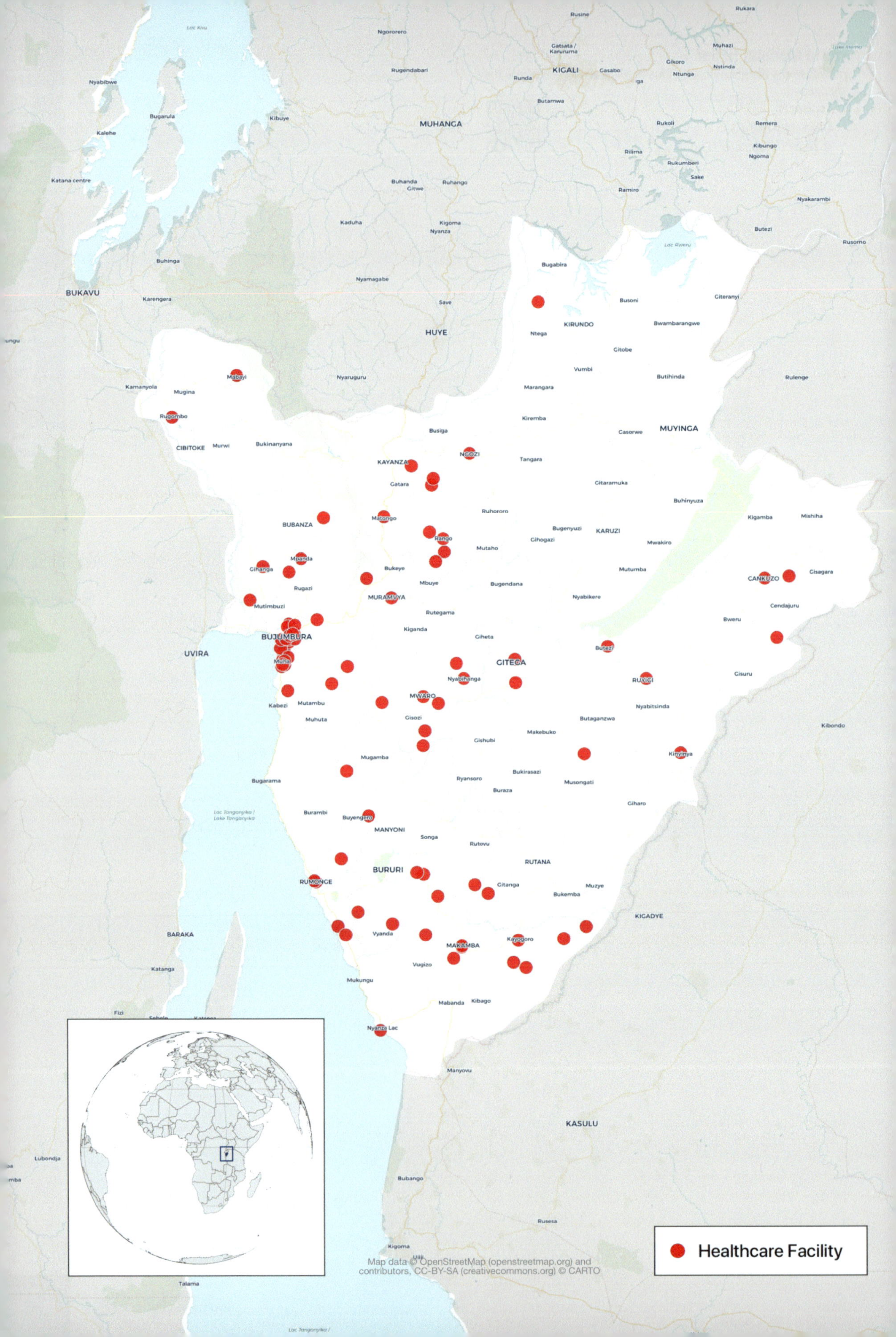

Lac Kivu
Ngororero
Rusine
Rukara
Gatsata / Karuruma
Muhazi
Lake Ihema
Nyabibwe
Rugendabari
Runda
KIGALI
Gasabo
Gikoro
Ntunga
Nstinda
Butamwa
Bugarula
Kibuye
MUHANGA
Rukoli
Remera
Kalehe
Rilima
Kibungo
Ngoma
Rukumberi
Katana centre
Buhanda
Gitwe
Ruhango
Sake
Ramiro
Nyakarambi
Kaduha
Kigoma
Nyanza
Butezi
Lac Rweru
Rusomo
Buhinga
Bugabira
Nyamagabe
BUKAVU
Karengera
Save
Busoni
Giteranyi
Ntega
KIRUNDO
Bwambarangwe
HUYE
Gitobe
Vumbi
Mabayi
Nyaruguru
Butihinda
Rulenge
Kamanyola
Mugina
Marangara
Rugombo
Kiremba
Busiga
Casorwe
MUYINGA
CIBITOKE
Murwi
Bukinanyana
NGOZI
KAYANZA
Tangara
Gatara
Gitaramuka
Buhinyuza
Ruhororo
Matongo
BUBANZA
Kigamba
Mishiha
Bugenyuzi
KARUZI
Rango
Gihogazi
Mutaho
Mwakiro
Mpanda
Gihanga
Bukeye
Mutumba
Cankuzo
Gisagara
Rugazi
Mbuye
Bugendana
MURAMVYA
Nyabikere
Mutimbuzi
Cendajuru
Rutegama
Bweru
BUJUMBURA
Kiganda
Giheta
UVIRA
Butezi
GITEGA
Muha
Nyabihanga
RUYIGI
Gisuru
MWARO
Kabezi
Mutambu
Nyabitsinda
Muhuta
Gisozi
Butaganzwa
Makebuko
Kibondo
Gishubi
Kinyinya
Mugamba
Bukirasazi
Ryansoro
Musongati
Bugarama
Buraza
Giharo
Lac Tanganyika / Lake Tanganyika
Buramb
Buyengero
MANYONI
Songa
Rutovu
RUTANA
BURURI
RUMONGE
Gitanga
Muzye
Bukemba
KIGADYE
BARAKA
Vyanda
Kayogoro
MAKAMBA
Katanga
Vugizo
Mukungu
Mabanda
Kibago
Fizi
Nyanza Lac
Manyovu
KASULU
Lubondja
Bubango
Rusesa
Kigoma
Healthcare Facility
Map data © OpenStreetMap (openstreetmap.org) and contributors, CC-BY-SA (creativecommons.org) © CARTO
Talama
Lac Tanganyika /

Burundi

Landlocked in the middle of Central-East Africa, the Republic of Burundi lies between Tanzania, Uganda, and the Democratic Republic of the Congo, and shares a long border with Lake Tanganyika. One of the last-standing African monarchies, whose kingship fell in 1966, Burundi has a population of 11.9 million. While small, Burundi is one of the most densely populated countries in Africa, with 470 inhabitants per square kilometer. The nation is 75 percent Christian and is unique for its linguistic homogeneity: Nearly the entire population speaks Kirundi.

Formerly a colony of Germany and Belgium, Burundi achieved independence in 1962, followed by decades of ethnic tension. The country has experienced both a civil war and a string of contentious elections. Ethnic friction between the usually-dominant Tutsi minority and the Hutu majority has further damaged the country's political stability and ability to control corruption. The majority of the population continues to live in poverty, with economic instability disproportionately affecting rural areas, where only 2 percent of households have access to electricity. In addition, food insecurity in Burundi is nearly double the average for sub-Saharan countries.

While life expectancy has increased and under-five mortality has decreased over time, communicable and non-communicable diseases continue to contribute to poor health indicators and a large burden of disease in the population. Illnesses causing the most deaths include diarrheal diseases, neonatal disorders, tuberculosis, malaria, lower respiratory infections, stroke, ischemic heart disease, congenital defects, HIV/AIDS, and protein-energy malnutrition, with significant increases in stroke and ischemic heart disease in recent years. Road injuries have also increased significantly in recent years and are a main contributor to disability.

11.9M
Population

$261
GDP Per Capita

61 years
Life Expectancy
↑ Improving

10	**79**	**548**
Doctors/100k	**Beds**/100k	**Deaths**/100k
Physician Density	Hospital Bed Density	Maternal Mortality

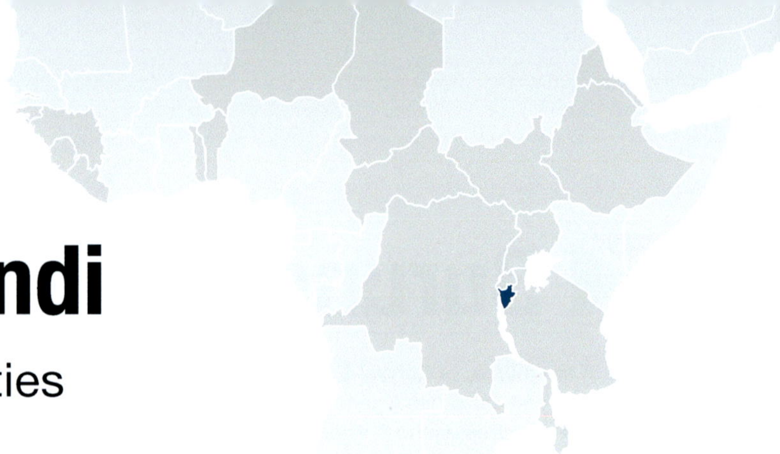

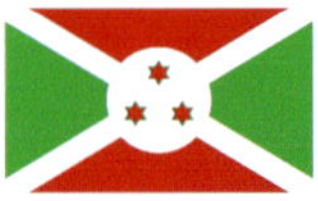

Burundi

Healthcare Facilities

Aluma
Boulevard de l'Unité,
Bujumbura, Bujumbura Mairie,
Burundi
🌐 https://vfapp.org/22a7

Banyagihugu 2
Avenue du Marche Kanyosha,
Kanyosha, Bujumbura Mairie,
Burundi
🌐 https://vfapp.org/2635

Bethel
7ème Avenue, Kanyosha,
Bujumbura Mairie, Burundi
🌐 https://vfapp.org/b33f

Bukiriro
RN 3, Kanyosha, Bujumbura
Mairie, Burundi
🌐 https://vfapp.org/a2f1

Bumerec
Avenue Ririkumutima,
Bujumbura, Bujumbura Mairie,
Burundi
🌐 https://vfapp.org/e57a

Cabara
RN 3, Kigwena, Rumonge,
Burundi
🌐 https://vfapp.org/8f3f

Cankuzo Hospital
RN 11, Cankuzo, Burundi
🌐 https://vfapp.org/28af

Cemadif
Rue Mugamba, Bujumbura,
Bujumbura Mairie, Burundi
🌐 https://vfapp.org/a4bd

Centre Medico Chirurgical de Kinindo (CMCK)
RN 3, Muha, Bujumbura Mairie,
Burundi
🌐 https://vfapp.org/7e17

Centre Médico -Technique de Ngozi
Ngozi, Burundi
🌐 https://vfapp.org/146c

Cibitoke District Hospital
RN 5, Cibitoke, Cibitoke,
Burundi
🌐 https://vfapp.org/b264

Croix Rouge Mwaro
RP 31, Mwaro, Mwaro, Burundi
🌐 https://vfapp.org/11ac

Dunga
RN 11, Makamba, Makamba,
Burundi
🌐 https://vfapp.org/d54f

Enfant Soleil
Chaussée du Peuple
Murundi, Bujumbura,
Bujumbura Mairie, Burundi
🌐 https://vfapp.org/4ec8

Gasenyi I
Rango, Kayanza, Burundi
🌐 https://vfapp.org/86d9

Gisenyi
Buyagira, Makamba, Burundi
🌐 https://vfapp.org/8984

Horizon
7ème Avenue, Kanyosha,
Bujumbura Mairie, Burundi
🌐 https://vfapp.org/4579

Hospital at Bisoro
Bisoro, Mwaro, Burundi
🌐 https://vfapp.org/22a9

Hospital at Bubera
Bubera, Rumonge, Burundi
🌐 https://vfapp.org/9e2f

Hospital at Buta
RN 17, Buta, Bururi, Burundi
🌐 https://vfapp.org/6abf

Hospital at Bwatemba
Bwatemba, Bururi, Burundi
🌐 https://vfapp.org/b964

Hospital at Gashirwe
Gashirwe, Cankuzo, Burundi
🌐 https://vfapp.org/c7f4

Hospital at Gatabo
Gatabo, Makamba, Burundi
🌐 https://vfapp.org/cfd5

Hospital at Gatakazi
Gatakazi, Musongati, Rutana,
Burundi
🌐 https://vfapp.org/32fb

Hospital at Gihanga
Gihanga, Burundi
🌐 https://vfapp.org/5b3c

Hospital at Gishiha
Gishiha, Makamba, Burundi
🌐 https://vfapp.org/2825

Hospital at Kanyosha
8ème Avenue, Kanyosha, Bujumbura Mairie, Burundi
https://vfapp.org/1a4a

Hospital at Kigwena
RN 3, Kigwena, Rumonge, Burundi
https://vfapp.org/4a92

Hospital at Makamba
Makamba, Burundi
https://vfapp.org/37d1

Hospital at Matara
RN7, Matara, Bujumbura Rural, Burundi
https://vfapp.org/34c7

Hospital at Matongo
RN 1, Matongo, Kayanza, Burundi
https://vfapp.org/5184

Hospital at Mugeni
Mugeni, Makamba, Burundi
https://vfapp.org/a8da

Hospital at Muhama
Muhama, Makamba, Burundi
https://vfapp.org/bb42

Hospital at Munini
RN 17, Munini, Bururi, Burundi
https://vfapp.org/ba6f

Hospital at Muramvya
RN 2, Muramvya, Muramvya, Burundi
https://vfapp.org/89b6

Hospital at Musenyi
Ngozi, Musenyi, Burundi
https://vfapp.org/b6c9

Hospital at Nyabihanga
Nyabihanga, Burundi
https://vfapp.org/cd2b

Hospital at Nyakararo
RN 18, Nyakararo, Mwaro, Burundi
https://vfapp.org/361f

Hospital at Nyakuguma
Nyakuguma, Rutana, Burundi
https://vfapp.org/83ab

Hospital at Nyarurama
Nyarurama, Burundi
https://vfapp.org/a976

Hospital at Rorero
Rorero, Burundi
https://vfapp.org/692d

Hospital at Rukago
RP 51, Rukago, Kayanza, Burundi
https://vfapp.org/34b9

Hospital Bwiza Jabe
Boulevard Ouest, Bujumbura, Bujumbura Mairie, Burundi
https://vfapp.org/7d61

Hospital Gaheta
Muramvya, Mbuye, Burundi
https://vfapp.org/3b1c

Hospital Gahombo
Kayanza, Gahombo, Burundi
https://vfapp.org/fc9b

Hospital Kankima
Bujumbura Rural, Mugongomanga, Burundi
https://vfapp.org/3195

Hospital Karehe
Muramvya, Mbuye, Burundi
https://vfapp.org/9176

Hospital Muramvya
Muramvya, Burundi
https://vfapp.org/3aeb

Hospital Mutaho
Mutaho, Muramvya, Burundi
https://vfapp.org/3b77

Hôpital de Kinyinya
RP 72, Kinyinya, Ruyigi, Burundi
https://vfapp.org/12b9

Hôpital de Rumonge
RN 3, Rumonge, Rumonge, Burundi
https://vfapp.org/addd

Hôpital Général de Mpanda
RN 9, Mpanda, Burundi
https://vfapp.org/529a

Hôpital Kibumbu
RN 18, Kibumbu, Mwaro, Burundi
https://vfapp.org/3968

Hôpital Mabayi
RN 10, Mabayi, Cibitoke, Burundi
https://vfapp.org/8421

Hôpital Militaire de Kamenge
Boulevard du 28 Novembre, Bujumbura, Burundi
https://vfapp.org/5e8e

Hôpital MSF de l'Arche
Avenue Kibezi, Bujumbura, Bujumbura Mairie, Burundi
https://vfapp.org/74e5

Hôpital Nyanzalac
RN 3, Nyanza Lac, Makamba, Burundi
https://vfapp.org/1895

Hôpital Prince Régent Charles (HPRC)
9 Avenue de l'Hôpital, Bujumbura, Burundi
https://vfapp.org/7519

Hôpital Roi Khaled
Vers ETS Kamenge, Bujumbura, Bujumbura Mairie, Burundi
https://vfapp.org/7dfe

Hôpital Régional de Gitega
Gitega, Burundi
https://vfapp.org/6d2c

Ibitalo ya Butezi
RP 201, Butezi, Ruyigi, Burundi
https://vfapp.org/68ea

Izere
RN 11, Makamba, Makamba, Burundi
https://vfapp.org/8e46

Kayogoro
RN 11, Makamba, Makamba, Burundi
https://vfapp.org/51ce

Kibezi
Bururi, Mugamba, Burundi
https://vfapp.org/b88c

Kibuye Hope Hospital (KHH)
Songa, Gitega, Burundi
https://vfapp.org/216c

Kigutu Hospital
Kirungu, Burundi
https://vfapp.org/afc3

Kinima
RN 3, Mena, Bujumbura Rural, Burundi
https://vfapp.org/7dcd

Kira Hospital
Boulevard de la Liberté, Bujumbura, Bujumbura Mairie, Burundi
https://vfapp.org/f933

La Charité
Boulevard Général Adolphe Nshimirimana, Bujumbura, Bujumbura Mairie, Burundi
https://vfapp.org/1752

Misericorde
Rue Gitaramuka, Bujumbura, Bujumbura Mairie, Burundi
https://vfapp.org/941d

Muberure
RN 1, Mirango, Bujumbura Mairie, Burundi
https://vfapp.org/75cf

Mugendo
Nyange, Kirundo, Burundi
https://vfapp.org/e17e

Muhweza
Rubimba, Bururi, Burundi
https://vfapp.org/18d1

Murengeza
R P 105, Murira, Bubanza, Burundi
https://vfapp.org/c2e8

Musigati
RN 9, Bubanza, Bubanza, Burundi
https://vfapp.org/a161

Muzenga I
RN 17, Kiremba, Bururi, Burundi
https://vfapp.org/a211

Muzenga II
Buyengero, Burundi
https://vfapp.org/24ca

Nyabiraba
RP 108, Vugizo, Bujumbura Rural, Burundi
https://vfapp.org/bc18

Nyakaraye
RP 32, Kavumu, Mwaro, Burundi
https://vfapp.org/147f

Parable
3ème Avenue, Muha, Bujumbura Mairie, Burundi
https://vfapp.org/4c2b

REMA Hospital
RN 13, Nyamutobo, Ruyigi, Burundi
https://vfapp.org/9cd4

Saint David
Boulevard Général Adolphe Nshimirimana, Bujumbura, Bujumbura Mairie, Burundi
https://vfapp.org/8d14

Saint Sauveur
RN 3, Rumonge, Rumonge, Burundi
https://vfapp.org/46a5

Santé Pour Tous
23e Avenue, Bujumbura, Bujumbura Mairie, Burundi
https://vfapp.org/15ca

Solidarité
22e Avenue, Bujumbura, Bujumbura Mairie, Burundi
https://vfapp.org/688b

Swaa-Burundi
Boulevard Mwambutsa, Bujumbura, Bujumbura Mairie, Burundi
https://vfapp.org/f283

Umuvyeyi
RN 3, Muha, Bujumbura Mairie, Burundi
https://vfapp.org/7f39

Burundi

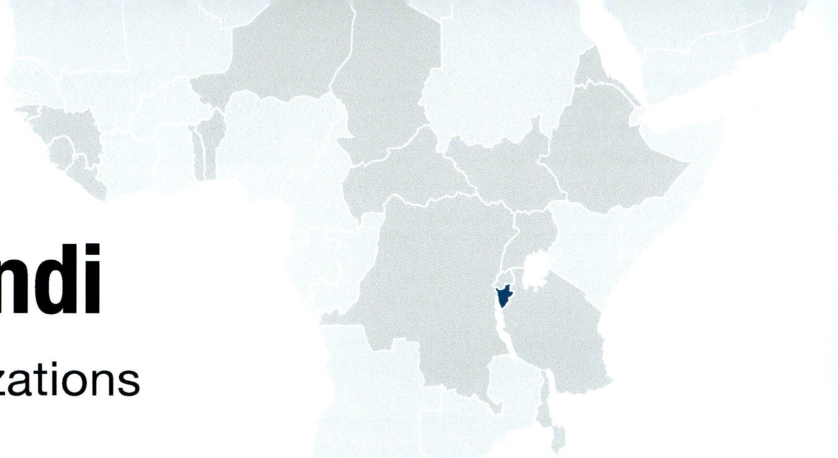

Nonprofit Organizations

Abt Associates
Seeks to improve the quality of life and economic well-being of people worldwide, while striving to meet and exceed the highest professional standards.

General, Logist-Op, MF Med, OB-GYN, Peds
+1 212-779-7700
https://vfapp.org/cec2

Africa CDC
Aims to strengthen the capacity and capability of Africa's public health institutions as well as partnerships to detect and respond quickly and effectively to disease threats and outbreaks, based on data-driven interventions and programs.

Infect Dis, Logist-Op, Pub Health
+251 11 551 7700
https://vfapp.org/339c

Africa Humanitarian Action (AHA)
Responds to crises, conflicts, and disasters in Africa, while informing and advising the international community, governments, civil society, and the private sector on humanitarian issues of concern to Africa. Supports institutional and organizational development efforts.

General, Infect Dis, MF Med, Nutr, OB-GYN
+251 11 660 4800
https://vfapp.org/3ca2

Africa Indoor Residual Spraying Project (AIRS)
Aims to protect millions of people in Africa from malaria by spraying insecticide on the walls, ceilings, and other indoor resting places of mosquitoes that transmit malaria.

Infect Dis
+1 301-347-5000
https://vfapp.org/9bd1

African Health Now
Promotes and provides information and access to sustainable primary healthcare to women, children, and families living across Sub-Saharan Africa.

Dent-OMFS, Endo, General, Infect Dis, MF Med, OB-GYN
https://vfapp.org/c766

Against Malaria Foundation
Helps protect people from malaria. Funds anti-malaria nets, specifically long-lasting insecticidal nets (LLINs), and works with distribution partners to ensure they are used. Tracks and reports on net use and malaria case data.

Infect Dis
+44 20 7371 8735
https://vfapp.org/337d

American Academy of Ophthalmology
Protects sight and empowers lives by serving as an advocate for patients and the public, leading ophthalmic education, and advancing the profession of ophthalmology.

Ophth-Opt
+1 415-561-8500
https://vfapp.org/89a2

Amref Health Africa
Serves millions of people across thirty-five countries in Sub-Saharan Africa, strengthening health systems, and training African health workers to respond to the continent's most critical health issues.

All-Immu, General, Infect Dis, Logist-Op, MF Med, OB-GYN, Path, Pub Health, Surg
+254 20 6993000
https://vfapp.org/6985

AO Alliance
Builds solutions to lessen the burden of injuries in low- and middle-income countries, while enhancing the care of the injured to reduce human suffering, disability, and poverty.

Ortho, Surg
https://vfapp.org/8cd5

Association for the Promotion of Human Health (APSH), Burundi
Promotes good health, education, and hope for children and underprivileged populations in Burundi.

CV Med, General, Infect Dis, OB-GYN
+257 71 29 66 75
https://vfapp.org/1e7c

Beta Humanitarian Help
Provides plastic surgery in underserved areas of the world.

Anesth, Plast
+49 228 909075778
https://vfapp.org/7221

Canadian Foundation for Women's Health
Seeks to advance the health of women in Canada and around the world through research, education, and advocacy in obstetrics and

gynecology.

MF Med, OB-GYN

+1 613-730-4192

https://vfapp.org/f41e

CARE

Works around the globe to save lives, defeat poverty, and achieve social justice.

ER Med, General

+1 800-422-7385

https://vfapp.org/7232

Carter Center, The

Seeks to prevent and resolve conflicts, enhance freedom and democracy, and improve health, while remaining committed to human rights and the alleviation of human suffering.

Infect Dis, MF Med, Ophth-Opt

+1 800-550-3560

https://vfapp.org/6556

Catholic Organization for Relief & Development Aid (CORDAID)

Provides humanitarian assistance and creates opportunities to improve security, healthcare, education, and inclusive economic growth in fragile and conflict-affected areas.

ER Med, Infect Dis, MF Med, OB-GYN, Peds, Psych

+31 70 313 6300

https://vfapp.org/8ae5

Center for Strategic and International Studies (CSIS) Commission on Strengthening America's Health Security

Brings together a distinguished and diverse group of high-level opinion leaders bridging security and health, with the core aim to chart a bold vision for the future of U.S. leadership in global health.

ER Med, Infect Dis, MF Med, Pub Health

+1 202-887-0200

https://vfapp.org/6d7f

Chain of Hope

Provides lifesaving heart operations for children around the world and supports the development of cardiac services in numerous developing and war-torn countries.

Anesth, CT Surg, CV Med, Crit-Care, Ped Surg, Peds, Pulm-Critic, Surg

+44 20 7351 1978

https://vfapp.org/1b1b

Christian Blind Mission (CBM)

Aims to improve the quality of life of persons with disabilities in the poorest countries, addressing poverty as a cause, and a consequence, of disability, and working in partnership to create a society for all.

ENT, General, Infect Dis, OB-GYN, Ophth-Opt, Ortho, Peds, Psych, Rehab, Surg

+49 6251 131131

https://vfapp.org/3824

Cleft Africa

Strives to provide underserved Africans with cleft lips and palates with access to the best possible treatment for their condition, so that they can live a life free of the health problems caused by cleft.

Anesth, Dent-OMFS, Ped Surg, Surg

https://vfapp.org/8298

Comitato Collaborazione Medica (CCM)

Supports development processes that safeguard and promote the right to health with a global approach, working on health needs and influencing socio-economic factors, identifying poverty as the main cause for the lack of health.

All-Immu, General, Infect Dis, MF Med, OB-GYN

+39 011 660 2793

https://vfapp.org/4272

Concern Worldwide

Seeks to permanently transform the lives of people living in extreme poverty, tackling its root causes, and building resilience.

Logist-Op, MF Med, Nutr, OB-GYN

+353 1 417 7700

https://vfapp.org/77e9

Core Group

Aims to improve and expand community health practices for underserved populations, especially women and children, through collaborative action and learning.

General, Infect Dis, MF Med, Medicine, OB-GYN, Peds, Pub Health

+1 202-380-3400

https://vfapp.org/9de3

Developing Country NGO Delegation: Global Fund to Fight AIDS, TB & Malaria

Works to strengthen the engagement of civil society actors and organizations in developing countries to contribute toward achieving a world in which AIDS, TB, and Malaria are no longer global, public health, and human rights threats.

Infect Dis, Pub Health

+254 20 2515790

https://vfapp.org/3149

Direct Relief

Improves the health and lives of people affected by poverty or emergency situations by mobilizing and providing essential medical resources needed for their care.

ER Med, Logist-Op

+1 805-964-4767

https://vfapp.org/58e5

Doctors Without Borders/Médecins Sans Frontières (MSF)

Responds to emergencies and provides lifesaving medical care where needed most, including during disasters, conflicts, and epidemics.

Anesth, Crit-Care, ER Med, General, Infect Dis, Nutr, OB-GYN, Ped Surg, Peds, Psych, Pub Health, Surg

+1 212-679-6800

https://vfapp.org/f363

Enabel

As the development agency of the Belgian federal government, charged with implementing Belgium's international development policy, carries out public service assignments in Belgium and abroad pursuant to the 2030 Agenda for Sustainable Development.

General, Infect Dis, Logist-Op, MF Med, OB-GYN, Peds, Pub Health

+32 2 505 37 00

https://vfapp.org/5af7

END Fund, The

Aims to control and eliminate the most prevalent neglected diseases among the world's poorest and most vulnerable people.

Infect Dis
📞 +1 646-690-9775
🌐 https://vfapp.org/2614

EngenderHealth
Works to implement high-quality, gender-equitable programs that advance sexual and reproductive health and rights.
General, MF Med, OB-GYN, Peds
📞 +1 202-902-2000
🌐 https://vfapp.org/1cb2

Episcopal Relief & Development
Provides relief in times of disaster and promotes sustainable development by identifying and addressing the root causes of suffering.
Infect Dis, MF Med, Neonat, Nutr, Peds
📞 +1 855-312-4325
🌐 https://vfapp.org/7cfa

Fracarita International
Provides support and services in the fields of mental healthcare, care for people with a disability, and education.
Psych, Rehab
🌐 https://vfapp.org/8d3c

Fred Hollows Foundation, The
Works toward a world in which no person is needlessly blind or vision impaired.
Ophth-Opt, Pub Health, Surg
📞 +1 646-374-0445
🌐 https://vfapp.org/73e5

Global Clubfoot Initiative (GCI)
Promotes and resources the treatment of children with clubfoot in developing countries using the Ponseti technique.
Ortho, Ped Surg
🌐 https://vfapp.org/f229

Global Ministries – The United Methodist Church
As the worldwide mission and development agency of The United Methodist Church, Global Ministries works with more than 300 hospitals and clinics around the world through its Global Health Unit.
Anesth, CT Surg, CV Med, Crit-Care, Dent-OMFS, Derm, ER Med, GI, General, Infect Dis, Logist-Op, MF Med, Medicine, Neonat, Nephro, Nutr, OB-GYN, Ophth-Opt, Ortho, Palliative, Peds, Pod, Psych, Pub Health, Rehab, Rheum, Surg, Urol
📞 +1 800-862-4246
🌐 https://vfapp.org/1723

Global Oncology (GO)
Brings the best in cancer care to underserved patients around the world and collaborates across geographic, professional, and academic borders to improve cancer care, research, and education.
Heme-Onc, Path, Rad-Onc
🌐 https://vfapp.org/fcb8

Health Equity Initiative
Aims to build and sustain a global community that engages across sectors and disciplines to advance health equity.
Pub Health
🌐 https://vfapp.org/e2e2

HealthNet TPO
Aims to facilitate and strengthen communities and help them to regain control and maintain their health and well-being, believing that even the most vulnerable people have the inner strength to rebuild a better future for themselves.
Crit-Care, General, Infect Dis, Logist-Op, Medicine, OB-GYN, Ophth-Opt, Peds, Psych, Pub Health, Surg
📞 +31 20 620 0005
🌐 https://vfapp.org/67d6

Healthy Developments
Provides Germany-supported health and social protection programs around the globe in a collaborative knowledge management process.
All-Immu, General, Infect Dis, Logist-Op, MF Med
🌐 https://vfapp.org/dc31

Hope and Healing International
Gives hope and healing to children and families trapped by poverty and disability.
General, Nutr, Ophth-Opt, Peds, Rehab
📞 +1 905-640-6464
🌐 https://vfapp.org/c638

Hope Walks
Frees children, families, and communities from the burden of clubfoot, inspired by the Christian faith.
Ortho, Ped Surg, Peds, Rehab
📞 +1 717-502-4400
🌐 https://vfapp.org/f6d4

ICAP at Columbia University
Serves as global leader in supporting the scale-up of multidisciplinary HIV/AIDS prevention, care, and treatment programs based on a family-focused approach.
General, Infect Dis, MF Med, Medicine, OB-GYN, Pub Health
📞 +1 212-342-0505
🌐 https://vfapp.org/a8ef

International Agency for the Prevention of Blindness (IAPB), The
Leads international efforts in blindness-prevention activities, works toward a world where no one is needlessly visually impaired, and ensures that everyone has access to the best possible standard of eye health.
Infect Dis, Ophth-Opt, Pub Health
🌐 https://vfapp.org/87a2

International Council of Ophthalmology
Works with ophthalmologic societies and others to enhance ophthalmic education and improve access to the highest quality eye care in order to preserve and restore vision for the people of the world.
Ophth-Opt
🌐 https://vfapp.org/ffd2

International Federation of Red Cross and Red Crescent Societies (IFRC)
Coordinates and directs international assistance following natural and man-made disasters in nonconflict situations through the world's largest humanitarian and development network. Provides disaster-preparedness programs, healthcare activities, and promotes humanitarian values.
ER Med, General, Infect Dis, Nutr
📞 +1 212-338-0161
🌐 https://vfapp.org/b4ee

International Medical and Surgical Aid (IMSA)
Aims to save lives and alleviate suffering through education, healthcare, surgical camps, and quality medical programs.
Anesth, General, Ped Surg, Surg
+44 7598 088806
https://vfapp.org/2561

International Medical Corps
Seeks to improve quality of life through health interventions and related activities that strengthen underserved communities worldwide, with the flexibility to respond rapidly to emergencies and offer medical services and training to people at the highest risk.
ER Med, General, Infect Dis, Nutr, OB-GYN, Peds, Pub Health, Surg
+1 310-826-7800
https://vfapp.org/a8a5

International Organization for Migration (IOM) – The UN Migration Agency
Promotes evidence-informed policies and holistic, preventive, and curative health programs that are beneficial, accessible, and equitable for vulnerable migrants.
General, Infect Dis, OB-GYN
+27 12 342 2789
https://vfapp.org/621a

International Planned Parenthood Federation (IPPF)
Leads a locally owned, globally connected civil society movement that provides and enables services and champions sexual and reproductive health and rights for all, especially the underserved.
Infect Dis, MF Med, OB-GYN
+44 20 7939 8200
https://vfapp.org/dc97

International Rescue Committee (IRC)
Responds to the world's worst humanitarian crises and helps people whose lives and livelihoods are shattered by conflict and disaster to survive, recover, and gain control of their future.
ER Med, General, Infect Dis, MF Med, Peds
+1 212-551-3000
https://vfapp.org/5d24

International Trachoma Initiative (iTi)
Works toward a world free from trachoma, a preventable cause of blindness, and provides comprehensive support to national ministries of health and governmental and nongovernmental organizations to implement a comprehensive approach to fight trachoma.
Infect Dis, Ophth-Opt
+1 404-371-0466
https://vfapp.org/3278

John Snow, Inc. (JSI)
Aims to improve the health and well-being of underserved and vulnerable people and communities throughout the world.
General, Infect Dis, Logist-Op, MF Med, OB-GYN, Peds, Psych, Pub Health
+1 617-482-9485
https://vfapp.org/ba78

Johns Hopkins Center for Global Health
Facilitates and focuses the extensive expertise and resources of the Johns Hopkins institutions together with global collaborators to effectively address and ameliorate the world's most pressing health issues.
General, Genetics, Logist-Op, MF Med, Peds, Psych, Pub Health, Pulm-Critic
+1 410-502-9872
https://vfapp.org/54ce

Joint United Nations Programme on HIV/AIDS (UNAIDS)
Aims to place people living with HIV and people affected by the virus at the decision-making table and at the center of designing, delivering, and monitoring the AIDS response.
Infect Dis
+41 22 791 36 66
https://vfapp.org/464a

Kibuye Hope Hospital (KHH)
Serves and treats surrounding communities through high-quality specialist doctors, a robust medical school, government support, and an expanding campus, inspired by the Christian faith.
Anesth, ER Med, Medicine, Ophth-Opt, Ophth-Opt, Path, Peds, Radiol, Surg
https://vfapp.org/bdf8

Lay Volunteers International Association (LVIA)
Fosters local and global change to help overcome extreme poverty, reinforce equitable and sustainable development, and enhance dialogue between Italian and African communities.
ER Med, Logist-Op, MF Med, Neonat, Nutr, OB-GYN, Peds
+39 0171 696975
https://vfapp.org/ecd4

Life for a Child
Supports the provision of the best possible health care, given local circumstances, to all children and youth with diabetes in less-resourced countries, through the strengthening of existing diabetes services.
Endo, Medicine, Peds
https://vfapp.org/d712

LifeNet International
Transforms African healthcare by equipping and empowering existing local health centers to provide quality, sustainable, and lifesaving care to patients.
General, Infect Dis, MF Med, Neonat, OB-GYN, Pub Health
+1 407-630-9518
https://vfapp.org/e5d2

Lions Clubs International
Empowers volunteers to serve their communities, meet humanitarian needs, encourage peace, and promote international understanding through Lions clubs.
Heme-Onc, Medicine, Nutr, Ophth-Opt
+1 630-571-5466
https://vfapp.org/7b12

Management Sciences for Health (MSH)
Works with countries and communities to save lives and improve the health of the world's poorest and most vulnerable people by building strong, resilient, sustainable health systems.
Infect Dis, Logist-Op, Pub Health
+1 617-250-9500
https://vfapp.org/6aa2

MAP International
Provides medicines and health supplies to those in need around the world so they might experience life to the fullest.
Logist-Op
+1 800-225-8550
https://vfapp.org/deed

MedShare
Aims to improve the quality of life of people, communities, and the planet by sourcing and directly delivering surplus medical supplies and equipment to communities in need around the world.
Logist-Op
+1 770-323-5858
https://vfapp.org/c8bc

Mercy Ships
Operates hospital ships staffed by volunteers to bring hope, healing, and healthcare to underserved communities worldwide.
Anesth, Dent-OMFS, Logist-Op, Neonat, OB-GYN, Ophth-Opt, Ortho, Palliative, Plast, Psych, Surg
+1 903-939-7000
https://vfapp.org/2e99

Mission Partners for Christ
Provides medication, treatment, screenings, and health education in underserved communities around the world, inspired by the Christian faith.
Dent-OMFS, General, Ophth-Opt
+1 312-307-5475
https://vfapp.org/eb25

NCD Alliance
Unites and strengthens civil society to stimulate collaborative advocacy, action, and accountability for NCD (noncommunicable disease) prevention and control.
All-Immu, CV Med, General, Heme-Onc, Medicine, Peds, Psych
+41 22 809 18 11
https://vfapp.org/abdd

Neglected Tropical Disease NGO Network
Works to create a global forum for non-governmental organizations working to control onchocerciasis, lymphatic filariasis, schistosomiasis, soil transmitted helminths, and trachoma.
Infect Dis, Logist-Op
+1 929-272-6227
https://vfapp.org/c511

Operation Fistula
Exists to end obstetric fistula by building models of care that serve every woman, everywhere.
MF Med, OB-GYN, Surg
+1 512-687-3479
https://vfapp.org/ce8e

Pact
Works on the ground to improve the lives of those who are challenged by poverty and marginalization, striving for a world where all people are heard, capable, and vibrant.
Infect Dis, Logist-Op, MF Med, Pub Health
+1 202-466-5666
https://vfapp.org/9a6c

Pan-African Academy of Christian Surgeons (PAACS)
Exists to train and support African surgeons to provide excellent, compassionate care to those most in need, inspired by the Christian faith.
Anesth, CT Surg, Neurosurg, OB-GYN, Ortho, Ped Surg, Plast, Surg
+1 847-571-9926
https://vfapp.org/85ba

Partners in Health
Responds to the moral imperative to provide high-quality healthcare globally to those who need it most, while striving to ease suffering by providing a comprehensive model of care that includes access to food, transportation, housing, and other key components of healing.
CT Surg, General, Heme-Onc, Infect Dis, MF Med, Neurosurg, OB-GYN, Ortho, Plast, Psych, Urol
+1 857-880-5600
https://vfapp.org/dc9c

Pathfinder International
Champions sexual and reproductive health and rights worldwide, mobilizing communities most in need to break through barriers and forge paths to a healthier future.
OB-GYN
+1 617-924-7200
https://vfapp.org/a7b3

PINCC Preventing Cervical Cancer
Seeks to prevent female-specific diseases in developing countries by utilizing low-cost and low-technology methods to create sustainable programs through patient education, medical personnel training, and facility outfitting.
OB-GYN
+1 830-708-6009
https://vfapp.org/9666

Project Concern International (PCI)
Drives innovation from the ground up to enhance health, end hunger, overcome hardship, and advance women and girls—resulting in meaningful and measurable change in people's lives.
Infect Dis, MF Med, Nutr, OB-GYN, Peds
+1 858-279-9690
https://vfapp.org/5ed7

PSI – Population Services International
Dedicates efforts to improving the health of people in the developing world by focusing on challenges such as a lack of family planning, HIV/AIDS, barriers to maternal health, and the greatest threats to children under the age of 5, including malaria, diarrhea, pneumonia, and malnutrition.
Infect Dis, MF Med, OB-GYN, Peds
+1 202-785-0072
https://vfapp.org/ffe3

RestoringVision
Empowers lives by restoring vision for millions of people in need.
Ophth-Opt
+1 209-980-7323
https://vfapp.org/e121

Rockefeller Foundation, The
Works to promote the well-being of humanity.

Logist-Op, Nutr, Pub Health
+1 212-869-8500
https://vfapp.org/5424

Rotary International
Provides service to others, improves lives, and advances world understanding, goodwill, and peace through its fellowship of business, professional, and community leaders.
ER Med, General, Infect Dis, MF Med, OB-GYN
https://vfapp.org/8fb5

Salvation Army International, The
Seeks to meet human needs through services in education, healthcare, community support, emergency response, and ministry development, inspired by the Christian faith.
Dent-OMFS, Derm, ER Med, Infect Dis, MF Med, Medicine, Nutr, OB-GYN, Ophth-Opt, Palliative, Psych, Rehab, Surg
+44 20 7332 0101
https://vfapp.org/8eb3

Samaritan's Purse International Disaster Relief
Provides spiritual and physical aid to hurting people around the world, such as victims of war, poverty, natural disasters, disease, and famine, based in Christian ministry.
Anesth, CT Surg, Crit-Care, Dent-OMFS, Derm, ENT, ER Med, Endo, GI, General, Heme-Onc, Infect Dis, MF Med, Neonat, Nephro, Neuro, Neurosurg, Nutr, OB-GYN, Ophth-Opt, Ortho, Path, Ped Surg, Peds, Plast, Psych, Pulm-Critic, Radiol, Rehab, Rheum, Surg, Urol, Vasc Surg
+1 800-528-1980
https://vfapp.org/87e3

Santé Communauté Développement
Promotes the health of communities in Burundi through information, education, and promotion of good practices leading to health and development.
General, OB-GYN
+257 22 27 90 25
https://vfapp.org/62d4

Save the Children
Gives children around the world a healthy start in life, the opportunity to learn, and protection from harm.
All-Immu, Crit-Care, ER Med, General, Infect Dis, MF Med, Medicine, Neonat, OB-GYN, Peds, Psych, Pub Health
+1 800-728-3843
https://vfapp.org/2e73

SEE International
Provides sustainable medical, surgical, and educational services through volunteer ophthalmic surgeons, with the objectives of restoring sight and preventing blindness to disadvantaged individuals worldwide.
Ophth-Opt, Surg
+1 805-963-3303
https://vfapp.org/6e1b

SIGN Fracture Care International
Builds orthopedic capacity around the world and provides the injured poor access to fracture surgery by donating orthopedic education and implant systems to surgeons in developing countries.
Ortho, Rehab, Surg
+1 509-371-1107
https://vfapp.org/123d

Smile Train
Seeks to give every child with a cleft the opportunity for a healthy, productive life by providing free cleft repair surgery and comprehensive cleft care in their own communities.
Dent-OMFS, ENT, Plast
+1 800-932-9541
https://vfapp.org/f21d

Solthis
Improves disease prevention and access to quality care by strengthening the health systems and services of the countries served.
General, Infect Dis, Logist-Op, MF Med, Neonat, Path
+33 1 81 70 17 90
https://vfapp.org/a71d

Swiss Tropical and Public Health Institute
Contributes to the improvement of the health of populations internationally, nationally, and locally through excellence in research, education, and services.
Infect Dis, Pub Health
+41 61 284 81 11
https://vfapp.org/2ee4

Task Force for Global Health, The
Consists of programs and focus areas that cover a range of global health issues including neglected tropical diseases, infectious diseases, vaccines, field epidemiology, public health informatics, health workforce development, and global health ethics.
Infect Dis, Logist-Op, Medicine, Ophth-Opt, Peds
+1 404-371-0466
https://vfapp.org/714c

Tearfund
Responds to crisis and partners with local churches to bring restoration to those living in poverty, inspired by the Christian faith.
ER Med, Logist-Op
+44 20 3906 3906
https://vfapp.org/f6cf

Terre Des Hommes
Works to improve the conditions of the most vulnerable children worldwide by improving the health of children under the age of 3, protecting migrant children, providing humanitarian aid to children and their families in times of crisis, and preventing child exploitation.
ER Med, MF Med, Neonat, OB-GYN, Ped Surg, Peds
+41 58 611 06 66
https://vfapp.org/2689

Union for International Cancer Control (UICC)
Unites and supports the cancer community to reduce the global cancer burden, promote greater equity, and ensure that cancer control continues to be a priority in the world health and development agenda.
Heme-Onc, Pub Health
+41 22 809 18 11
https://vfapp.org/88b1

United Nations Children's Fund (UNICEF)
Works in over 190 countries and territories to save children's lives, to defend their rights, and to help them fulfill their potential, from early childhood through adolescence.
All-Immu, Infect Dis, MF Med, Neonat, Nutr, OB-GYN, Ped Surg, Peds, Pub Health
https://vfapp.org/42d7

United Nations Development Programme (UNDP)
Helps countries achieve the simultaneous eradication of extreme poverty and significant reduction of inequalities and exclusion using a sustainable human development approach.

Infect Dis, Logist-Op, Pub Health

🌐 https://vfapp.org/935c

United Nations High Commissioner for Refugees (UNHCR)
Safeguards the rights and well-being of people who have been forced to flee, ensuring that everybody has the right to seek asylum and find safe refuge in another country, with the goal of seeking lasting solutions.

General, MF Med, Medicine, OB-GYN, Peds, Psych, Pub Health

🌐 https://vfapp.org/6636

United Nations Office for the Coordination of Humanitarian Affairs (OCHA)
Contributes to principled and effective humanitarian response through coordination, advocacy, policy, information management, and humanitarian financing tools and services, by leveraging functional expertise throughout the organization.

Logist-Op

🌐 https://vfapp.org/22b8

United Nations Population Fund (UNFPA)
Supports reproductive healthcare for women and youth in more than 150 countries, focusing on delivering a world where every pregnancy is wanted, every childbirth is safe, and every young person's potential is fulfilled.

Infect Dis, MF Med, Neonat, OB-GYN, Peds, Pub Health

📞 +1 212-963-6008

🌐 https://vfapp.org/c969

United States Agency for International Development (USAID)
Promotes and demonstrates democratic values abroad and advances a free, peaceful, and prosperous world. Leads the U.S. government's international development and disaster assistance through partnerships and investments that save lives.

ER Med, Infect Dis, MF Med, OB-GYN, Peds

📞 +1 202-712-0000

🌐 https://vfapp.org/9a99

USAID: EQUIP Health
Exists as an effective, efficient response mechanism to achieving global HIV epidemic control by delivering the right intervention at the right place and in the right way.

Infect Dis

📞 +27 11 276 8850

🌐 https://vfapp.org/d76a

USAID: Health Finance and Governance Project
Uses research to implement strategies to help countries develop robust governance systems, increase their domestic resources for health, manage those resources more effectively, and make wise purchasing decisions.

Logist-Op

📞 +1 202-712-0000

🌐 https://vfapp.org/8652

USAID: Human Resources for Health 2030 (HRH2030)
Helps low- and middle-income countries develop the health workforce needed to prevent maternal and child deaths, support the goals of Family Planning 2020, control the HIV/AIDS epidemic, and protect communities from infectious diseases.

Logist-Op

📞 +1 202-955-3300

🌐 https://vfapp.org/9ea8

Village Health Works
Provides quality, compassionate healthcare in a dignified environment while also addressing the root causes of illness, poverty, violence, and neglect.

Anesth, General, Infect Dis, MF Med, Medicine, OB-GYN, Peds, Psych, Surg

📞 +1 917-546-9219

🌐 https://vfapp.org/56b5

Vision for the Poor
Reduces human suffering and improves quality of life through the recovery of sight by building sustainable eye hospitals in developing countries, empowering local eye specialists, funding essential ophthalmic infrastructure, and partnering with like-minded agencies.

Ophth-Opt

📞 +1 814-823-4486

🌐 https://vfapp.org/528e

Vision Outreach International
Advocates for helping the blind in underserved regions of the world and empowers the poor through sight restoration.

Ophth-Opt

📞 +1 269-428-3300

🌐 https://vfapp.org/9721

Vitamin Angels
Helps at-risk populations in need—specifically pregnant women, new mothers, and children under age five—to gain access to life-changing vitamins and minerals.

General, Nutr

📞 +1 805-564-8400

🌐 https://vfapp.org/7da1

Wings of Hope for Africa Foundation
Aims to support family welfare, empowers communities, and develops self-sufficiency programs to end poverty in Burundi and Rwanda, East Africa, and in Calgary, Canada.

Infect Dis, Medicine, Peds

📞 +1 403-815-0037

🌐 https://vfapp.org/8d4e

Women's Refugee Commission
Seeks to improve lives by protecting the rights of women, children, and youth displaced by conflict and crisis through researching their needs, identifying solutions, and advocating for programs and policies to strengthen their resilience.

General, MF Med, Neonat, OB-GYN, Peds, Psych

📞 +1 212-551-3115

🌐 https://vfapp.org/3d8f

World Gospel Mission
Mobilizes volunteers to help transform communities through healthcare and education, based in Christian ministry.

ER Med, General

📞 +1 765-664-7331

https://vfapp.org/efa4

World Health Organization, The (WHO)
The United Nations' agency for health provides leadership on global health matters, shapes the health research agenda, setting norms and standards, articulates evidence-based policy options, provides technical support and monitoring to countries, and assesses health trends.

ER Med, General, Infect Dis, Logist-Op, MF Med, OB-GYN, Peds, Psych, Pub Health

+41 22 791 21 11

https://vfapp.org/c476

World Relief
Brings sustainable solutions to the world's greatest problems: disasters, extreme poverty, violence, oppression, and mass displacement.

ER Med, Nutr, Psych, Pub Health

+1 800-535-5433

https://vfapp.org/fbcd

World Vision International
Works with vulnerable communities around the world to overcome poverty and injustice with child-focused programs.

ER Med, General, Infect Dis, MF Med, Nutr, OB-GYN, Peds

+1 626-303-8811

https://vfapp.org/2642

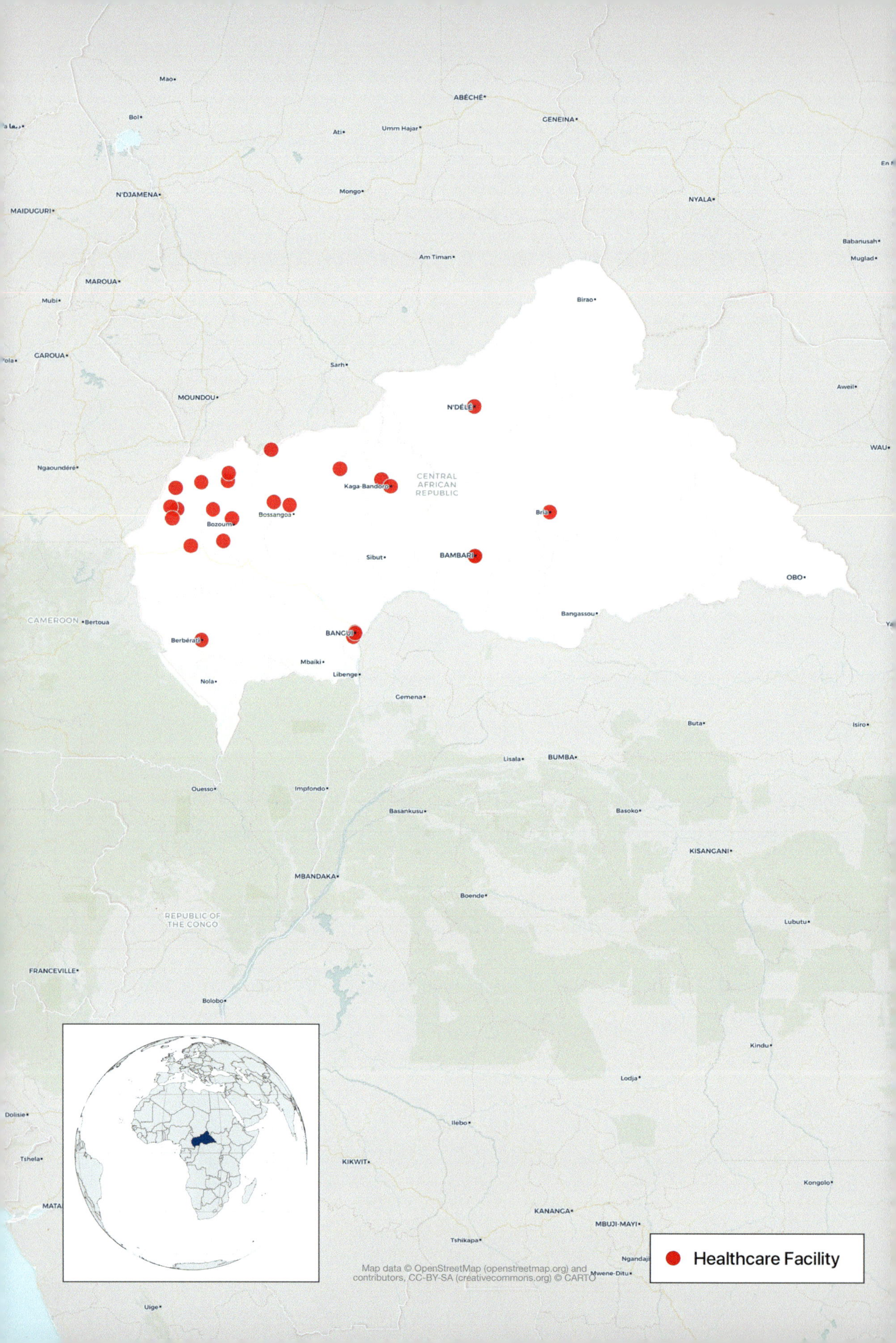

Mao
Bol
ABÉCHÉ
GENEINA
Ati
Umm Hajar
N'DJAMENA
MAIDUGURI
Mongo
NYALA
Am Timan
Babanusah
Muglad
MAROUA
Mubi
Birao
GAROUA
Sarh
MOUNDOU
Aweil
N'DÉLÉ
WAU
Ngaoundéré
CENTRAL
AFRICAN
REPUBLIC
Kaga-Bandoro
Bossangoa
Bozoum
Bria
Sibut
BAMBARI
OBO
Bangassou
CAMEROON
Bertoua
Berbérati
BANGUI
Mbaïki
Libenge
Nola
Gemena
Buta
Isiro
Lisala
BUMBA
Ouesso
Impfondo
Basankusu
Basoko
KISANGANI
MBANDAKA
Boende
REPUBLIC OF
THE CONGO
Lubutu
FRANCEVILLE
Bolobo
Kindu
Lodja
Dolisie
Ilebo
Tshela
KIKWIT
Kongolo
KANANGA
MBUJI-MAYI
Tshikapa
Ngandajika
Mwene-Ditu
Uige
Healthcare Facility
Map data © OpenStreetMap (openstreetmap.org) and contributors, CC-BY-SA (creativecommons.org) © CARTO

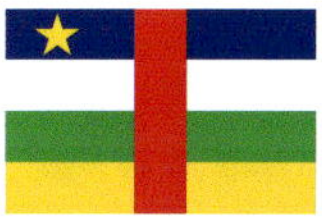

Central African Republic

Located in the middle of the African continent is the Central African Republic (CAR), whose neighbors include Chad, Sudan, South Sudan, the Democratic Republic of the Congo, the Republic of the Congo, and Cameroon. Known for its exceptional natural beauty and wildlife, the CAR is home to a young population of 6 million people living primarily in the western and central areas of the country and around the capital city of Bangui. The majority of the population is Christian and culturally falls into several ethnic groups including the Baya, Banda, Mandjia, Sara, and M'Baka-bantu. The national language is Sangho, but French is also spoken in an official capacity.

The Central African Republic achieved independence from France in 1960 and has since experienced decades of misrule, military coups, contentious elections, and rebellion. The country's most recent state of turmoil was the result of a violent takeover of power in 2013 and an uprising that displaced 25 percent of the population. In February 2018, progress was made when the country signed an African Union–mediated peace agreement with 14 armed groups; however, fighting between rebel groups continues. Today the CAR is one of the world's poorest and least developed countries. About 71 percent of the population lives below the international poverty line.

As a result of conflict and economic turmoil, more than half the country requires humanitarian assistance, with over one million in acute need. Health indicators include an alarming maternal mortality rate and an average life expectancy of 53 years. Leading causes of death include tuberculosis, diarrheal diseases, lower respiratory infections, HIV/AIDS, neonatal disorders, and malaria. In recent years, congenital defects and stroke have also become more significant contributors to death, as have road injuries.

6M
Population

$468
GDP Per Capita

53 years
Life Expectancy
↑ Improving

7.2	100	829
Doctors/100k	**Beds**/100k	**Deaths**/100k
Physician Density	Hospital Bed Density	Maternal Mortality

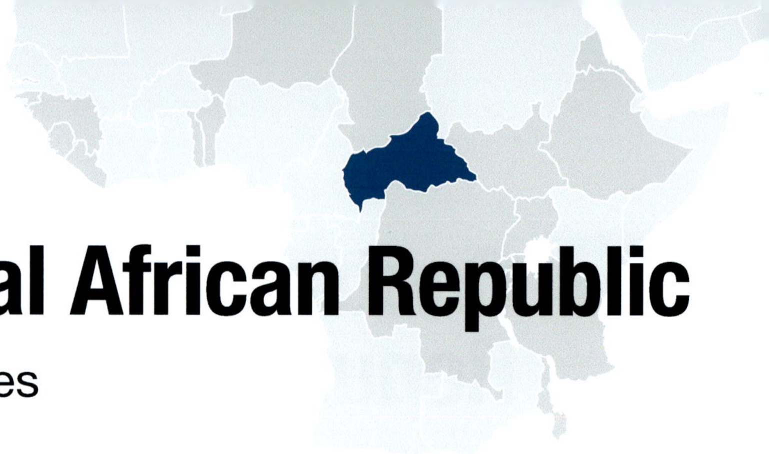

Central African Republic

Healthcare Facilities

ACABEF Antenne Ouaka
Ouaka, Bambari, Centre Ville, Central African Republic
https://vfapp.org/e851

Hospital at Batangafo
Batangafo, Central African Republic
https://vfapp.org/5bd8

Hospital at Dohiya
Nana-Mambere, Bouar, Niem-Yelewa, Dohiya, Central African Republic
https://vfapp.org/fcb7

Hospital at Kella Moelle
Ouham-Pende, Koui, Kella Moelle, Central African Republic
https://vfapp.org/6fcc

Hospital at Kokol
RR 6, Bétara, Ouham-Pendé, Central African Republic
https://vfapp.org/613c

Hospital at Kounpala
Ouham-Pende, Bocaranga, Loura, Kounpala, Central African Republic
https://vfapp.org/869e

Hospital at Kounpo
Kounpo, Ouham-Pendé, Central African Republic
https://vfapp.org/d822

Hospital at Yelewa
Nana-Mambere, Bouar, Niem-Yelewa, Yelewa, Central African Republic
https://vfapp.org/546b

Hôpital Communautaire
Avenue des Martyrs, Bangui, Central African Republic
https://vfapp.org/25ef

Hôpital de Bimbo
Bimbo, Central African Republic
https://vfapp.org/2f15

Hôpital de l'Amitié
1359 RN 2, Bangî – Bangui, Central African Republic
https://vfapp.org/c52e

Hôpital Préfectoral
RN 3, Bouar, Nana-Mambéré, Central African Republic
https://vfapp.org/af1b

Hôpital Préfectoral
RN 8, N'Délé, Bamingui-Bangoran, Central African Republic
https://vfapp.org/7cef

Hôpital Préfectoral de Kaga-Bandoro
Nana-Gribizi, Kaga-Bandoro, Centre-ville, Central African Republic
https://vfapp.org/eb73

Hôpital Régional de Berbérati
RN 6, Berbérati, Mambéré-Kadéï, Central African Republic
https://vfapp.org/9e55

Hôpital Régional de Bria
RN 5, Bria, Haute-Kotto, Central African Republic
https://vfapp.org/d69c

Hôpital Universitaire Régional de Bambari
RN2, Bambari, Central African Republic
https://vfapp.org/5517

PS Bodouk
RN 1, Bokongo 1, Ouham, Central African Republic
https://vfapp.org/a48c

PS de Boyali Yaho
Boyali Yaho, Ouham-Pendé, Central African Republic
https://vfapp.org/2dd3

PS de Oda-Kete
Oda-Kota, Ouham, Central African Republic
https://vfapp.org/2fbb

PS de Patcho
RR 10, Boumbala 2, Nana-Grébizi, Central African Republic
https://vfapp.org/eaf8

PS de Tolle
RR 4, Gouni, Ouham-Pendé, Central African Republic
https://vfapp.org/ac99

PS Gbade
Route Gbade – Bobili, Boyongo, Ouham, Central African Republic
https://vfapp.org/ea1b

PS Pendé
RR 4, Kalandao, Ouham-Pendé, Central African Republic
https://vfapp.org/1c35

Sanguere Lim
Ouham-Pende, Koui, Koui,
Sanguere Lim, Central African Republic
https://vfapp.org/f737

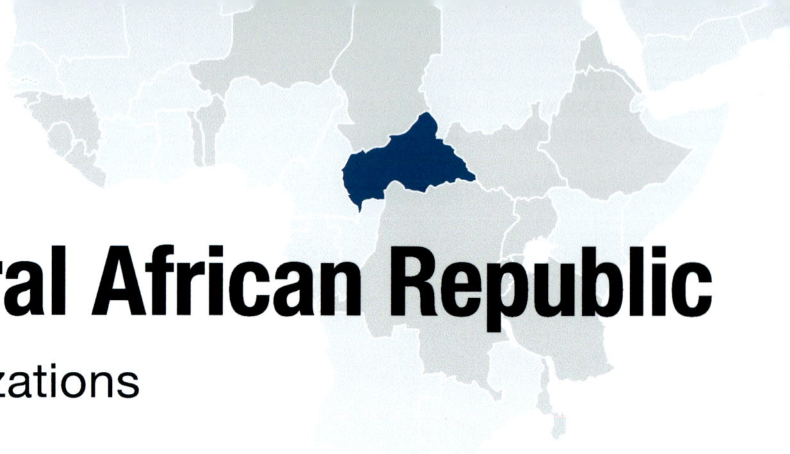

Central African Republic

Nonprofit Organizations

Action Against Hunger
Aims to end life-threatening hunger for good through treating and preventing malnutrition across more than forty-five countries.
📞 +1 212-967-7800
🌐 https://vfapp.org/2dbc

Africa CDC
Aims to strengthen the capacity and capability of Africa's public health institutions as well as partnerships to detect and respond quickly and effectively to disease threats and outbreaks, based on data-driven interventions and programs.
Infect Dis, Logist-Op, Pub Health
📞 +251 11 551 7700
🌐 https://vfapp.org/339c

Africa Inland Mission International
Seeks to establish churches and community development programs including health care projects, based in Christian ministry.
Anesth, Dent-OMFS, ER Med, General, MF Med, Medicine, OB-GYN, OB-GYN, Ophth-Opt, Ped Surg, Peds, Rehab
🌐 https://vfapp.org/f2f6

Alliance for International Medical Action, The (ALIMA)
Provides quality medical care to vulnerable populations, partnering with and developing national medical organizations and conducting medical research to bring innovation to twelve African countries where ALIMA works.
ER Med, General, Infect Dis, Logist-Op, MF Med, OB-GYN, Path, Peds, Psych, Pub Health
📞 +1 646-619-9074
🌐 https://vfapp.org/1c11

American Academy of Pediatrics
Seeks to attain optimal physical, mental, and social health and well-being for all infants, children, adolescents, and young adults.
Anesth, Crit-Care, Neonat, Ped Surg
📞 +1 800-433-9016
🌐 https://vfapp.org/9633

Carter Center, The
Seeks to prevent and resolve conflicts, enhance freedom and democracy, and improve health, while remaining committed to human rights and the alleviation of human suffering.
Infect Dis, MF Med, Ophth-Opt
📞 +1 800-550-3560
🌐 https://vfapp.org/6556

Catholic Organization for Relief & Development Aid (CORDAID)
Provides humanitarian assistance and creates opportunities to improve security, healthcare, education, and inclusive economic growth in fragile and conflict-affected areas.
ER Med, Infect Dis, MF Med, OB-GYN, Peds, Psych
📞 +31 70 313 6300
🌐 https://vfapp.org/8ae5

Concern Worldwide
Seeks to permanently transform the lives of people living in extreme poverty, tackling its root causes, and building resilience.
Logist-Op, MF Med, Nutr, OB-GYN
📞 +353 1 417 7700
🌐 https://vfapp.org/77e9

Dental Hope for Children
Seeks to provide dental services to children in underserved areas, based in Christian ministry.
Dent-OMFS
🌐 https://vfapp.org/1426

Doctors with Africa (CUAMM)
Advocates for the universal right to health and promotes the values of international solidarity, justice, and peace. Works to protect and improve the well-being and health of vulnerable communities in Africa with a long-term development perspective.
ER Med, Infect Dis, MF Med, Neonat, OB-GYN, Peds
🌐 https://vfapp.org/d2fb

Doctors Without Borders/Médecins Sans Frontières (MSF)
Responds to emergencies and provides lifesaving medical care where needed most, including during disasters, conflicts, and epidemics.
Anesth, Crit-Care, ER Med, General, Infect Dis, Nutr, OB-GYN, Ped Surg, Peds, Psych, Pub Health, Surg
📞 +1 212-679-6800
🌐 https://vfapp.org/f363

Dream Sant'Egidio

Seeks to counter HIV/AIDS in Africa by eliminating the transmission of HIV from mother to child, with a focus on women because of the importance of their role in the community.

Infect Dis, MF Med, Neonat, OB-GYN, Path, Peds

+39 06 899 2225

https://vfapp.org/f466

EMERGENCY

Provides free, high-quality healthcare to victims of war, poverty, and landmines. Also builds hospitals and trains local staff, while pursuing human-rights-based medicine.

ER Med, Neonat, OB-GYN, Ophth-Opt, Ped Surg

+39 02 881881

https://vfapp.org/c361

Enabel

As the development agency of the Belgian federal government, charged with implementing Belgium's international development policy, carries out public service assignments in Belgium and abroad pursuant to the 2030 Agenda for Sustainable Development.

General, Infect Dis, Logist-Op, MF Med, OB-GYN, Peds, Pub Health

+32 2 505 37 00

https://vfapp.org/5af7

END Fund, The

Aims to control and eliminate the most prevalent neglected diseases among the world's poorest and most vulnerable people.

Infect Dis

+1 646-690-9775

https://vfapp.org/2614

Finn Church Aid

Supports people in the most vulnerable situations within fragile and disaster-affected regions in three thematic priority areas: right to peace, livelihood, and education.

ER Med, Psych, Pub Health

+358 20 7871201

https://vfapp.org/9623

Fondation Follereau

Promotes the quality of life of the most vulnerable African communities. Alongside trusted partners, the foundation supports local initiatives in healthcare and education.

General, Infect Dis, OB-GYN

+352 44 66 06 34

https://vfapp.org/bcc7

Fracarita International

Provides support and services in the fields of mental healthcare, care for people with a disability, and education.

Psych, Rehab

https://vfapp.org/8d3c

Global Ministries – The United Methodist Church

As the worldwide mission and development agency of The United Methodist Church, Global Ministries works with more than 300 hospitals and clinics around the world through its Global Health Unit.

Anesth, CT Surg, CV Med, Crit-Care, Dent-OMFS, Derm, ER Med, GI, General, Infect Dis, Logist-Op, MF Med, Medicine, Neonat, Nephro, Nutr, OB-GYN, Ophth-Opt, Ortho, Palliative, Peds, Pod, Psych, Pub Health, Rehab, Rheum, Surg, Urol

+1 800-862-4246

https://vfapp.org/1723

Global Oncology (GO)

Brings the best in cancer care to underserved patients around the world and collaborates across geographic, professional, and academic borders to improve cancer care, research, and education.

Heme-Onc, Path, Rad-Onc

https://vfapp.org/fcb8

Grassroot Soccer

Leverages the power of soccer to educate, inspire, and mobilize at risk youth in developing countries to overcome their greatest health challenges, live healthier more productive lives, and be agents for change in their communities.

Infect Dis

+1 603-277-9685

https://vfapp.org/3521

HumaniTerra

Helps countries and populations emerging from economic and human crisis to rebuild their healthcare system in a sustainable way. Committed to three fundamental and complementary actions: operating, training, and rebuilding.

Anesth, ENT, ER Med, MF Med, OB-GYN, Ortho, Plast, Surg

+33 4 91 42 10 00

https://vfapp.org/b371

International Agency for the Prevention of Blindness (IAPB), The

Leads international efforts in blindness-prevention activities, works toward a world where no one is needlessly visually impaired, and ensures that everyone has access to the best possible standard of eye health.

Infect Dis, Ophth-Opt, Pub Health

https://vfapp.org/87a2

International Federation of Red Cross and Red Crescent Societies (IFRC)

Coordinates and directs international assistance following natural and man-made disasters in nonconflict situations through the world's largest humanitarian and development network. Provides disaster-preparedness programs, healthcare activities, and promotes humanitarian values.

ER Med, General, Infect Dis, Nutr

+1 212-338-0161

https://vfapp.org/b4ee

International Medical Corps

Seeks to improve quality of life through health interventions and related activities that strengthen underserved communities worldwide, with the flexibility to respond rapidly to emergencies and offer medical services and training to people at the highest risk.

ER Med, General, Infect Dis, Nutr, OB-GYN, Peds, Pub Health, Surg

+1 310-826-7800

https://vfapp.org/a8a5

International Organization for Migration (IOM) – The UN Migration Agency

Promotes evidence-informed policies and holistic, preventive, and curative health programs that are beneficial, accessible, and equitable for vulnerable migrants.

General, Infect Dis, OB-GYN

📞 +27 12 342 2789
🌐 https://vfapp.org/621a

International Planned Parenthood Federation (IPPF)

Leads a locally owned, globally connected civil society movement that provides and enables services and champions sexual and reproductive health and rights for all, especially the underserved.

Infect Dis, MF Med, OB-GYN
📞 +44 20 7939 8200
🌐 https://vfapp.org/dc97

International Rescue Committee (IRC)

Responds to the world's worst humanitarian crises and helps people whose lives and livelihoods are shattered by conflict and disaster to survive, recover, and gain control of their future.

ER Med, General, Infect Dis, MF Med, Peds
📞 +1 212-551-3000
🌐 https://vfapp.org/5d24

International Trachoma Initiative (iTi)

Works toward a world free from trachoma, a preventable cause of blindness, and provides comprehensive support to national ministries of health and governmental and nongovernmental organizations to implement a comprehensive approach to fight trachoma.

Infect Dis, Ophth-Opt
📞 +1 404-371-0466
🌐 https://vfapp.org/3278

Islamic Medical Association of North America

Fosters health promotion, disease prevention, and health maintenance in communities around the world through direct patient care and health programs.

Anesth, Dent-OMFS, ER Med, General, Logist-Op, Ophth-Opt, Peds, Plast, Surg
📞 +1 630-932-0000
🌐 https://vfapp.org/a157

Joint United Nations Programme on HIV/AIDS (UNAIDS)

Aims to place people living with HIV and people affected by the virus at the decision-making table and at the center of designing, delivering, and monitoring the AIDS response.

Infect Dis
📞 +41 22 791 36 66
🌐 https://vfapp.org/464a

Life for a Child

Supports the provision of the best possible health care, given local circumstances, to all children and youth with diabetes in less-resourced countries, through the strengthening of existing diabetes services.

Endo, Medicine, Peds
🌐 https://vfapp.org/d712

Lions Clubs International

Empowers volunteers to serve their communities, meet humanitarian needs, encourage peace, and promote international understanding through Lions clubs.

Heme-Onc, Medicine, Nutr, Ophth-Opt
📞 +1 630-571-5466
🌐 https://vfapp.org/7b12

London School of Hygiene & Tropical Medicine: Health in Humanitarian Crises Centre

Advances health and health equity in crisis-affected countries through research, education, and translation of knowledge into policy and practice.

ER Med, Infect Dis, Pub Health
📞 +44 20 7636 8636
🌐 https://vfapp.org/96ad

MAP International

Provides medicines and health supplies to those in need around the world so they might experience life to the fullest.

Logist-Op
📞 +1 800-225-8550
🌐 https://vfapp.org/deed

Massachusetts General Hospital Global Surgery Initiative

Aims to improve surgical education and access to advanced surgical care in resource-limited settings around the world by performing surgical operations as visitors, training local surgeons, and sharing medical technology through international partnerships across disciplines.

Anesth, Crit-Care, ER Med, Heme-Onc, Peds, Surg
📞 +1 617-724-4093
🌐 https://vfapp.org/31b1

Médecins du Monde/Doctors of the World

Provides care, bears witness, and supports social change worldwide with innovative medical programs and evidence-based advocacy initiatives.

ER Med, General, Infect Dis, MF Med, Neonat, OB-GYN, Peds, Pub Health
📞 +33 1 44 92 15 15
🌐 https://vfapp.org/a43d

MENTOR Initiative

Saves lives in emergencies through tropical disease control, and helps people recover from crisis with dignity, working side by side with communities, health workers, and health authorities to leave a lasting impact.

ER Med, Infect Dis
📞 +44 1444 412171
🌐 https://vfapp.org/3bd5

Mercy Ships

Operates hospital ships staffed by volunteers to bring hope, healing, and healthcare to underserved communities worldwide.

Anesth, Dent-OMFS, Logist-Op, Neonat, OB-GYN, Ophth-Opt, Ortho, Palliative, Plast, Psych, Surg
📞 +1 903-939-7000
🌐 https://vfapp.org/2e99

Neglected Tropical Disease NGO Network

Works to create a global forum for non-governmental organizations working to control onchocerciasis, lymphatic filariasis, schistosomiasis, soil transmitted helminths, and trachoma.

Infect Dis, Logist-Op
📞 +1 929-272-6227
🌐 https://vfapp.org/c511

Première Urgence International

Helps civilians who are marginalized or excluded as a result of natural disasters, war, or economic collapse.

ER Med, General, MF Med, Peds, Psych

📞 +53 119997400027
🌐 https://vfapp.org/62ba

RestoringVision
Empowers lives by restoring vision for millions of people in need.
Ophth-Opt
📞 +1 209-980-7323
🌐 https://vfapp.org/e121

Rotary International
Provides service to others, improves lives, and advances world understanding, goodwill, and peace through its fellowship of business, professional, and community leaders.
ER Med, General, Infect Dis, MF Med, OB-GYN
🌐 https://vfapp.org/8fb5

Sanofi Espoir Foundation
Contributes to reducing health inequalities among populations that need it most by applying a socially responsible approach focused on fighting childhood cancers in low-income countries, improving maternal and newborn health, and improving access to care.
ER Med, OB-GYN, Peds
📞 +33 1 53 77 91 38
🌐 https://vfapp.org/943b

Smile Train
Seeks to give every child with a cleft the opportunity for a healthy, productive life by providing free cleft repair surgery and comprehensive cleft care in their own communities.
Dent-OMFS, ENT, Plast
📞 +1 800-932-9541
🌐 https://vfapp.org/f21d

Swiss Tropical and Public Health Institute
Contributes to the improvement of the health of populations internationally, nationally, and locally through excellence in research, education, and services.
Infect Dis, Pub Health
📞 +41 61 284 81 11
🌐 https://vfapp.org/2ee4

Task Force for Global Health, The
Consists of programs and focus areas that cover a range of global health issues including neglected tropical diseases, infectious diseases, vaccines, field epidemiology, public health informatics, health workforce development, and global health ethics.
Infect Dis, Logist-Op, Medicine, Ophth-Opt, Peds
📞 +1 404-371-0466
🌐 https://vfapp.org/714c

Tearfund
Responds to crisis and partners with local churches to bring restoration to those living in poverty, inspired by the Christian faith.
ER Med, Logist-Op
📞 +44 20 3906 3906
🌐 https://vfapp.org/f6cf

United Nations Children's Fund (UNICEF)
Works in over 190 countries and territories to save children's lives, to defend their rights, and to help them fulfill their potential, from early childhood through adolescence.
All-Immu, Infect Dis, MF Med, Neonat, Nutr, OB-GYN, Ped Surg, Peds, Pub Health
🌐 https://vfapp.org/42d7

United Nations Development Programme (UNDP)
Helps countries achieve the simultaneous eradication of extreme poverty and significant reduction of inequalities and exclusion using a sustainable human development approach.
Infect Dis, Logist-Op, Pub Health
🌐 https://vfapp.org/935c

United Nations High Commissioner for Refugees (UNHCR)
Safeguards the rights and well-being of people who have been forced to flee, ensuring that everybody has the right to seek asylum and find safe refuge in another country, with the goal of seeking lasting solutions.
General, MF Med, Medicine, OB-GYN, Peds, Psych, Pub Health
🌐 https://vfapp.org/6636

United Nations Office for the Coordination of Humanitarian Affairs (OCHA)
Contributes to principled and effective humanitarian response through coordination, advocacy, policy, information management, and humanitarian financing tools and services, by leveraging functional expertise throughout the organization.
Logist-Op
🌐 https://vfapp.org/22b8

United Nations Population Fund (UNFPA)
Supports reproductive healthcare for women and youth in more than 150 countries, focusing on delivering a world where every pregnancy is wanted, every childbirth is safe, and every young person's potential is fulfilled.
Infect Dis, MF Med, Neonat, OB-GYN, Peds, Pub Health
📞 +1 212-963-6008
🌐 https://vfapp.org/c969

United States Agency for International Development (USAID)
Promotes and demonstrates democratic values abroad and advances a free, peaceful, and prosperous world. Leads the U.S. government's international development and disaster assistance through partnerships and investments that save lives.
ER Med, Infect Dis, MF Med, OB-GYN, Peds
📞 +1 202-712-0000
🌐 https://vfapp.org/9a99

University of Virginia: Anesthesiology Department Global Health Initiatives
Educates and trains physicians, to help people achieve healthy productive lives, and advances knowledge in the medical sciences.
Anesth, Pub Health
📞 +1 434-924-2283
🌐 https://vfapp.org/1b8b

Vitamin Angels
Helps at-risk populations in need—specifically pregnant women, new mothers, and children under age five—to gain access to life-changing vitamins and minerals.

General, Nutr
+1 805-564-8400
https://vfapp.org/7da1

World Health Organization, The (WHO)
The United Nations' agency for health provides leadership on global health matters, shapes the health research agenda, setting norms and standards, articulates evidence-based policy options, provides technical support and monitoring to countries, and assesses health trends.
ER Med, General, Infect Dis, Logist-Op, MF Med, OB-GYN, Peds, Psych, Pub Health
+41 22 791 21 11
https://vfapp.org/c476

World Vision International
Works with vulnerable communities around the world to overcome poverty and injustice with child-focused programs.
ER Med, General, Infect Dis, MF Med, Nutr, OB-GYN, Peds
+1 626-303-8811
https://vfapp.org/2642

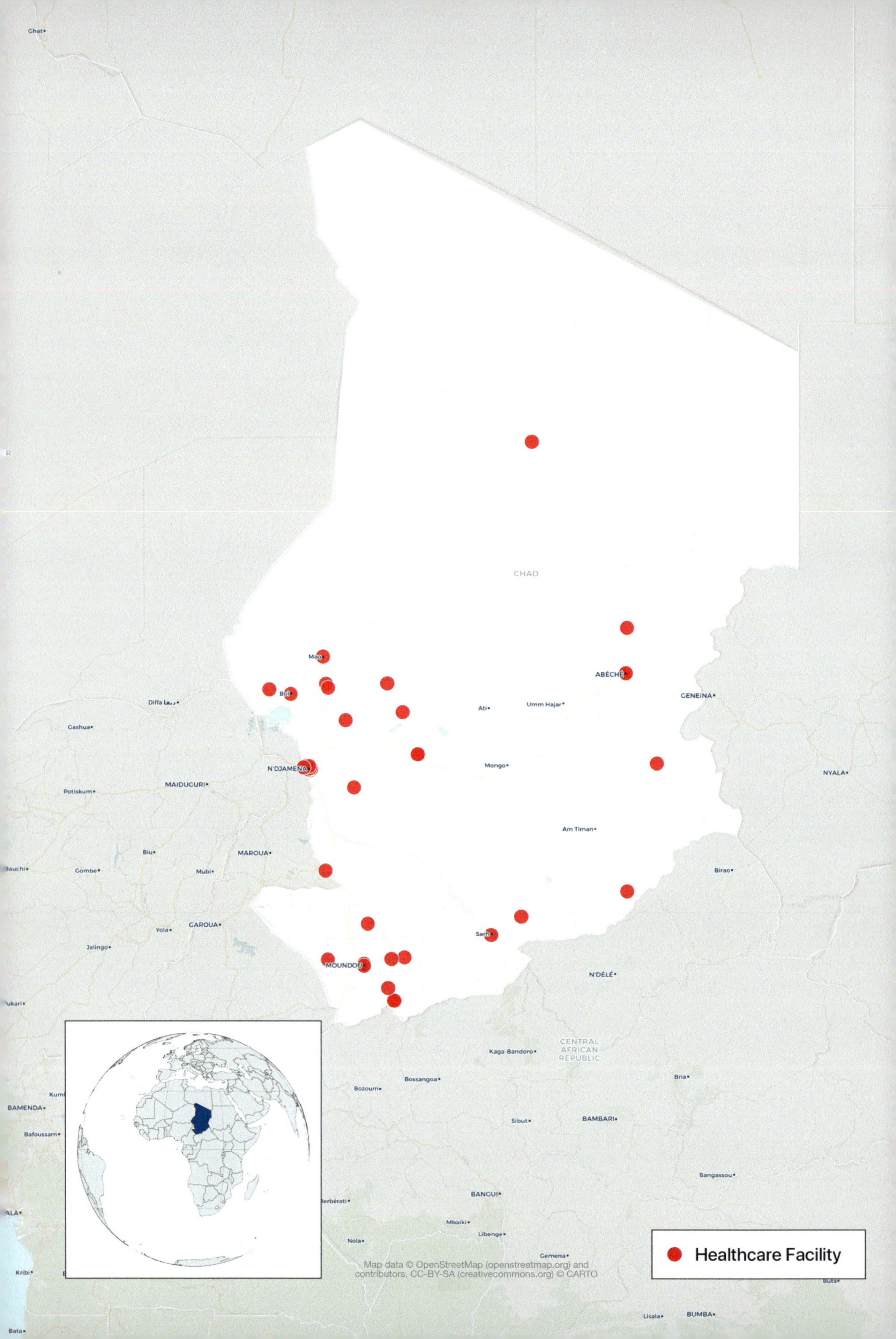

Ghat
CHAD
Mao
Bol
ABÉCHÉ
GENEINA
Ati
Umm Hajar
Diffa
Gashua
N'DJAMENA
Mongo
NYALA
MAIDUGURI
Potiskum
Am Timan
Biu
MAROUA
Bauchi
Gombe
Mubi
Birao
Yola
GAROUA
Jalingo
Sarh
MOUNDOU
N'DÉLÉ
Kaga-Bandoro
CENTRAL AFRICAN REPUBLIC
Bossangoa
Bozoum
Bria
BAMENDA
Bafoussam
Sibut
BAMBARI
Bangassou
BANGUI
Berbérati
Mbaiki
Libenge
Nola
Gemena
Kribi
Buta
Lisala
BUMBA
Bata
Healthcare Facility
Map data © OpenStreetMap (openstreetmap.org) and contributors, CC-BY-SA (creativecommons.org) © CARTO

Chad

The Republic of Chad, a landlocked country in central Africa, is home to more than 16.9 million people. Its capital city, N'Djamena, is known for a blend of modern and historical architecture and culture. Apart from its capital, Chad is largely rural. With about 200 ethnic groups, Chad has a diverse cultural history and population; upward of 120 languages and dialects are spoken, with French, Arabic, and Sara recognized as the official languages.

Chad gained its independence in 1960, and has since experienced conflict with bordering countries, invasions, civil warfare, and recurring rebellions. Decades of instability have left much of the population struggling: 66.2 percent of Chadians live in extreme poverty. Chad's limited resources and poor infrastructure must also accommodate more than 450,000 refugees from Sudan, the Central African Republic, and Nigeria. Previously a primarily agrarian economy, Chad became heavily dependent on oil after its discovery in 2013. Compounding an already dangerous socioeconomic situation is the impact of climate change and rapid desertification of Lake Chad.

Poverty, conflict, and instability have in turn affected the health of the Chadian population, many of whom experience food insecurity and hunger. About 43 percent of children under five are stunted, and 2.2 million are malnourished. Chad has one of the highest maternal mortality rates in central Africa due to inadequate access to health services. In addition to high maternal mortality, diarrheal diseases, lower respiratory infections, malaria, tuberculosis, stroke, ischemic heart disease, congenital defects, HIV/AIDS, and meningitis contribute most to deaths in the country. Death caused by neonatal disorders is also of notable significance and has increased substantially in recent years. The majority of physicians are concentrated in one region, near N'Djamena; the entire country urgently needs a larger and more evenly distributed healthcare workforce and a more developed healthcare infrastructure. The average life expectancy at birth is 54.

16.9M
Population

$710
GDP Per Capita

54 years
Life Expectancy
↑ Improving

4.3
Doctors/100k
Physician Density

40
Beds/100k
Hospital Bed Density

1,140
Deaths/100k
Maternal Mortality

Chad

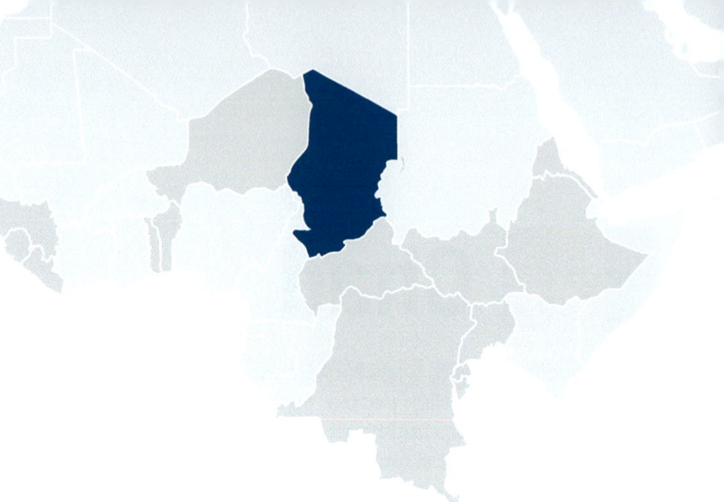

Healthcare Facilities

Adventist Hospital at Moundou
Moundou, Chad
https://vfapp.org/3284

Ancien Hôpital de Goré
Yanmodo, Logone Oriental, Chad
https://vfapp.org/9d71

Bere Adventist Hospital
Bere, Chad
https://vfapp.org/db32

Bokoro Hospital
Bokoro, Chad
https://vfapp.org/2371

Centre de Sante Roi Fayca
N'Djamena, Chad
https://vfapp.org/713f

Health District Administration
Sarh – Kyabe – Am Timan, كيابي Kyabé, Moyen-Chari شاري الأوسط, Chad / تشاد
https://vfapp.org/513d

Hôpital Chinois
Rond Point Gaoui دوار غاوي, N'Djaména انجمينا, N'Djaména انجمينا, Chad / تشاد
https://vfapp.org/4ceb

Hospital Alima
Ngouri, Chad
https://vfapp.org/eded

Hospital at Abéché
Abéché, Chad
https://vfapp.org/a2ab

Hospital at Dourbali
Dourbali/Abouguerne, Chad
https://vfapp.org/d37c

Hospital at Kochan
Kochan, Biltine, Chad
https://vfapp.org/3efe

Hospital at Timberi
Timberi, Chad
https://vfapp.org/ef85

Hospital Bokoro
RN N'Djamena-Bokoro, Bokoro-Hadjer-Lamis, Chad
https://vfapp.org/2461

Hospital District de Massakory
Ndjamena – Massakory – Faya Largeau National Road, Massakory ماساكوري, Hadjer-Lamis حجر لميس, Chad / تشاد
https://vfapp.org/1ca5

Hospital Kouga
Kouga-Chad, Chad
https://vfapp.org/b1b2

Hospital Moussoro
Moussoro, Chad
https://vfapp.org/7968

Hôpital Central
زنقة العقيد مول Rue du Colonel Moll, Djambal Bor جامبال بحر, N'Djaména انجمينا, Chad / تشاد
https://vfapp.org/5b67

Hôpital Central de Sarh
Sarh, Chad
https://vfapp.org/4efd

Hôpital de District de Beinamar
Palagamian, لوقون الغربية Logone Occidental, Chad / تشاد
https://vfapp.org/bb4a

Hôpital de Farcha Zarafa
1er Arrondissement طريق فارشا/ الدائرة الأولى, N'Djamena, 1er Arrondissement / الدائرة الأولى, BP41, Chad / تشاد
https://vfapp.org/d1bc

Hôpital de Faya
Chari Chifini شارع شيفيني, Faya-Largeau فايا لارجو, Borkou بوركو, Chad / تشاد
https://vfapp.org/9d9b

Hôpital de Goré
Yanmodo يانمودو, Logone Oriental لوقون الشرقية, Chad / تشاد
https://vfapp.org/aab3

Hôpital de Gozator
N'Djamena, Chad
https://vfapp.org/68e1

Hôpital de Guinebor II
شارع أبو رتشا, N'Djaména انجمينا, N'Djaména انجمينا, Chad / تشاد
https://vfapp.org/d632

Hôpital de Kindjiria
Massakory-N'Gouri-Bol-Niger Border, Délékerie Kangara, Hadjer-Lamis حجر لميس, Chad / تشاد
https://vfapp.org/48c4

Hôpital de l'Union
N'Djamena – Moundou, N'Djaména انجمينا, N'Djaména انجمينا, Chad / تشاد
https://vfapp.org/82b4

Hôpital de la Paix
N'Djamena, Chad
https://vfapp.org/ed6d

Hôpital de la Renaissance
شارع بيرميل, N'Djaména انجمينا, N'Djaména انجمينا, Chad / تشاد
https://vfapp.org/2cea

Hôpital de Mao
Mao ماو, Kanem كانم, Chad / تشاد
https://vfapp.org/dbc5

Hôpital du Distric Sanitaire de Baga Sola
Baga Sola, Chad
https://vfapp.org/b178

Hôpital Garnison
3015 زنقة, N'Djaména انجمينا, N'Djaména انجمينا, Chad / تشاد
https://vfapp.org/7f44

Hôpital Général de Doba
Moundou – Doba National Road, Ndoubeu Aeroport, Logone Oriental لوقون الشرقية, Chad / تشاد
https://vfapp.org/4851

Hôpital Mère et Enfant
Rue du Cherif شارع الشريف, N'Djaména انجمينا, N'Djaména انجمينا, Chad / تشاد
https://vfapp.org/63aa

Hôpital Provincial de Moussoro
Ndjamena – Massakory – Faya Largeau National Road, Moussoro موسورو, Barh el Gazel بحر الغزال, Chad / تشاد
https://vfapp.org/bd69

Hôpital Régional d'Abéché
Abéché, Chad
https://vfapp.org/678a

Hôpital Régional de Bol
Bol بول, Lac البحيرة, Chad / تشاد
https://vfapp.org/be1c

Hôpital Régional de Bongor
Djamena-Moundou, Bongor, Chad
https://vfapp.org/da14

Hôpital Régional de Goz Beida
مسار جبل, Goz Beïda قوز بيضة, Sila سيلا, Chad / تشاد
https://vfapp.org/414d

Hôpital Saint Joseph
Bébédja, Chad
https://vfapp.org/66f7

Le Bon Samaritain Hospital
Pont de Chagoua, N'Djaména انجمينا, N'Djaména انجمينا, Chad / تشاد
https://vfapp.org/283d

National General Reference Hospital
Rond Point Mairie دوار دار البلدية, N'Djaména انجمينا, N'Djaména انجمينا, Chad / تشاد
https://vfapp.org/1bb1

Ordre de Malte
Chari-mongo -شارع شاري مونقو, N'Djaména انجمينا, N'Djaména انجمينا, Chad / تشاد
https://vfapp.org/378d

Singamong
Avenue Tombalbaye, Doumbeur 1, Logone Occidental, Chad
https://vfapp.org/bd98

Chad

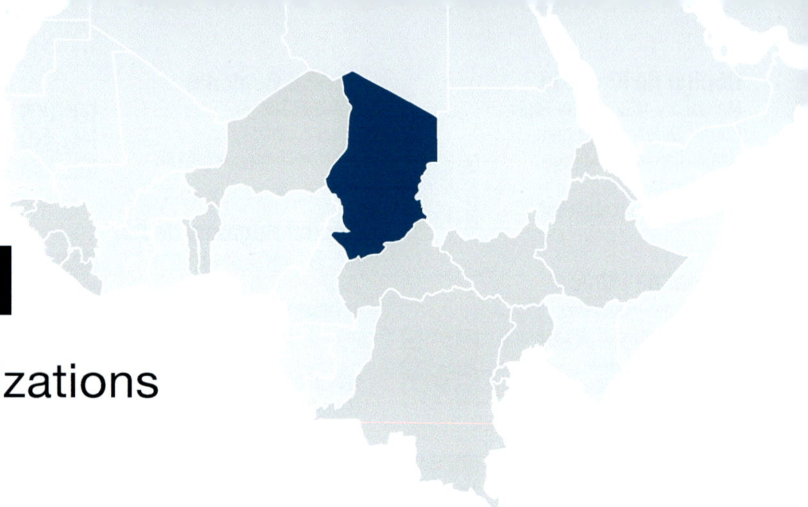

Nonprofit Organizations

Action Against Hunger
Aims to end life-threatening hunger for good through treating and preventing malnutrition across more than forty-five countries.
+1 212-967-7800
https://vfapp.org/2dbc

Adventist Health International
Focuses on upgrading and managing mission hospitals by providing governance, consultation, and technical assistance to a number of affiliated Seventh-Day Adventist hospitals throughout Africa, Asia, and the Americas.
Dent-OMFS, General, Pub Health
+1 909-558-5610
https://vfapp.org/16aa

Africa CDC
Aims to strengthen the capacity and capability of Africa's public health institutions as well as partnerships to detect and respond quickly and effectively to disease threats and outbreaks, based on data-driven interventions and programs.
Infect Dis, Logist-Op, Pub Health
+251 11 551 7700
https://vfapp.org/339c

Africa Humanitarian Action (AHA)
Responds to crises, conflicts, and disasters in Africa, while informing and advising the international community, governments, civil society, and the private sector on humanitarian issues of concern to Africa. Supports institutional and organizational development efforts.
General, Infect Dis, MF Med, Nutr, OB-GYN
+251 11 660 4800
https://vfapp.org/3ca2

Africa Inland Mission International
Seeks to establish churches and community development programs including health care projects, based in Christian ministry.
Anesth, Dent-OMFS, ER Med, General, MF Med, Medicine, OB-GYN, OB-GYN, Ophth-Opt, Ped Surg, Peds, Rehab
https://vfapp.org/f2f6

Alliance for International Medical Action, The (ALIMA)
Provides quality medical care to vulnerable populations, partnering with and developing national medical organizations and conducting medical research to bring innovation to twelve African countries where ALIMA works.
ER Med, General, Infect Dis, Logist-Op, MF Med, OB-GYN, Path, Peds, Psych, Pub Health
+1 646-619-9074
https://vfapp.org/1c11

Americares
Saves lives and improves health for people affected by poverty or disaster and responds with life-changing medicine, medical supplies, and health programs including domestic and global medical clinics.
All-Immu, ER Med, General, Infect Dis, MF Med, Nutr
+1 203-658-9500
https://vfapp.org/e567

AO Alliance
Builds solutions to lessen the burden of injuries in low- and middle-income countries, while enhancing the care of the injured to reduce human suffering, disability, and poverty.
Ortho, Surg
https://vfapp.org/8cd5

CARE
Works around the globe to save lives, defeat poverty, and achieve social justice.
ER Med, General
+1 800-422-7385
https://vfapp.org/7232

Carter Center, The
Seeks to prevent and resolve conflicts, enhance freedom and democracy, and improve health, while remaining committed to human rights and the alleviation of human suffering.
Infect Dis, MF Med, Ophth-Opt
+1 800-550-3560
https://vfapp.org/6556

Christian Aid Ministries
Strives to be a trustworthy and efficient channel for Amish, Mennonite, and other conservative Anabaptist groups and individuals to minister to physical and spiritual needs around the world.
CT Surg, ER Med, Logist-Op, Ortho, Pub Health
+1 330-893-2428
https://vfapp.org/7b33

Christian Blind Mission (CBM)
Aims to improve the quality of life of persons with disabilities in the poorest countries, addressing poverty as a cause, and a consequence, of disability, and working in partnership to create a society for all.

ENT, General, Infect Dis, OB-GYN, Ophth-Opt, Ortho, Peds, Psych, Rehab, Surg

📞 +49 6251 131131

🌐 https://vfapp.org/3824

Christian Connections for International Health (CCIH)
Promotes global health and wholeness from a Christian perspective.

All-Immu, General, Infect Dis, MF Med, Neonat, OB-GYN, Psych

📞 +1 703-923-8960

🌐 https://vfapp.org/fa5d

Christian Health Service Corps
Brings Christian doctors, health professionals, and health educators who are committed to serving the poor to places that have little or no access to healthcare.

Anesth, Dent-OMFS, General, Medicine, Peds, Surg

📞 +1 903-962-4000

🌐 https://vfapp.org/da57

Concern Worldwide
Seeks to permanently transform the lives of people living in extreme poverty, tackling its root causes, and building resilience.

Logist-Op, MF Med, Nutr, OB-GYN

📞 +353 1 417 7700

🌐 https://vfapp.org/77e9

Direct Relief
Improves the health and lives of people affected by poverty or emergency situations by mobilizing and providing essential medical resources needed for their care.

ER Med, Logist-Op

📞 +1 805-964-4767

🌐 https://vfapp.org/58e5

Doctors Without Borders/Médecins Sans Frontières (MSF)
Responds to emergencies and provides lifesaving medical care where needed most, including during disasters, conflicts, and epidemics.

Anesth, Crit-Care, ER Med, General, Infect Dis, Nutr, OB-GYN, Ped Surg, Peds, Psych, Pub Health, Surg

📞 +1 212-679-6800

🌐 https://vfapp.org/f363

eHealth Africa
Builds stronger health systems in Africa through the design and implementation of data-driven solutions, responding to local needs and providing underserved communities with the necessary tools to lead healthier lives.

Logist-Op, Path

🌐 https://vfapp.org/db6a

END Fund, The
Aims to control and eliminate the most prevalent neglected diseases among the world's poorest and most vulnerable people.

Infect Dis

📞 +1 646-690-9775

🌐 https://vfapp.org/2614

eRanger
Provides sustainable solutions to transportation and medical provision such as ambulances and mobile clinics in developing countries.

ER Med, General, Logist-Op

📞 +27 40 654 3207

🌐 https://vfapp.org/4c18

Evangelical Alliance Mission, The (TEAM)
Provides services in the areas of church planting, community development, healthcare, social justice, business as mission, and more.

Dent-OMFS, General, Ophth-Opt

📞 +1 800-343-3144

🌐 https://vfapp.org/9faa

Fistula Foundation
Aims to engage the support of people worldwide who are eager to see the day when no woman suffers from obstetric fistula. Raises and directs funds to doctors and hospitals providing life-transforming surgery to women in need.

OB-GYN

📞 +1 408-249-9596

🌐 https://vfapp.org/e958

Global Oncology (GO)
Brings the best in cancer care to underserved patients around the world and collaborates across geographic, professional, and academic borders to improve cancer care, research, and education.

Heme-Onc, Path, Rad-Onc

🌐 https://vfapp.org/fcb8

Health Equity Initiative
Aims to build and sustain a global community that engages across sectors and disciplines to advance health equity.

Pub Health

🌐 https://vfapp.org/e2e2

Hope and Healing International
Gives hope and healing to children and families trapped by poverty and disability.

General, Nutr, Ophth-Opt, Peds, Rehab

📞 +1 905-640-6464

🌐 https://vfapp.org/c638

Humanity & Inclusion
Works alongside people with disabilities and vulnerable populations, taking action and bearing witness in order to respond to their essential needs, improve their living conditions and health, and promote respect for their dignity and fundamental rights.

General, Infect Dis, MF Med, Medicine, Ortho, Peds, Psych, Pub Health, Rehab

📞 +1 301-891-2138

🌐 https://vfapp.org/16b7

Humanity First
Provides aid and assistance to those in need, offering sustainable development solutions to society while providing and empowering local communities with the resources to help themselves.

ER Med, General, MF Med, Ophth-Opt

📞 +44 20 8417 0082

🌐 https://vfapp.org/13cc

International Agency for the Prevention of Blindness (IAPB), The

Leads international efforts in blindness-prevention activities, works toward a world where no one is needlessly visually impaired, and ensures that everyone has access to the best possible standard of eye health.

Infect Dis, Ophth-Opt, Pub Health

https://vfapp.org/87a2

International Federation of Red Cross and Red Crescent Societies (IFRC)

Coordinates and directs international assistance following natural and man-made disasters in nonconflict situations through the world's largest humanitarian and development network. Provides disaster-preparedness programs, healthcare activities, and promotes humanitarian values.

ER Med, General, Infect Dis, Nutr

+1 212-338-0161

https://vfapp.org/b4ee

International Medical and Surgical Aid (IMSA)

Aims to save lives and alleviate suffering through education, healthcare, surgical camps, and quality medical programs.

Anesth, General, Ped Surg, Surg

+44 7598 088806

https://vfapp.org/2561

International Organization for Migration (IOM) – The UN Migration Agency

Promotes evidence-informed policies and holistic, preventive, and curative health programs that are beneficial, accessible, and equitable for vulnerable migrants.

General, Infect Dis, OB-GYN

+27 12 342 2789

https://vfapp.org/621a

International Planned Parenthood Federation (IPPF)

Leads a locally owned, globally connected civil society movement that provides and enables services and champions sexual and reproductive health and rights for all, especially the underserved.

Infect Dis, MF Med, OB-GYN

+44 20 7939 8200

https://vfapp.org/dc97

International Rescue Committee (IRC)

Responds to the world's worst humanitarian crises and helps people whose lives and livelihoods are shattered by conflict and disaster to survive, recover, and gain control of their future.

ER Med, General, Infect Dis, MF Med, Peds

+1 212-551-3000

https://vfapp.org/5d24

International Trachoma Initiative (iTi)

Works toward a world free from trachoma, a preventable cause of blindness, and provides comprehensive support to national ministries of health and governmental and nongovernmental organizations to implement a comprehensive approach to fight trachoma.

Infect Dis, Ophth-Opt

+1 404-371-0466

https://vfapp.org/3278

International Union Against Tuberculosis and Lung Disease

Develops, implements, and assesses anti-tuberculosis, lung health, and noncommunicable disease programs.

Infect Dis, Pub Health, Pulm-Critic

+33 1 44 32 03 60

https://vfapp.org/3e82

Intersos

Provides emergency medical assistance to victims of armed conflicts, natural disasters, and extreme exclusion, with particular attention to the protection of the most vulnerable people.

ER Med, General, Nutr

+39 06 853 7431

https://vfapp.org/dbac

Islamic Medical Association of North America

Fosters health promotion, disease prevention, and health maintenance in communities around the world through direct patient care and health programs.

Anesth, Dent-OMFS, ER Med, General, Logist-Op, Ophth-Opt, Peds, Plast, Surg

+1 630-932-0000

https://vfapp.org/a157

Jhpiego

Creates and delivers transformative healthcare solutions that save lives in partnership with national governments, health experts, and local communities.

General, Infect Dis, OB-GYN, Surg

+1 410-537-1800

https://vfapp.org/45b8

Joint United Nations Programme on HIV/AIDS (UNAIDS)

Aims to place people living with HIV and people affected by the virus at the decision-making table and at the center of designing, delivering, and monitoring the AIDS response.

Infect Dis

+41 22 791 36 66

https://vfapp.org/464a

Lions Clubs International

Empowers volunteers to serve their communities, meet humanitarian needs, encourage peace, and promote international understanding through Lions clubs.

Heme-Onc, Medicine, Nutr, Ophth-Opt

+1 630-571-5466

https://vfapp.org/7b12

Management Sciences for Health (MSH)

Works with countries and communities to save lives and improve the health of the world's poorest and most vulnerable people by building strong, resilient, sustainable health systems.

Infect Dis, Logist-Op, Pub Health

+1 617-250-9500

https://vfapp.org/6aa2

MAP International

Provides medicines and health supplies to those in need around the world so they might experience life to the fullest.

Logist-Op

+1 800-225-8550

https://vfapp.org/deed

MENTOR Initiative

Saves lives in emergencies through tropical disease control, and helps people recover from crisis with dignity, working side by side with communities, health workers, and health authorities to leave a lasting impact.

ER Med, Infect Dis

+44 1444 412171

https://vfapp.org/3bd5

Mission Africa

Brings medical care, training, and compassion to underserved communities in Africa, based in Christian ministry.

Dent-OMFS, General, Infect Dis

+44 28 9040 2850

https://vfapp.org/df4d

Operation Fistula

Exists to end obstetric fistula by building models of care that serve every woman, everywhere.

MF Med, OB-GYN, Surg

+1 512-687-3479

https://vfapp.org/ce8e

Première Urgence International

Helps civilians who are marginalized or excluded as a result of natural disasters, war, or economic collapse.

ER Med, General, MF Med, Peds, Psych

+53 119997400027

https://vfapp.org/62ba

RestoringVision

Empowers lives by restoring vision for millions of people in need.

Ophth-Opt

+1 209-980-7323

https://vfapp.org/e121

Rockefeller Foundation, The

Works to promote the well-being of humanity.

Logist-Op, Nutr, Pub Health

+1 212-869-8500

https://vfapp.org/5424

Rotary International

Provides service to others, improves lives, and advances world understanding, goodwill, and peace through its fellowship of business, professional, and community leaders.

ER Med, General, Infect Dis, MF Med, OB-GYN

https://vfapp.org/8fb5

Sightsavers

Prevents avoidable blindness in some of the poorest parts of the world by treating debilitating eye diseases.

Infect Dis, Ophth-Opt, Surg

+1 800-707-9746

https://vfapp.org/aa52

SIGN Fracture Care International

Builds orthopedic capacity around the world and provides the injured poor access to fracture surgery by donating orthopedic education and implant systems to surgeons in developing countries.

Ortho, Rehab, Surg

+1 509-371-1107

https://vfapp.org/123d

Smile Train

Seeks to give every child with a cleft the opportunity for a healthy, productive life by providing free cleft repair surgery and comprehensive cleft care in their own communities.

Dent-OMFS, ENT, Plast

+1 800-932-9541

https://vfapp.org/f21d

Solthis

Improves disease prevention and access to quality care by strengthening the health systems and services of the countries served.

General, Infect Dis, Logist-Op, MF Med, Neonat, Path

+33 1 81 70 17 90

https://vfapp.org/a71d

Swiss Tropical and Public Health Institute

Contributes to the improvement of the health of populations internationally, nationally, and locally through excellence in research, education, and services.

Infect Dis, Pub Health

+41 61 284 81 11

https://vfapp.org/2ee4

Task Force for Global Health, The

Consists of programs and focus areas that cover a range of global health issues including neglected tropical diseases, infectious diseases, vaccines, field epidemiology, public health informatics, health workforce development, and global health ethics.

Infect Dis, Logist-Op, Medicine, Ophth-Opt, Peds

+1 404-371-0466

https://vfapp.org/714c

Tearfund

Responds to crisis and partners with local churches to bring restoration to those living in poverty, inspired by the Christian faith.

ER Med, Logist-Op

+44 20 3906 3906

https://vfapp.org/f6cf

Union for International Cancer Control (UICC)

Unites and supports the cancer community to reduce the global cancer burden, promote greater equity, and ensure that cancer control continues to be a priority in the world health and development agenda.

Heme-Onc, Pub Health

+41 22 809 18 11

https://vfapp.org/88b1

United Nations Children's Fund (UNICEF)

Works in over 190 countries and territories to save children's lives, to defend their rights, and to help them fulfill their potential, from early childhood through adolescence.

All-Immu, Infect Dis, MF Med, Neonat, Nutr, OB-GYN, Ped Surg, Peds, Pub Health

https://vfapp.org/42d7

United Nations Development Programme (UNDP)

Helps countries achieve the simultaneous eradication of extreme poverty and significant reduction of inequalities and exclusion using a sustainable human development approach.

Infect Dis, Logist-Op, Pub Health

https://vfapp.org/935c

United Nations High Commissioner for Refugees (UNHCR)

Safeguards the rights and well-being of people who have been forced to flee, ensuring that everybody has the right to seek asylum and find safe refuge in another country, with the goal of seeking lasting solutions.

General, MF Med, Medicine, OB-GYN, Peds, Psych, Pub Health

https://vfapp.org/6636

United Nations Office for the Coordination of Humanitarian Affairs (OCHA)

Contributes to principled and effective humanitarian response through coordination, advocacy, policy, information management, and humanitarian financing tools and services, by leveraging functional expertise throughout the organization.

Logist-Op

https://vfapp.org/22b8

United Nations Population Fund (UNFPA)

Supports reproductive healthcare for women and youth in more than 150 countries, focusing on delivering a world where every pregnancy is wanted, every childbirth is safe, and every young person's potential is fulfilled.

Infect Dis, MF Med, Neonat, OB-GYN, Peds, Pub Health

+1 212-963-6008

https://vfapp.org/c969

United States Agency for International Development (USAID)

Promotes and demonstrates democratic values abroad and advances a free, peaceful, and prosperous world. Leads the U.S. government's international development and disaster assistance through partnerships and investments that save lives.

ER Med, Infect Dis, MF Med, OB-GYN, Peds

+1 202-712-0000

https://vfapp.org/9a99

United Surgeons for Children (USFC)

Pursues greater health and opportunity for children in the most neglected pockets of the world, with a specific focus and expertise in surgery.

Anesth, CT Surg, Neonat, Neurosurg, OB-GYN, Peds, Radiol, Surg

https://vfapp.org/3b4c

Women's Refugee Commission

Seeks to improve lives by protecting the rights of women, children, and youth displaced by conflict and crisis through researching their needs, identifying solutions, and advocating for programs and policies to strengthen their resilience.

General, MF Med, Neonat, OB-GYN, Peds, Psych

+1 212-551-3115

https://vfapp.org/3d8f

World Health Organization, The (WHO)

The United Nations' agency for health provides leadership on global health matters, shapes the health research agenda, setting norms and standards, articulates evidence-based policy options, provides technical support and monitoring to countries, and assesses health trends.

ER Med, General, Infect Dis, Logist-Op, MF Med, OB-GYN, Peds, Psych, Pub Health

+41 22 791 21 11

https://vfapp.org/c476

World Vision International

Works with vulnerable communities around the world to overcome poverty and injustice with child-focused programs.

ER Med, General, Infect Dis, MF Med, Nutr, OB-GYN, Peds

+1 626-303-8811

https://vfapp.org/2642

Worldwide Healing Hands

Works to improve the quality of healthcare for women and children in the most underserved areas of the world and to stop the preventable deaths of mothers.

General, MF Med, Neonat, OB-GYN

+1 707-279-8733

https://vfapp.org/b331

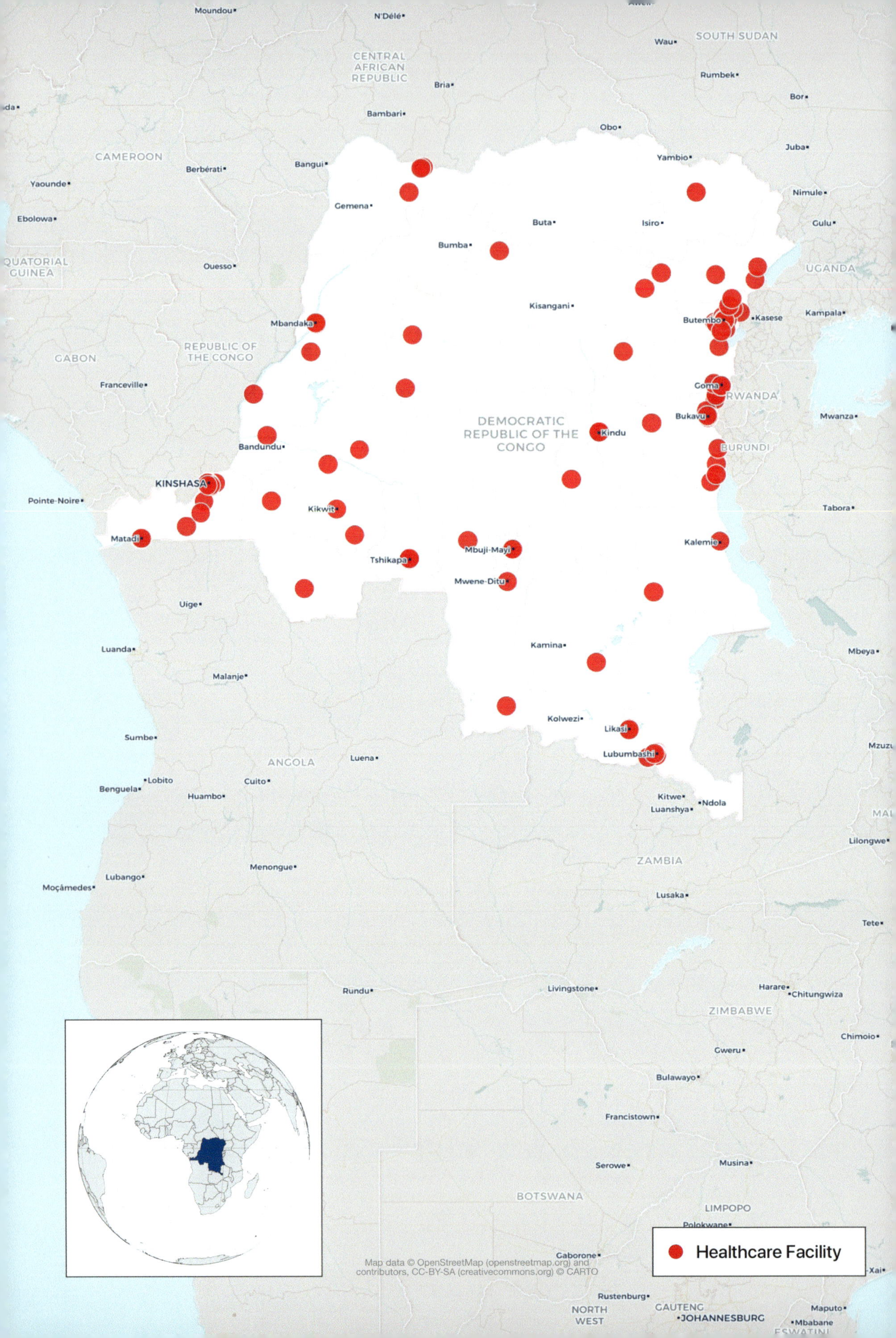
Moundou
N'Délé
SOUTH SUDAN
Wau
CENTRAL AFRICAN REPUBLIC
Rumbek
Bria
Bor
Bambari
Obo
Juba
CAMEROON
Yambio
Berbérati
Bangui
Yaounde
Nimule
Gemena
Ebolowa
Buta
Isiro
Gulu
Bumba
Ouesso
UGANDA
Kisangani
Kampala
Kasese
Butembo
Mbandaka
REPUBLIC OF THE CONGO
GABON
Franceville
Goma
RWANDA
Bukavu
Mwanza
DEMOCRATIC REPUBLIC OF THE CONGO
Kindu
Bandundu
BURUNDI
KINSHASA
Pointe-Noire
Kikwit
Tabora
Matadi
Kalemie
Mbuji-Mayi
Tshikapa
Mwene-Ditu
Uige
Luanda
Kamina
Mbeya
Malanje
Kolwezi
Likasi
Sumbe
Lubumbashi
ANGOLA
Luena
Lobito
Cuito
Benguela
Huambo
Kitwe
Ndola
Luanshya
Lilongwe
ZAMBIA
Menongue
Lubango
Moçâmedes
Lusaka
Tete
Rundu
Livingstone
Harare
Chitungwiza
ZIMBABWE
Chimoio
Gweru
Bulawayo
Francistown
Serowe
Musina
BOTSWANA
LIMPOPO
Polokwane
Healthcare Facility
Map data © OpenStreetMap (openstreetmap.org) and contributors, CC-BY-SA (creativecommons.org) © CARTO
Gaborone
Xai
Rustenburg
NORTH WEST
GAUTENG
JOHANNESBURG
Maputo
Mbabane

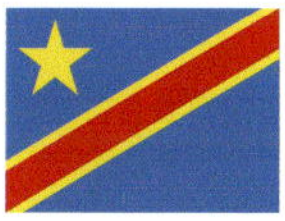

Democratic Republic of the Congo

The Democratic Republic of the Congo (DRC) is the largest country in sub-Saharan Africa, with an area equivalent to Western Europe. A beautiful country, the DRC is home to vast reserves of resources ranging from diamonds to hydroelectric potential. The population of more than 101.8 million comprises more than 200 ethnic groups, most of which are Bantu. As much as 45 percent of the population lives in urban areas, predominantly in the cities in the northeast and in the capital, Kinshasa. French is the official language of the DRC; many people communicate using Lingala, the lingua franca.

The Democratic Republic of Congo won its independence from Belgium in 1960, followed by years of political and social instability. The country has experienced conflict stemming from decades of civil war and corruption, which still exists today. And while the economic situation in the DRC has improved over the past two decades, in 2018, 72 percent of the population lived in extreme poverty. Less than half of the population has access to clean drinking water, and only 20 percent has access to sanitation.

The country's largely rural population faces a high burden of communicable and non-communicable diseases, as well as injuries. Significant causes of death include malaria, tuberculosis, lower respiratory infections, neonatal disorders, diarrheal diseases, stroke, ischemic heart disease, road injuries, hypertensive heart disease, cirrhosis, congenital defects, and HIV/AIDS. A number of Ebola outbreaks has also burdened the DRC. Fears of epidemic coupled with violence across the country has contributed to a growing public health challenge: poor mental health and depressive disorders. Unfortunately, maternal and child health indicators have not improved significantly since the beginning of the century.

101.8M
Population

$545
GDP Per Capita

60 years
Life Expectancy
↑ Improving

7.4
Doctors/100k
Physician Density

80
Beds/100k
Hospital Bed Density

473
Deaths/100k
Maternal Mortality

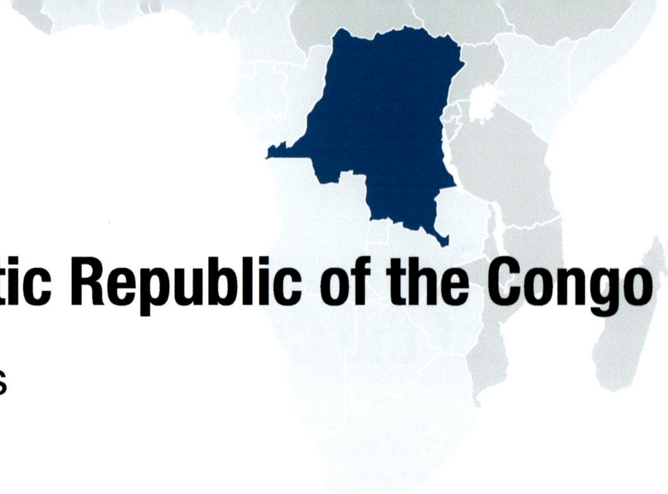

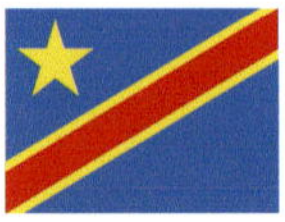

Democratic Republic of the Congo

Healthcare Facilities

Bribano Médical
Avenue Tumba, Kingabwa, Kinshasa, Democratic Republic of the Congo
🌐 https://vfapp.org/2925

Bugarula
Bugarula, Sud-Kivu, Democratic Republic of the Congo
🌐 https://vfapp.org/363a

CH Anuarite
RN4, Paida, Nord-Kivu, Democratic Republic of the Congo
🌐 https://vfapp.org/4792

CH Baraka
Route Kitulu, Butembo, Nord-Kivu, Democratic Republic of the Congo
🌐 https://vfapp.org/83cc

CH Butuhe
RS534, Butuhe, Nord-Kivu, Democratic Republic of the Congo
🌐 https://vfapp.org/f659

CH Cbca
Avenue des Martyrs, Butembo, Nord-Kivu, Democratic Republic of the Congo
🌐 https://vfapp.org/cc62

CH Cemebu
RS1032, Katwa, Nord-Kivu, Democratic Republic of the Congo
🌐 https://vfapp.org/e819

CH de Gloria
RN44, Beni, Nord-Kivu, Democratic Republic of the Congo
🌐 https://vfapp.org/aae6

CH Dieu Merci
Route Kitulu, Butembo, Nord-Kivu, Democratic Republic of the Congo
🌐 https://vfapp.org/ecfb

CH Don Beni
RN2, Butembo, Nord-Kivu, Democratic Republic of the Congo
🌐 https://vfapp.org/a53a

Ch Fepsi
Avenue du Centre, Butembo, Nord-Kivu, Democratic Republic of the Congo
🌐 https://vfapp.org/1d45

CH Kasinga
RS534, Butuhe, Nord-Kivu, Democratic Republic of the Congo
🌐 https://vfapp.org/3953

CH Maboya
RN2, Maboya, Nord-Kivu, Democratic Republic of the Congo
🌐 https://vfapp.org/76cc

CH Mahamba
RN2, Butembo, Nord-Kivu, Democratic Republic of the Congo
🌐 https://vfapp.org/654e

CH Makasi
RN2, Butembo, Nord-Kivu, Democratic Republic of the Congo
🌐 https://vfapp.org/ffd9

CH Mama Muyisa
Avenue du Marché, Butembo, Nord-Kivu, Democratic Republic of the Congo
🌐 https://vfapp.org/6e72

CH Matanda
RN2, Butembo, Nord-Kivu, Democratic Republic of the Congo
🌐 https://vfapp.org/61d2

CH Muchanga
RN2, Butembo, Nord-Kivu, Democratic Republic of the Congo
🌐 https://vfapp.org/bbcc

CH Mukongo
Butembo, Nord-Kivu, Democratic Republic of the Congo
🌐 https://vfapp.org/5188

CH Mukuna
Route Kitulu, Butembo, Nord-Kivu, Democratic Republic of the Congo
🌐 https://vfapp.org/5566

CH Rughenda
Route Kitulu, Butembo, Nord-Kivu, Democratic Republic of the Congo
🌐 https://vfapp.org/e857

CH Rwenzori
RN2, Butembo, Nord-Kivu, Democratic Republic of the Congo
🌐 https://vfapp.org/49f9

CH Saint Luc
Route Kitulu, Butembo, Nord-Kivu, Democratic Republic of the Congo
🌐 https://vfapp.org/2e77

CH Sainte Famille
Route Kitulu, Butembo, Nord-Kivu, Democratic Republic of the Congo
🌐 https://vfapp.org/9dea

CH Sainte Stella
RN2, Lubero, Nord-Kivu, Democratic Republic of the Congo
🌐 https://vfapp.org/34ca

CH Tumaini
Butembo, Nord-Kivu, Democratic Republic of the Congo
🌐 https://vfapp.org/69f5

CH Uor
RN2, Butembo, Nord-Kivu, Democratic Republic of the Congo
🌐 https://vfapp.org/9bed

CH Vighole
RS1032, Katwa, Nord-Kivu, Democratic Republic of the Congo
🌐 https://vfapp.org/7b48

CHU de Mbandaka
Avenue Cimetière, Mbandaka, Équateur, Democratic Republic of the Congo
🌐 https://vfapp.org/1cf2

CHU de Ruwenzori
Route Kitulu, Butembo, Nord-Kivu, Democratic Republic of the Congo
🌐 https://vfapp.org/312e

Clinique Ngaliema
Avenue des Cliniques, Cliniques, Kinshasa, Democratic Republic of the Congo
🌐 https://vfapp.org/e9c4

CPN Espoir
Avenue de l'Est, Kingabwa, Kinshasa, Democratic Republic of the Congo
🌐 https://vfapp.org/3653

HGR Beni
RN2, Beni, Nord-Kivu, Democratic Republic of the Congo
🌐 https://vfapp.org/ca65

HGR Bukama
Avenue de la Prison, Bukama, Haut-Lomami, Democratic Republic of the Congo
🌐 https://vfapp.org/b4c3

HGR Charite Maternelle
Goma, Democratic Republic of the Congo
🌐 https://vfapp.org/68bd

HGR de Kasaji
RN39, Kasaji, Lualaba, Democratic Republic of the Congo
🌐 https://vfapp.org/3678

HGR de Vuhovi
Vuhovi, Nord-Kivu, Democratic Republic of the Congo
🌐 https://vfapp.org/b1ec

HGR Katwa
RS1032, Katwa, Nord-Kivu, Democratic Republic of the Congo
🌐 https://vfapp.org/b5d9

HGR Kitatumba
29756, Butembo, Nord-Kivu, Democratic Republic of the Congo
🌐 https://vfapp.org/4a7e

HGR Le Roi
RN2, Butembo, Nord-Kivu, Democratic Republic of the Congo
🌐 https://vfapp.org/14f2

HGR Lubero
RN2, Lubero, Nord-Kivu, Democratic Republic of the Congo
🌐 https://vfapp.org/4bd2

HGR Masereka
Butembo, Nord-Kivu, Democratic Republic of the Congo
🌐 https://vfapp.org/b1d6

HJ Hospital
Petit Boulevard Industriel, Industriel, Kinshasa, Democratic Republic of the Congo
🌐 https://vfapp.org/9546

Hospital at Beni
Beni, Democratic Republic of the Congo
🌐 https://vfapp.org/cff2

Hospital at Monkole
Kasangulu, Democratic Republic of the Congo
🌐 https://vfapp.org/8de8

Hospital Gecamines Kambove
Kambove-Likasi, Democratic Republic of the Congo
🌐 https://vfapp.org/4a74

Hospital General de Mukongola
Kabare, Democratic Republic of the Congo
🌐 https://vfapp.org/1db9

Hospital Mtaa Wa Kivu Kusini
Mtaa Wa Kivu Kusini, Goma, Democratic Republic of the Congo
🌐 https://vfapp.org/2a93

Hospital Saint Joseph
N1, Kinshasa, Democratic Republic of the Congo
🌐 https://vfapp.org/c959

Hôpital Catholique Tonga
Avenue Etonga, Bahumbu, Kinshasa, Democratic Republic of the Congo
🌐 https://vfapp.org/927a

Hôpital de Baraka
Piste d'aviation, Baraka, Sud-Kivu, Democratic Republic of the Congo
🌐 https://vfapp.org/e564

Hôpital de Dungu
RP420, Dungu, Haut-Uele, Democratic Republic of the Congo
https://vfapp.org/c9ef

Hôpital de Gungu
RP231, Gungu, Kwilu, Democratic Republic of the Congo
https://vfapp.org/32a3

Hôpital de Kayna
RN2, Kayna, Nord-Kivu, Democratic Republic of the Congo
https://vfapp.org/1d7e

Hôpital de Kenge
RP242, Kenge, Kwango, Democratic Republic of the Congo
https://vfapp.org/e5f6

Hôpital de Kirotshe
RN2, Kalehe, Democratic Republic of the Congo
https://vfapp.org/8dbe

Hôpital de la Rive
Avenue des Touristes, Kinshasa, Kinshasa, Democratic Republic of the Congo
https://vfapp.org/5b6c

Hôpital de Référence de Kiamvu
Matadi, Kongo-Central, Democratic Republic of the Congo
https://vfapp.org/1187

Hôpital de Référence de Makala
Rue Dua, Selembao, Kinshasa, Democratic Republic of the Congo
https://vfapp.org/e87c

Hôpital de Référence de Matete
Avenue Diwaz, Vivi, Kinshasa, Democratic Republic of the Congo
https://vfapp.org/2365

Hôpital du Cinquantenaire
Avenue de la Libération, ONL, Kinshasa, Democratic Republic of the Congo
https://vfapp.org/f685

Hôpital General de Reference de Lubutu
RN3, Lubutu, Maniema, Democratic Republic of the Congo
https://vfapp.org/e1ce

Hôpital General de Référence de Bafwasende
Bafwasende, Democratic Republic of the Congo
https://vfapp.org/fead

Hôpital General de Référence de Kalemie
59, Avenue Lumumba, District du Tanganyika, Province du Katanga, Democratic Republic of the Congo
https://vfapp.org/55ad

Hôpital Gécamines de Kipushi
Kipushi, Democratic Republic of the Congo
https://vfapp.org/42eb

Hôpital Gécamines Sud
Route de Kipushi, Mampala, Haut-Katanga, Democratic Republic of the Congo
https://vfapp.org/16a4

Hôpital Général de Shabunda
Avenue Aeroport, Shabunda, Sud-Kivu, Democratic Republic of the Congo
https://vfapp.org/e798

Hôpital Général de Bikoro
RN21, Bikoro, Équateur, Democratic Republic of the Congo
https://vfapp.org/4462

Hôpital Général de Dipumba
Avenue de la Kanshi, Nzaba, Bipemba, Democratic Republic of the Congo
https://vfapp.org/f792

Hôpital Général de Fizi
RP527, Rtnc, Sud-Kivu, Democratic Republic of the Congo
https://vfapp.org/be33

Hôpital Général de Mandima
N4, Mambasa, Democratic Republic of the Congo
https://vfapp.org/93c2

Hôpital Général de Nia-Nia
RN4, Nia-Nia, Ituri, Democratic Republic of the Congo
https://vfapp.org/9cbb

Hôpital Général de Référence
RP628, Manono, Tanganyika, Democratic Republic of the Congo
https://vfapp.org/c65e

Hôpital Général de Référence d'Oshwe
RS212, Oshwe, Mai-Ndombe, Democratic Republic of the Congo
https://vfapp.org/f63f

Hôpital Général de Référence d'Uvira
RN5, Shishi, Sud-Kivu, Democratic Republic of the Congo
https://vfapp.org/ec76

Hôpital Général de Référence de Geti
Gety, Ituri, Democratic Republic of the Congo
https://vfapp.org/4477

Hôpital Général de Référence de Kikwit
Avenue Lukengo, Kikwit, Kwilu, Democratic Republic of the Congo
https://vfapp.org/636a

Hôpital Général de Référence de Kindu/HGR
Avenue de l'Hopital, CAMP SNCC/KINDU, Maniema, Democratic Republic of the Congo
https://vfapp.org/7f6b

Hôpital Général de Référence de Mbandaka
Avenue Mundji, Mbandaka, Équateur, Democratic Republic of the Congo
https://vfapp.org/ff53

Hôpital Général de Référence de Monkoto
RS315, Monkoto, Tshuapa, Democratic Republic of the Congo
https://vfapp.org/2ed6

Hôpital Général de Référence de Mushie
Rue Mahenge, Mushie, Mai-Ndombe, Democratic Republic of the Congo
⊕ https://vfapp.org/6337

Hôpital Général de Référence de Mutwanga
Mutwanga, Nord-Kivu, Democratic Republic of the Congo
⊕ https://vfapp.org/d5eb

Hôpital Général de Référence de Nundu
RN5, Mboko, Sud-Kivu, Democratic Republic of the Congo
⊕ https://vfapp.org/af92

Hôpital Général de Référence de Panzi
Bukavu, Democratic Republic of the Congo
⊕ https://vfapp.org/862b

Hôpital Général de Référence de Sia
RP219, Sia, Kwilu, Democratic Republic of the Congo
⊕ https://vfapp.org/1815

Hôpital Général de Référence de Tshikapa
RN1, Tshikapa, Kasaï, Democratic Republic of the Congo
⊕ https://vfapp.org/7fd5

Hôpital Général de Référence du Nord Kivu
RN2, Les Volcans, Nord-Kivu, Democratic Republic of the Congo
⊕ https://vfapp.org/a2a1

Hôpital Général de Référence Tunda
RP511, Djele, Maniema, Democratic Republic of the Congo
⊕ https://vfapp.org/45f1

Hôpital Général de Référence Wangata
Wangata, Équateur, Democratic Republic of the Congo
⊕ https://vfapp.org/514b

Hôpital Général de Référence Yalimbongo
RP405, Yalimbongo, Tshopo, Democratic Republic of the Congo
⊕ https://vfapp.org/c156

Hôpital Général de Yumbi
Avenue Martyr, Yumbi, Mai-Ndombe, Democratic Republic of the Congo
⊕ https://vfapp.org/2379

Hôpital Général du Cinquantenaire
Avenue Muela, Munua, Haut-Katanga, Democratic Republic of the Congo
⊕ https://vfapp.org/491a

Hôpital Géréral de Référence de Panzi
RP239, Panzi, Kwango, Democratic Republic of the Congo
⊕ https://vfapp.org/e63f

Hôpital Kimbanguiste
Avenue de la IIème République, Kutu, Kinshasa, Democratic Republic of the Congo
⊕ https://vfapp.org/4675

Hôpital Militaire Régional de Kinshasa Camp Kokolo
Avenue de la Libération, La Voix du Peuple, Kinshasa, Democratic Republic of the Congo
⊕ https://vfapp.org/6915

Hôpital Moderne – Lopitálo ya motindo mwa sika
RN8, Boende, Tshuapa, Democratic Republic of the Congo
⊕ https://vfapp.org/5896

Hôpital Monkole 3
Avenue Monkole, Kinshasa, Kinshasa, Democratic Republic of the Congo
⊕ https://vfapp.org/915c

Hôpital Mutombo
Boulevard Lumumba, Sans Fil, Kinshasa, Democratic Republic of the Congo
⊕ https://vfapp.org/5893

Hôpital PNC/Camp Soyo
Matadi – Ango Ango, Matadi, Kongo-Central, Democratic Republic of the Congo
⊕ https://vfapp.org/9571

Hôpital Provincial Général de Reférence de Bukavu
Bukavu, Democratic Republic of the Congo
⊕ https://vfapp.org/8bca

Hôpital Provincial Général de Référence de Kinshasa
Avenue de l'Hôpital, Golf, Kinshasa, Democratic Republic of the Congo
⊕ https://vfapp.org/82e1

Hôpital Pédiatrique de Kalembelembe
Avenue Kalembelembe, Lokole, Kinshasa, Democratic Republic of the Congo
⊕ https://vfapp.org/32b3

Hôpital Radem
Avenue Changalele III, Gambela 1, Haut-Katanga, Democratic Republic of the Congo
⊕ https://vfapp.org/9899

Hôpital Saint Luc de Kisantu
RN16, Kisantu, Kongo-Central, Democratic Republic of the Congo
⊕ https://vfapp.org/bc83

Hôpital Saint-Jean-Baptiste de Bonzola
Mbuji-Mayi, Democratic Republic of the Congo
⊕ https://vfapp.org/21cb

Hôpital SNCC/KINDU
Avenue Industrielle, CAMP SNCC/KINDU, Maniema, Democratic Republic of the Congo
⊕ https://vfapp.org/f4ba

Hôpital SS Mabanga
Rue Lubaya, Yolo-Sud 1, Kinshasa, Democratic Republic of the Congo
⊕ https://vfapp.org/dd6b

Hôpital Tshiamala
RN1, Mwene-Ditu, Lomami,

Democratic Republic of the Congo
🌐 https://vfapp.org/9bfb

IME Loko
Lisala-Gbadolite, Wodzo, Nord-Ubangi, Democratic Republic of the Congo
🌐 https://vfapp.org/4634

Jukayi
Kabuluanda, Kananga, Kasaï-Central, Democratic Republic of the Congo
🌐 https://vfapp.org/2942

Kawembe General Referral Hospital
Mbuji-Mayi, Democratic Republic of the Congo
🌐 https://vfapp.org/ccfd

Kihumba
Kihumba, Sud-Kivu, Democratic Republic of the Congo
🌐 https://vfapp.org/e238

Kinshasa General Hospital
Avenue de l'Hopital, Kinshasa, Democratic Republic of the Congo
🌐 https://vfapp.org/e2ca

Kitumaini
Avenue de Kambove, Kiwele, Haut-Katanga, Democratic Republic of the Congo
🌐 https://vfapp.org/4922

Les Aiglons
3ème Rue, Malemba, Kinshasa, Democratic Republic of the Congo
🌐 https://vfapp.org/fc99

Ma Famille
20 Boulevard Lumumba, Quartier 12, Kinshasa, Democratic Republic of the Congo
🌐 https://vfapp.org/f34b

Mbanza-Ngungu Hospital
R115, Mbanza-Ngungu, Democratic Republic of the Congo
🌐 https://vfapp.org/fb2a

Mobayi Mbongo General Reference Hospital
RN24, Beseli, Nord-Ubangi, Democratic Republic of the Congo
🌐 https://vfapp.org/e2e9

MSF – Bon Marché
Bigo, Bunia, Ituri, Democratic Republic of the Congo
🌐 https://vfapp.org/26ca

ORT Foyer
Avenue Upemba, Kisale, Haut-Katanga, Democratic Republic of the Congo
🌐 https://vfapp.org/9958

Panzi Hospital
Mushununu, Q. Panzi, Bukavu 266, Democratic Republic of the Congo
🌐 https://vfapp.org/b627

Railroad Hospital
Avenue De Lukafu, SNCC, Haut-Katanga, Democratic Republic of the Congo
🌐 https://vfapp.org/42ef

TVC Medical
77 Kenge, Diomi, Kinshasa, Democratic Republic of the Congo
🌐 https://vfapp.org/eebf

TVC Medical Mobayi
Mobayi-Mbongo, Democratic Republic of the Congo
🌐 https://vfapp.org/6961

Vanga Evangelical Hospital
Tshikapa, Democratic Republic of the Congo
🌐 https://vfapp.org/2445

Yolo Medical
Avenue Yolo, Mososo, Kinshasa, Democratic Republic of the Congo
🌐 https://vfapp.org/2211

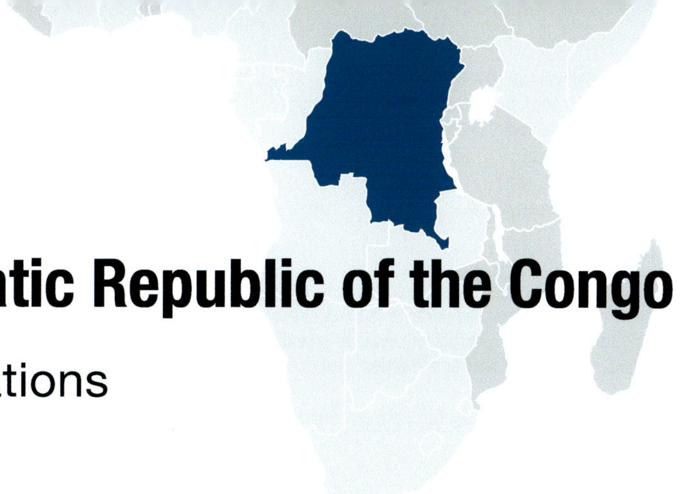

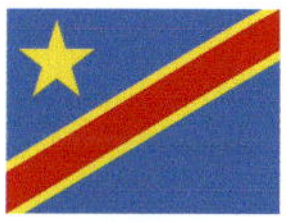

Democratic Republic of the Congo

Nonprofit Organizations

A.F.R.I.C.A.N. Foundation
Aims to improve cardiovascular health in sub-Saharan Africa.

CV Med, Crit-Care
+243 815 815 336
https://vfapp.org/517e

Abt Associates
Seeks to improve the quality of life and economic well-being of people worldwide, while striving to meet and exceed the highest professional standards.

General, Logist-Op, MF Med, OB-GYN, Peds
+1 212-779-7700
https://vfapp.org/cec2

Accomplish Children's Trust
Provides education and medical care to children with disabilities. Also addresses the financial implications of caring for a child with disabilities by helping families to earn an income.

Neuro, Peds, Rehab
https://vfapp.org/de84

Action Against Hunger
Aims to end life-threatening hunger for good through treating and preventing malnutrition across more than forty-five countries.

+1 212-967-7800
https://vfapp.org/2dbc

Advance Family Planning
Aims to achieve global expansion and access to quality contraceptive information, services, and supplies through financial investment and political commitment.

General, MF Med, Pub Health
+1 410-502-8715
https://vfapp.org/7478

Africa CDC
Aims to strengthen the capacity and capability of Africa's public health institutions as well as partnerships to detect and respond quickly and effectively to disease threats and outbreaks, based on data-driven interventions and programs.

Infect Dis, Logist-Op, Pub Health
+251 11 551 7700
https://vfapp.org/339c

Africa Humanitarian Action (AHA)
Responds to crises, conflicts, and disasters in Africa, while informing and advising the international community, governments, civil society, and the private sector on humanitarian issues of concern to Africa. Supports institutional and organizational development efforts.

General, Infect Dis, MF Med, Nutr, OB-GYN
+251 11 660 4800
https://vfapp.org/3ca2

Africa Indoor Residual Spraying Project (AIRS)
Aims to protect millions of people in Africa from malaria by spraying insecticide on the walls, ceilings, and other indoor resting places of mosquitoes that transmit malaria.

Infect Dis
+1 301-347-5000
https://vfapp.org/9bd1

African Field Epidemiology Network (AFENET)
Strengthens field epidemiology and public health laboratory capacity to contribute effectively to addressing epidemics and other major public health problems in Africa.

All-Immu, Infect Dis, Path, Pub Health
https://vfapp.org/df2e

Africa Inland Mission International
Seeks to establish churches and community development programs including health care projects, based in Christian ministry.

Anesth, Dent-OMFS, ER Med, General, MF Med, Medicine, OB-GYN, OB-GYN, Ophth-Opt, Ped Surg, Peds, Rehab
https://vfapp.org/f2f6

Against Malaria Foundation
Helps protect people from malaria. Funds anti-malaria nets, specifically long-lasting insecticidal nets (LLINs), and works with distribution partners to ensure they are used. Tracks and reports on net use and malaria case data.

Infect Dis
+44 20 7371 8735
https://vfapp.org/337d

AISPO
Implements international initiatives in the healthcare sector and remains involved in a variety of projects to combat poverty, social

injustice, and disease in the world.

All-Immu, ER Med, GI, General, Infect Dis, Logist-Op, MF Med, Neonat, OB-GYN, Peds, Psych, Pub Health, Radiol

+39 02 2643 4481

https://vfapp.org/c9e6

ALIGHT

Works closely with refugees, trafficked persons, economic migrants, and other displaced persons to co-design solutions that help them build full and fulfilling lives by providing healthcare, clean water, shelter protection, and economic opportunity.

ER Med, General, Infect Dis, MF Med, Neonat, Peds

+1 800-875-7060

https://vfapp.org/5993

Alliance for International Medical Action, The (ALIMA)

Provides quality medical care to vulnerable populations, partnering with and developing national medical organizations and conducting medical research to bring innovation to twelve African countries where ALIMA works.

ER Med, General, Infect Dis, Logist-Op, MF Med, OB-GYN, Path, Peds, Psych, Pub Health

+1 646-619-9074

https://vfapp.org/1c11

Alliance for Smiles

Improves the lives of children and communities impacted by cleft by providing free comprehensive treatment while building local capacity for long-term care.

Dent-OMFS, Ped Surg, Plast, Surg

+1 415-647-4481

https://vfapp.org/bb32

American Academy of Pediatrics

Seeks to attain optimal physical, mental, and social health and well-being for all infants, children, adolescents, and young adults.

Anesth, Crit-Care, Neonat, Ped Surg

+1 800-433-9016

https://vfapp.org/9633

American Foundation for Children with AIDS

Provides critical comprehensive services to infected and affected HIV-positive children and their caregivers.

Infect Dis, Nutr, Pub Health

+1 888-683-8323

https://vfapp.org/6258

Americares

Saves lives and improves health for people affected by poverty or disaster and responds with life-changing medicine, medical supplies, and health programs including domestic and global medical clinics.

All-Immu, ER Med, General, Infect Dis, MF Med, Nutr

+1 203-658-9500

https://vfapp.org/e567

Amref Health Africa

Serves millions of people across thirty-five countries in Sub-Saharan Africa, strengthening health systems, and training African health workers to respond to the continent's most critical health issues.

All-Immu, General, Infect Dis, Logist-Op, MF Med, OB-GYN, Path, Pub Health, Surg

+254 20 6993000

https://vfapp.org/6985

AO Alliance

Builds solutions to lessen the burden of injuries in low- and middle-income countries, while enhancing the care of the injured to reduce human suffering, disability, and poverty.

Ortho, Surg

https://vfapp.org/8cd5

Association of Medical Doctors of Asia (AMDA)

Strives to support people affected by disasters and economic distress on their road to recovery, establishing a true partnership with special emphasis on local initiative.

ER Med, Logist-Op, Pub Health

+81 86-252-6051

https://vfapp.org/e3d4

Canada-Africa Community Health Alliance

Sends Canadian volunteer teams on two- to three-week missions to African communities to work hand-in-hand with local partners.

General, Infect Dis, MF Med, OB-GYN, Peds, Surg

+1 613-234-9992

https://vfapp.org/4c94

Canadian Foundation for Women's Health

Seeks to advance the health of women in Canada and around the world through research, education, and advocacy in obstetrics and gynecology.

MF Med, OB-GYN

+1 613-730-4192

https://vfapp.org/f41e

CARE

Works around the globe to save lives, defeat poverty, and achieve social justice.

ER Med, General

+1 800-422-7385

https://vfapp.org/7232

Carter Center, The

Seeks to prevent and resolve conflicts, enhance freedom and democracy, and improve health, while remaining committed to human rights and the alleviation of human suffering.

Infect Dis, MF Med, Ophth-Opt

+1 800-550-3560

https://vfapp.org/6556

Catholic Organization for Relief & Development Aid (CORDAID)

Provides humanitarian assistance and creates opportunities to improve security, healthcare, education, and inclusive economic growth in fragile and conflict-affected areas.

ER Med, Infect Dis, MF Med, OB-GYN, Peds, Psych

+31 70 313 6300

https://vfapp.org/8ae5

Catholic World Mission

Works to rebuild communities worldwide by helping to alleviate poverty and empower underserved areas, while spreading the message of the Catholic Church.

ER Med, General, Nutr, Peds

+1 770-828-4966

https://vfapp.org/7b5f

Center for Strategic and International Studies (CSIS) Commission on Strengthening America's Health Security

Brings together a distinguished and diverse group of high-level opinion leaders bridging security and health, with the core aim to chart a bold vision for the future of U.S. leadership in global health.

ER Med, Infect Dis, MF Med, Pub Health

+1 202-887-0200

https://vfapp.org/6d7f

Central Congo Partnership

Collaborates with Partners in Mission to work with other clinical leadership in the Congo, providing assessment of the medical needs of underserved communities to develop strategic responses.

General, Ophth-Opt, Surg

https://vfapp.org/2eb4

Chain of Hope (La Chaîne de l'Espoir)

Helps underprivileged children around the world by providing them with access to healthcare.

Anesth, CT Surg, Crit-Care, ER Med, Neurosurg, Ortho, Ped Surg, Surg, Vasc Surg

+33 1 44 12 66 66

https://vfapp.org/e871

Christian Blind Mission (CBM)

Aims to improve the quality of life of persons with disabilities in the poorest countries, addressing poverty as a cause, and a consequence, of disability, and working in partnership to create a society for all.

ENT, General, Infect Dis, OB-GYN, Ophth-Opt, Ortho, Peds, Psych, Rehab, Surg

+49 6251 131131

https://vfapp.org/3824

Christian Connections for International Health (CCIH)

Promotes global health and wholeness from a Christian perspective.

All-Immu, General, Infect Dis, MF Med, Neonat, OB-GYN, Psych

+1 703-923-8960

https://vfapp.org/fa5d

Christian Health Service Corps

Brings Christian doctors, health professionals, and health educators who are committed to serving the poor to places that have little or no access to healthcare.

Anesth, Dent-OMFS, General, Medicine, Peds, Surg

+1 903-962-4000

https://vfapp.org/da57

Clinton Health Access Initiative (CHAI)

Aims to save lives and reduce the burden of disease in low- and middle-income countries. Works with partners to strengthen the capabilities of governments and the private sector to create and sustain high-quality health systems.

General, Heme-Onc, Infect Dis, Logist-Op, MF Med, Medicine, Neonat, Nutr, OB-GYN, Path, Peds, Rad-Onc

+1 617-774-0110

https://vfapp.org/9ed7

Concern Worldwide

Seeks to permanently transform the lives of people living in extreme poverty, tackling its root causes, and building resilience.

Logist-Op, MF Med, Nutr, OB-GYN

+353 1 417 7700

https://vfapp.org/77e9

Core Group

Aims to improve and expand community health practices for underserved populations, especially women and children, through collaborative action and learning.

General, Infect Dis, MF Med, Medicine, OB-GYN, Peds, Pub Health

+1 202-380-3400

https://vfapp.org/9de3

Cura for the World

Seeks to heal, nourish, and embrace the neglected by building medical clinics in remote communities in dire need of medical care.

ER Med, General, Peds

https://vfapp.org/c55f

Dikembe Mutombo Foundation

Strives to improve the health, education, and quality of life for the people of the Democratic Republic of the Congo through an emphasis on primary healthcare and disease prevention, the promotion of health policy, health research, and increased access to healthcare education.

All-Immu, Dent-OMFS, OB-GYN, Ophth-Opt, Ortho, Ped Surg, Surg

+1 404-262-2109

https://vfapp.org/85d4

Direct Relief

Improves the health and lives of people affected by poverty or emergency situations by mobilizing and providing essential medical resources needed for their care.

ER Med, Logist-Op

+1 805-964-4767

https://vfapp.org/58e5

Doctors Without Borders/Médecins Sans Frontières (MSF)

Responds to emergencies and provides lifesaving medical care where needed most, including during disasters, conflicts, and epidemics.

Anesth, Crit-Care, ER Med, General, Infect Dis, Nutr, OB-GYN, Ped Surg, Peds, Psych, Pub Health, Surg

+1 212-679-6800

https://vfapp.org/f363

Drugs for Neglected Diseases Initiative

Develops lifesaving medicines for people with neglected diseases around the world, having developed eight treatments for five deadly diseases and saving millions of lives since 2003.

Infect Dis, Pub Health

+41 22 906 92 30

https://vfapp.org/969c

Effect: Hope (The Leprosy Mission Canada)

Connects like-minded Canadians to people suffering in isolation from debilitating neglected tropical diseases like leprosy, lymphatic filariasis, Buruli ulcer, and STH.

General, Infect Dis

+1 888-537-7679

https://vfapp.org/f12a

eHealth Africa
Builds stronger health systems in Africa through the design and implementation of data-driven solutions, responding to local needs and providing underserved communities with the necessary tools to lead healthier lives.
Logist-Op, Path
https://vfapp.org/db6a

Elizabeth Glaser Pediatric AIDS Foundation
Seeks to end global pediatric HIV/AIDS through prevention and treatment programs, research, and advocacy.
Infect Dis, Nutr, OB-GYN, Peds
+1 888-499-4673
https://vfapp.org/d6ec

Enabel
As the development agency of the Belgian federal government, charged with implementing Belgium's international development policy, carries out public service assignments in Belgium and abroad pursuant to the 2030 Agenda for Sustainable Development.
General, Infect Dis, Logist-Op, MF Med, OB-GYN, Peds, Pub Health
+32 2 505 37 00
https://vfapp.org/5af7

END Fund, The
Aims to control and eliminate the most prevalent neglected diseases among the world's poorest and most vulnerable people.
Infect Dis
+1 646-690-9775
https://vfapp.org/2614

EngenderHealth
Works to implement high-quality, gender-equitable programs that advance sexual and reproductive health and rights.
General, MF Med, OB-GYN, Peds
+1 202-902-2000
https://vfapp.org/1cb2

Episcopal Relief & Development
Provides relief in times of disaster and promotes sustainable development by identifying and addressing the root causes of suffering.
Infect Dis, MF Med, Neonat, Nutr, Peds
+1 855-312-4325
https://vfapp.org/7cfa

eRanger
Provides sustainable solutions to transportation and medical provision such as ambulances and mobile clinics in developing countries.
ER Med, General, Logist-Op
+27 40 654 3207
https://vfapp.org/4c18

USAID: Fistula Care Plus
A fistula repair and prevention project from USAID that builds on, enhances, and expands the work undertaken by the previous Fistula Care project (2007–2013), with attention to new areas of focus so that obstetric fistula can become a rare event for future generations.
MF Med, OB-GYN, Surg
+1 202-902-2000
https://vfapp.org/a7cd

Fistula Foundation
Aims to engage the support of people worldwide who are eager to see the day when no woman suffers from obstetric fistula. Raises and directs funds to doctors and hospitals providing life-transforming surgery to women in need.
OB-GYN
+1 408-249-9596
https://vfapp.org/e958

Fondation Follereau
Promotes the quality of life of the most vulnerable African communities. Alongside trusted partners, the foundation supports local initiatives in healthcare and education.
General, Infect Dis, OB-GYN
+352 44 66 06 34
https://vfapp.org/bcc7

Fracarita International
Provides support and services in the fields of mental healthcare, care for people with a disability, and education.
Psych, Rehab
https://vfapp.org/8d3c

Gift of Life International
Provides lifesaving cardiac treatment to children in developing countries while developing sustainable pediatric cardiac programs by implementing screening, surgical, and training missions.
Anesth, CT Surg, CV Med, Crit-Care, Ped Surg, Peds, Pulm-Critic
+1 855-734-3278
https://vfapp.org/f2f9

Global Alliance to Prevent Prematurity and Stillbirth (GAPPS)
Seeks to improve birth outcomes worldwide by reducing the burden of premature birth and stillbirth.
All-Immu, Infect Dis, MF Med, Neonat, Neonat, OB-GYN
+1 206-413-7954
https://vfapp.org/3f74

Global Clubfoot Initiative (GCI)
Promotes and resources the treatment of children with clubfoot in developing countries using the Ponseti technique.
Ortho, Ped Surg
https://vfapp.org/f229

Global Ministries – The United Methodist Church
As the worldwide mission and development agency of The United Methodist Church, Global Ministries works with more than 300 hospitals and clinics around the world through its Global Health Unit.
Anesth, CT Surg, CV Med, Crit-Care, Dent-OMFS, Derm, ER Med, GI, General, Infect Dis, Logist-Op, MF Med, Medicine, Neonat, Nephro, Nutr, OB-GYN, Ophth-Opt, Ortho, Palliative, Peds, Pod, Psych, Pub Health, Rehab, Rheum, Surg, Urol
+1 800-862-4246
https://vfapp.org/1723

Global Offsite Care
Aims to be a catalyst for increasing access to specialized healthcare for all, and provides technology platforms to doctors and clinics around the world through rotary club–sponsored telemedicine projects.

Crit-Care, ER Med, General, Pulm-Critic
+1 707-827-1524
https://vfapp.org/61b5

Global Oncology (GO)
Brings the best in cancer care to underserved patients around the world and collaborates across geographic, professional, and academic borders to improve cancer care, research, and education.
Heme-Onc, Path, Rad-Onc
https://vfapp.org/fcb8

Global Outreach Doctors
Provides global health medical services in developing countries affected by famine, infant mortality, and chronic health issues.
All-Immu, Anesth, ER Med, General, Infect Dis, MF Med, Peds, Surg
+1 505-473-9333
https://vfapp.org/8514

Global Strategies
Empowers communities in the most neglected areas of the world to improve the lives of women and children through healthcare.
MF Med, Neonat, OB-GYN, Peds
+1 415-451-1814
https://vfapp.org/ef92

Grassroot Soccer
Leverages the power of soccer to educate, inspire, and mobilize at risk youth in developing countries to overcome their greatest health challenges, live healthier more productive lives, and be agents for change in their communities.
Infect Dis
+1 603-277-9685
https://vfapp.org/3521

HandUp Congo
Responds to community requests by providing the tools and training to help Congolese communities generate income to improve education, health, and well-being.
Crit-Care, ER Med, General, MF Med, Ophth-Opt, Pub Health
+61 417 272 101
https://vfapp.org/7a8b

HEAL Africa
Compassionately serves vulnerable people and communities in the Democratic Republic of the Congo through a holistic approach to healthcare, education, community action, and leadership development in response to changing needs.
Medicine, OB-GYN, Ortho, Peds, Surg
+1 816-536-3751
https://vfapp.org/cf5d

Heineman Medical Outreach
Provides medical and educational assistance globally to promote sustainable healthcare and enhanced living standards in underserved communities through the International Medical Outreach (IMO) program, a collaborative partnership between Heineman Medical Outreach and Atrium Health.
Anesth, CT Surg, CV Med, ER Med, General, Heme-Onc, Logist-Op, Medicine, Neonat, OB-GYN, Ped Surg, Peds, Surg, Vasc Surg
+1 704-374-0505
https://vfapp.org/389b

Hope and Healing International
Gives hope and healing to children and families trapped by poverty and disability.
General, Nutr, Ophth-Opt, Peds, Rehab
+1 905-640-6464
https://vfapp.org/c638

Hope Walks
Frees children, families, and communities from the burden of clubfoot, inspired by the Christian faith.
Ortho, Ped Surg, Peds, Rehab
+1 717-502-4400
https://vfapp.org/f6d4

Humanity First
Provides aid and assistance to those in need, offering sustainable development solutions to society while providing and empowering local communities with the resources to help themselves.
ER Med, General, MF Med, Ophth-Opt
+44 20 8417 0082
https://vfapp.org/13cc

ICAP at Columbia University
Serves as global leader in supporting the scale-up of multidisciplinary HIV/AIDS prevention, care, and treatment programs based on a family-focused approach.
General, Infect Dis, MF Med, Medicine, OB-GYN, Pub Health
+1 212-342-0505
https://vfapp.org/a8ef

IMA World Health
Works to build healthier communities by collaborating with key partners to serve vulnerable people with a focus on health, healing, and well-being for all.
Infect Dis, MF Med, Nutr, OB-GYN, Pub Health
+1 202-888-6200
https://vfapp.org/8316

Imaging the World
Develops sustainable models for ultrasound imaging in the world's lowest resource settings and uses a technology-enabled solution to improve healthcare access, integrating lifesaving ultrasound and training programs in rural communities.
Logist-Op, OB-GYN, Radiol
https://vfapp.org/59e4

International Agency for the Prevention of Blindness (IAPB), The
Leads international efforts in blindness-prevention activities, works toward a world where no one is needlessly visually impaired, and ensures that everyone has access to the best possible standard of eye health.
Infect Dis, Ophth-Opt, Pub Health
https://vfapp.org/87a2

International Council of Ophthalmology
Works with ophthalmologic societies and others to enhance ophthalmic education and improve access to the highest quality eye care in order to preserve and restore vision for the people of the world.
Ophth-Opt
https://vfapp.org/ffd2

International Federation of Red Cross and Red Crescent Societies (IFRC)
Coordinates and directs international assistance following natural

and man-made disasters in nonconflict situations through the world's largest humanitarian and development network. Provides disaster-preparedness programs, healthcare activities, and promotes humanitarian values.

ER Med, General, Infect Dis, Nutr

+1 212-338-0161

https://vfapp.org/b4ee

International Medical Corps

Seeks to improve quality of life through health interventions and related activities that strengthen underserved communities worldwide, with the flexibility to respond rapidly to emergencies and offer medical services and training to people at the highest risk.

ER Med, General, Infect Dis, Nutr, OB-GYN, Peds, Pub Health, Surg

+1 310-826-7800

https://vfapp.org/a8a5

International Organization for Migration (IOM) – The UN Migration Agency

Promotes evidence-informed policies and holistic, preventive, and curative health programs that are beneficial, accessible, and equitable for vulnerable migrants.

General, Infect Dis, OB-GYN

+27 12 342 2789

https://vfapp.org/621a

International Pediatric Nephrology Association (IPNA)

Leads the global efforts to successfully address the care for all children with kidney disease through advocacy, education, and training.

Medicine, Nephro, Peds

https://vfapp.org/b59d

International Planned Parenthood Federation (IPPF)

Leads a locally owned, globally connected civil society movement that provides and enables services and champions sexual and reproductive health and rights for all, especially the underserved.

Infect Dis, MF Med, OB-GYN

+44 20 7939 8200

https://vfapp.org/dc97

International Rescue Committee (IRC)

Responds to the world's worst humanitarian crises and helps people whose lives and livelihoods are shattered by conflict and disaster to survive, recover, and gain control of their future.

ER Med, General, Infect Dis, MF Med, Peds

+1 212-551-3000

https://vfapp.org/5d24

International Trachoma Initiative (iTi)

Works toward a world free from trachoma, a preventable cause of blindness, and provides comprehensive support to national ministries of health and governmental and nongovernmental organizations to implement a comprehensive approach to fight trachoma.

Infect Dis, Ophth-Opt

+1 404-371-0466

https://vfapp.org/3278

International Union Against Tuberculosis and Lung Disease

Develops, implements, and assesses anti-tuberculosis, lung health, and noncommunicable disease programs.

Infect Dis, Pub Health, Pulm-Critic

+33 1 44 32 03 60

https://vfapp.org/3e82

Intersos

Provides emergency medical assistance to victims of armed conflicts, natural disasters, and extreme exclusion, with particular attention to the protection of the most vulnerable people.

ER Med, General, Nutr

+39 06 853 7431

https://vfapp.org/dbac

InterSurgeon

Fosters collaborative partnerships in the field of global surgery that will advance clinical care, teaching, training, research, and the provision and maintenance of medical equipment.

ENT, Neurosurg, Ortho, Ped Surg, Plast, Surg, Urol

https://vfapp.org/6f8a

IntraHealth International

Improves the performance of health workers and strengthens the systems in which they work.

CV Med, Endo, General, Infect Dis, MF Med, Neonat, Nutr, OB-GYN

+1 919-313-3554

https://vfapp.org/ddc8

Ipas

Focuses efforts on women and girls who want contraception or abortion, and builds programs around their needs and how best to support them.

OB-GYN

https://vfapp.org/8e39

Jericho Road Community Health Center

Provides holistic healthcare for underserved and marginalized communities around the world, inspired by the Christian faith.

Anesth, General, Heme-Onc, Infect Dis, Medicine, OB-GYN, Ped Surg, Peds, Psych, Surg

+1 716-348-3000

https://vfapp.org/3d6b

Jewish World Watch

Brings help and healing to survivors of mass atrocities around the globe and seeks to inspire people of all faiths and cultures to join the ongoing fight against genocide.

ER Med, Logist-Op, OB-GYN, Peds

+1 818-501-1836

https://vfapp.org/8c92

Jhpiego

Creates and delivers transformative healthcare solutions that save lives in partnership with national governments, health experts, and local communities.

General, Infect Dis, OB-GYN, Surg

+1 410-537-1800

https://vfapp.org/45b8

John Snow, Inc. (JSI)
Aims to improve the health and well-being of underserved and vulnerable people and communities throughout the world.

General, Infect Dis, Logist-Op, MF Med, OB-GYN, Peds, Psych, Pub Health

+1 617-482-9485

https://vfapp.org/ba78

Johns Hopkins Center for Communication Programs
Believes in the power of communication to save lives, by empowering people to adopt healthy behaviors for themselves, their families, and their communities.

General, Infect Dis, Logist-Op, OB-GYN, Pub Health

+1 410-659-6300

https://vfapp.org/1bf9

Johns Hopkins Center for Global Health
Facilitates and focuses the extensive expertise and resources of the Johns Hopkins institutions together with global collaborators to effectively address and ameliorate the world's most pressing health issues.

General, Genetics, Logist-Op, MF Med, Peds, Psych, Pub Health, Pulm-Critic

+1 410-502-9872

https://vfapp.org/54ce

Joint United Nations Programme on HIV/AIDS (UNAIDS)
Aims to place people living with HIV and people affected by the virus at the decision-making table and at the center of designing, delivering, and monitoring the AIDS response.

Infect Dis

+41 22 791 36 66

https://vfapp.org/464a

Kids Care Everywhere
Seeks to empower physicians in under-resourced environments with multimedia, state-of-the-art medical software, and to inspire young professionals to become future global healthcare leaders.

Logist-Op, Ped Surg, Peds

https://vfapp.org/bc23

Last Mile Health
Links community health workers with frontline health workers—nurses, doctors, and midwives at community clinics—and supports them to bring lifesaving services to the doorsteps of people living far from care.

General, Logist-Op, OB-GYN, Pub Health

+1 617-880-6163

https://vfapp.org/37da

Leja Bulela
Supports internally displaced persons living in Tshibombo Tshimuangi and the residents of Kasai-Oriental Province with initiatives that promote adequate healthcare, educational opportunities, and agricultural opportunities.

General, OB-GYN, Peds

https://vfapp.org/afee

Life for a Child
Supports the provision of the best possible health care, given local circumstances, to all children and youth with diabetes in less-resourced countries, through the strengthening of existing diabetes services.

Endo, Medicine, Peds

https://vfapp.org/d712

LifeNet International
Transforms African healthcare by equipping and empowering existing local health centers to provide quality, sustainable, and lifesaving care to patients.

General, Infect Dis, MF Med, Neonat, OB-GYN, Pub Health

+1 407-630-9518

https://vfapp.org/e5d2

Light for the World
Contributes to a world in which persons with disabilities fully exercise their rights and assists persons with disabilities living in poverty.

Ophth-Opt, Rehab

+43 1 8101300

https://vfapp.org/3ff6

London School of Hygiene & Tropical Medicine: Health in Humanitarian Crises Centre
Advances health and health equity in crisis-affected countries through research, education, and translation of knowledge into policy and practice.

ER Med, Infect Dis, Pub Health

+44 20 7636 8636

https://vfapp.org/96ad

MAGNA International
Helps those who are suffering or recovering from conflicts and disasters by reducing the risks of diseases and treating them immediately.

ER Med, General, Infect Dis, Peds, Surg

+421 2/381 046 69

https://vfapp.org/58f4

Malaika
Operates in the Democratic Republic of Congo with the mission of empowering girls and their communities through education and health.

General, Infect Dis

+1 212-726-1089

https://vfapp.org/94ad

Management Sciences for Health (MSH)
Works with countries and communities to save lives and improve the health of the world's poorest and most vulnerable people by building strong, resilient, sustainable health systems.

Infect Dis, Logist-Op, Pub Health

+1 617-250-9500

https://vfapp.org/6aa2

MAP International
Provides medicines and health supplies to those in need around the world so they might experience life to the fullest.

Logist-Op

+1 800-225-8550

https://vfapp.org/deed

Marie Stopes International
Provides the contraception and safe abortion services that enable women all over the world to choose their own futures.

Infect Dis, MF Med, Neonat, OB-GYN, Pub Health

+44 20 7636 6200

https://vfapp.org/9525

Medair
Works to relieve human suffering in some of the world's most remote and devasted places, saving lives in emergencies and helping people in crises survive and recover, inspired by the Christian faith.
ER Med, General, Logist-Op, MF Med, Pub Health
+41 21 694 35 35
https://vfapp.org/5b33

Médecins du Monde/Doctors of the World
Provides care, bears witness, and supports social change worldwide with innovative medical programs and evidence-based advocacy initiatives.
ER Med, General, Infect Dis, MF Med, Neonat, OB-GYN, Peds, Pub Health
+33 1 44 92 15 15
https://vfapp.org/a43d

Medical Benevolence Foundation (MBF)
Works with partners in developing countries to build sustainable healthcare for those most in need through faith-based global medical missions.
General, Logist-Op, MF Med, OB-GYN, Surg
+1 800-547-7627
https://vfapp.org/c3e8

Medical Care Development International (MCD International)
Works to strengthen health systems through innovative, sustainable interventions.
Infect Dis, Logist-Op, OB-GYN, Pub Health
+1 301-562-1920
https://vfapp.org/dc5c

MedShare
Aims to improve the quality of life of people, communities, and the planet by sourcing and directly delivering surplus medical supplies and equipment to communities in need around the world.
Logist-Op
+1 770-323-5858
https://vfapp.org/c8bc

MENTOR Initiative
Saves lives in emergencies through tropical disease control, and helps people recover from crisis with dignity, working side by side with communities, health workers, and health authorities to leave a lasting impact.
ER Med, Infect Dis
+44 1444 412171
https://vfapp.org/3bd5

Mercy Ships
Operates hospital ships staffed by volunteers to bring hope, healing, and healthcare to underserved communities worldwide.
Anesth, Dent-OMFS, Logist-Op, Neonat, OB-GYN, Ophth-Opt, Ortho, Palliative, Plast, Psych, Surg
+1 903-939-7000
https://vfapp.org/2e99

MiracleFeet
Brings low-cost treatment to every child on the planet born with clubfoot, a leading cause of physical disability.
Ortho, Peds, Rehab
+1 919-240-5572
https://vfapp.org/bda8

Mission Bambini
Helps to support children living in poverty, sickness, and without education, giving them the opportunity and hope of a better life.
CT Surg, CV Med, Crit-Care, ER Med, Ped Surg, Peds
+39 02 210 0241
https://vfapp.org/dc1a

MPACT for Mankind
Transforms communities by improving health outcomes, enhancing knowledge, and providing hope while promoting sustainable growth.
ER Med, General
+1 469-998-1381
https://vfapp.org/1c61

MSD for Mothers
Designs scalable solutions that help end preventable maternal deaths.
MF Med, OB-GYN, Pub Health
https://vfapp.org/9f99

Norwegian People's Aid
Aims to improve living conditions, to create a democratic, just, and safe society.
ER Med, Logist-Op
+47 22 03 77 00
https://vfapp.org/2d8e

Nurses with Purpose
Supports nurses who have a passion to serve in their communities and abroad through medical mission trips in several different medical specialties.
General
+1 704-907-8901
https://vfapp.org/384a

Operation Fistula
Exists to end obstetric fistula by building models of care that serve every woman, everywhere.
MF Med, OB-GYN, Surg
+1 512-687-3479
https://vfapp.org/ce8e

Operation Smile
Treats patients with cleft lip and cleft palate, and creates solutions that deliver safe surgery to people where it's needed most.
Anesth, Dent-OMFS, ENT, Ped Surg, Plast
+1 757-321-7645
https://vfapp.org/5c29

Operation Walk
Provides the gift of mobility through life-changing joint replacement surgeries at no cost for those in need in the U.S. and globally.
Anesth, Ortho, Rehab, Surg
+1 310-493-8073
https://vfapp.org/bafe

Options
Believes in a world where women and children can access the high-quality health services they need, without financial burden.
Logist-Op, MF Med, Neonat, OB-GYN

☎ +44 20 7430 1900
🌐 https://vfapp.org/3a48

Pact
Works on the ground to improve the lives of those who are challenged by poverty and marginalization, striving for a world where all people are heard, capable, and vibrant.
Infect Dis, Logist-Op, MF Med, Pub Health
☎ +1 202-466-5666
🌐 https://vfapp.org/9a6c

Panzi Hospital and Foundations
Creates a safe space that supports women's physical healing, fosters their emotional recovery, and helps rebuild livelihoods and communities for survivors of sexual violence.
Derm, ENT, GI, Infect Dis, Medicine, OB-GYN, Ophth-Opt, Peds, Rehab, Rheum, Urol
☎ +1 301-541-8375
🌐 https://vfapp.org/1686

PATH
Advances health equity through innovation and partnerships so people, communities, and economies can thrive.
All-Immu, CV Med, Endo, Heme-Onc, Infect Dis, MF Med, Neonat, Nutr, OB-GYN, Path, Peds, Pulm-Critic
☎ +1 202-822-0033
🌐 https://vfapp.org/b4db

Pathfinder International
Champions sexual and reproductive health and rights worldwide, mobilizing communities most in need to break through barriers and forge paths to a healthier future.
OB-GYN
☎ +1 617-924-7200
🌐 https://vfapp.org/a7b3

Paul Carlson Partnership
Works together with partners in Africa to invest in local efforts in medical and economic development.
ER Med, General
☎ +1 773-907-3302
🌐 https://vfapp.org/cef2

Philips Foundation
Aims to reduce healthcare inequality by providing access to quality healthcare for disadvantaged communities.
CV Med, OB-GYN, Ped Surg, Peds, Surg, Urol
🌐 https://vfapp.org/bacb

Première Urgence International
Helps civilians who are marginalized or excluded as a result of natural disasters, war, or economic collapse.
ER Med, General, MF Med, Peds, Psych
☎ +53 119997400027
🌐 https://vfapp.org/62ba

Project SOAR
Conducts HIV operations research around the world to identify practical solutions to improve HIV prevention, care, and treatment services.
ER Med, General, MF Med, OB-GYN, Psych
☎ +1 202-237-9400
🌐 https://vfapp.org/1a77

RestoringVision
Empowers lives by restoring vision for millions of people in need.
Ophth-Opt
☎ +1 209-980-7323
🌐 https://vfapp.org/e121

Rockefeller Foundation, The
Works to promote the well-being of humanity.
Logist-Op, Nutr, Pub Health
☎ +1 212-869-8500
🌐 https://vfapp.org/5424

Rotary International
Provides service to others, improves lives, and advances world understanding, goodwill, and peace through its fellowship of business, professional, and community leaders.
ER Med, General, Infect Dis, MF Med, OB-GYN
🌐 https://vfapp.org/8fb5

ROW Foundation
Works to improve the quality of training for healthcare providers, and the diagnosis and treatment available to people with epilepsy and associated psychiatric disorders in under-resourced areas of the world.
Neuro, Psych
☎ +1 630-791-0247
🌐 https://vfapp.org/25eb

Salvation Army International, The
Seeks to meet human needs through services in education, healthcare, community support, emergency response, and ministry development, inspired by the Christian faith.
Dent-OMFS, Derm, ER Med, Infect Dis, MF Med, Medicine, Nutr, OB-GYN, Ophth-Opt, Palliative, Psych, Rehab, Surg
☎ +44 20 7332 0101
🌐 https://vfapp.org/8eb3

Sanofi Espoir Foundation
Contributes to reducing health inequalities among populations that need it most by applying a socially responsible approach focused on fighting childhood cancers in low-income countries, improving maternal and newborn health, and improving access to care.
ER Med, OB-GYN, Peds
☎ +33 1 53 77 91 38
🌐 https://vfapp.org/943b

Save the Children
Gives children around the world a healthy start in life, the opportunity to learn, and protection from harm.
All-Immu, Crit-Care, ER Med, General, Infect Dis, MF Med, Medicine, Neonat, OB-GYN, Peds, Psych, Pub Health
☎ +1 800-728-3843
🌐 https://vfapp.org/2e73

SEE International
Provides sustainable medical, surgical, and educational services through volunteer ophthalmic surgeons, with the objectives of restoring sight and preventing blindness to disadvantaged individuals worldwide.
Ophth-Opt, Surg
☎ +1 805-963-3303
🌐 https://vfapp.org/6e1b

Sightsavers
Prevents avoidable blindness in some of the poorest parts of the world by treating debilitating eye diseases.
Infect Dis, Ophth-Opt, Surg
+1 800-707-9746
https://vfapp.org/aa52

SIGN Fracture Care International
Builds orthopedic capacity around the world and provides the injured poor access to fracture surgery by donating orthopedic education and implant systems to surgeons in developing countries.
Ortho, Rehab, Surg
+1 509-371-1107
https://vfapp.org/123d

Smile Train
Seeks to give every child with a cleft the opportunity for a healthy, productive life by providing free cleft repair surgery and comprehensive cleft care in their own communities.
Dent-OMFS, ENT, Plast
+1 800-932-9541
https://vfapp.org/f21d

Solthis
Improves disease prevention and access to quality care by strengthening the health systems and services of the countries served.
General, Infect Dis, Logist-Op, MF Med, Neonat, Path
+33 1 81 70 17 90
https://vfapp.org/a71d

Surgical Healing of Africa's Youth Foundation, The (S.H.A.Y.)
Provides volunteer reconstructive surgery to children in need, including treating congenital anomalies such as cleft lip/palate and general reconstruction.
Anesth, Dent-OMFS, Peds, Plast
+1 310-860-0646
https://vfapp.org/41a7

Sustainable Cardiovascular Health Equity Development Alliance
Fights cardiovascular disease in underserved populations globally via education, training, and increasing interventional capacity.
CV Med, Pub Health, Radiol
+1 608-338-3357
https://vfapp.org/799c

Sustainable Kidney Care Foundation (SKCF)
Works to provide treatment for kidney injury where none exists, and aims to reduce mortality from treatable acute kidney injury (AKI).
Infect Dis, Medicine, Nephro
https://vfapp.org/1926

Sustainable Medical Missions
Trains and supports Indigenous healthcare and faith leaders in underdeveloped communities to treat neglected tropical diseases (NTDs) and other endemic conditions affecting the poorest community members by pairing faith-based solutions with best practices.
Infect Dis, Pub Health
+1 513-543-2896
https://vfapp.org/9165

Swiss Tropical and Public Health Institute
Contributes to the improvement of the health of populations internationally, nationally, and locally through excellence in research, education, and services.
Infect Dis, Pub Health
+41 61 284 81 11
https://vfapp.org/2ee4

T1International
Supports local communities by giving them the tools needed to stand up for the right to better access to insulin and diabetes supplies.
Endo, General, Medicine, Pub Health
https://vfapp.org/d7d4

Task Force for Global Health, The
Consists of programs and focus areas that cover a range of global health issues including neglected tropical diseases, infectious diseases, vaccines, field epidemiology, public health informatics, health workforce development, and global health ethics.
Infect Dis, Logist-Op, Medicine, Ophth-Opt, Peds
+1 404-371-0466
https://vfapp.org/714c

Tearfund
Responds to crisis and partners with local churches to bring restoration to those living in poverty, inspired by the Christian faith.
ER Med, Logist-Op
+44 20 3906 3906
https://vfapp.org/f6cf

Turing Foundation
Aims to contribute toward a better world and a better society by focusing on efforts such as health, art, education, and nature.
Infect Dis
+31 20 520 0010
https://vfapp.org/6bcc

U.S. President's Malaria Initiative (PMI)
Supports low-income countries to help control and eliminate malaria through cost-effective, lifesaving malaria interventions.
Infect Dis, MF Med, OB-GYN
+1 202-712-0000
https://vfapp.org/dc8b

Union for International Cancer Control (UICC)
Unites and supports the cancer community to reduce the global cancer burden, promote greater equity, and ensure that cancer control continues to be a priority in the world health and development agenda.
Heme-Onc, Pub Health
+41 22 809 18 11
https://vfapp.org/88b1

United Nations Children's Fund (UNICEF)
Works in over 190 countries and territories to save children's lives, to defend their rights, and to help them fulfill their potential, from early childhood through adolescence.

All-Immu, Infect Dis, MF Med, Neonat, Nutr, OB-GYN, Ped Surg, Peds, Pub Health
🌐 https://vfapp.org/42d7

United Nations Development Programme (UNDP)
Helps countries achieve the simultaneous eradication of extreme poverty and significant reduction of inequalities and exclusion using a sustainable human development approach.
Infect Dis, Logist-Op, Pub Health
🌐 https://vfapp.org/935c

United Nations High Commissioner for Refugees (UNHCR)
Safeguards the rights and well-being of people who have been forced to flee, ensuring that everybody has the right to seek asylum and find safe refuge in another country, with the goal of seeking lasting solutions.
General, MF Med, Medicine, OB-GYN, Peds, Psych, Pub Health
🌐 https://vfapp.org/6636

United Nations Office for the Coordination of Humanitarian Affairs (OCHA)
Contributes to principled and effective humanitarian response through coordination, advocacy, policy, information management, and humanitarian financing tools and services, by leveraging functional expertise throughout the organization.
Logist-Op
🌐 https://vfapp.org/22b8

United Nations Population Fund (UNFPA)
Supports reproductive healthcare for women and youth in more than 150 countries, focusing on delivering a world where every pregnancy is wanted, every childbirth is safe, and every young person's potential is fulfilled.
Infect Dis, MF Med, Neonat, OB-GYN, Peds, Pub Health
📞 +1 212-963-6008
🌐 https://vfapp.org/c969

United States Agency for International Development (USAID)
Promotes and demonstrates democratic values abroad and advances a free, peaceful, and prosperous world. Leads the U.S. government's international development and disaster assistance through partnerships and investments that save lives.
ER Med, Infect Dis, MF Med, OB-GYN, Peds
📞 +1 202-712-0000
🌐 https://vfapp.org/9a99

United States President's Emergency Plan for AIDS Relief (PEPFAR)
The U.S. global HIV/AIDS response works to prevent new HIV infections and accelerate progress to control the global epidemic in more than 50 countries, by partnering with governments to support sustainable, integrated, and country-led responses to HIV/AIDS.
Infect Dis, Pub Health
🌐 https://vfapp.org/a57c

University of California, Los Angeles: UCLA-DRC Health Research and Training Program
Aims to strengthen local and international capacity to rapidly identify and respond to disease outbreaks, conduct critical infectious disease research, and develop innovative prevention and control strategies.
All-Immu, Infect Dis, MF Med, Path, Pub Health
📞 +1 310-825-2096
🌐 https://vfapp.org/84ab

University of California: Global Health Institute
Mobilizes people and resources across the University of California to advance global health research, education, and collaboration.
General, OB-GYN, Pub Health
🌐 https://vfapp.org/ee7f

Upright Africa
Empowers the people of the Democratic Republic of Congo to build a sustainable future for themselves by sharing practical procedures and techniques with Congolese medical professionals. Also provides daily necessities to those without access.
General, Infect Dis, Nutr, Ped Surg, Surg
📞 +1 254-307-1941
🌐 https://vfapp.org/74cd

USAID: Maternal and Child Survival Program
Works to prevent child and maternal deaths.
Infect Dis, MF Med, Neonat, OB-GYN, Peds
🌐 https://vfapp.org/6fcf

USAID: EQUIP Health
Exists as an effective, efficient response mechanism to achieving global HIV epidemic control by delivering the right intervention at the right place and in the right way.
Infect Dis
📞 +27 11 276 8850
🌐 https://vfapp.org/d76a

USAID: Health Finance and Governance Project
Uses research to implement strategies to help countries develop robust governance systems, increase their domestic resources for health, manage those resources more effectively, and make wise purchasing decisions.
Logist-Op
📞 +1 202-712-0000
🌐 https://vfapp.org/8652

USAID: Health Policy Initiative
Provides field-level programming in health policy development and implementation.
General, Infect Dis, MF Med, OB-GYN, Peds
🌐 https://vfapp.org/8f84

USAID: Leadership, Management and Governance Project
Improves leadership, management, and governance practices to strengthen health systems and improve health for all, including vulnerable populations worldwide.
Logist-Op
🌐 https://vfapp.org/d35e

USAID: Maternal and Child Health Integrated Program
Works to improve the health of women and their families, including programs for maternal, newborn, and child health, immunization, family planning, nutrition, malaria, and HIV/AIDS.
All-Immu, General, Infect Dis, MF Med
📞 +1 202-835-3136
🌐 https://vfapp.org/4415

Vitamin Angels

Helps at-risk populations in need—specifically pregnant women, new mothers, and children under age five—to gain access to life-changing vitamins and minerals.

General, Nutr

+1 805-564-8400

https://vfapp.org/7da1

Watsi

Uses technology to make healthcare a reality for those who might not otherwise be able to afford it.

Pub Health, Surg

+1 256-792-8747

https://vfapp.org/41a3

Women for Women International

Supports the most marginalized women to earn and save money, improve health and well-being, influence decisions in their home and community, and connect to networks for support.

MF Med, OB-GYN

+1 202-737-7705

https://vfapp.org/768c

Women Orthopaedist Global Outreach (WOGO)

Provides free, life-altering orthopedic surgery that eliminates debilitating arthritis and restores disabled joints so that women can reclaim their ability to care for themselves, their families, and their communities.

Anesth, Ortho, Rehab, Surg

+1 844-588-9646

https://vfapp.org/6386

Women's Refugee Commission

Seeks to improve lives by protecting the rights of women, children, and youth displaced by conflict and crisis through researching their needs, identifying solutions, and advocating for programs and policies to strengthen their resilience.

General, MF Med, Neonat, OB-GYN, Peds, Psych

+1 212-551-3115

https://vfapp.org/3d8f

World Health Organization, The (WHO)

The United Nations' agency for health provides leadership on global health matters, shapes the health research agenda, setting norms and standards, articulates evidence-based policy options, provides technical support and monitoring to countries, and assesses health trends.

ER Med, General, Infect Dis, Logist-Op, MF Med, OB-GYN, Peds, Psych, Pub Health

+41 22 791 21 11

https://vfapp.org/c476

World Hope International

Empowers the poorest individuals around the world so they can become agents of change within their communities, by offering resources and knowledge.

Infect Dis, Logist-Op, MF Med, OB-GYN, Peds

+1 703-923-9414

https://vfapp.org/a4b8

World Relief

Brings sustainable solutions to the world's greatest problems: disasters, extreme poverty, violence, oppression, and mass displacement.

ER Med, Nutr, Psych, Pub Health

+1 800-535-5433

https://vfapp.org/fbcd

World Vision International

Works with vulnerable communities around the world to overcome poverty and injustice with child-focused programs.

ER Med, General, Infect Dis, MF Med, Nutr, OB-GYN, Peds

+1 626-303-8811

https://vfapp.org/2642

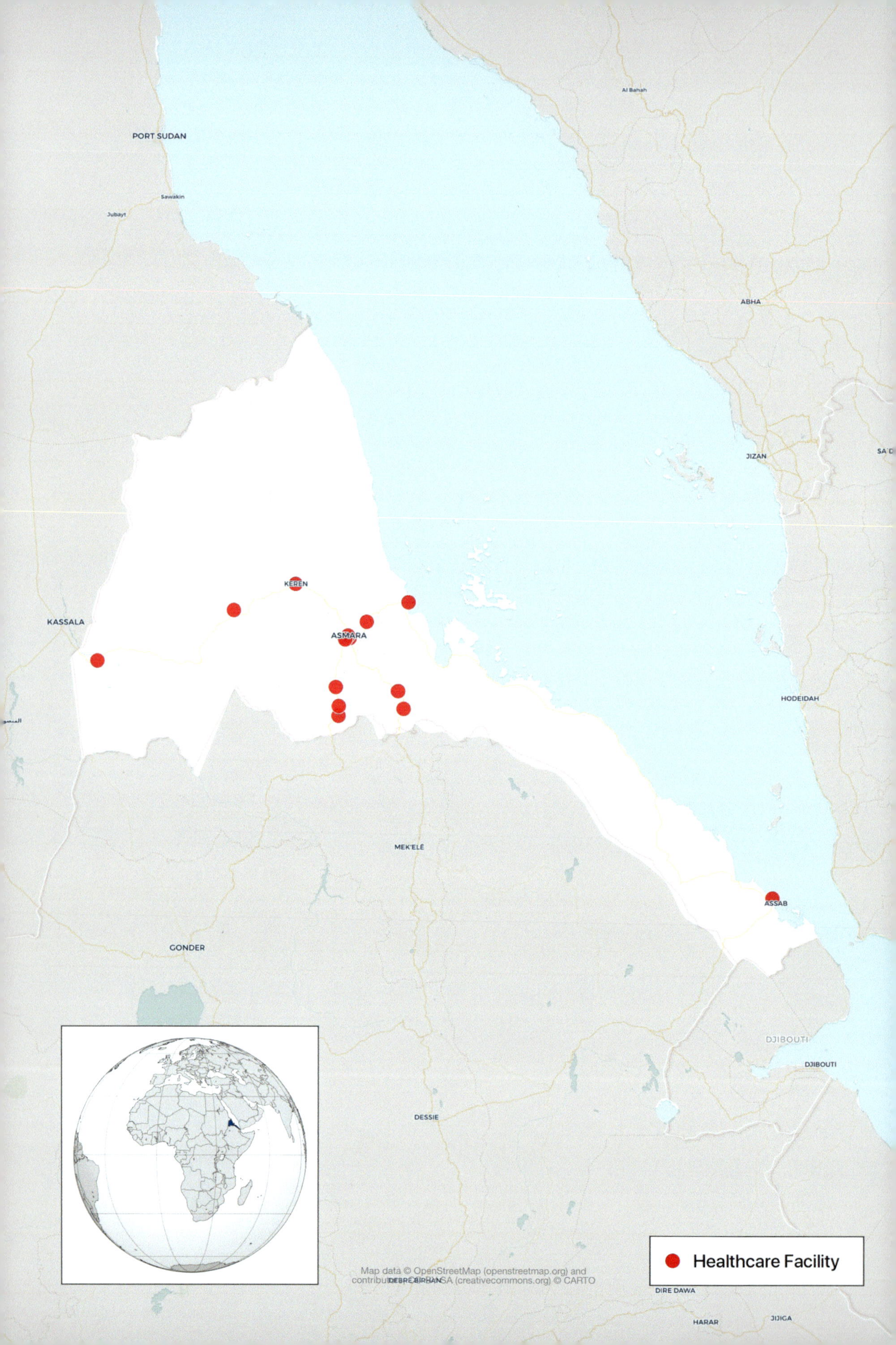

PORT SUDAN
Sawakin
Jubayt
Al Bahah
ABHA
JIZAN
KEREN
KASSALA
ASMARA
HODEIDAH
MEK'ELE
ASSAB
GONDER
DJIBOUTI
DJIBOUTI
DESSIE
Healthcare Facility
Map data © OpenStreetMap (openstreetmap.org) and contributors, CC-BY-SA (creativecommons.org) © CARTO
DEBRE BIRHAN
DIRE DAWA
HARAR
JIJIGA

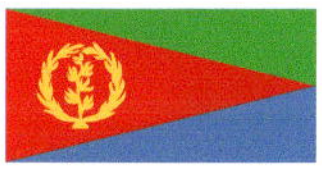

Eritrea

A small country in the Horn of Africa, the State of Eritrea is bordered by Sudan to the north and west, and Ethiopia and the Republic of Djibouti to the south. Home to a historically important trade route, Eritrea was at times colonized by Italy and Ethiopia. As such, the country's cultural legacies are still apparent and interesting to experience.The majority of Eritrea's 6.1 million people belong to the Tigrinya and Tigre ethnic groups. Most of the population live in the middle of the country around urban centers like Asmara, the capital, and cities such as Keren. Overall, around 40 percent of the population is urban.

After a 30-year war for liberation from Ethiopia, Eritrea became independent in 1993. A brief period of stability was followed by a border war with Ethiopia, in 1998, which ended in 2000. Since then, Eritrea has been in a state of transitional political arrangements. The highly militarized one-party state has been ranked by the Committee to Protect Journalists as the most censored country in the world. Eritrea's contentious history has left it as one of the poorest countries in Africa, facing economic and political strife.

Eritrea's political struggles have affected the overall health of the population, with preventable diseases making up around 70 percent of all disease. The country's impoverished population faces significant levels of death due to tuberculosis, lower respiratory infections, diarrheal diseases, neonatal disorders, HIV/AIDS, road injuries, protein-energy malnutrition, and measles. In recent years, death due to non-communicable diseases such as stroke, ischemic heart disease, cirrhosis, and diabetes has also increased significantly.

6.1M
Population

$643
GDP Per Capita

66 years
Life Expectancy
↑ Improving

6.3
Doctors/100k
Physician Density

70
Beds/100k
Hospital Bed Density

480
Deaths/100k
Maternal Mortality

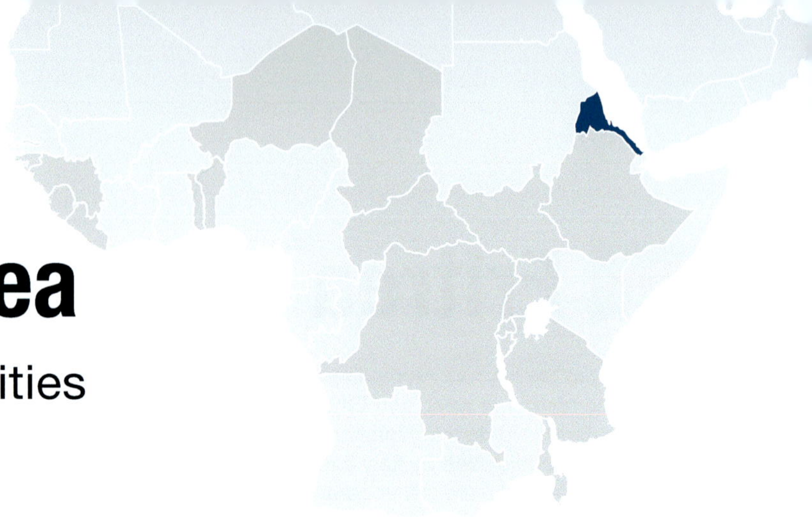

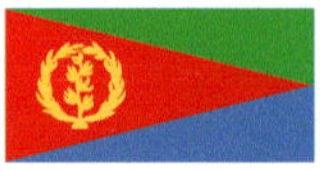

Eritrea

Healthcare Facilities

Adi Quala Hospital
Adi Quala, Eritrea
https://vfapp.org/dcff

Adikeyh Hospital
Adi Keyh, Eritrea
https://vfapp.org/a1f9

Āssab Hospital
Āssab, Eritrea
https://vfapp.org/75c2

Halibet Referral Hospital
ጎደና ሳሕል, ኣስመራ
Asmara أسمرة, ዞባ ማእከል
المنطقة المركزية, Eritrea
https://vfapp.org/c883

Keren Hospital
ጽርግያ طريق أغوردات – كرن
ከረን አቑርደት, ከረን Keren
كرن, ዞባ ዓንሰባ Anseba
عنسبا, Eritrea
https://vfapp.org/74c7

Massawa Hospital
ጽርግያ ኣስመራ ምጽዋዕ
Asmara Massawa Road طريق
أسمرة – مصوع, ምጽዋዕ
Massawa, ዞባ ሰሜናዊ
ቀይሕ ባሕሪ Northern Red
Sea Zone شمال البحر الأحمر,
Eritrea
https://vfapp.org/6d74

Mekane Hiwot Hospital
172-2 Street, Asmara,
Zoba Center Central District,
Eritrea
https://vfapp.org/9edf

Mendefera Referral Hospital
Mendefera, Eritrea
https://vfapp.org/239f

Mini Hospital
P-4, Adewuhi, Adi Awhi,
Eritrea
https://vfapp.org/465a

Sanafi Hospital
Asmara Zalambesa Road, Adi
Qiih/Adi Keyh, Eritrea
https://vfapp.org/1a4e

Sembel Hospital
Asmara, Eritrea
https://vfapp.org/34dd

St. Mary's Psychiatric Hospital Sembel
Zoba Center Street, Asmara,
Asmara, Eritrea
https://vfapp.org/3bf7

Tessenei Hospital
Teseney, Eritrea
https://vfapp.org/97b1

Zonal Referral Hospital Ghinda
Asmara-Massawa Road,
Dengolo, Northern Red Sea
Zone, Eritrea
https://vfapp.org/fa46

Āk'ordat Hospital
Barentu – Ak'ordat Road
/ طريق بارنتو – أغوردات,
ኣቑርደት Akordat أغوردات,
ጋሽ-ባርካ Gash Barka القاش
وبركة, Eritrea
https://vfapp.org/4451

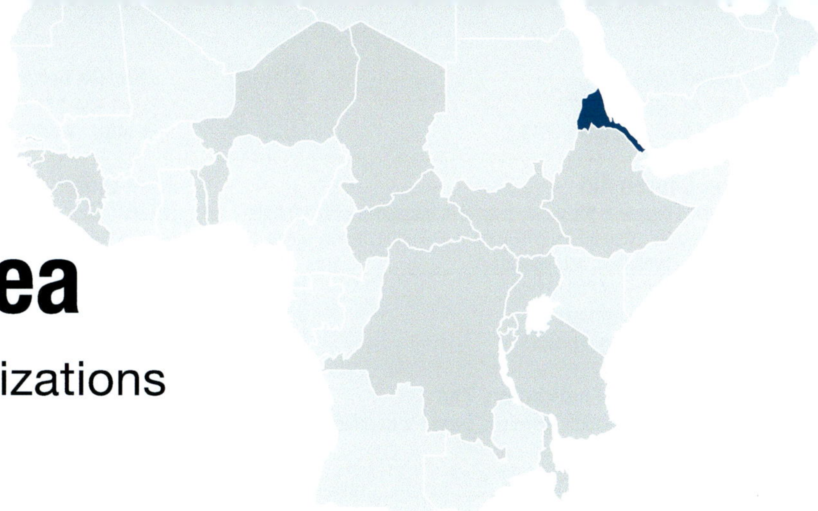

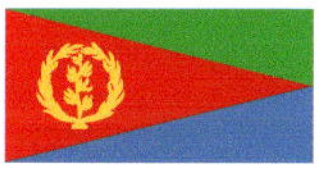

Eritrea

Nonprofit Organizations

Africa CDC
Aims to strengthen the capacity and capability of Africa's public health institutions as well as partnerships to detect and respond quickly and effectively to disease threats and outbreaks, based on data-driven interventions and programs.
Infect Dis, Logist-Op, Pub Health
☎ +251 11 551 7700
🌐 https://vfapp.org/339c

Americares
Saves lives and improves health for people affected by poverty or disaster and responds with life-changing medicine, medical supplies, and health programs including domestic and global medical clinics.
All-Immu, ER Med, General, Infect Dis, MF Med, Nutr
☎ +1 203-658-9500
🌐 https://vfapp.org/e567

Amref Health Africa
Serves millions of people across thirty-five countries in Sub-Saharan Africa, strengthening health systems, and training African health workers to respond to the continent's most critical health issues.
All-Immu, General, Infect Dis, Logist-Op, MF Med, OB-GYN, Path, Pub Health, Surg
☎ +254 20 6993000
🌐 https://vfapp.org/6985

Carter Center, The
Seeks to prevent and resolve conflicts, enhance freedom and democracy, and improve health, while remaining committed to human rights and the alleviation of human suffering.
Infect Dis, MF Med, Ophth-Opt
☎ +1 800-550-3560
🌐 https://vfapp.org/6556

Center for Strategic and International Studies (CSIS) Commission on Strengthening America's Health Security
Brings together a distinguished and diverse group of high-level opinion leaders bridging security and health, with the core aim to chart a bold vision for the future of U.S. leadership in global health.
ER Med, Infect Dis, MF Med, Pub Health
☎ +1 202-887-0200
🌐 https://vfapp.org/6d7f

Chain of Hope
Provides lifesaving heart operations for children around the world and supports the development of cardiac services in numerous developing and war-torn countries.
Anesth, CT Surg, CV Med, Crit-Care, Ped Surg, Peds, Pulm-Critic, Surg
☎ +44 20 7351 1978
🌐 https://vfapp.org/1b1b

Christian Aid Ministries
Strives to be a trustworthy and efficient channel for Amish, Mennonite, and other conservative Anabaptist groups and individuals to minister to physical and spiritual needs around the world.
CT Surg, ER Med, Logist-Op, Ortho, Pub Health
☎ +1 330-893-2428
🌐 https://vfapp.org/7b33

Developing Country NGO Delegation: Global Fund to Fight AIDS, TB & Malaria
Works to strengthen the engagement of civil society actors and organizations in developing countries to contribute toward achieving a world in which AIDS, TB, and Malaria are no longer global, public health, and human rights threats.
Infect Dis, Pub Health
☎ +254 20 2515790
🌐 https://vfapp.org/3149

Direct Relief
Improves the health and lives of people affected by poverty or emergency situations by mobilizing and providing essential medical resources needed for their care.
ER Med, Logist-Op
☎ +1 805-964-4767
🌐 https://vfapp.org/58e5

EMERGENCY
Provides free, high-quality healthcare to victims of war, poverty, and landmines. Also builds hospitals and trains local staff, while pursuing human-rights-based medicine.
ER Med, Neonat, OB-GYN, Ophth-Opt, Ped Surg
☎ +39 02 881881
🌐 https://vfapp.org/c361

END Fund, The
Aims to control and eliminate the most prevalent neglected diseases among the world's poorest and most vulnerable people.

Infect Dis
+1 646-690-9775
https://vfapp.org/2614

Finn Church Aid
Supports people in the most vulnerable situations within fragile and disaster-affected regions in three thematic priority areas: right to peace, livelihood, and education.
ER Med, Psych, Pub Health
+358 20 7871201
https://vfapp.org/9623

Fred Hollows Foundation, The
Works toward a world in which no person is needlessly blind or vision impaired.
Ophth-Opt, Pub Health, Surg
+1 646-374-0445
https://vfapp.org/73e5

Global Oncology (GO)
Brings the best in cancer care to underserved patients around the world and collaborates across geographic, professional, and academic borders to improve cancer care, research, and education.
Heme-Onc, Path, Rad-Onc
https://vfapp.org/fcb8

Health Equity Initiative
Aims to build and sustain a global community that engages across sectors and disciplines to advance health equity.
Pub Health
https://vfapp.org/e2e2

International Agency for the Prevention of Blindness (IAPB), The
Leads international efforts in blindness-prevention activities, works toward a world where no one is needlessly visually impaired, and ensures that everyone has access to the best possible standard of eye health.
Infect Dis, Ophth-Opt, Pub Health
https://vfapp.org/87a2

International Federation of Gynecology and Obstetrics (FIGO)
Implements global projects on specific women's health issues.
MF Med, Medicine, Neonat, OB-GYN, Surg, Urol
+44 20 7928 1166
https://vfapp.org/c4b4

International Federation of Red Cross and Red Crescent Societies (IFRC)
Coordinates and directs international assistance following natural and man-made disasters in nonconflict situations through the world's largest humanitarian and development network. Provides disaster-preparedness programs, healthcare activities, and promotes humanitarian values.
ER Med, General, Infect Dis, Nutr
+1 212-338-0161
https://vfapp.org/b4ee

International Trachoma Initiative (iTi)
Works toward a world free from trachoma, a preventable cause of blindness, and provides comprehensive support to national ministries of health and governmental and nongovernmental organizations to implement a comprehensive approach to fight trachoma.

Infect Dis, Ophth-Opt
+1 404-371-0466
https://vfapp.org/3278

Joint United Nations Programme on HIV/AIDS (UNAIDS)
Aims to place people living with HIV and people affected by the virus at the decision-making table and at the center of designing, delivering, and monitoring the AIDS response.
Infect Dis
+41 22 791 36 66
https://vfapp.org/464a

Life for a Child
Supports the provision of the best possible health care, given local circumstances, to all children and youth with diabetes in less-resourced countries, through the strengthening of existing diabetes services.
Endo, Medicine, Peds
https://vfapp.org/d712

MedShare
Aims to improve the quality of life of people, communities, and the planet by sourcing and directly delivering surplus medical supplies and equipment to communities in need around the world.
Logist-Op
+1 770-323-5858
https://vfapp.org/c8bc

Mercy Ships
Operates hospital ships staffed by volunteers to bring hope, healing, and healthcare to underserved communities worldwide.
Anesth, Dent-OMFS, Logist-Op, Neonat, OB-GYN, Ophth-Opt, Ortho, Palliative, Plast, Psych, Surg
+1 903-939-7000
https://vfapp.org/2e99

Mission Bambini
Helps to support children living in poverty, sickness, and without education, giving them the opportunity and hope of a better life.
CT Surg, CV Med, Crit-Care, ER Med, Ped Surg, Peds
+39 02 210 0241
https://vfapp.org/dc1a

Operation Fistula
Exists to end obstetric fistula by building models of care that serve every woman, everywhere.
MF Med, OB-GYN, Surg
+1 512-687-3479
https://vfapp.org/ce8e

Optometry Giving Sight
Delivers eye exams and low or no-cost glasses, provides training for local eye care professionals, and establishes optometry schools, vision centers and optical labs.
Ophth-Opt
+1 303-526-0430
https://vfapp.org/33ea

People to People Canada (P2P)
Contributes to the fight against preventable diseases and addresses the full range of determinants of health (physical, social, economic, and cultural) affecting vulnerable communities.
Infect Dis, Psych, Pub Health

☏ +1 416-690-8005
⊕ https://vfapp.org/67d8

RestoringVision
Empowers lives by restoring vision for millions of people in need.
Ophth-Opt
☏ +1 209-980-7323
⊕ https://vfapp.org/e121

Rockefeller Foundation, The
Works to promote the well-being of humanity.
Logist-Op, Nutr, Pub Health
☏ +1 212-869-8500
⊕ https://vfapp.org/5424

Rotary International
Provides service to others, improves lives, and advances world understanding, goodwill, and peace through its fellowship of business, professional, and community leaders.
ER Med, General, Infect Dis, MF Med, OB-GYN
⊕ https://vfapp.org/8fb5

SATMED
Serves non-governmental organizations, hospitals, medical universities, and other healthcare providers active in resource-poor areas, by providing open-access e-health services for the health community.
Logist-Op
⊕ https://vfapp.org/b8d5

Save A Child's Heart
Provides lifesaving cardiac treatment to children in developing countries, and trains healthcare professionals from these countries to deliver quality care in their communities.
CT Surg, CV Med, Crit-Care, Ped Surg, Peds
☏ +1 240-223-3940
⊕ https://vfapp.org/1bef

Surgeons for Smiles
Brings first-class medical and dental care to those in need in developing countries around the world.
Anesth, Dent-OMFS, OB-GYN, Ped Surg, Plast, Surg
☏ +1 301-352-6311
⊕ https://vfapp.org/3427

Task Force for Global Health, The
Consists of programs and focus areas that cover a range of global health issues including neglected tropical diseases, infectious diseases, vaccines, field epidemiology, public health informatics, health workforce development, and global health ethics.
Infect Dis, Logist-Op, Medicine, Ophth-Opt, Peds
☏ +1 404-371-0466
⊕ https://vfapp.org/714c

United Nations Children's Fund (UNICEF)
Works in over 190 countries and territories to save children's lives, to defend their rights, and to help them fulfill their potential, from early childhood through adolescence.
All-Immu, Infect Dis, MF Med, Neonat, Nutr, OB-GYN, Ped Surg, Peds, Pub Health
⊕ https://vfapp.org/42d7

United Nations Development Programme (UNDP)
Helps countries achieve the simultaneous eradication of extreme poverty and significant reduction of inequalities and exclusion using a sustainable human development approach.
Infect Dis, Logist-Op, Pub Health
⊕ https://vfapp.org/935c

United Nations High Commissioner for Refugees (UNHCR)
Safeguards the rights and well-being of people who have been forced to flee, ensuring that everybody has the right to seek asylum and find safe refuge in another country, with the goal of seeking lasting solutions.
General, MF Med, Medicine, OB-GYN, Peds, Psych, Pub Health
⊕ https://vfapp.org/6636

United Nations Office for the Coordination of Humanitarian Affairs (OCHA)
Contributes to principled and effective humanitarian response through coordination, advocacy, policy, information management, and humanitarian financing tools and services, by leveraging functional expertise throughout the organization.
Logist-Op
⊕ https://vfapp.org/22b8

United Nations Population Fund (UNFPA)
Supports reproductive healthcare for women and youth in more than 150 countries, focusing on delivering a world where every pregnancy is wanted, every childbirth is safe, and every young person's potential is fulfilled.
Infect Dis, MF Med, Neonat, OB-GYN, Peds, Pub Health
☏ +1 212-963-6008
⊕ https://vfapp.org/c969

University of Pennsylvania Perelman School of Medicine Center for Global Health
Aims to improve health equity worldwide – through enhanced public health awareness and access to care, discovery and outcomes based research, and comprehensive educational programs grounded in partnership.
Heme-Onc, Infect Dis, OB-GYN
☏ +1 215-898-0848
⊕ https://vfapp.org/cb57

Women's Refugee Commission
Seeks to improve lives by protecting the rights of women, children, and youth displaced by conflict and crisis through researching their needs, identifying solutions, and advocating for programs and policies to strengthen their resilience.
General, MF Med, Neonat, OB-GYN, Peds, Psych
☏ +1 212-551-3115
⊕ https://vfapp.org/3d8f

World Health Organization, The (WHO)
The United Nations' agency for health provides leadership on global health matters, shapes the health research agenda, setting norms and standards, articulates evidence-based policy options, provides technical support and monitoring to countries, and assesses health trends.
ER Med, General, Infect Dis, Logist-Op, MF Med, OB-GYN, Peds, Psych, Pub Health
☏ +41 22 791 21 11
⊕ https://vfapp.org/c476

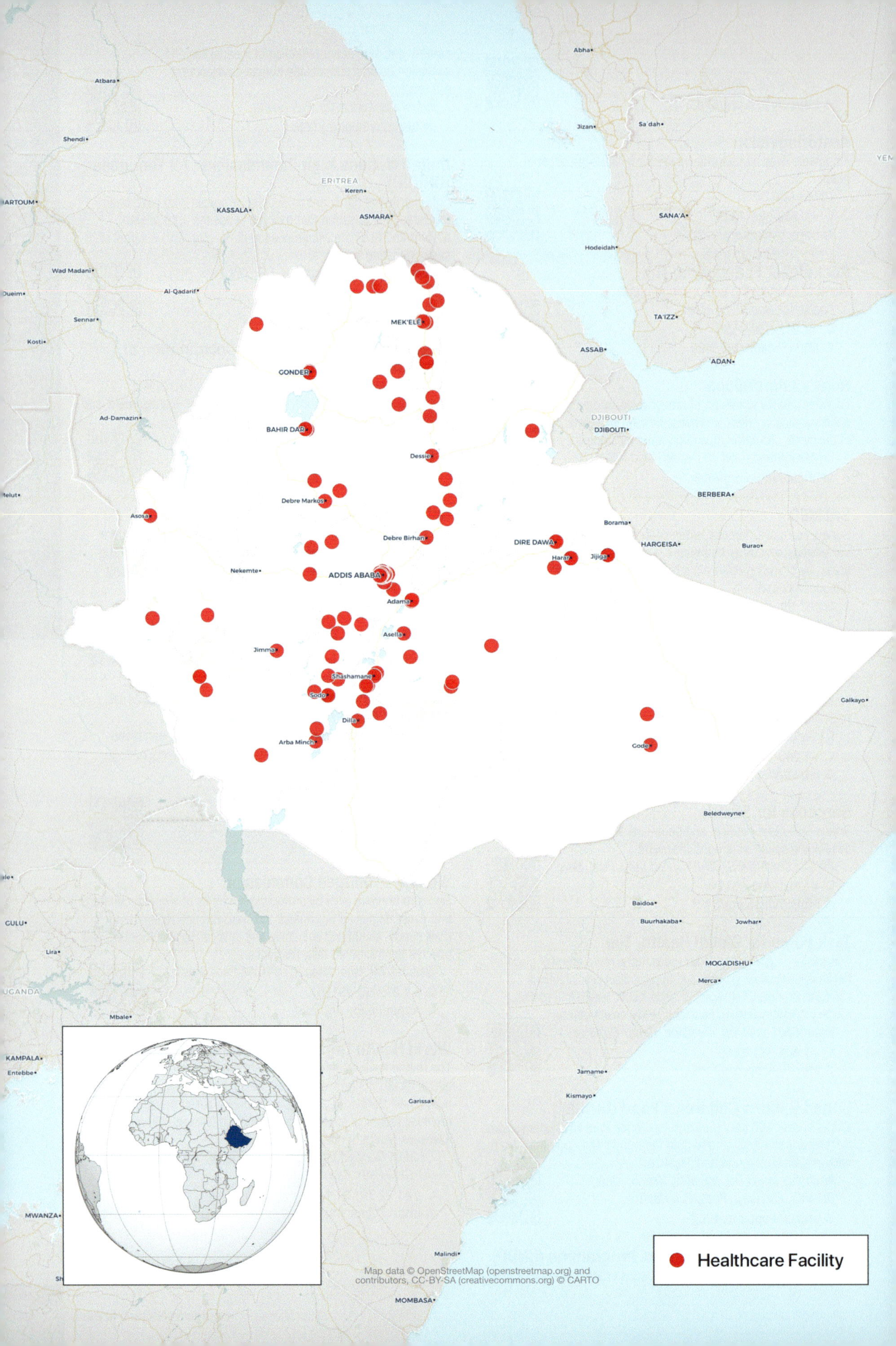

Abha
Atbara
Jizan
Sa'dah
Shendi
ERITREA
Keren
KASSALA
ASMARA
SANA'A
Hodeidah
Wad Madani
Al-Qadarif
Sennar
MEK'ELE
TA'IZZ
Kosti
ASSAB
ADAN
GONDER
Ad-Damazin
DJIBOUTI
BAHIR DAR
Dessie
BERBERA
Debre Markos
Asosa
Borama
Debre Birhan
DIRE DAWA
HARGEISA
Burao
Harar
Jijiga
Nekemte
ADDIS ABABA
Adama
Asella
Jimma
Shashamane
Galkayo
Sodo
Dilla
Arba Minch
Gode
Beledweyne
Baidoa
GULU
Buurhakaba
Jowhar
Lira
MOGADISHU
UGANDA
Merca
Mbale
KAMPALA
Entebbe
Jamame
Garissa
Kismayo
MWANZA
Malindi
MOMBASA
Healthcare Facility
Map data © OpenStreetMap (openstreetmap.org) and contributors, CC-BY-SA (creativecommons.org) © CARTO

Ethiopia

Located in the Horn of Africa, the Federal Democratic Republic of Ethiopia has a population of 108.1 million that is 43.8 percent Ethiopian Orthodox, 31.3 percent Muslim, and 22.8 percent Protestant. Eighty different ethnic groups, speaking 200 different native dialects, live there. Most of Ethiopia's population can be found in the highlands of the north and middle geographies of the country, particularly around the capital city of Addis Ababa. Ethiopia is often called the "Cradle of Mankind." Fossils of some of humankind's earliest ancestors can be found in Ethiopia, as well as nine UNESCO World Heritage Sites, more than any other country in Africa.

Ethiopia is the only country in sub-Saharan Africa to never be colonized, although it did experience Italian occupation from 1936–1941. But the country has faced decades of conflict with neighbors, environmental disasters, famine, forced population resettlement due to overworked land, and political instability. As a result, Ethiopia remains in a vulnerable state and has been ranked as one of the poorest countries in the world.

Poverty has resulted in poor health and a weak healthcare system that can't keep up with the population's needs. Maternal mortality, malaria, tuberculosis, and HIV/AIDS are all areas of concern. Significant malnutrition results in 50 percent of children having stunted growth by age five. The largest contributors to death include neonatal disorders, diarrheal disease, lower respiratory infections, HIV/AIDS, malaria, meningitis, and measles. Additional significant causes of death include non-communicable diseases, such as congenital defects as well as stroke, ischemic heart disease, and cirrhosis, which have increased substantially in recent years.

108.1M
Population

$858
GDP Per Capita

66 years
Life Expectancy
↑ Improving

7.7
Doctors/100k
Physician Density

33
Beds/100k
Hospital Bed Density

401
Deaths/100k
Maternal Mortality

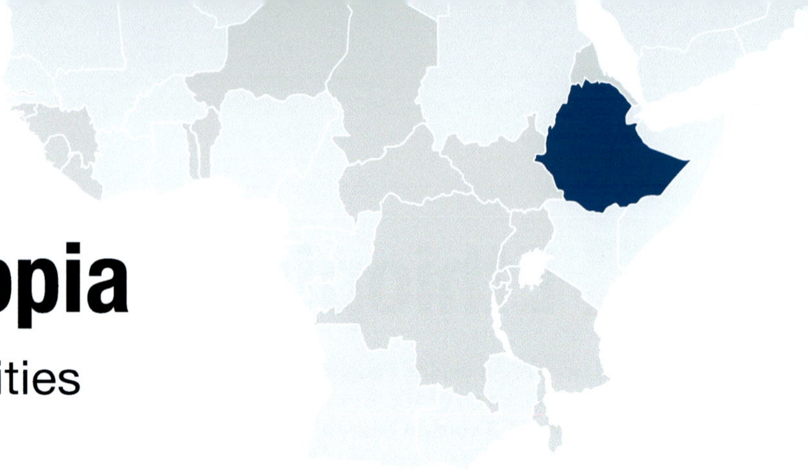

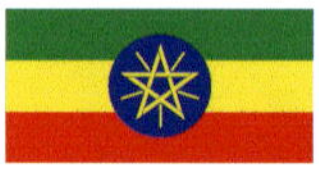

Ethiopia

Healthcare Facilities

AaBET Hospital
1271 Dej. Zewdu Aba Koran St., Addis Ababa, Ethiopia
🌐 https://vfapp.org/d59c

Adama Referral Hospital
Adama, Ethiopia
🌐 https://vfapp.org/1aa5

Addis Ababa Fistula Hospital
Addis Ababa, Ethiopia
🌐 https://vfapp.org/7fa3

Addis Cardiac Hospital
Ring Road, Addis Ababa, Ethiopia
🌐 https://vfapp.org/87b4

Addis Hiwot General Hospital
Addis Ababa, Ethiopia
🌐 https://vfapp.org/a981

Adigrat Ras Sibhat Hospital
Adigrat, Ethiopia
🌐 https://vfapp.org/fd4c

Aflagat General Hospital
Route 3, Bahir Dar, Ethiopia
🌐 https://vfapp.org/ea43

Aksum K'Idist Maryam Hospital
Bole Road, Axum, Tigray, Ethiopia
🌐 https://vfapp.org/bdd3

Alert Hospital
Ring Road, Addis Ababa, Ethiopia
🌐 https://vfapp.org/bb78

Amanuel Hospital
Congo Street, Addis Ababa, Ethiopia
🌐 https://vfapp.org/8782

Amdework Hospital
Amdework, Ethiopia
🌐 https://vfapp.org/8c8c

Amin General Hospital
Dejazmach Balcha Aba Nefso Street, Addis Ababa, Ethiopia
🌐 https://vfapp.org/b8c7

Arba Minch Hospital
Arba Minch, Ethiopia
🌐 https://vfapp.org/c762

Art Hospital
Dire Dawa, Ethiopia
🌐 https://vfapp.org/f92e

Asaita Referral Hospital
Asaita, Afar, Ethiopia
🌐 https://vfapp.org/461f

Asella Hospital
09, Assela, Ethiopia
🌐 https://vfapp.org/659c

Assosa Hospital
Asosa – Kurmuk/Guba Road, Benishngul-Gumuz, Ethiopia
🌐 https://vfapp.org/4bac

Atsbi Hospital
Tigray, Adigrat, Ethiopia
🌐 https://vfapp.org/67cc

Attat Hospital
Welkite Gurage, Emdibir, Southern Nations Nationalities Peoples, Ethiopia
🌐 https://vfapp.org/2e88

Ayder Referral Hospital
Mek'ele-Weldiya Road, Adi Gura, Tigray, Ethiopia
🌐 https://vfapp.org/1c2b

B.G.M. Hospital
Addis Ababa, Ethiopia
🌐 https://vfapp.org/6f27

Balcha Hospital
Liberia Street, Addis Ababa, Ethiopia
🌐 https://vfapp.org/ef86

Bekoji Hospital
Bekoji, Ethiopia
🌐 https://vfapp.org/731f

Bethel 2 Hospital
Addis Ababa, Ethiopia
🌐 https://vfapp.org/3cc4

Bethel Teaching
Addis Ababa, Ethiopia
🌐 https://vfapp.org/535f

Bethezata Hospital
Ras Mekonnen Avenue, Addis Ababa, Addis Ababa, Ethiopia
🌐 https://vfapp.org/4d33

Betsegah Obstetrics and Gynecology Special Hospital
Ghana Street, Addis Ababa, Ethiopia
⊕ https://vfapp.org/6877

Bilal Hospital
Dire Dawa, Ethiopia
⊕ https://vfapp.org/fdd4

Bishoftu
Bishoftu, Oromia, Ethiopia
⊕ https://vfapp.org/ea6b

Black Lion Hospital Cancer Center
Burundi Street, Addis Ababa, Ethiopia
⊕ https://vfapp.org/4e89

Bona General Hospital
Bona Qabelanka, Ethiopia
⊕ https://vfapp.org/3183

Brass MCH Hospital
Ring Road, Addis Ababa, Ethiopia
⊕ https://vfapp.org/27a1

Brooke Hospital
South Africa Street, Addis Ababa, Addis Ababa, Ethiopia
⊕ https://vfapp.org/19a8

Butajira General Hospital
Butajira, Ethiopia
⊕ https://vfapp.org/faa8

Chencha Hospital
Chencha, Ethiopia
⊕ https://vfapp.org/7772

CURE Ethiopia Children's Hospital
Hamle 19 Public Park, Addis Ababa, Ethiopia
⊕ https://vfapp.org/5b13

Debre Berhan Referral Hospital
ደብረ ብርሃን / Debre Birhan, Ethiopia
⊕ https://vfapp.org/1ebb

Debre Birhan Referral Hospital
Debre Birhan, Ethiopia
⊕ https://vfapp.org/6f3e

Debre Markos Referral Hospital
Debre Markos, Ethiopia
⊕ https://vfapp.org/9f27

Dembecha Hospital
Dembecha, Ethiopia
⊕ https://vfapp.org/c1d1

Dessie Hospital
ደሴ / Dessie, Ethiopia
⊕ https://vfapp.org/63e1

Dilla Referral Hospital
Addis Ababa to Nairobi road, ዲላ / Dilla, ኦሮሚያ ክልል / Oromia, Ethiopia
⊕ https://vfapp.org/a646

Effesson Regional Hospital
Ataye, Ethiopia
⊕ https://vfapp.org/135f

Eka Kotebe General Hospital
Fikre Mariam Aba Techan Street, Addis Ababa, Ethiopia
⊕ https://vfapp.org/b49c

Ethio Wise Hospital
Fitawrari Habte Giorgis Street, Addis Ababa, Ethiopia
⊕ https://vfapp.org/63bf

Ethio-Tebebe MCH Hospital
Sefere Selam, Addis Ababa, Ethiopia
⊕ https://vfapp.org/c59a

Ethiopian Federal Police Commission Referral Hospital
Chad Street, Addis Ababa, Ethiopia
⊕ https://vfapp.org/aac4

Fatsi Hospital
Fatsi/Tigray, Ethiopia
⊕ https://vfapp.org/1a84

Felege Hiwot Referral Hospital
Bahir Dar Zuria, Ethiopia
⊕ https://vfapp.org/d678

Gambella Hospital
Gambela – Gore, ጋምቤላ / Gambela, ጋምቤላ ሕዝቦች ክልል / Gambela, Ethiopia
⊕ https://vfapp.org/931a

Gambi General Hospital
Haile Silase Road, Grass Village, Ethiopia
⊕ https://vfapp.org/fc68

Harar General Hospital
Harar, Ethiopia
⊕ https://vfapp.org/3335

Genet General Hospital
Genet General Hospital PLC, Addis Ababa, Ethiopia
⊕ https://vfapp.org/9a9a

Gesund
Addis Ababa, Ethiopia
⊕ https://vfapp.org/89c1

Ghandi Hospital
Ras Desta Damtew Street, Addis Ababa, Ethiopia
⊕ https://vfapp.org/13c6

Gindeberet Hospital
Kachise, Oromia, Ethiopia
⊕ https://vfapp.org/9155

Girawa
Girawa, Ethiopia
⊕ https://vfapp.org/c9f4

Girum General Hospital
Addis Ketema Sub City, Addis Ababa, Ethiopia
⊕ https://vfapp.org/37f2

Goba Hospital
Goba, Ethiopia
⊕ https://vfapp.org/be1b

Gode Hospital
Gode – Walakhere Highway, ጎዴ / Gode, ሶማሌ ክልል / Somali, Ethiopia
⊕ https://vfapp.org/13a9

Gonder University Hospital
Bahir Dar – Gonder Road, ጎንደር / Gonder, Ethiopia
https://vfapp.org/b136

Haleluya General Hospital
Debre Zeit Road, Addis Ababa, Ethiopia
https://vfapp.org/377c

Hamlin Fistula Hospital
Ring Road, Addis Ababa, Ethiopia
https://vfapp.org/b548

Hiwot Fana Referral Hospital
Harar, Ethiopia
https://vfapp.org/f68d

Haro Miriam Hospital
Cheliya, Ethiopia
https://vfapp.org/6cb9

Hawaria H.C.
Ezhana Welene, Ethiopia
https://vfapp.org/d197

Hawassa University Referral Hospital
Addis Ababa to Nairobi Road, Afarara, ኦሮሚያ ክልል / Oromia, Ethiopia
https://vfapp.org/e931

Hayat Hospital
Addis Ababa, Ethiopia
https://vfapp.org/cadd

Hoospitaala Rifti Vaalii
Oromia Street, ናዳማ / Nazret, ኦሮሚያ ክልል / Oromia, Ethiopia
https://vfapp.org/deb1

Hospital at Bahir Dar
Bezavit Road, Bete Mengistu Rd, ባሕር-ዳር / Bahir Dar, Ethiopia
https://vfapp.org/ce3b

Hospital at Denan
Denan, ሶማሌ ክልል / Somali, Ethiopia
https://vfapp.org/59a7

Hospital at Edaga Hamus town
Saesi Tsaedaemba, Ethiopia
https://vfapp.org/6bfc

Hospital at Hawassa
Addis Ababa to Nairobi Road, Afarara, ኦሮሚያ ክልል / Oromia, Ethiopia
https://vfapp.org/1d56

Hospital at Jinka
Jinka, Gazer, Ethiopia
https://vfapp.org/27a3

Hospital at Kembolcha
Kombosha, Oromia, Ethiopia
https://vfapp.org/7dc7

Hospital at Kemse
Kemse, Ethiopia
https://vfapp.org/1e67

Hospital at Mekele
Mekele, Ethiopia
https://vfapp.org/5cba

Hospital at Metu
Metu, Ethiopia
https://vfapp.org/e828

Hospital at Nazret
College Road, ናዳማ /Nazret, ኦሮሚያ ክልል / Oromia, Ethiopia
https://vfapp.org/e832

Hospital at Sanja
Sanja, Ethiopia
https://vfapp.org/67a1

Hospital at Shashamene
Shashemene, Ethiopia
https://vfapp.org/f639

Hospital at Shoa Robit
Shoa Robit, Ethiopia
https://vfapp.org/8b99

Hospital at Tigray
Godena Eyassu Street, Mek'elē, Tigray, Ethiopia
https://vfapp.org/bc42

Hospital at Weldiya
Weldiya, Ethiopia
https://vfapp.org/a4be

Hospital at Wukro Maray
3, ኣኽሱም / Axum, Tigray, Ethiopia
https://vfapp.org/582b

Hospital Emmanuel Cathedrale of Robe
8, Robe, Oromia, Ethiopia
https://vfapp.org/a1ee

Hospital Sheik Hussein
Sheikh Hussein, Gololcha, Ethiopia
https://vfapp.org/7775

Hospital Wacha
Tepi – Shishinda, Tepi, Southern Nations Nationalities Peoples, Ethiopia
https://vfapp.org/f47c

Hulsehet Referral Hospital
Churchill Avenue, Addis Ababa, Ethiopia
https://vfapp.org/cd87

Ibex Hospital
Yohannis Church, Gonder, Ethiopia
https://vfapp.org/e899

ICMC Hospital
Addis Ababa, Ethiopia
https://vfapp.org/644a

JJU Meles Zenawi Memorial Referral Hospital
Jijiga, Ethiopia
https://vfapp.org/4625

Jugal Hospital
Amir Uga, ሐረር / Harar, ሀረሪ ሁስኒ / Harar, Ethiopia
https://vfapp.org/bab6

Kadisco General Hospital
Road to Gergi Giorgis, Addis Ababa / አዲስ አበባ, አዲስ አበባ / Addis Ababa, Ethiopia
https://vfapp.org/3b8e

Karamara General Hospital
4, Jijiga, Somali Region, Ethiopia
🌐 https://vfapp.org/d75b

Kidus Gebriel Hospital
Addis Ababa, Ethiopia
🌐 https://vfapp.org/35ad

Kindo Koyisha Hospital
Chida-Sodo, Bale, ደቡብ ብሔሮች ብሔረሰቦችና ሕዝቦች ክልል / Southern Nations Nationalities Peoples, Ethiopia
🌐 https://vfapp.org/4fd5

Kobo Hospital
Mek'ele-Weldiya Road, Kobo, Ethiopia
🌐 https://vfapp.org/428d

Kuyi Hospital
Geter Kuy Road, Kuyi, Ethiopia
🌐 https://vfapp.org/3f43

Kwante
Zizencio Guakepece, Zizencio, ደቡብ ብሔሮች ብሔረሰቦችና ሕዝቦች ክልል / Southern Nations Nationalities Peoples, Ethiopia
🌐 https://vfapp.org/9458

Lalibela Hospital
Lalibela-Geshena-Road, Akotola, Ethiopia
🌐 https://vfapp.org/692e

Land Mark Hospital
Mozambique Street, Addis Ababa, Ethiopia
🌐 https://vfapp.org/d169

Lena Carl Hospital
Mek'ele-Weldiya Road, Maychew, Tigray, Ethiopia
🌐 https://vfapp.org/bb38

Machew Hospital
Endamehoni, Ethiopia
🌐 https://vfapp.org/69bd

Markos Hospital
Old Italian Road, መቐለ / Mek'elē, ትግራይ / Tigray, Ethiopia
🌐 https://vfapp.org/d233

MCM
Egzabheraab To Mebrathail, Addis Ababa, Ethiopia
🌐 https://vfapp.org/d414

Mekelle Hospital
Witten Germany Street, Mek'elē, Tigray, Ethiopia
🌐 https://vfapp.org/6aea

Meles Zenawi Memorial Referral Hospital
Jijiga, Ethiopia
🌐 https://vfapp.org/9f2b

Menelik II Referral Hospital
Yeka, Addis Ababa, Ethiopia
🌐 https://vfapp.org/68f9

Mizan-Aman Teaching Hospital
Mizan – Maji, Greater Aman, ደቡብ ብሔሮች ብሔረሰቦችና ሕዝቦች ክልል / Southern Nations Nationalities Peoples, Ethiopia
🌐 https://vfapp.org/5745

Nain Specialized Maternal and Child Hospital
Mauritius Street, Addis Ababa / አዲስ አበባ, አዲስ አበባ / Addis Ababa, Ethiopia
🌐 https://vfapp.org/79f6

NEMMG Hospital Hossana
Welkite Gurage, Hossana, ደቡብ ብሔሮች ብሔረሰቦችና ሕዝቦች ክልል / Southern Nations Nationalities Peoples, Ethiopia
🌐 https://vfapp.org/3d3f

Number One Health Station
Awash – Assab, Awragoda, Dire Dawa, Ethiopia
🌐 https://vfapp.org/151f

Ras Desta Hospital
Addis Ababa, Ethiopia
🌐 https://vfapp.org/d62e

Rim and Men's Hospital
Witten Germany Street, Mek'elē, Tigray, Ethiopia
🌐 https://vfapp.org/73ce

Shanan Gibe General Hospital
Jimma, Ethiopia
🌐 https://vfapp.org/e9f2

Shashamane Hospital
Kuyera Dedeba, Ethiopia
🌐 https://vfapp.org/d8de

Shiek Hassan Referral Hospital
Jijiga, Ethiopia
🌐 https://vfapp.org/f618

Shinshiro Primary Hospital
Shinshicho, Southern Nations, Nationalities and Peoples, Ethiopia
🌐 https://vfapp.org/a1cb

Shone Hospital
41, ሾኔ / Shone, ደቡብ ብሔሮች ብሔረሰቦችና ሕዝቦች ክልል / Southern Nations Nationalities Peoples, Ethiopia
🌐 https://vfapp.org/a3e3

Silk Road Hospital
Egypt Street, Addis Ababa, Addis Ababa, Ethiopia
🌐 https://vfapp.org/bb16

Sister Aquila Hospital
Darartu Tulu Street, Adama, Nazret, Oromia, Ethiopia
🌐 https://vfapp.org/667b

Soddo Christian Hospital
Sodo to Arba Minch, Sodo, Southern Nations Nationalities Peoples, Ethiopia
🌐 https://vfapp.org/8ceb

St. Petros Specialized TB Hospital
Intoto Road, Addis Ababa, Ethiopia
🌐 https://vfapp.org/d142

St. Paul's Hospital
Swaziland St, Addis Ababa, Ethiopia
🌐 https://vfapp.org/638a

St. Yared Hospital
Fikre Mariam Aba Techan Street, Addis Ababa, Ethiopia
🌐 https://vfapp.org/6cf9

Suhul Referral Hospital
3, Shire, Tigray, Ethiopia
https://vfapp.org/221c

Tefera Hailu Memorial Hospital
Sekota, Ethiopia
https://vfapp.org/e7e1

Tekelehaymanot Hospital
Gobena Aba Tigu Street, Addis Ababa, Ethiopia
https://vfapp.org/9bbc

Tepi General Hospital
Tepi – Shishinda, Southern Nations, Nationalities and Peoples Region, Ethiopia
https://vfapp.org/d11a

Tezena
Ring Road, Addis Ababa, Ethiopia
https://vfapp.org/a54d

Tikur Anbass General Specialized Hospital
Wereda 03, Ethiopia
https://vfapp.org/a797

Tirunesh Dibaba Hospital
Addis Ababa, Ethiopia
https://vfapp.org/df54

Tor Hailoch
Smuts Av, Addis Ababa, Ethiopia
https://vfapp.org/c75d

Tuber Clouses
Fitawrari Habte Giorgis Street, Addis Ababa, Ethiopia
https://vfapp.org/c528

Tzna Hospital
TZNA General Hospital, Addis Ababa, Ethiopia
https://vfapp.org/e5e1

Wanted Life Hospital
Belay Zeleke, Bahir Dar, Ethiopia
https://vfapp.org/6a82

Wolayita Sodo University Hospital
Hawassa Sodo, Southern Nations, Nationalities and Peoples Region, Ethiopia
https://vfapp.org/8811

Wukro General Hospital
Wukro, Tigray, Ethiopia
https://vfapp.org/ae5d

Yekatit 12 Hospital
Weatherall Street, Addis Ababa, Ethiopia
https://vfapp.org/d5aa

Yemariam Work Hospital
Awash – Assab Awragoda, Dire Dawa, Ethiopia
https://vfapp.org/76ee

Yerer Hospital
Road to Gergi Giorgis, Addis Ababa, Ethiopia
https://vfapp.org/add9

Yirga Alem Hospital
Yirgalem General Hospital, Sidama Zone, Southern Ethiopia
https://vfapp.org/9941

Yordanos Orthopaedic Hospital
Tesema Aba Kemaw Street, Addis Ababa, Ethiopia
https://vfapp.org/d112

Zewditu Memorial Hospital
Wendimeneh Street, Addis Ababa, Ethiopia
https://vfapp.org/63e8

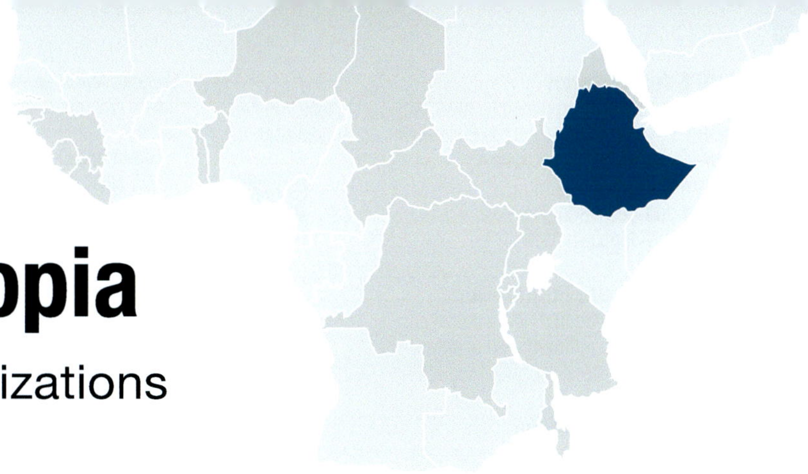

Ethiopia

Nonprofit Organizations

Abt Associates
Seeks to improve the quality of life and economic well-being of people worldwide, while striving to meet and exceed the highest professional standards.
General, Logist-Op, MF Med, OB-GYN, Peds
+1 212-779-7700
https://vfapp.org/cec2

Aceso Global
Provides strategic healthcare advisory services in low- and middle-income countries to design and deliver highly customized, evidence-based solutions that address the complex nature of healthcare systems, with a goal to strengthen and provide affordable, high-quality care to all.
Logist-Op, Pub Health
+1 202-758-2636
https://vfapp.org/b3b7

Action Against Hunger
Aims to end life-threatening hunger for good through treating and preventing malnutrition across more than forty-five countries.
+1 212-967-7800
https://vfapp.org/2dbc

Addis Clinic, The
Utilizes telemedicine to care for people living in medically underserved areas, connects volunteer physicians with global health challenges, and provides support to local partner organizations and frontline health workers.
General, Infect Dis
+1 339-225-9886
https://vfapp.org/f82f

Advance Family Planning
Aims to achieve global expansion and access to quality contraceptive information, services, and supplies through financial investment and political commitment.
General, MF Med, Pub Health
+1 410-502-8715
https://vfapp.org/7478

Adventist Health International
Focuses on upgrading and managing mission hospitals by providing governance, consultation, and technical assistance to a number of affiliated Seventh-Day Adventist hospitals throughout Africa, Asia, and the Americas.
Dent-OMFS, General, Pub Health
+1 909-558-5610
https://vfapp.org/16aa

Africa CDC
Aims to strengthen the capacity and capability of Africa's public health institutions as well as partnerships to detect and respond quickly and effectively to disease threats and outbreaks, based on data-driven interventions and programs.
Infect Dis, Logist-Op, Pub Health
+251 11 551 7700
https://vfapp.org/339c

Africa Humanitarian Action (AHA)
Responds to crises, conflicts, and disasters in Africa, while informing and advising the international community, governments, civil society, and the private sector on humanitarian issues of concern to Africa. Supports institutional and organizational development efforts.
General, Infect Dis, MF Med, Nutr, OB-GYN
+251 11 660 4800
https://vfapp.org/3ca2

Africa Indoor Residual Spraying Project (AIRS)
Aims to protect millions of people in Africa from malaria by spraying insecticide on the walls, ceilings, and other indoor resting places of mosquitoes that transmit malaria.
Infect Dis
+1 301-347-5000
https://vfapp.org/9bd1

African Field Epidemiology Network (AFENET)
Strengthens field epidemiology and public health laboratory capacity to contribute effectively to addressing epidemics and other major public health problems in Africa.
All-Immu, Infect Dis, Path, Pub Health
https://vfapp.org/df2e

Against Malaria Foundation
Helps protect people from malaria. Funds anti-malaria nets, specifically long-lasting insecticidal nets (LLINs), and works with distribution partners to ensure they are used. Tracks and reports on net use and malaria case data.
Infect Dis
+44 20 7371 8735
https://vfapp.org/337d

AHOPE for Children
Aims to help children orphaned by AIDS, especially those infected with HIV. Provides medical care to children including administering lifesaving antiretroviral medication.
General, Infect Dis
+1 703-683-7500
https://vfapp.org/8538

AIDS Healthcare Foundation
Provides cutting-edge HIV/AIDS medical care and advocacy to over one million people in forty-three countries.
Infect Dis
+1 323-860-5200
https://vfapp.org/b27c

Al-Ihsan Foundation
Aims to establish and maintain a (global) society that serves and empowers all those in need.
ER Med, General, MF Med, Nutr, Ophth-Opt, Peds, Surg
+61 1300 998 444
https://vfapp.org/fff2

AMARI (African Mental Health Research Initiative)
Seeks to build an Africa-led network of future leaders in mental, neurological, and substance use (MNS) research in Ethiopia, Malawi, South Africa, and Zimbabwe.
Neuro, Psych
+263 24 2708020
https://vfapp.org/5e9d

American Academy of Ophthalmology
Protects sight and empowers lives by serving as an advocate for patients and the public, leading ophthalmic education, and advancing the profession of ophthalmology.
Ophth-Opt
+1 415-561-8500
https://vfapp.org/89a2

American Academy of Pediatrics
Seeks to attain optimal physical, mental, and social health and well-being for all infants, children, adolescents, and young adults.
Anesth, Crit-Care, Neonat, Ped Surg
+1 800-433-9016
https://vfapp.org/9633

American International Health Alliance (AIHA)
Strengthens health systems and workforce capacity worldwide through locally-driven, peer-to-peer institutional partnerships.
CV Med, ER Med, Infect Dis, Medicine, OB-GYN
+1 202-789-1136
https://vfapp.org/69fd

Americares
Saves lives and improves health for people affected by poverty or disaster and responds with life-changing medicine, medical supplies, and health programs including domestic and global medical clinics.
All-Immu, ER Med, General, Infect Dis, MF Med, Nutr
+1 203-658-9500
https://vfapp.org/e567

Amref Health Africa
Serves millions of people across thirty-five countries in Sub-Saharan Africa, strengthening health systems, and training African health workers to respond to the continent's most critical health issues.
All-Immu, General, Infect Dis, Logist-Op, MF Med, OB-GYN, Path, Pub Health, Surg
+254 20 6993000
https://vfapp.org/6985

Amsterdam Institute for Global Health and Development (AIGHD)
Provides sustainable solutions to major health problems across our planet by forging synergies between disciplines, healthcare delivery, research, and education.
Infect Dis
+31 20 210 3960
https://vfapp.org/d73d

Anania Mothers and Children Specialized Medical Center
Provides comprehensive and compassionate women's healthcare for mothers and children in Addis Ababa and the surrounding cities.
ER Med, General, OB-GYN, Peds
+251 11 156 5045
https://vfapp.org/a13e

AO Alliance
Builds solutions to lessen the burden of injuries in low- and middle-income countries, while enhancing the care of the injured to reduce human suffering, disability, and poverty.
Ortho, Surg
https://vfapp.org/8cd5

Aslan Project, The
Seeks to elevate standards of pediatric cancer care and increase survival rates in limited-resource countries.
Anesth, Heme-Onc, Ped Surg, Peds, Psych, Rad-Onc, Rehab
+1 202-507-9671
https://vfapp.org/e633

Assist International
Designs and implements humanitarian programs that build capacity, develop opportunities, and save lives around the world.
Infect Dis, Ped Surg, Peds
+1 831-438-4582
https://vfapp.org/9a3b

Australian Doctors for Africa
Develops healthier environments and builds capacity through the provision of voluntary medical assistance, while training and teaching doctors, nurses, and allied health workers and improving infrastructure and providing medical equipment.
Anesth, ENT, GI, Logist-Op, MF Med, OB-GYN, Ortho, Ped Surg, Peds, Urol
+61 8 6478 8951
https://vfapp.org/f769

Benjamin H. Josephson, MD Fund
Provides healthcare professionals with the financial resources necessary to deliver medical services for those in need throughout the world.
General, OB-GYN
+1 908-522-2853
https://vfapp.org/6acc

BethanyKids

Transforms the lives of African children with surgical conditions and disabilities through pediatric surgery, rehabilitation, public education, spiritual ministry, and training health professionals.

Neurosurg, Nutr, Ortho, Ped Surg, Peds, Rehab, Surg

https://vfapp.org/db4e

BFIRST – British Foundation for International Reconstructive Surgery & Training

Supports projects across the developing world to train surgeons in their local environment to effectively manage devastating injuries.

Anesth, Plast, Surg

+44 20 7831 5161

https://vfapp.org/ad4f

Bill & Melinda Gates Foundation

Focuses on global issues, from poverty to health, to education, offering the opportunity to dramatically improve the quality of life for billions of people, by building partnerships that bring together resources, expertise, and vision to identify issues, find answers, and drive change.

All-Immu, General, Infect Dis, MF Med, Neonat, OB-GYN, Pub Health

https://vfapp.org/7cf2

Boston Cardiac Foundation, The

Provides advanced medical technologies and cardiac care such as pacemaker implantation to patients around the world who would otherwise not have access to these services.

Anesth, CT Surg, CV Med, Crit-Care

+1 781-662-6404

https://vfapp.org/8fd3

Boston Children's Hospital: Global Health Program

Helps solve pediatric global health care challenges by transferring expertise through long-term partnerships with scalable impact, while working in the field to strengthen healthcare systems, advocate, research and provide care delivery or education as a way of sustainably improving the health of children worldwide.

Anesth, CV Med, Crit-Care, ER Med, Heme-Onc, Infect Dis, Medicine, Nutr, Palliative, Ped Surg, Peds

+1 617-919-6438

https://vfapp.org/f9f8

Bridge to Health Medical and Dental

Seeks to provide health care to those who need it most based on a philosophy of partnership, education, and community development. Strives to bring solutions to global health issues in underserved communities through clinical outreach and medical and dental training.

Dent-OMFS, General, Infect Dis, MF Med, OB-GYN, Ophth-Opt, Ortho, Pub Health, Radiol

https://vfapp.org/bb2c

BroadReach

Collaborates with governments, multinational health organizations, donors, and private sector companies to affect healthcare reform and solve the world's biggest health challenges.

Logist-Op

+27 21 514 8300

https://vfapp.org/7812

Burn Care International

Seeks to improve the lives of burn survivors around the world through effective rehabilitation.

Derm, Nutr, Psych, Surg

+1 843-662-6717

https://vfapp.org/78d1

Canadian Network for International Surgery, The

Aims to improve maternal health, increase safety, and build local capacity in low-income countries by creating and providing surgical and midwifery courses, training domestically, and transferring skills.

Logist-Op, Surg

+1 877-217-8856

https://vfapp.org/86ff

Cancer Care Ethiopia

Aims to provide a quality and standardized system of cancer care in Ethiopia for poor cancer patients by helping them get appropriate treatment, making their lives more comfortable, improving prevention, early detection, treatment, and palliative care, and raising awareness in society.

Heme-Onc, Nutr, Palliative

+251 93 822 2222

https://vfapp.org/ad6f

CARE

Works around the globe to save lives, defeat poverty, and achieve social justice.

ER Med, General

+1 800-422-7385

https://vfapp.org/7232

Carter Center, The

Seeks to prevent and resolve conflicts, enhance freedom and democracy, and improve health, while remaining committed to human rights and the alleviation of human suffering.

Infect Dis, MF Med, Ophth-Opt

+1 800-550-3560

https://vfapp.org/6556

Catherine Hamlin Fistula Foundation

Works to eradicate obstetric fistula by holistically treating women with obstetric fistulas in Ethiopia, as the global reference organization and leader in this effort.

MF Med, OB-GYN, Rehab, Surg

+61 2 9440 7001

https://vfapp.org/ab72

Catholic Organization for Relief & Development Aid (CORDAID)

Provides humanitarian assistance and creates opportunities to improve security, healthcare, education, and inclusive economic growth in fragile and conflict-affected areas.

ER Med, Infect Dis, MF Med, OB-GYN, Peds, Psych

+31 70 313 6300

https://vfapp.org/8ae5

Centre for Global Mental Health

Closes the care gap and reduces human rights abuses experienced by people living with mental, neurological, and substance use conditions, particularly in low-resource settings.

Neuro, OB-GYN, Palliative, Peds, Psych

https://vfapp.org/a96d

Chain of Hope

Provides lifesaving heart operations for children around the world and supports the development of cardiac services in numerous developing and war-torn countries.

Anesth, CT Surg, CV Med, Crit-Care, Ped Surg, Peds, Pulm-Critic, Surg
📞 +44 20 7351 1978
🌐 https://vfapp.org/1b1b

CharityVision International
Focuses on restoring curable sight impairment worldwide by empowering local physicians and creating sustainable solutions.
Logist-Op, Ophth-Opt, Surg
📞 +1 435-200-4910
🌐 https://vfapp.org/6231

ChildFund Australia
Works to reduce poverty for children in many of the world's most disadvantaged communities.
ER Med, General, Peds
📞 +1 800023600
🌐 https://vfapp.org/13df

Children's Surgery International
Provides free medical and surgical services to children in need around the world, and instruction and training to local surgeons and other medical providers such as doctors, anesthesiologists, nurses, and technicians.
Anesth, Dent-OMFS, Ortho, Ped Surg, Peds, Plast, Surg
📞 +1 612-746-4082
🌐 https://vfapp.org/26d3

Christian Aid Ministries
Strives to be a trustworthy and efficient channel for Amish, Mennonite, and other conservative Anabaptist groups and individuals to minister to physical and spiritual needs around the world.
CT Surg, ER Med, Logist-Op, Ortho, Pub Health
📞 +1 330-893-2428
🌐 https://vfapp.org/7b33

Christian Blind Mission (CBM)
Aims to improve the quality of life of persons with disabilities in the poorest countries, addressing poverty as a cause, and a consequence, of disability, and working in partnership to create a society for all.
ENT, General, Infect Dis, OB-GYN, Ophth-Opt, Ortho, Peds, Psych, Rehab, Surg
📞 +49 6251 131131
🌐 https://vfapp.org/3824

Christian Health Service Corps
Brings Christian doctors, health professionals, and health educators who are committed to serving the poor to places that have little or no access to healthcare.
Anesth, Dent-OMFS, General, Medicine, Peds, Surg
📞 +1 903-962-4000
🌐 https://vfapp.org/da57

Clinton Health Access Initiative (CHAI)
Aims to save lives and reduce the burden of disease in low- and middle-income countries. Works with partners to strengthen the capabilities of governments and the private sector to create and sustain high-quality health systems.
General, Heme-Onc, Infect Dis, Logist-Op, MF Med, Medicine, Neonat, Nutr, OB-GYN, Path, Peds, Rad-Onc
📞 +1 617-774-0110
🌐 https://vfapp.org/9ed7

Columbia University: Columbia Office of Global Surgery (COGS)
Helps to increase access to safe and affordable surgical care, as a means to reduce health disparities and the global burden of disease.
Anesth, CT Surg, Crit-Care, Dent-OMFS, ENT, ER Med, Infect Dis, MF Med, Neurosurg, OB-GYN, Ophth-Opt, Ortho, Ped Surg, Plast, Plast, Pub Health, Surg, Urol
🌐 https://vfapp.org/4349

Columbia University: Global Mental Health Programs
Pioneers research initiatives, promotes mental health, and aims to reduce the burden of mental illness worldwide.
Psych
📞 +1 646-774-5308
🌐 https://vfapp.org/c5cd

Comitato Collaborazione Medica (CCM)
Supports development processes that safeguard and promote the right to health with a global approach, working on health needs and influencing socio-economic factors, identifying poverty as the main cause for the lack of health.
All-Immu, General, Infect Dis, MF Med, OB-GYN
📞 +39 011 660 2793
🌐 https://vfapp.org/4272

Concern Worldwide
Seeks to permanently transform the lives of people living in extreme poverty, tackling its root causes, and building resilience.
Logist-Op, MF Med, Nutr, OB-GYN
📞 +353 1 417 7700
🌐 https://vfapp.org/77e9

Core Group
Aims to improve and expand community health practices for underserved populations, especially women and children, through collaborative action and learning.
General, Infect Dis, MF Med, Medicine, OB-GYN, Peds, Pub Health
📞 +1 202-380-3400
🌐 https://vfapp.org/9de3

CURE
Operates charitable hospitals and programs in underserved countries worldwide where patients receive surgical treatment, based in Christian ministry.
Anesth, Neurosurg, Ortho, Ped Surg, Peds, Rehab, Surg
📞 +1 616-512-3105
🌐 https://vfapp.org/aa16

CureCervicalCancer
Focuses on the early detection and prevention of cervical cancer around the globe for the women who need it most.
Heme-Onc, OB-GYN
📞 +1 310-601-3002
🌐 https://vfapp.org/ace1

D-tree Digital Global Health
Demonstrates and advocates for the potential of digital technology to transform health systems and improve health and wellbeing for all.
Logist-Op, MF Med, OB-GYN, Peds, Pub Health

📞 +1 978-238-9122
🌐 https://vfapp.org/1f79

Dentaid
Seeks to treat, equip, train, and educate people in need of dental care.

Dent-OMFS
📞 +44 1794 324249
🌐 https://vfapp.org/a183

Direct Relief
Improves the health and lives of people affected by poverty or emergency situations by mobilizing and providing essential medical resources needed for their care.

ER Med, Logist-Op
📞 +1 805-964-4767
🌐 https://vfapp.org/58e5

Doctors with Africa (CUAMM)
Advocates for the universal right to health and promotes the values of international solidarity, justice, and peace. Works to protect and improve the well-being and health of vulnerable communities in Africa with a long-term development perspective.

ER Med, Infect Dis, MF Med, Neonat, OB-GYN, Peds
🌐 https://vfapp.org/d2fb

Doctors Without Borders/Médecins Sans Frontières (MSF)
Responds to emergencies and provides lifesaving medical care where needed most, including during disasters, conflicts, and epidemics.

Anesth, Crit-Care, ER Med, General, Infect Dis, Nutr, OB-GYN, Ped Surg, Peds, Psych, Pub Health, Surg
📞 +1 212-679-6800
🌐 https://vfapp.org/f363

Drugs for Neglected Diseases Initiative
Develops lifesaving medicines for people with neglected diseases around the world, having developed eight treatments for five deadly diseases and saving millions of lives since 2003.

Infect Dis, Pub Health
📞 +41 22 906 92 30
🌐 https://vfapp.org/969c

Duke University: Global Health Institute
Sparks innovation in global health research and education, and brings together knowledge and resources to address the most important global health issues of our time.

All-Immu, Infect Dis, MF Med, OB-GYN, Pub Health
📞 +1 919-681-7760
🌐 https://vfapp.org/c4cd

Elton John Aids Foundation
Seeks to address and overcome the stigma, discrimination, and neglect that prevents ending AIDS by funding local experts to challenge discrimination, prevent infections, and provide treatment.

Infect Dis, Pub Health
📞 +1 212-219-0670
🌐 https://vfapp.org/9d31

Emory University School of Medicine
Aims to provide residents/fellows from clinical departments with knowledge and practical experience in global health by building ongoing collaborations between Emory University and academic instituions abroad.

Anesth, CV Med, General, Infect Dis, Pulm-Critic, Rheum, Surg
📞 +1 404-778-7777
🌐 https://vfapp.org/a6f7

Emory University School of Medicine: Global Surgery Program
A leading institution with the highest standards in education, biomedical research, and patient care.

Anesth, Dent-OMFS, ER Med, Pub Health, Surg, Urol
📞 +1 404-727-5660
🌐 https://vfapp.org/2b26

END Fund, The
Aims to control and eliminate the most prevalent neglected diseases among the world's poorest and most vulnerable people.

Infect Dis
📞 +1 646-690-9775
🌐 https://vfapp.org/2614

EngenderHealth
Works to implement high-quality, gender-equitable programs that advance sexual and reproductive health and rights.

General, MF Med, OB-GYN, Peds
📞 +1 202-902-2000
🌐 https://vfapp.org/1cb2

eRanger
Provides sustainable solutions to transportation and medical provision such as ambulances and mobile clinics in developing countries.

ER Med, General, Logist-Op
📞 +27 40 654 3207
🌐 https://vfapp.org/4c18

Ethiopia Act
Aims to help those who suffer from diseases such as HIV/AIDS, cervical cancer, and tuberculosis. Based in Christian ministry, also aims to see gospel-centered churches planted that serve people in need.

General, Infect Dis, Medicine, OB-GYN
📞 +251 11 844 8841
🌐 https://vfapp.org/945a

Ethiopia Healthcare Network
Provides healthcare to women and children in Ethiopia without access to services.

General, Infect Dis, MF Med, OB-GYN, Peds
📞 +251 11 828 4122
🌐 https://vfapp.org/b892

Ethiopia Medical Project (EMP)
Supports Buccama Health Centre in rural Ethiopia and focuses on preventing, raising awareness of, and treating podoconiosis and uterine prolapse.

Derm, General, OB-GYN, Ortho, Pod, Rehab
🌐 https://vfapp.org/d9a1

Ethiopia Mission Trip
Aspires to create sustainable change that brings hope, health, opportunity, progress, and education.

General, Ophth-Opt
+1 626-794-3953
https://vfapp.org/a7ba

Ethiopia Urban Health Extension Program (USAID)
Aims to support at scale the implementation and monitoring of the Government of Ethiopia's UHEP (GoE/UHEP), and to improve access to and demand for health services.
Infect Dis, MF Med, Pub Health
+1 617-482-9485
https://vfapp.org/2f2a

Ethiopiaid
Aims to transform lives in Ethiopia and break the cycle of poverty by enabling the poorest and most vulnerable and their communities to live with dignity, to build resilience, and achieve real and sustainable solutions to the challenges they face.
ER Med, MF Med, Nutr, OB-GYN, Ortho, Palliative, Peds, Pub Health
+44 1225 476385
https://vfapp.org/5e59

Ethiopian Children's Fund, The
Works to uplift children and adolescents in extreme poverty, and to do so sustainably through education, nutrition, and primary healthcare.
General, Peds
+251 91 146 5239
https://vfapp.org/4ea5

Evidence Project, The
Improves family-planning policies, programs, and practices through the strategic generation, translation, and use of evidence.
General, MF Med
+1 202-237-9400
https://vfapp.org/f9e7

Eye Foundation of America
Works toward a world without childhood blindness.
Ophth-Opt
+1 304-599-0705
https://vfapp.org/a7eb

Eyes for Africa
Works to make a difference by treating preventable blindness and restoring sight, resulting in improved lives and livelihoods.
Anesth, Ophth-Opt
+61 412 254 417
https://vfapp.org/9223

Facing Africa – NOMA
Helps Ethiopian children with noma (cancrum oris) and other severe facial deformities to get surgical treatment and start new lives.
Anesth, Dent-OMFS, Ped Surg, Plast, Surg
+44 1380 827038
https://vfapp.org/82d7

Fistula Foundation
Aims to engage the support of people worldwide who are eager to see the day when no woman suffers from obstetric fistula. Raises and directs funds to doctors and hospitals providing life-transforming surgery to women in need.
OB-GYN
+1 408-249-9596
https://vfapp.org/e958

Flying Doctors of America
Brings together teams of physicians, dentists, nurses, and other healthcare professionals to care for people who would not receive medical care.
Dent-OMFS, GI, General, Surg
+1 208-952-4684
https://vfapp.org/58b6

Foundation For International Education In Neurological Surgery (FIENS), The
Provides hands-on training and education to neurosurgeons around the world.
Neuro, Neurosurg, Surg
https://vfapp.org/bab8

Foundation for Special Surgery
Provides high-quality, complex surgical care by increasing surgical expertise in Africa through the participation of surgeons across various specialties to provide premium care and skills transfer/education to benefit patients.
Anesth, CT Surg, ENT, Endo, Neurosurg, Plast, Surg, Urol
+1 301-787-8914
https://vfapp.org/53db

Fracarita International
Provides support and services in the fields of mental healthcare, care for people with a disability, and education.
Psych, Rehab
https://vfapp.org/8d3c

Fred Hollows Foundation, The
Works toward a world in which no person is needlessly blind or vision impaired.
Ophth-Opt, Pub Health, Surg
+1 646-374-0445
https://vfapp.org/73e5

Free to Smile Foundation
Serves impoverished and underserved children suffering from cleft lip/palate deformities around the world.
Anesth, Dent-OMFS, ENT, Ped Surg, Plast
+1 614-307-7567
https://vfapp.org/218b

Friends of UNFPA
Promotes the health, dignity, and rights of women and girls around the world by supporting the lifesaving work of UNFPA, the United Nations reproductive health and rights agency, through education, advocacy, and fundraising.
MF Med, OB-GYN
+1 646-649-9100
https://vfapp.org/2a3a

Gift of Life International
Provides lifesaving cardiac treatment to children in developing countries while developing sustainable pediatric cardiac programs by implementing screening, surgical, and training missions.
Anesth, CT Surg, CV Med, Crit-Care, Ped Surg, Peds, Pulm-Critic
+1 855-734-3278
https://vfapp.org/f2f9

Global Alliance to Prevent Prematurity and Stillbirth (GAPPS)
Seeks to improve birth outcomes worldwide by reducing the burden of premature birth and stillbirth.
All-Immu, Infect Dis, MF Med, Neonat, Neonat, OB-GYN
+1 206-413-7954
https://vfapp.org/3f74

Global Clubfoot Initiative (GCI)
Promotes and resources the treatment of children with clubfoot in developing countries using the Ponseti technique.
Ortho, Ped Surg
https://vfapp.org/f229

Global ENT Outreach
Saves lives and prevents avoidable deafness from ear disease for those affected by poverty and lack of care so they can reach their full human potential.
ENT, Surg
+1 360-678-1383
https://vfapp.org/ef5c

Global Eye Mission
Strives to bring hope and healing to the lives of those living in underserved regions of the world by providing high-quality eye care to help the blind see, and improving the quality of life for individuals and entire communities.
Ophth-Opt, Surg
+1 952-484-9710
https://vfapp.org/197e

Global Medical Foundation Australia
Provides medical, surgical, dental, and educational welfare to underprivileged communities and gives them access to the basics that are often take for granted.
Dent-OMFS, ER Med, General, OB-GYN, Ortho, Surg
https://vfapp.org/fa56

Global Medical Missions Alliance
Brings and promotes Christian-centered missional life to the body of healthcare professionals and its partners.
Dent-OMFS, ER Med, Pub Health, Rehab, Surg
+1 714-444-3032
https://vfapp.org/29c7

Global NeuroCare
Aims to improve neurological care in developing countries by working with local partners to improve patient care, train physicians, and advance medical research.
Neuro, Neurosurg
https://vfapp.org/d76c

Global Oncology (GO)
Brings the best in cancer care to underserved patients around the world and collaborates across geographic, professional, and academic borders to improve cancer care, research, and education.
Heme-Onc, Path, Rad-Onc
https://vfapp.org/fcb8

Global Outreach Doctors
Provides global health medical services in developing countries affected by famine, infant mortality, and chronic health issues.
All-Immu, Anesth, ER Med, General, Infect Dis, MF Med, Peds, Surg
+1 505-473-9333
https://vfapp.org/8514

GOAL
Works with the most vulnerable communities to help them respond to and recover from humanitarian crises, and to assist them in building transcendent solutions to mitigate poverty and vulnerability.
ER Med, General, Pub Health
+353 1 280 9779
https://vfapp.org/bbea

Grace for Impact
Provides high-quality healthcare and education to the rural poor, where it is needed most, in Sub-Saharan Africa and Southeast Asia.
Dent-OMFS, General, Ophth-Opt
+1 214-646-8055
https://vfapp.org/3ed1

Grassroot Soccer
Leverages the power of soccer to educate, inspire, and mobilize at risk youth in developing countries to overcome their greatest health challenges, live healthier more productive lives, and be agents for change in their communities.
Infect Dis
+1 603-277-9685
https://vfapp.org/3521

Hamlin Fistula Ethiopia
Focuses on free treatment and prevention of childbirth injuries such as obstetric fistulas in the main hospital in Addis and the five outreach centers (Bahir Dar, Mekele, Yirgalem, Harar, and Mutu). Also supports prevention through training at Hamlin College of Midwives and rehabilitation.
MF Med, OB-GYN, Path, Surg
+251 11 371 6544
https://vfapp.org/3e56

Healing the Children
Helps underserved children around the world secure the medical care they need to lead more fulfilling lives.
Anesth, Dent-OMFS, ENT, General, Medicine, Ophth-Opt, Ped Surg, Peds, Plast, Surg
+1 509-327-4281
https://vfapp.org/d4ee

Healing the Children Northeast
Helps underserved children around the world secure the medical care they need to lead more fulfilling lives.
Anesth, Dent-OMFS, ENT, General, Medicine, Ophth-Opt, Ped Surg, Peds, Plast
+1 860-355-1828
https://vfapp.org/16ba

Health Equity Initiative
Aims to build and sustain a global community that engages across sectors and disciplines to advance health equity.
Pub Health
https://vfapp.org/e2e2

Health Poverty Action
Works in partnership with people around the world who are pursuing change in their own communities to demand health

justice and challenge power imbalances.
ER Med, General, Infect Dis, Psych, Pub Health
+44 20 7840 3777
https://vfapp.org/ee58

Health[e] Foundation
Supports health professionals and community workers in the world's most vulnerable societies to ensure quality health for everyone in need by providing digital education and information, using e-learning and m-health.
Logist-Op
https://vfapp.org/b73b

Healthy Developments
Provides Germany-supported health and social protection programs around the globe in a collaborative knowledge management process.
All-Immu, General, Infect Dis, Logist-Op, MF Med
https://vfapp.org/dc31

HelpAge International
Works to ensure that people everywhere understand how much older people contribute to society and that they must enjoy their right to healthcare, social services, economic, and physical security.
General, Geri, Infect Dis, Medicine, Pub Health
+44 20 7148 7623
https://vfapp.org/5d91

Himalayan Cataract Project
Works to cure needless blindness with the highest quality care at the lowest cost.
Anesth, Ophth-Opt, Surg
+1 888-287-8530
https://vfapp.org/3b3d

Hope and Healing International
Gives hope and healing to children and families trapped by poverty and disability.
General, Nutr, Ophth-Opt, Peds, Rehab
+1 905-640-6464
https://vfapp.org/c638

Hope Walks
Frees children, families, and communities from the burden of clubfoot, inspired by the Christian faith.
Ortho, Ped Surg, Peds, Rehab
+1 717-502-4400
https://vfapp.org/f6d4

Horn of Africa Neonatal Development Services (HANDS)
Focuses on saving infants' lives in Ethiopia by facilitating the implementation of skilled medical care by local medical professionals.
MF Med, Neonat, Peds
https://vfapp.org/8f47

Humanity & Inclusion
Works alongside people with disabilities and vulnerable populations, taking action and bearing witness in order to respond to their essential needs, improve their living conditions and health, and promote respect for their dignity and fundamental rights.
General, Infect Dis, MF Med, Medicine, Ortho, Peds, Psych, Pub Health, Rehab
+1 301-891-2138
https://vfapp.org/16b7

Hunger Project, The
Aims to end hunger and poverty by pioneering sustainable, grassroots, women-centered strategies and advocating for their widespread adoption in countries throughout the world.
Infect Dis, Nutr, OB-GYN, Pub Health
+1 212-251-9100
https://vfapp.org/3a49

Hunt Foundation, The
Organizes teams of medical professionals to travel to countries around the globe with the goal of healing individuals in need, while educating, training, and demonstrating proper medical and surgical techniques.
Neurosurg, Ortho, Surg
+1 310-423-9834
https://vfapp.org/cee2

ICAP at Columbia University
Serves as global leader in supporting the scale-up of multidisciplinary HIV/AIDS prevention, care, and treatment programs based on a family-focused approach.
General, Infect Dis, MF Med, Medicine, OB-GYN, Pub Health
+1 212-342-0505
https://vfapp.org/a8ef

Institute for Healthcare Improvement (IHI)
Aims to improve health and healthcare worldwide by working with health professionals to strengthen systems.
Crit-Care, Infect Dis, MF Med, Medicine, Neonat, OB-GYN, Pub Health
+1 617-301-4800
https://vfapp.org/ecae

International Agency for the Prevention of Blindness (IAPB), The
Leads international efforts in blindness-prevention activities, works toward a world where no one is needlessly visually impaired, and ensures that everyone has access to the best possible standard of eye health.
Infect Dis, Ophth-Opt, Pub Health
https://vfapp.org/87a2

International Children's Heart Foundation
Provides free surgical care, medical training, and technology to save the lives of children with congenital heart disease in developing countries.
Anesth, CT Surg, CV Med, Crit-Care, Ped Surg, Peds, Pulm-Critic
+1 901-869-4243
https://vfapp.org/86c1

International Children's Heart Fund
Aims to promote the international growth and quality of cardiac surgery, particularly in children and young adults.
CT Surg, Ped Surg
https://vfapp.org/33fb

International Council of Ophthalmology
Works with ophthalmologic societies and others to enhance ophthalmic education and improve access to the highest quality eye care in order to preserve and restore vision for the people of the world.
Ophth-Opt
https://vfapp.org/ffd2

International Eye Foundation (IEF)
Eliminates preventable and treatable blindness by making quality sustainable eye care services accessible and affordable worldwide.

Infect Dis, Logist-Op, Ophth-Opt

+1 240-290-0263

https://vfapp.org/e839

International Federation of Gynecology and Obstetrics (FIGO)
Implements global projects on specific women's health issues.

MF Med, Medicine, Neonat, OB-GYN, Surg, Urol

+44 20 7928 1166

https://vfapp.org/c4b4

International Federation of Red Cross and Red Crescent Societies (IFRC)
Coordinates and directs international assistance following natural and man-made disasters in nonconflict situations through the world's largest humanitarian and development network. Provides disaster-preparedness programs, healthcare activities, and promotes humanitarian values.

ER Med, General, Infect Dis, Nutr

+1 212-338-0161

https://vfapp.org/b4ee

International Learning Movement (ILM UK)
Supports some of the world's poorest people in developing countries with core projects in education, safe drinking water, and healthcare.

General, Ophth-Opt

+44 1254 265451

https://vfapp.org/b974

International Medical and Surgical Aid (IMSA)
Aims to save lives and alleviate suffering through education, healthcare, surgical camps, and quality medical programs.

Anesth, General, Ped Surg, Surg

+44 7598 088806

https://vfapp.org/2561

International Medical Corps
Seeks to improve quality of life through health interventions and related activities that strengthen underserved communities worldwide, with the flexibility to respond rapidly to emergencies and offer medical services and training to people at the highest risk.

ER Med, General, Infect Dis, Nutr, OB-GYN, Peds, Pub Health, Surg

+1 310-826-7800

https://vfapp.org/a8a5

International Organization for Migration (IOM) – The UN Migration Agency
Promotes evidence-informed policies and holistic, preventive, and curative health programs that are beneficial, accessible, and equitable for vulnerable migrants.

General, Infect Dis, OB-GYN

+27 12 342 2789

https://vfapp.org/621a

International Pediatric Nephrology Association (IPNA)
Leads the global efforts to successfully address the care for all children with kidney disease through advocacy, education, and training.

Medicine, Nephro, Peds

https://vfapp.org/b59d

International Planned Parenthood Federation (IPPF)
Leads a locally owned, globally connected civil society movement that provides and enables services and champions sexual and reproductive health and rights for all, especially the underserved.

Infect Dis, MF Med, OB-GYN

+44 20 7939 8200

https://vfapp.org/dc97

International Rescue Committee (IRC)
Responds to the world's worst humanitarian crises and helps people whose lives and livelihoods are shattered by conflict and disaster to survive, recover, and gain control of their future.

ER Med, General, Infect Dis, MF Med, Peds

+1 212-551-3000

https://vfapp.org/5d24

International Trachoma Initiative (iTi)
Works toward a world free from trachoma, a preventable cause of blindness, and provides comprehensive support to national ministries of health and governmental and nongovernmental organizations to implement a comprehensive approach to fight trachoma.

Infect Dis, Ophth-Opt

+1 404-371-0466

https://vfapp.org/3278

InterSurgeon
Fosters collaborative partnerships in the field of global surgery that will advance clinical care, teaching, training, research, and the provision and maintenance of medical equipment.

ENT, Neurosurg, Ortho, Ped Surg, Plast, Surg, Urol

https://vfapp.org/6f8a

IntraHealth International
Improves the performance of health workers and strengthens the systems in which they work.

CV Med, Endo, General, Infect Dis, MF Med, Neonat, Nutr, OB-GYN

+1 919-313-3554

https://vfapp.org/ddc8

Ipas
Focuses efforts on women and girls who want contraception or abortion, and builds programs around their needs and how best to support them.

OB-GYN

https://vfapp.org/8e39

Jackson Hill Taye Foundation
Provides healthcare services for women and children in Ethiopia using state-of-the-art innovations, techniques, and equipment.

General, MF Med, OB-GYN, Peds

+1 808-895-8586

https://vfapp.org/c289

Jhpiego
Creates and delivers transformative healthcare solutions that save

lives in partnership with national governments, health experts, and local communities.

General, Infect Dis, OB-GYN, Surg

+1 410-537-1800

https://vfapp.org/45b8

John Snow, Inc. (JSI)

Aims to improve the health and well-being of underserved and vulnerable people and communities throughout the world.

General, Infect Dis, Logist-Op, MF Med, OB-GYN, Peds, Psych, Pub Health

+1 617-482-9485

https://vfapp.org/ba78

Johns Hopkins Center for Communication Programs

Believes in the power of communication to save lives, by empowering people to adopt healthy behaviors for themselves, their families, and their communities.

General, Infect Dis, Logist-Op, OB-GYN, Pub Health

+1 410-659-6300

https://vfapp.org/1bf9

Johns Hopkins Center for Global Health

Facilitates and focuses the extensive expertise and resources of the Johns Hopkins institutions together with global collaborators to effectively address and ameliorate the world's most pressing health issues.

General, Genetics, Logist-Op, MF Med, Peds, Psych, Pub Health, Pulm-Critic

+1 410-502-9872

https://vfapp.org/54ce

Joint United Nations Programme on HIV/AIDS (UNAIDS)

Aims to place people living with HIV and people affected by the virus at the decision-making table and at the center of designing, delivering, and monitoring the AIDS response.

Infect Dis

+41 22 791 36 66

https://vfapp.org/464a

Kids Care Everywhere

Seeks to empower physicians in under-resourced environments with multimedia, state-of-the-art medical software, and to inspire young professionals to become future global healthcare leaders.

Logist-Op, Ped Surg, Peds

https://vfapp.org/bc23

Kind Cuts for Kids

Aims to improve medical services for children in developing countries through education, demonstration, and skill transfer to local healthcare professionals.

Anesth, Medicine, Ped Surg, Surg

+61 3 9364 2930

https://vfapp.org/e3d7

Kletjian Foundation

Works toward a world in which all people have access to safe, sustainable, and high-quality medical care, building collaborative networks and supporting entrepreneurial leaders that promote global health equity.

CT Surg, ENT, General, Ortho, Surg

https://vfapp.org/12c2

Last Mile Health

Links community health workers with frontline health workers—nurses, doctors, and midwives at community clinics—and supports them to bring lifesaving services to the doorsteps of people living far from care.

General, Logist-Op, OB-GYN, Pub Health

+1 617-880-6163

https://vfapp.org/37da

Lay Volunteers International Association (LVIA)

Fosters local and global change to help overcome extreme poverty, reinforce equitable and sustainable development, and enhance dialogue between Italian and African communities.

ER Med, Logist-Op, MF Med, Neonat, Nutr, OB-GYN, Peds

+39 0171 696975

https://vfapp.org/ecd4

Leprosy Mission England and Wales, The

Leads the fight against leprosy by supporting people living with leprosy today and serving future generations by working to end the transmission of the disease.

Infect Dis, Pub Health

https://vfapp.org/4c67

Leprosy Mission: Northern Ireland, The

Leads the fight against leprosy by supporting people living with leprosy today and serving future generations by working to end the transmission of the disease.

General, Infect Dis

+44 28 9262 9500

https://vfapp.org/e265

Life for a Child

Supports the provision of the best possible health care, given local circumstances, to all children and youth with diabetes in less-resourced countries, through the strengthening of existing diabetes services.

Endo, Medicine, Peds

https://vfapp.org/d712

Lifebox

Seeks to provide safer surgery and anesthesia in low-resource countries by investing in tools, training, and partnerships for safe surgery.

Anesth, Crit-Care, Surg

+44 20 3286 0402

https://vfapp.org/2d4d

Light for the World

Contributes to a world in which persons with disabilities fully exercise their rights and assists persons with disabilities living in poverty.

Ophth-Opt, Rehab

+43 1 8101300

https://vfapp.org/3ff6

Lions Clubs International

Empowers volunteers to serve their communities, meet humanitarian needs, encourage peace, and promote international understanding through Lions clubs.

Heme-Onc, Medicine, Nutr, Ophth-Opt

+1 630-571-5466

https://vfapp.org/7b12

London School of Hygiene & Tropical Medicine: International Centre for Eye Health
Works to improve eye health and eliminate avoidable visual impairment and blindness with a focus on low-income populations.
Logist-Op, Ophth-Opt, Pub Health
+44 20 7958 8316
https://vfapp.org/6f5f

Management Sciences for Health (MSH)
Works with countries and communities to save lives and improve the health of the world's poorest and most vulnerable people by building strong, resilient, sustainable health systems.
Infect Dis, Logist-Op, Pub Health
+1 617-250-9500
https://vfapp.org/6aa2

MAP International
Provides medicines and health supplies to those in need around the world so they might experience life to the fullest.
Logist-Op
+1 800-225-8550
https://vfapp.org/deed

Marie Stopes International
Provides the contraception and safe abortion services that enable women all over the world to choose their own futures.
Infect Dis, MF Med, Neonat, OB-GYN, Pub Health
+44 20 7636 6200
https://vfapp.org/9525

Massachusetts General Hospital Global Surgery Initiative
Aims to improve surgical education and access to advanced surgical care in resource-limited settings around the world by performing surgical operations as visitors, training local surgeons, and sharing medical technology through international partnerships across disciplines.
Anesth, Crit-Care, ER Med, Heme-Onc, Peds, Surg
+1 617-724-4093
https://vfapp.org/31b1

Maternity Foundation
Works to ensure safer childbirth for women and newborns everywhere through innovative mobile health solutions such as the Safe Delivery App, a mobile training tool for skilled birth attendants.
MF Med, OB-GYN, Pub Health
https://vfapp.org/ff4f

Maternity Worldwide
Works with communities and partners to identify and develop appropriate and effective ways to reduce maternal and newborn mortality and morbidity, facilitate communities to access quality skilled maternity care, and support the provision of quality skilled care.
MF Med, OB-GYN
+44 1273 234033
https://vfapp.org/822b

Maverick Collective
Aims to build a global community of strategic philanthropists and informed advocates who use their intellectual and financial resources to create change.
Infect Dis, MF Med, OB-GYN
+1 202-785-0072
https://vfapp.org/ea49

McGill University Health Centre: Centre for Global Surgery
Works to reduce the impact of injury by advancing surgical care through research and education in resource-limited settings.
ER Med, Logist-Op, Ped Surg, Surg
+1 514-934-1934
https://vfapp.org/7246

MCM General Hospital
Provides advanced medical services to Ethiopians unable to get proper medical care, inspired by the Christian faith.
Anesth, Dent-OMFS, Medicine, Neurosurg, Nutr, OB-GYN, Ophth-Opt, Ortho, Peds, Radiol, Surg
+1 918-605-0965
https://vfapp.org/6283

Médecins du Monde/Doctors of the World
Provides care, bears witness, and supports social change worldwide with innovative medical programs and evidence-based advocacy initiatives.
ER Med, General, Infect Dis, MF Med, Neonat, OB-GYN, Peds, Pub Health
+33 1 44 92 15 15
https://vfapp.org/a43d

Medical Ministry International
Provides compassionate healthcare in areas of need, inspired by the Christian faith.
CT Surg, Dent-OMFS, ENT, General, OB-GYN, Ophth-Opt, Ortho, Plast, Rehab, Surg, Urol, Vasc Surg
+1 905-545-4400
https://vfapp.org/5da6

Medical Missions Outreach
Visits developing countries to provide quality, ethical healthcare and outreach to those in need, based in Christian ministry.
Dent-OMFS, Ophth-Opt, Ortho, Surg
+1 410-391-7000
https://vfapp.org/1197

MedShare
Aims to improve the quality of life of people, communities, and the planet by sourcing and directly delivering surplus medical supplies and equipment to communities in need around the world.
Logist-Op
+1 770-323-5858
https://vfapp.org/c8bc

MicroResearch: Africa/Asia
Seeks to improve health outcomes in Africa by training, mentoring, and supporting local multidisciplinary health professional researchers.
Infect Dis, Nutr, OB-GYN, Psych
https://vfapp.org/13e7

Mission Bambini
Helps to support children living in poverty, sickness, and without education, giving them the opportunity and hope of a better life.

CT Surg, CV Med, Crit-Care, ER Med, Ped Surg, Peds
+39 02 210 0241
https://vfapp.org/dc1a

Mission Vision
Seeks to decrease blindness and other eye-related disabilities, as well as to increase academic performance and general quality of life.
Ophth-Opt
+1 724-553-3114
https://vfapp.org/83d8

Morbidity Management and Disability Prevention Project (MMPD)
Helps countries provide high-quality treatment and care for people suffering from the debilitating effects of trachoma and lymphatic filariasis, complementing other major initiatives supporting disease elimination through mass drug administration.
Heme-Onc, Infect Dis, Ophth-Opt
https://vfapp.org/387e

Mossy Foot Project, The
Works to provide mossy foot patients in Ethiopia with life-changing support through education, prevention, medical treatment, vocational training, and a message of hope.
Heme-Onc, Infect Dis, Ortho, Rehab
https://vfapp.org/2f5c

MSD for Mothers
Designs scalable solutions that help end preventable maternal deaths.
MF Med, OB-GYN, Pub Health
https://vfapp.org/9f99

Multi-Agency International Training and Support (MAITS)
Improves the lives of some of the world's poorest people living with disabilities through better access to quality health and education services and support.
Neuro, Psych, Rehab
+44 20 7258 8443
https://vfapp.org/9dcd

NCD Alliance
Unites and strengthens civil society to stimulate collaborative advocacy, action, and accountability for NCD (noncommunicable disease) prevention and control.
All-Immu, CV Med, General, Heme-Onc, Medicine, Peds, Psych
+41 22 809 18 11
https://vfapp.org/abdd

Nordic Medical Centre (NMC)
Contributes to health and well-being by providing high level care to all patients through integrated clinical practice and health education.
ER Med, General, Medicine, Surg
+251 92 910 5653
https://vfapp.org/7919

NTD Advocacy Learning Action (NALA)
Breaks the poverty cycle by eradicating neglected tropical diseases (NTDs) and other diseases of poverty.
Infect Dis, Pub Health
https://vfapp.org/be81

NuVasive Spine Foundation (NSF)
Partners with leading spine surgeons, nonprofits, and in-country medical professionals/facilities to bring life-changing spine surgery to under-resourced communities around the world.
Logist-Op, Ortho, Ped Surg, Rehab, Surg
+1 800-455-1476
https://vfapp.org/6ccc

Operation Fistula
Exists to end obstetric fistula by building models of care that serve every woman, everywhere.
MF Med, OB-GYN, Surg
+1 512-687-3479
https://vfapp.org/ce8e

Operation Smile
Treats patients with cleft lip and cleft palate, and creates solutions that deliver safe surgery to people where it's needed most.
Anesth, Dent-OMFS, ENT, Ped Surg, Plast
+1 757-321-7645
https://vfapp.org/5c29

Options
Believes in a world where women and children can access the high-quality health services they need, without financial burden.
Logist-Op, MF Med, Neonat, OB-GYN
+44 20 7430 1900
https://vfapp.org/3a48

Optometry Giving Sight
Delivers eye exams and low or no-cost glasses, provides training for local eye care professionals, and establishes optometry schools, vision centers and optical labs.
Ophth-Opt
+1 303-526-0430
https://vfapp.org/33ea

Orbis International
Works to prevent and treat blindness through hands-on training and improved access to quality eye care.
Anesth, Ophth-Opt, Surg
+1 646-674-5500
https://vfapp.org/f2b2

Oxford University Global Surgery Group (OUGSG)
Aims to contribute to the provision of high-quality surgical care globally, particularly in low- and middle-income countries (LMICs) while bringing together students, researchers, and clinicians with an interest in global surgery, anaesthesia, and obstetrics and gynecology.
Anesth, MF Med, OB-GYN, Ortho, Surg
+44 1865 737543
https://vfapp.org/c624

Pact
Works on the ground to improve the lives of those who are challenged by poverty and marginalization, striving for a world where all people are heard, capable, and vibrant.
Infect Dis, Logist-Op, MF Med, Pub Health
+1 202-466-5666
https://vfapp.org/9a6c

Pan-African Academy of Christian Surgeons (PAACS)
Exists to train and support African surgeons to provide excellent,

compassionate care to those most in need, inspired by the Christian faith.

Anesth, CT Surg, Neurosurg, OB-GYN, Ortho, Ped Surg, Plast, Surg

+1 847-571-9926

https://vfapp.org/85ba

PATH

Advances health equity through innovation and partnerships so people, communities, and economies can thrive.

All-Immu, CV Med, Endo, Heme-Onc, Infect Dis, MF Med, Neonat, Nutr, OB-GYN, Path, Peds, Pulm-Critic

+1 202-822-0033

https://vfapp.org/b4db

Pathfinder International

Champions sexual and reproductive health and rights worldwide, mobilizing communities most in need to break through barriers and forge paths to a healthier future.

OB-GYN

+1 617-924-7200

https://vfapp.org/a7b3

People to People

Aims to build a bridge linking the diaspora with Ethiopian institutions for effective human resource development, healthcare, and education.

Crit-Care, ENT, ER Med, Infect Dis, Logist-Op, MF Med, Medicine, Neonat, Neuro, OB-GYN, Ophth-Opt, Peds, Pub Health, Urol

+1 606-780-9591

https://vfapp.org/2431

People to People Canada (P2P)

Contributes to the fight against preventable diseases and addresses the full range of determinants of health (physical, social, economic, and cultural) affecting vulnerable communities.

Infect Dis, Psych, Pub Health

+1 416-690-8005

https://vfapp.org/67d8

Population Council

Conducts research to address critical health and development issues, helping deliver solutions to improve lives around the world.

Logist-Op, Pub Health

+1 212-339-0500

https://vfapp.org/1777

Project Concern International (PCI)

Drives innovation from the ground up to enhance health, end hunger, overcome hardship, and advance women and girls—resulting in meaningful and measurable change in people's lives.

Infect Dis, MF Med, Nutr, OB-GYN, Peds

+1 858-279-9690

https://vfapp.org/5ed7

Project HOPE

Works on the front lines of the world's health challenges, partnering hand-in-hand with communities, healthcare workers, and public health systems to ensure sustainable change.

CV Med, ER Med, Endo, General, Infect Dis, MF Med, Peds

+1 844-349-0188

https://vfapp.org/2bd7

Project Mercy

Provides community development and famine relief in Ethiopia.

MF Med, Medicine, OB-GYN, Peds, Surg

+1 260-747-2559

https://vfapp.org/23ea

Project SOAR

Conducts HIV operations research around the world to identify practical solutions to improve HIV prevention, care, and treatment services.

ER Med, General, MF Med, OB-GYN, Psych

+1 202-237-9400

https://vfapp.org/1a77

PSI – Population Services International

Dedicates efforts to improving the health of people in the developing world by focusing on challenges such as a lack of family planning, HIV/AIDS, barriers to maternal health, and the greatest threats to children under the age of 5, including malaria, diarrhea, pneumonia, and malnutrition.

Infect Dis, MF Med, OB-GYN, Peds

+1 202-785-0072

https://vfapp.org/ffe3

RAD-AID International

Improves and optimizes access to medical imaging and radiology in low-resource regions of the world.

Rad-Onc, Radiol

https://vfapp.org/537f

Rainbow Humanitarian Caretaker Foundation

Provides support for the urban poor and homeless women and children in Addis Ababa and for the rural community of Debre Musa, Ethiopia.

General, Peds

https://vfapp.org/155f

Resolute Health Outreach

Builds the capacity of Ethiopian healthcare workers through training, equipment, and outcomes research.

Anesth, ENT, Endo, Logist-Op, Neuro, Ortho, Path, Plast, Surg, Vasc Surg

https://vfapp.org/a811

RestoringVision

Empowers lives by restoring vision for millions of people in need.

Ophth-Opt

+1 209-980-7323

https://vfapp.org/e121

Rockefeller Foundation, The

Works to promote the well-being of humanity.

Logist-Op, Nutr, Pub Health

+1 212-869-8500

https://vfapp.org/5424

Rose Charities International

Aims to support communities to improve quality of life and reduce the effects of poverty through innovative, self-sustaining projects and partnerships.

ENT, ER Med, General, Infect Dis, Neonat, OB-GYN, Ophth-Opt, Ped Surg, Peds, Rehab, Urol

+1 604-733-0442

https://vfapp.org/53df

Rotary International
Provides service to others, improves lives, and advances world understanding, goodwill, and peace through its fellowship of business, professional, and community leaders.
ER Med, General, Infect Dis, MF Med, OB-GYN
https://vfapp.org/8fb5

Rotaplast International
Helps children and families worldwide by eliminating the burden of cleft lip and/or palate, burn scarring, and other deformities by sending medical teams to provide free reconstructive surgery, ancillary treatment, and training.
Anesth, Dent-OMFS, ENT, Ped Surg, Plast, Surg
+1 415-252-1111
https://vfapp.org/78b3

ROW Foundation
Works to improve the quality of training for healthcare providers, and the diagnosis and treatment available to people with epilepsy and associated psychiatric disorders in under-resourced areas of the world.
Neuro, Psych
+1 630-791-0247
https://vfapp.org/25eb

Rutgers New Jersey Medical School
Seeks to support and promote the global health efforts of the faculty, staff, and learners in the areas of education, research, and service through The Rutgers New Jersey Medical School's Office of Global Health.
Anesth, CV Med, Crit-Care, Neurosurg, OB-GYN, Psych
+1 732-445-4636
https://vfapp.org/8e67

Samaritan's Purse International Disaster Relief
Provides spiritual and physical aid to hurting people around the world, such as victims of war, poverty, natural disasters, disease, and famine, based in Christian ministry.
Anesth, CT Surg, Crit-Care, Dent-OMFS, Derm, ENT, ER Med, Endo, GI, General, Heme-Onc, Infect Dis, MF Med, Neonat, Nephro, Neuro, Neurosurg, Nutr, OB-GYN, Ophth-Opt, Ortho, Path, Ped Surg, Peds, Plast, Psych, Pulm-Critic, Radiol, Rehab, Rheum, Surg, Urol, Vasc Surg
+1 800-528-1980
https://vfapp.org/87e3

Save A Child's Heart
Provides lifesaving cardiac treatment to children in developing countries, and trains healthcare professionals from these countries to deliver quality care in their communities.
CT Surg, CV Med, Crit-Care, Ped Surg, Peds
+1 240-223-3940
https://vfapp.org/1bef

Save the Children
Gives children around the world a healthy start in life, the opportunity to learn, and protection from harm.
All-Immu, Crit-Care, ER Med, General, Infect Dis, MF Med, Medicine, Neonat, OB-GYN, Peds, Psych, Pub Health
+1 800-728-3843
https://vfapp.org/2e73

SEVA
Delivers vital eye care services to the world's most vulnerable, including women, children, and Indigenous peoples.
Ophth-Opt, Surg
+1 510-845-7382
https://vfapp.org/1e87

Sightsavers
Prevents avoidable blindness in some of the poorest parts of the world by treating debilitating eye diseases.
Infect Dis, Ophth-Opt, Surg
+1 800-707-9746
https://vfapp.org/aa52

SIGN Fracture Care International
Builds orthopedic capacity around the world and provides the injured poor access to fracture surgery by donating orthopedic education and implant systems to surgeons in developing countries.
Ortho, Rehab, Surg
+1 509-371-1107
https://vfapp.org/123d

Simavi
Strives for a world in which all women and girls are socially and economically empowered and pursue their rights to live a healthy life, free from discrimination, coercion, and violence.
MF Med, OB-GYN
+31 88 313 1500
https://vfapp.org/b57b

Simien Mountains Mobile Medical Service
Aims to deliver free, essential medical care to remote villages in Ethiopia's Simien Mountains.
General, Infect Dis, OB-GYN, Peds
+44 20 3286 8975
https://vfapp.org/3d48

Smile Train
Seeks to give every child with a cleft the opportunity for a healthy, productive life by providing free cleft repair surgery and comprehensive cleft care in their own communities.
Dent-OMFS, ENT, Plast
+1 800-932-9541
https://vfapp.org/f21d

Soddo Christian Hospital
Provides medical care based in Christian ministry to the people of southern Ethiopia, where there is limited healthcare available for a population of more than 10 million people.
Dent-OMFS, General, MF Med, Ophth-Opt, Ortho, Peds, Radiol, Surg
+1 630-510-2222
https://vfapp.org/af11

SOS Children's Villages International
Supports children through alternative care and family strengthening.
ER Med, Peds
+43 1 36824570
https://vfapp.org/aca1

Stand By Me
Helps children facing terrible circumstances and provides the care, love, and attention they need to thrive through children's homes and schools.
Peds

📞 +44 1708 442271
🌐 https://vfapp.org/a224

Stanford University School of Medicine: Weiser Lab Global Surgery
Integrates research, education, patient care and community service.
Logist-Op, Pub Health, Surg
📞 +1 650-723-4000
🌐 https://vfapp.org/9153

Sustainable Cardiovascular Health Equity Development Alliance
Fights cardiovascular disease in underserved populations globally via education, training, and increasing interventional capacity.
CV Med, Pub Health, Radiol
📞 +1 608-338-3357
🌐 https://vfapp.org/799c

Sustainable Kidney Care Foundation (SKCF)
Works to provide treatment for kidney injury where none exists, and aims to reduce mortality from treatable acute kidney injury (AKI).
Infect Dis, Medicine, Nephro
🌐 https://vfapp.org/1926

Swiss Tropical and Public Health Institute
Contributes to the improvement of the health of populations internationally, nationally, and locally through excellence in research, education, and services.
Infect Dis, Pub Health
📞 +41 61 284 81 11
🌐 https://vfapp.org/2ee4

Task Force for Global Health, The
Consists of programs and focus areas that cover a range of global health issues including neglected tropical diseases, infectious diseases, vaccines, field epidemiology, public health informatics, health workforce development, and global health ethics.
Infect Dis, Logist-Op, Medicine, Ophth-Opt, Peds
📞 +1 404-371-0466
🌐 https://vfapp.org/714c

Tearfund
Responds to crisis and partners with local churches to bring restoration to those living in poverty, inspired by the Christian faith.
ER Med, Logist-Op
📞 +44 20 3906 3906
🌐 https://vfapp.org/f6cf

THET Partnerships for Global Health
Trains and educates health workers in Africa and Asia, working in partnership with organizations and volunteers from across the UK.
General
📞 +44 20 7290 3891
🌐 https://vfapp.org/f937

Third World Eye Care Society (TWECS)
Collects old, unused eyeglasses and distributes them in conjunction with eye exams given by properly trained individuals.
Logist-Op, Ophth-Opt
📞 +1 604-874-2733
🌐 https://vfapp.org/8618

Three Roots International
Cultivates community development and economic capacity by empowering families through education, health, and income-generating activities.
General, Infect Dis, Peds
🌐 https://vfapp.org/bb33

Tomorrow Come Foundation
Helps provide a safe home, to support a healthy life, and to foster growth through education for the children in and around the New Hope Center for Children and Handicapped.
General, Rehab, Surg
📞 +1 406-272-2366
🌐 https://vfapp.org/1123

U.S. President's Malaria Initiative (PMI)
Supports low-income countries to help control and eliminate malaria through cost-effective, lifesaving malaria interventions.
Infect Dis, MF Med, OB-GYN
📞 +1 202-712-0000
🌐 https://vfapp.org/dc8b

Union for International Cancer Control (UICC)
Unites and supports the cancer community to reduce the global cancer burden, promote greater equity, and ensure that cancer control continues to be a priority in the world health and development agenda.
Heme-Onc, Pub Health
📞 +41 22 809 18 11
🌐 https://vfapp.org/88b1

United Nations Children's Fund (UNICEF)
Works in over 190 countries and territories to save children's lives, to defend their rights, and to help them fulfill their potential, from early childhood through adolescence.
All-Immu, Infect Dis, MF Med, Neonat, Nutr, OB-GYN, Ped Surg, Peds, Pub Health
🌐 https://vfapp.org/42d7

United Nations Development Programme (UNDP)
Helps countries achieve the simultaneous eradication of extreme poverty and significant reduction of inequalities and exclusion using a sustainable human development approach.
Infect Dis, Logist-Op, Pub Health
🌐 https://vfapp.org/935c

United Nations High Commissioner for Refugees (UNHCR)
Safeguards the rights and well-being of people who have been forced to flee, ensuring that everybody has the right to seek asylum and find safe refuge in another country, with the goal of seeking lasting solutions.
General, MF Med, Medicine, OB-GYN, Peds, Psych, Pub Health
🌐 https://vfapp.org/6636

United Nations Office for the Coordination of Humanitarian Affairs (OCHA)
Contributes to principled and effective humanitarian response through coordination, advocacy, policy, information management,

and humanitarian financing tools and services, by leveraging functional expertise throughout the organization.

Logist-Op

https://vfapp.org/22b8

United Nations Population Fund (UNFPA)

The United Nations sexual and reproductive health agency is focused on delivering a world where every pregnancy is wanted, every childbirth is safe, and every young person's potential is fulfilled.

Infect Dis, MF Med, Neonat, OB-GYN, Peds, Pub Health

+1 212-963-6008

https://vfapp.org/c969

United States Agency for International Development (USAID)

Promotes and demonstrates democratic values abroad and advances a free, peaceful, and prosperous world. Leads the U.S. government's international development and disaster assistance through partnerships and investments that save lives.

ER Med, Infect Dis, MF Med, OB-GYN, Peds

+1 202-712-0000

https://vfapp.org/9a99

United States President's Emergency Plan for AIDS Relief (PEPFAR)

The U.S. global HIV/AIDS response works to prevent new HIV infections and accelerate progress to control the global epidemic in more than 50 countries, by partnering with governments to support sustainable, integrated, and country-led responses to HIV/AIDS.

Infect Dis, Pub Health

https://vfapp.org/a57c

University of Illinois at Chicago: Center for Global Health

Aims to improve the health of populations around the world and reduce health disparities by collaboratively conducting trans-disciplinary research, training the next generations of global health leaders, and building the capacities of global and local partners.

Pub Health

+1 312-355-4116

https://vfapp.org/b749

University of British Columbia - Faculty of Medicine: Branch for International Surgical Care

Aims to advance sustainable improvements in the delivery of surgical care in the world's most underserved countries by building capacity within the field of surgery through the provision of care in low-resource settings.

Anesth, ER Med, Neurosurg, Surg, Urol

+1 604-875-4111

https://vfapp.org/4164

University of California, Berkeley: Bixby Center for Population, Health & Sustainability

Aims to help manage population growth, improve maternal health, and address the unmet need for family planning within a human rights framework.

OB-GYN

+1 510-642-6915

https://vfapp.org/ff2b

University of California: Global Health Institute

Mobilizes people and resources across the University of California to advance global health research, education, and collaboration.

General, OB-GYN, Pub Health

https://vfapp.org/ee7f

University of California Los Angeles: David Geffen School of Medicine Global Health Program

Catalyzes opportunities to improve health globally by engaging in multi-disciplinary and innovative education programs, research initiatives, and bilateral partnerships that provide opportunities for trainees, faculty, and staff to contribute to sustainable health initiatives and to address health inequities facing the world today.

All-Immu, Infect Dis, Logist-Op, MF Med, Medicine, Neonat, OB-GYN, Ortho, Ped Surg, Peds, Radiol

+1 310-312-0531

https://vfapp.org/f1a4

University of California San Francisco: Francis I. Proctor Foundation for Ophthalmology

Aims to prevent blindness worldwide through research and teaching focused on infectious and inflammatory eye disease.

Ophth-Opt, Pub Health

+1 415-476-1442

https://vfapp.org/cf47

University of Colorado: Global Emergency Care Initiative

Strives to sustainably improve emergency care outcomes in low- and middle-income communities worldwide by linking cutting-edge academics with excellent on-the-ground implementation.

ER Med

https://vfapp.org/417a

University of Michigan Medical School Global REACH

Aims to facilitate health research, education, and collaboration among Michigan Medicine learners and faculty with our global partners to reduce health disparities for the benefit of communities worldwide.

ENT, General, Ophth-Opt, Peds, Psych, Pub Health, Urol

+1 734-615-5692

https://vfapp.org/5f19

University of Michigan: Department of Surgery Global Health

Improves the health of patients, populations and communities through excellence in education, patient care, community service, research and technology development, and through leadership activities.

Anesth, Ortho, Surg

+1 734-936-5732

https://vfapp.org/2fd8

University of New Mexico School of Medicine: Project Echo

Seeks to improve health outcomes worldwide through the use of a technology called telementoring, a guided-practice model in which the participating clinician retains responsibility for managing the patient.

General, Infect Dis, MF Med, OB-GYN, Path, Peds

+1 505-750-3246
https://vfapp.org/6c9a

University of Pennsylvania Perelman School of Medicine Center for Global Health

Aims to improve health equity worldwide – through enhanced public health awareness and access to care, discovery and outcomes based research, and comprehensive educational programs grounded in partnership.

Heme-Onc, Infect Dis, OB-GYN

+1 215-898-0848
https://vfapp.org/cb57

University of Toledo: Global Health Program

Aims to be a transformative force in medical education, biomedical research, and healthcare delivery.

CV Med, CV Med, ER Med, Infect Dis, Medicine, Neuro, Neurosurg, OB-GYN, Ophth-Opt, Ortho, Peds, Plast, Psych, Surg

+1 419-530-2549
https://vfapp.org/71f2

University of Toronto: Global Surgery

Focuses on excellent clinical care, outstanding research productivity and the delivery of state of the art educational programs.

Surg

+1 416-978-2623
https://vfapp.org/1ad5

University of Virginia: Anesthesiology Department Global Health Initiatives

Educates and trains physicians, to help people achieve healthy productive lives, and advances knowledge in the medical sciences.

Anesth, Pub Health

+1 434-924-2283
https://vfapp.org/1b8b

University of Wisconsin-Madison: Department of Surgery

Provides comprehensive educational experiences, groundbreaking research and superb patient care.

Anesth, ENT, ER Med, Endo, Peds, Plast, Pub Health, Surg

+1 608-265-8854
https://vfapp.org/64c2

USAID: Maternal and Child Survival Program

Works to prevent child and maternal deaths.

Infect Dis, MF Med, Neonat, OB-GYN, Peds

https://vfapp.org/6fcf

USAID: Deliver Project

Builds a global supply chain to deliver lifesaving health products to people in order to enable countries to provide family planning, protect against malaria, and limit the spread of pandemic threats.

Infect Dis, Logist-Op, MF Med

+1 202-712-0000
https://vfapp.org/374e

USAID: Health Finance and Governance Project

Uses research to implement strategies to help countries develop robust governance systems, increase their domestic resources for health, manage those resources more effectively, and make wise purchasing decisions.

Logist-Op

+1 202-712-0000
https://vfapp.org/8652

USAID: Leadership, Management and Governance Project

Improves leadership, management, and governance practices to strengthen health systems and improve health for all, including vulnerable populations worldwide.

Logist-Op

https://vfapp.org/d35e

USAID: Maternal and Child Health Integrated Program

Works to improve the health of women and their families, including programs for maternal, newborn, and child health, immunization, family planning, nutrition, malaria, and HIV/AIDS.

All-Immu, General, Infect Dis, MF Med

+1 202-835-3136
https://vfapp.org/4415

Vision Aid Overseas

Enables people living in poverty to access affordable glasses and eye care.

Ophth-Opt

+44 1293 535016
https://vfapp.org/c695

Vision Outreach International

Advocates for helping the blind in underserved regions of the world and empowers the poor through sight restoration.

Ophth-Opt

+1 269-428-3300
https://vfapp.org/9721

Vital Strategies

Helps governments strengthen their public health systems to contend with the most important and difficult health challenges, while accelerating progress on the world's most pressing health problems.

CV Med, Infect Dis, Peds

+1 212-500-5720
https://vfapp.org/fe25

Vitamin Angels

Helps at-risk populations in need—specifically pregnant women, new mothers, and children under age five—to gain access to life-changing vitamins and minerals.

General, Nutr

+1 805-564-8400
https://vfapp.org/7da1

Voluntary Service Overseas (VSO)

Works with health workers, communities, and governments to improve health services and rights for women, babies, youth, people with disabilities, and prisoners.

General, MF Med, OB-GYN

+44 20 8780 7500
https://vfapp.org/213d

Watsi

Uses technology to make healthcare a reality for those who might not otherwise be able to afford it.

Pub Health, Surg

📞 +1 256-792-8747
🌐 https://vfapp.org/41a3

Wax and Gold
Develops and implements scalable education programs capable of being duplicated in facilities nationwide.
MF Med, Neonat, Peds
🌐 https://vfapp.org/dbd8

WEEMA International
Partners with rural communities in southwestern Ethiopia to provide safe water, lifesaving healthcare, quality education, and economic opportunities.
MF Med, Ophth-Opt, Peds, Pub Health
📞 +1 617-682-0101
🌐 https://vfapp.org/974c

Wings of Healing
Provides medical aid and education to African countries through medical mission programs and long-term educational partnerships.
Anesth, MF Med, Neonat, OB-GYN, Surg
🌐 https://vfapp.org/f1e4

Women and Children First
Pioneers approaches that support communities to solve problems themselves.
MF Med, Neonat, OB-GYN, Peds
📞 +44 20 7700 6309
🌐 https://vfapp.org/cdc9

Women's Refugee Commission
Seeks to improve lives by protecting the rights of women, children, and youth displaced by conflict and crisis through researching their needs, identifying solutions, and advocating for programs and policies to strengthen their resilience.
General, MF Med, Neonat, OB-GYN, Peds, Psych
📞 +1 212-551-3115
🌐 https://vfapp.org/3d8f

World Blind Union (WBU)
Represents those experiencing blindness, speaking to governments and international bodies on issues concerning visual impairments.
Ophth-Opt
🌐 https://vfapp.org/2bd3

World Health Organization, The (WHO)
The United Nations' agency for health provides leadership on global health matters, shapes the health research agenda, setting norms and standards, articulates evidence-based policy options, provides technical support and monitoring to countries, and assesses health trends.
ER Med, General, Infect Dis, Logist-Op, MF Med, OB-GYN, Peds, Psych, Pub Health
📞 +41 22 791 21 11
🌐 https://vfapp.org/c476

World Medical Relief
Facilitates the distribution of surplus medical resources where they are needed.
Logist-Op
📞 +1 313-866-5333
🌐 https://vfapp.org/72dc

World Surgical Foundation
Provides charitable surgical healthcare to the world's poor and underserved in developing nations.
Ped Surg, Surg
📞 +1 717-232-1404
🌐 https://vfapp.org/c162

World Telehealth Initiative
Provides medical expertise to the world's most vulnerable communities to build local capacity and deliver core health services through a network of volunteer healthcare professionals supported with state-of-the-art technology.
Derm, Infect Dis, MF Med, Medicine, Neuro, OB-GYN, Peds, Pulm-Critic
🌐 https://vfapp.org/fa91

World Vision International
Works with vulnerable communities around the world to overcome poverty and injustice with child-focused programs.
ER Med, General, Infect Dis, MF Med, Nutr, OB-GYN, Peds
📞 +1 626-303-8811
🌐 https://vfapp.org/2642

Worldwide Fistula Fund
Protects and restores the health and dignity of the world's most vulnerable women by preventing and treating devastating childbirth injuries.
OB-GYN
📞 +1 847-592-2438
🌐 https://vfapp.org/8813

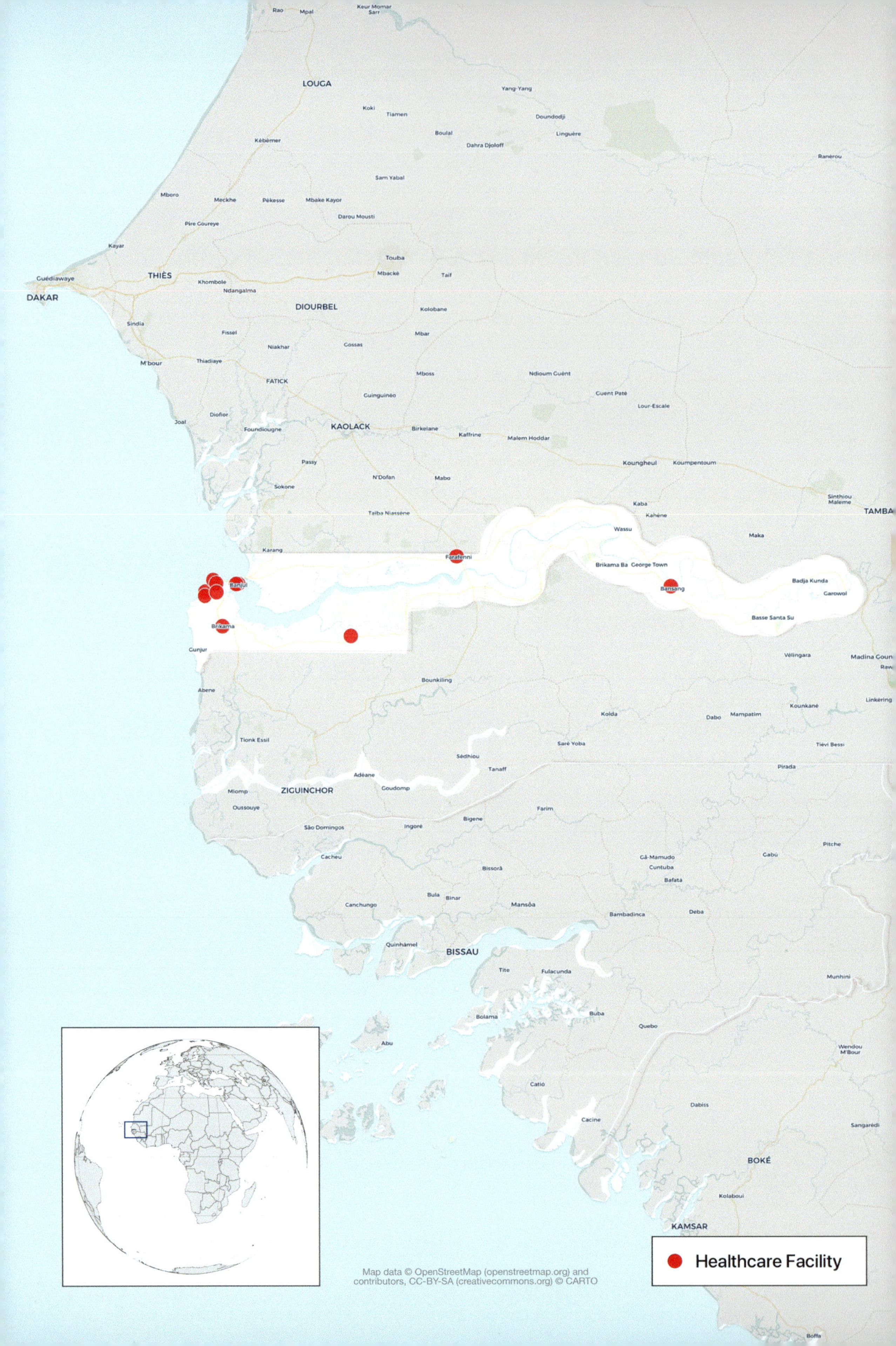
DAKAR
THIÈS
LOUGA
DIOURBEL
FATICK
KAOLACK
ZIGUINCHOR
BISSAU
BOKÉ
KAMSAR
TAMBA
Banjul
Brikama
Farafenni
Bansang
Gunjur
Basse Santa Su
Healthcare Facility
Map data © OpenStreetMap (openstreetmap.org) and contributors, CC-BY-SA (creativecommons.org) © CARTO

The Gambia

The Republic of The Gambia is a small West African country surrounded by Senegal on all sides except along its short coast. Referred to as the "smiling coast of Africa," The Gambia's long and winding shape was determined by British and French territory divisions established in the 19th century and follows the outline of the Gambia River. The majority of its more than 2.2 million person population is Muslim. It is one of the most densely populated countries in Africa, with about 57 percent of The Gambia's population concentrated in urban and peri-urban centers. The most commonly spoken language is English, in addition to several local languages representative of a variety of Gambian ethnic groups.

Since the country's independence from Britain in 1965, The Gambia has remained politically stable. Stability has not directly translated into prosperity, as nearly half of the population lives in poverty and almost 10 percent faces food insecurity. Two-thirds of the population earns their livelihood from the agricultural sector, but the overall output of the sector is low relative to the amount of arable land.

The poor socioeconomic situation in The Gambia is reflected in the health indicators of the country as well. Poverty in addition to a deteriorating infrastructure, a shortage of healthcare personnel, and an inadequate referral system contribute to a population in poor health. The top causes of death include lower respiratory infections, neonatal disorders, HIV/AIDS, tuberculosis, malaria, diarrheal diseases, maternal disorders, and increasingly, non-communicable diseases such as ischemic heart disease, stroke, liver cancer, and cirrhosis. Despite a precarious health situation in the country, some progress has been made: Life expectancy has continued to improve over the past few decades, as well as the under-five mortality rate, which is now nearly half of what it was in 1990.

2.2M
Population

$751
GDP Per Capita

62 years
Life Expectancy
↑ Improving

10.2
Doctors/100k
Physician Density

110
Beds/100k
Hospital Bed Density

597
Deaths/100k
Maternal Mortality

The Gambia

Healthcare Facilities

Africmed
AU Summit Highway, Sukuta, West Coast, The Gambia
https://vfapp.org/dd3a

Ahmadiyya Hospital
Kombo Sillah Drive, Serrekunda, The Gambia
https://vfapp.org/e7f8

Bansang Hospital Appeal
South Bank Road, Manneh Kunda, Upper River, The Gambia
https://vfapp.org/bcb6

Bijilo Medical Center/ Hospital BMC
Bijilo, Serrekunda, The Gambia
https://vfapp.org/6da4

Brikama District Hospital
Kombo Central, The Gambia
https://vfapp.org/93b2

Bwiam General Hospital
South Bank Road, Bwiam, West Coast, The Gambia
https://vfapp.org/b8c9

Edward Francis Small Teaching Hospital (EFSTH)
Marina Parade, Banjul, Banjul, The Gambia
https://vfapp.org/caeb

Farafenni Hospital
North Bank Road, Yallal Tankonjala, North Bank, The Gambia
https://vfapp.org/17f6

Medical Research Council
Garba Jahumpa Road, Serrekunda, Kanifing, The Gambia
https://vfapp.org/75e6

Psychiatric Hospital
Miniru Savage Rd, Banjul, Banjul, The Gambia
https://vfapp.org/1aa8

Serekunda General Hospital
Jimpex Road, Kanifing, Kanifing, The Gambia
https://vfapp.org/54e1

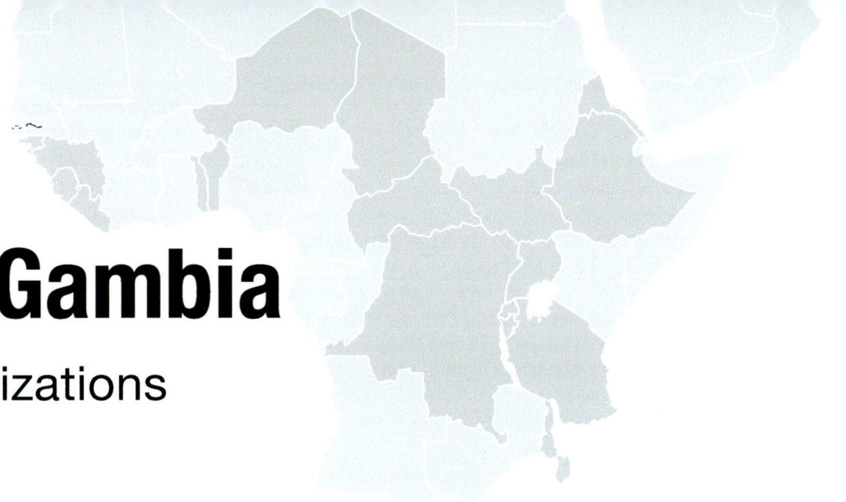

The Gambia

Nonprofit Organizations

Africa CDC
Aims to strengthen the capacity and capability of Africa's public health institutions as well as partnerships to detect and respond quickly and effectively to disease threats and outbreaks, based on data-driven interventions and programs.

Infect Dis, Logist-Op, Pub Health
📞 +251 11 551 7700
🌐 https://vfapp.org/339c

African Cultural Exchange, Inc., The
Enriches lives through humanitarian programs in culture, development, education, and healthcare.

General
📞 +1 888-748-0843
🌐 https://vfapp.org/f238

African Field Epidemiology Network (AFENET)
Strengthens field epidemiology and public health laboratory capacity to contribute effectively to addressing epidemics and other major public health problems in Africa.

All-Immu, Infect Dis, Path, Pub Health
🌐 https://vfapp.org/df2e

Against Malaria Foundation
Helps protect people from malaria. Funds anti-malaria nets, specifically long-lasting insecticidal nets (LLINs), and works with distribution partners to ensure they are used. Tracks and reports on net use and malaria case data.

Infect Dis
📞 +44 20 7371 8735
🌐 https://vfapp.org/337d

AO Alliance
Builds solutions to lessen the burden of injuries in low- and middle-income countries, while enhancing the care of the injured to reduce human suffering, disability, and poverty.

Ortho, Surg
🌐 https://vfapp.org/8cd5

Basic Foundations
Supports local projects and organizations that seek to meet the basic human needs of others in their community.

ER Med, General, Peds, Rehab,Surg
🌐 https://vfapp.org/c4be

Bijilo Medical Center/Hospital (BMC)
Provides comprehensive and affordable quality medical services to all in the Gambia.

General, OB-GYN, Path, Peds, Radiol, Rehab, Surg
📞 +220 666 5555
🌐 https://vfapp.org/776d

Bill & Melinda Gates Foundation
Focuses on global issues, from poverty to health, to education, offering the opportunity to dramatically improve the quality of life for billions of people, by building partnerships that bring together resources, expertise, and vision to identify issues, find answers, and drive change.

All-Immu, General, Infect Dis, MF Med, Neonat, OB-GYN, Pub Health
🌐 https://vfapp.org/7cf2

BroadReach
Collaborates with governments, multinational health organizations, donors, and private sector companies to affect healthcare reform and solve the world's biggest health challenges.

Logist-Op
📞 +27 21 514 8300
🌐 https://vfapp.org/7812

Center for Strategic and International Studies (CSIS) Commission on Strengthening America's Health Security
Brings together a distinguished and diverse group of high-level opinion leaders bridging security and health, with the core aim to chart a bold vision for the future of U.S. leadership in global health.

ER Med, Infect Dis, MF Med, Pub Health
📞 +1 202-887-0200
🌐 https://vfapp.org/6d7f

Chain of Hope
Provides lifesaving heart operations for children around the world and supports the development of cardiac services in numerous developing and war-torn countries.

Anesth, CT Surg, CV Med, Crit-Care, Ped Surg, Peds, Pulm-Critic, Surg
📞 +44 20 7351 1978
🌐 https://vfapp.org/1b1b

Child Aid Gambia
Alleviates poverty among children and their families living in The Gambia and Senegal, and works to improve quality of life for

children through specific projects for nutrition, education, and health.

Logist-Op, Nutr, OB-GYN, Peds

+44 1296 615989

https://vfapp.org/77a1

Developing Country NGO Delegation: Global Fund to Fight AIDS, TB & Malaria

Works to strengthen the engagement of civil society actors and organizations in developing countries to contribute toward achieving a world in which AIDS, TB, and Malaria are no longer global, public health, and human rights threats.

Infect Dis, Pub Health

+254 20 2515790

https://vfapp.org/3149

Dimbayaa Fertility for Africa

Provides infertility support through counseling, diagnosis, and treatment using artificial reproductive technology.

MF Med, OB-GYN

+220 214 5056

https://vfapp.org/d2c5

Direct Relief

Improves the health and lives of people affected by poverty or emergency situations by mobilizing and providing essential medical resources needed for their care.

ER Med, Logist-Op

+1 805-964-4767

https://vfapp.org/58e5

Gift of Life International

Provides lifesaving cardiac treatment to children in developing countries while developing sustainable pediatric cardiac programs by implementing screening, surgical, and training missions.

Anesth, CT Surg, CV Med, Crit-Care, Ped Surg, Peds, Pulm-Critic

+1 855-734-3278

https://vfapp.org/f2f9

Global Oncology (GO)

Brings the best in cancer care to underserved patients around the world and collaborates across geographic, professional, and academic borders to improve cancer care, research, and education.

Heme-Onc, Path, Rad-Onc

https://vfapp.org/fcb8

Health Equity Initiative

Aims to build and sustain a global community that engages across sectors and disciplines to advance health equity.

Pub Health

https://vfapp.org/e2e2

Heart to Heart International

Strengthens communities through improving health access, providing humanitarian development, and administering crisis relief worldwide. Engages volunteers, collaborates with partners, and deploys resources to achieve this mission.

Anesth, ER Med, General, Logist-Op, Medicine, Path, Path, Peds, Psych, Pub Health, Surg

+1 913-764-5200

https://vfapp.org/aacb

HelpMeSee

Trains local cataract specialists in Manual Small Incision Cataract Surgery (MSICS) in significant numbers, to meet the increasing demand for surgical services in the communities most impacted by cataract blindness.

Anesth, Ophth-Opt, Surg

+1 844-435-7638

https://vfapp.org/973c

Horizons Trust UK

Provides quality healthcare for those who desperately need it but have no financial means, and aims to build and manage a high-quality medical facility for those who can afford private treatment.

General, Infect Dis, MF Med

+44 1224 438094

https://vfapp.org/12ef

Humanity First

Provides aid and assistance to those in need, offering sustainable development solutions to society while providing and empowering local communities with the resources to help themselves.

ER Med, General, MF Med, Ophth-Opt

+44 20 8417 0082

https://vfapp.org/13cc

International Agency for the Prevention of Blindness (IAPB), The

Leads international efforts in blindness-prevention activities, works toward a world where no one is needlessly visually impaired, and ensures that everyone has access to the best possible standard of eye health.

Infect Dis, Ophth-Opt, Pub Health

https://vfapp.org/87a2

International Federation of Red Cross and Red Crescent Societies (IFRC)

Coordinates and directs international assistance following natural and man-made disasters in nonconflict situations through the world's largest humanitarian and development network. Provides disaster-preparedness programs, healthcare activities, and promotes humanitarian values.

ER Med, General, Infect Dis, Nutr

+1 212-338-0161

https://vfapp.org/b4ee

International Learning Movement (ILM UK)

Supports some of the world's poorest people in developing countries with core projects in education, safe drinking water, and healthcare.

General, Ophth-Opt

+44 1254 265451

https://vfapp.org/b974

International Medical Relief

Provides sustainable education, training, medical and dental care, and disaster relief and response in vulnerable communities worldwide.

Dent-OMFS, General, Infect Dis, Medicine, OB-GYN

+1 970-635-0110

https://vfapp.org/b3ed

International Mental Health Collaborating Network

Promotes and advocates for the human rights of people with mental health issues and gathers and shares the experiences and knowledge of good practices in community mental health from its membership network.

Psych

+44 1392 256286
https://vfapp.org/1551

International Organization for Migration (IOM) – The UN Migration Agency
Promotes evidence-informed policies and holistic, preventive, and curative health programs that are beneficial, accessible, and equitable for vulnerable migrants.
General, Infect Dis, OB-GYN
+27 12 342 2789
https://vfapp.org/621a

International Trachoma Initiative (iTi)
Works toward a world free from trachoma, a preventable cause of blindness, and provides comprehensive support to national ministries of health and governmental and nongovernmental organizations to implement a comprehensive approach to fight trachoma.
Infect Dis, Ophth-Opt
+1 404-371-0466
https://vfapp.org/3278

Islamic Medical Association of North America
Fosters health promotion, disease prevention, and health maintenance in communities around the world through direct patient care and health programs.
Anesth, Dent-OMFS, ER Med, General, Logist-Op, Ophth-Opt, Peds, Plast, Surg
+1 630-932-0000
https://vfapp.org/a157

John Snow, Inc. (JSI)
Aims to improve the health and well-being of underserved and vulnerable people and communities throughout the world.
General, Infect Dis, Logist-Op, MF Med, OB-GYN, Peds, Psych, Pub Health
+1 617-482-9485
https://vfapp.org/ba78

Lions Clubs International
Empowers volunteers to serve their communities, meet humanitarian needs, encourage peace, and promote international understanding through Lions clubs.
Heme-Onc, Medicine, Nutr, Ophth-Opt
+1 630-571-5466
https://vfapp.org/7b12

London School of Hygiene & Tropical Medicine
Seeks to improve health and health equity in the UK and worldwide, working in partnership to achieve excellence in public and global health research, education and translation of knowledge into policy and practice.
Infect Dis, Pub Health
+44 20 7636 8636
https://vfapp.org/349a

Management Sciences for Health (MSH)
Works with countries and communities to save lives and improve the health of the world's poorest and most vulnerable people by building strong, resilient, sustainable health systems.
Infect Dis, Logist-Op, Pub Health
+1 617-250-9500
https://vfapp.org/6aa2

MAP International
Provides medicines and health supplies to those in need around the world so they might experience life to the fullest.
Logist-Op
+1 800-225-8550
https://vfapp.org/deed

Maternal & Childhealth Advocacy International
Seeks to save and improve the lives of babies, children, and pregnant women in areas of extreme poverty by empowering and enabling in-country partners to strengthen emergency healthcare.
MF Med, Neonat, OB-GYN, Peds
+44 1445 781354
https://vfapp.org/ea67

Maternity Worldwide
Works with communities and partners to identify and develop appropriate and effective ways to reduce maternal and newborn mortality and morbidity, facilitate communities to access quality skilled maternity care, and support the provision of quality skilled care.
MF Med, OB-GYN
+44 1273 234033
https://vfapp.org/822b

Medics for Humanity
Advocates the universal right to health and promotes the values of international solidarity, justice, and peace.
Endo, General, Medicine, Nephro
+27 11 083 9713
https://vfapp.org/91f6

MedShare
Aims to improve the quality of life of people, communities, and the planet by sourcing and directly delivering surplus medical supplies and equipment to communities in need around the world.
Logist-Op
+1 770-323-5858
https://vfapp.org/c8bc

Mercy Ships
Operates hospital ships staffed by volunteers to bring hope, healing, and healthcare to underserved communities worldwide.
Anesth, Dent-OMFS, Logist-Op, Neonat, OB-GYN, Ophth-Opt, Ortho, Palliative, Plast, Psych, Surg
+1 903-939-7000
https://vfapp.org/2e99

MiracleFeet
Brings low-cost treatment to every child on the planet born with clubfoot, a leading cause of physical disability.
Ortho, Peds, Rehab
+1 919-240-5572
https://vfapp.org/bda8

OneSight
Brings eye exams and glasses to the people who lack access to vision care.
Ophth-Opt
+1 888-935-4589
https://vfapp.org/3ecc

Operation Fistula
Exists to end obstetric fistula by building models of care that serve every woman, everywhere.
MF Med, OB-GYN, Surg
+1 512-687-3479
https://vfapp.org/ce8e

Options
Believes in a world where women and children can access the high-quality health services they need, without financial burden.
Logist-Op, MF Med, Neonat, OB-GYN
+44 20 7430 1900
https://vfapp.org/3a48

PATH
Advances health equity through innovation and partnerships so people, communities, and economies can thrive.
All-Immu, CV Med, Endo, Heme-Onc, Infect Dis, MF Med, Neonat, Nutr, OB-GYN, Path, Peds, Pulm-Critic
+1 202-822-0033
https://vfapp.org/b4db

People for Change
Helps to eliminate the scarcity of access to basic healthcare, improve children's educational prospects in underdeveloped areas, and improve communities' sustainable access to wholesome food.
General, Infect Dis, Nutr, Peds
+44 7448 230967
https://vfapp.org/7499

Power Up Gambia
Hopes to improve healthcare delivery in The Gambia by providing proven, reliable, and sustainable electricity through solar energy.
General
https://vfapp.org/a671

Practical Tools Initiative
Provides or assists in the provision of education, training, healthcare projects and all the necessary support designed to enable individuals to generate a sustainable income.
General, Logist-Op, MF Med
+44 1329 829121
https://vfapp.org/16b6

Project Aid The Gambia
Provides development efforts in areas of education, health, and agriculture in targeted rural communities, including the operating of Jahaly Health Centre, a kindergarten, and support of the Ministry of Health with medical equipment and advice for rural healthcare.
General, Infect Dis, Logist-Op, MF Med, OB-GYN, Peds
+49 234 9418322
https://vfapp.org/96bd

RAD-AID International
Improves and optimizes access to medical imaging and radiology in low-resource regions of the world.
Rad-Onc, Radiol
https://vfapp.org/537f

RestoringVision
Empowers lives by restoring vision for millions of people in need.
Ophth-Opt
+1 209-980-7323
https://vfapp.org/e121

Riders for Health International
Aids in the last mile of healthcare delivery, by ensuring that healthcare reaches everyone, everywhere.
ER Med, Infect Dis, Logist-Op, Pub Health
+231 77 704 4287
https://vfapp.org/85aa

Rockefeller Foundation, The
Works to promote the well-being of humanity.
Logist-Op, Nutr, Pub Health
+1 212-869-8500
https://vfapp.org/5424

Rotary International
Provides service to others, improves lives, and advances world understanding, goodwill, and peace through its fellowship of business, professional, and community leaders.
ER Med, General, Infect Dis, MF Med, OB-GYN
https://vfapp.org/8fb5

Safe Anaesthesia Worldwide
Provides anesthesia to those in need in low-income countries to enable lifesaving surgery.
Anesth, Plast
+44 7527 506969
https://vfapp.org/134a

Save A Child's Heart
Provides lifesaving cardiac treatment to children in developing countries, and trains healthcare professionals from these countries to deliver quality care in their communities.
CT Surg, CV Med, Crit-Care, Ped Surg, Peds
+1 240-223-3940
https://vfapp.org/1bef

Sightsavers
Prevents avoidable blindness in some of the poorest parts of the world by treating debilitating eye diseases.
Infect Dis, Ophth-Opt, Surg
+1 800-707-9746
https://vfapp.org/aa52

SIGN Fracture Care International
Builds orthopedic capacity around the world and provides the injured poor access to fracture surgery by donating orthopedic education and implant systems to surgeons in developing countries.
Ortho, Rehab, Surg
+1 509-371-1107
https://vfapp.org/123d

Sound Seekers
Supports people with hearing loss by enabling access to healthcare and education.
ENT
+44 7305 433250
https://vfapp.org/ef1c

Sustainable Cardiovascular Health Equity Development Alliance
Fights cardiovascular disease in underserved populations globally via education, training, and increasing interventional

capacity.
CV Med, Pub Health, Radiol
+1 608-338-3357
https://vfapp.org/799c

Swiss Tropical and Public Health Institute
Contributes to the improvement of the health of populations internationally, nationally, and locally through excellence in research, education, and services.
Infect Dis, Pub Health
+41 61 284 81 11
https://vfapp.org/2ee4

T1International
Supports local communities by giving them the tools needed to stand up for the right to better access to insulin and diabetes supplies.
Endo, General, Medicine, Pub Health
https://vfapp.org/d7d4

Task Force for Global Health, The
Consists of programs and focus areas that cover a range of global health issues including neglected tropical diseases, infectious diseases, vaccines, field epidemiology, public health informatics, health workforce development, and global health ethics.
Infect Dis, Logist-Op, Medicine, Ophth-Opt, Peds
+1 404-371-0466
https://vfapp.org/714c

United Nations Children's Fund (UNICEF)
Works in over 190 countries and territories to save children's lives, to defend their rights, and to help them fulfill their potential, from early childhood through adolescence.
All-Immu, Infect Dis, MF Med, Neonat, Nutr, OB-GYN, Ped Surg, Peds, Pub Health
https://vfapp.org/42d7

United Nations Development Programme (UNDP)
Helps countries achieve the simultaneous eradication of extreme poverty and significant reduction of inequalities and exclusion using a sustainable human development approach.
Infect Dis, Logist-Op, Pub Health
https://vfapp.org/935c

United Nations High Commissioner for Refugees (UNHCR)
Safeguards the rights and well-being of people who have been forced to flee, ensuring that everybody has the right to seek asylum and find safe refuge in another country, with the goal of seeking lasting solutions.
General, MF Med, Medicine, OB-GYN, Peds, Psych, Pub Health
https://vfapp.org/6636

United Nations Population Fund (UNFPA)
Supports reproductive healthcare for women and youth in more than 150 countries, focusing on delivering a world where every pregnancy is wanted, every childbirth is safe, and every young person's potential is fulfilled.
Infect Dis, MF Med, Neonat, OB-GYN, Peds, Pub Health
+1 212-963-6008
https://vfapp.org/c969

USAID: Human Resources for Health 2030 (HRH2030)
Helps low- and middle-income countries develop the health workforce needed to prevent maternal and child deaths, support the goals of Family Planning 2020, control the HIV/AIDS epidemic, and protect communities from infectious diseases.
Logist-Op
+1 202-955-3300
https://vfapp.org/9ea8

Vision Care
Restores sight and helps patients get regular treatment at short-term eye camps and long-term base clinics by having doctors, missionaries, volunteers, and sponsors work together.
Ophth-Opt
+1 212-769-3056
https://vfapp.org/9d7c

Vitamin Angels
Helps at-risk populations in need—specifically pregnant women, new mothers, and children under age five—to gain access to life-changing vitamins and minerals.
General, Nutr
+1 805-564-8400
https://vfapp.org/7da1

World Health Organization, The (WHO)
The United Nations' agency for health provides leadership on global health matters, shapes the health research agenda, setting norms and standards, articulates evidence-based policy options, provides technical support and monitoring to countries, and assesses health trends.
ER Med, General, Infect Dis, Logist-Op, MF Med, OB-GYN, Peds, Psych, Pub Health
+41 22 791 21 11
https://vfapp.org/c476

World Medical Relief
Facilitates the distribution of surplus medical resources where they are needed.
Logist-Op
+1 313-866-5333
https://vfapp.org/72dc

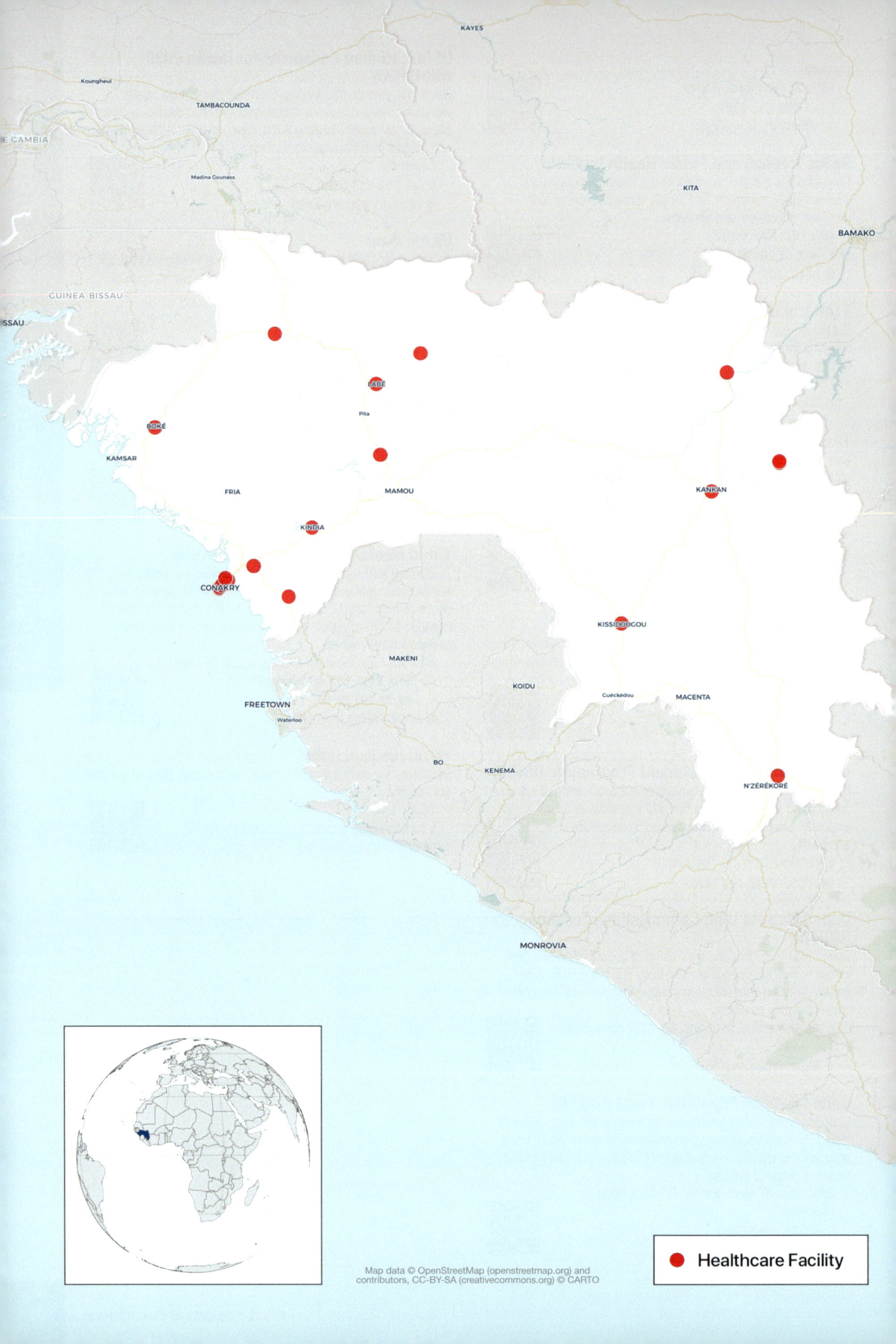
KAYES
Koungheul
TAMBACOUNDA
GAMBIA
Madina Gounass
KITA
BAMAKO
GUINEA-BISSAU
SSAU
LABÉ
Pita
BOKÉ
KAMSAR
FRIA
MAMOU
KANKAN
KINDIA
CONAKRY
KISSIDOUGOU
MAKENI
KOIDU
Guéckédou
MACENTA
FREETOWN
Waterloo
BO
KENEMA
N'ZÉRÉKORÉ
MONROVIA
Healthcare Facility
Map data © OpenStreetMap (openstreetmap.org) and contributors, CC-BY-SA (creativecommons.org) © CARTO

Guinea

The Republic of Guinea is a West African country bordered by Guinea-Bissau, Senegal, and Mali to the north, and Sierra Leone, Liberia, and Côte d'Ivoire to the south. Home to the Gambia, the Niger, and the Sénégal rivers, Guinea is known for its lovely landscapes and captivating waterfalls. The country has a predominantly Muslim population of over 12.5 million, with the highest density in the south and west of the country. As many as 40 different languages are spoken throughout the country, although French is the most widely used.

Formerly part of both the Ghana Empire and the Mali Empire, Guinea achieved independence from French West Africa in 1958. What followed was a period of political instability as rival groups fought for political power. Guinea is rich in resources including gold, diamonds, and a large portion of the world's bauxite. Agriculture is the nation's primary source of employment and income, but this way of life is threatened by climate change as annual rainfall totals decline and temperatures rise. Over half of the population lives in poverty.

Widespread poverty is reflected in the population's overall health. In addition to poor healthcare infrastructure, the country was also the origin of the 2014 Ebola outbreak, which devastated Guinea and spread to neighboring nations. Leading causes of death include lower respiratory infections, malaria, neonatal disorders, diarrheal diseases, stroke, ischemic heart disease, tuberculosis, HIV/AIDS, meningitis, congenital defects, and measles. Death from measles has decreased substantially, but it still remains a significant health threat and a top cause of death.

12.5M
Population

$1,064
GDP Per Capita

61 years
Life Expectancy
↑ Improving

8.3 Doctors/100k
Physician Density

30 Beds/100k
Hospital Bed Density

576 Deaths/100k
Maternal Mortality

Guinea

Healthcare Facilities

CHU de Donka
Route Donka, Dixinn, Conakry, Guinea
🌐 https://vfapp.org/5d71

CHU Ignace Deen
5e Avenue, Kaloum, Conakry, Guinea
🌐 https://vfapp.org/5513

CMC Bernard Kouchner de Coronthie
10e Boulevard, Kaloum, Conakry, Guinea
🌐 https://vfapp.org/755a

Hospital Prefectural de Dalaba
N5, Dalaba, Mamou, Guinea
🌐 https://vfapp.org/36fe

Hôpital de Gaoual Prefectoral
N24, Gaoual, Boké, Guinea
🌐 https://vfapp.org/3a2a

Hôpital de Kissidougou
N2, Kissidougou, Faranah, Guinea
🌐 https://vfapp.org/3baa

Hôpital de l'Amitié Sino-Guinéenne
Rue RO. 209, Ratoma, Conakry, Guinea
🌐 https://vfapp.org/9e85

Hôpital de Mandiana
Mandiana, Kankan, Guinea
🌐 https://vfapp.org/3283

Hôpital Indo Guinéen
Rue MO.258, Matoto, Conakry, Guinea
🌐 https://vfapp.org/154e

Hôpital Jean-Paul 2
Rue RO. 095, Ratoma, Conakry, Guinea
🌐 https://vfapp.org/69ca

Hôpital Karakoro
Forecariah, Guinea
🌐 https://vfapp.org/fad5

Hôpital Préfectoral de Koubia
Koubia, Labé, Guinea
🌐 https://vfapp.org/4af2

Hôpital Préfectoral de Mandiana
Mandiana, Kankan, Guinea
🌐 https://vfapp.org/f11e

Hôpital Préfectoral de Siguiri
N30, Siguiri, Kankan, Guinea
🌐 https://vfapp.org/9614

Hôpital Préfectorale de Coyah
N1, Coyah, Kindia, Guinea
🌐 https://vfapp.org/4629

Hôpital Régional Alpha Oumar Diallo
Place des Martyrs, Kindia, Kindia, Guinea
🌐 https://vfapp.org/e775

Hôpital Régional de Boké
N3, Boké-Centre, Boké, Guinea
🌐 https://vfapp.org/d95c

Hôpital Régional de Kankan
N1, Kankan-Centre, Kankan, Guinea
🌐 https://vfapp.org/bd5a

Hôpital Régional de Labé
N8, Labé-Centre, Labé, Guinea
🌐 https://vfapp.org/3e97

Regional Hospital at Nzérékoré
Nzérékoré, Guinea
🌐 https://vfapp.org/9312

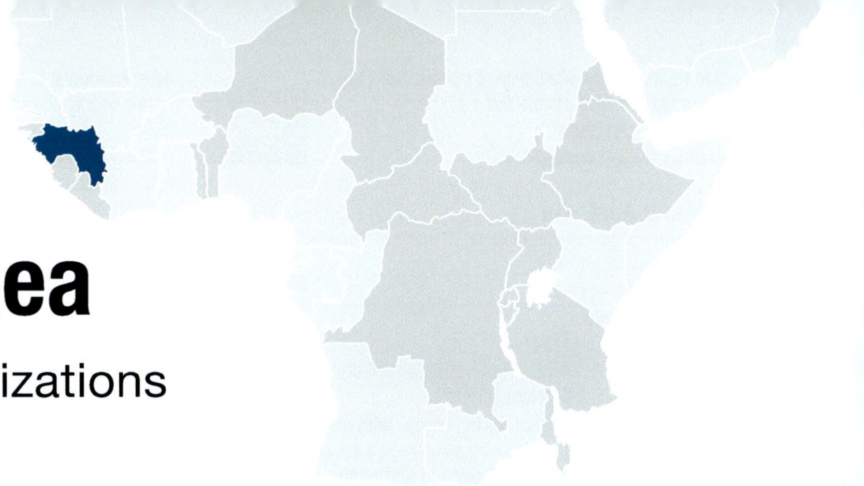

Guinea

Nonprofit Organizations

Abt Associates
Seeks to improve the quality of life and economic well-being of people worldwide, while striving to meet and exceed the highest professional standards.

General, Logist-Op, MF Med, OB-GYN, Peds

☎ +1 212-779-7700

🌐 https://vfapp.org/cec2

Advance Family Planning
Aims to achieve global expansion and access to quality contraceptive information, services, and supplies through financial investment and political commitment.

General, MF Med, Pub Health

☎ +1 410-502-8715

🌐 https://vfapp.org/7478

Africa CDC
Aims to strengthen the capacity and capability of Africa's public health institutions as well as partnerships to detect and respond quickly and effectively to disease threats and outbreaks, based on data-driven interventions and programs.

Infect Dis, Logist-Op, Pub Health

☎ +251 11 551 7700

🌐 https://vfapp.org/339c

Africa Humanitarian Action (AHA)
Responds to crises, conflicts, and disasters in Africa, while informing and advising the international community, governments, civil society, and the private sector on humanitarian issues of concern to Africa. Supports institutional and organizational development efforts.

General, Infect Dis, MF Med, Nutr, OB-GYN

☎ +251 11 660 4800

🌐 https://vfapp.org/3ca2

African Aid International
Works to improve the lives of those most in need in practical and sustainable ways.

Dent-OMFS

🌐 https://vfapp.org/9372

Against Malaria Foundation
Helps protect people from malaria. Funds anti-malaria nets, specifically long-lasting insecticidal nets (LLINs), and works with distribution partners to ensure they are used. Tracks and reports on net use and malaria case data.

Infect Dis

☎ +44 20 7371 8735

🌐 https://vfapp.org/337d

Alliance for International Medical Action, The (ALIMA)
Provides quality medical care to vulnerable populations, partnering with and developing national medical organizations and conducting medical research to bring innovation to twelve African countries where ALIMA works.

ER Med, General, Infect Dis, Logist-Op, MF Med, OB-GYN, Path, Peds, Psych, Pub Health

☎ +1 646-619-9074

🌐 https://vfapp.org/1c11

Amref Health Africa
Serves millions of people across thirty-five countries in Sub-Saharan Africa, strengthening health systems, and training African health workers to respond to the continent's most critical health issues.

All-Immu, General, Infect Dis, Logist-Op, MF Med, OB-GYN, Path, Pub Health, Surg

☎ +254 20 6993000

🌐 https://vfapp.org/6985

AO Alliance
Builds solutions to lessen the burden of injuries in low- and middle-income countries, while enhancing the care of the injured to reduce human suffering, disability, and poverty.

Ortho, Surg

🌐 https://vfapp.org/8cd5

Asclepius Snakebite Foundation
Seeks to reverse the cycle of tragic snakebite outcomes through a combination of innovative research, clinical medicine, and education-based public health initiatives.

Infect Dis, Pub Health

🌐 https://vfapp.org/d37d

BroadReach
Collaborates with governments, multinational health organizations, donors, and private sector companies to affect healthcare reform and solve the world's biggest health challenges.

Logist-Op

☎ +27 21 514 8300

🌐 https://vfapp.org/7812

Carter Center, The
Seeks to prevent and resolve conflicts, enhance freedom and democracy, and improve health, while remaining committed to

human rights and the alleviation of human suffering.
Infect Dis, MF Med, Ophth-Opt
+1 800-550-3560
https://vfapp.org/6556

ChildFund Australia
Works to reduce poverty for children in many of the world's most disadvantaged communities.
ER Med, General, Peds
+1 800023600
https://vfapp.org/13df

Christian Blind Mission (CBM)
Aims to improve the quality of life of persons with disabilities in the poorest countries, addressing poverty as a cause, and a consequence, of disability, and working in partnership to create a society for all.
ENT, General, Infect Dis, OB-GYN, Ophth-Opt, Ortho, Peds, Psych, Rehab, Surg
+49 6251 131131
https://vfapp.org/3824

Core Group
Aims to improve and expand community health practices for underserved populations, especially women and children, through collaborative action and learning.
General, Infect Dis, MF Med, Medicine, OB-GYN, Peds, Pub Health
+1 202-380-3400
https://vfapp.org/9de3

Dentaid
Seeks to treat, equip, train, and educate people in need of dental care.
Dent-OMFS
+44 1794 324249
https://vfapp.org/a183

Direct Relief
Improves the health and lives of people affected by poverty or emergency situations by mobilizing and providing essential medical resources needed for their care.
ER Med, Logist-Op
+1 805-964-4767
https://vfapp.org/58e5

Doctors Without Borders/Médecins Sans Frontières (MSF)
Responds to emergencies and provides lifesaving medical care where needed most, including during disasters, conflicts, and epidemics.
Anesth, Crit-Care, ER Med, General, Infect Dis, Nutr, OB-GYN, Ped Surg, Peds, Psych, Pub Health, Surg
+1 212-679-6800
https://vfapp.org/f363

Dream Sant'Egidio
Seeks to counter HIV/AIDS in Africa by eliminating the transmission of HIV from mother to child, with a focus on women because of the importance of their role in the community.
Infect Dis, MF Med, Neonat, OB-GYN, Path, Peds
+39 06 899 2225
https://vfapp.org/f466

Drugs for Neglected Diseases Initiative
Develops lifesaving medicines for people with neglected diseases around the world, having developed eight treatments for five deadly diseases and saving millions of lives since 2003.
Infect Dis, Pub Health
+41 22 906 92 30
https://vfapp.org/969c

Enabel
As the development agency of the Belgian federal government, charged with implementing Belgium's international development policy, carries out public service assignments in Belgium and abroad pursuant to the 2030 Agenda for Sustainable Development.
General, Infect Dis, Logist-Op, MF Med, OB-GYN, Peds, Pub Health
+32 2 505 37 00
https://vfapp.org/5af7

Episcopal Relief & Development
Provides relief in times of disaster and promotes sustainable development by identifying and addressing the root causes of suffering.
Infect Dis, MF Med, Neonat, Nutr, Peds
+1 855-312-4325
https://vfapp.org/7cfa

eRanger
Provides sustainable solutions to transportation and medical provision such as ambulances and mobile clinics in developing countries.
ER Med, General, Logist-Op
+27 40 654 3207
https://vfapp.org/4c18

Fistula Foundation
Aims to engage the support of people worldwide who are eager to see the day when no woman suffers from obstetric fistula. Raises and directs funds to doctors and hospitals providing life-transforming surgery to women in need.
OB-GYN
+1 408-249-9596
https://vfapp.org/e958

Fondation Follereau
Promotes the quality of life of the most vulnerable African communities. Alongside trusted partners, the foundation supports local initiatives in healthcare and education.
General, Infect Dis, OB-GYN
+352 44 66 06 34
https://vfapp.org/bcc7

Gift of Life International
Provides lifesaving cardiac treatment to children in developing countries while developing sustainable pediatric cardiac programs by implementing screening, surgical, and training missions.
Anesth, CT Surg, CV Med, Crit-Care, Ped Surg, Peds, Pulm-Critic
+1 855-734-3278
https://vfapp.org/f2f9

Global Ministries – The United Methodist Church
As the worldwide mission and development agency of The United Methodist Church, Global Ministries works with more than 300 hospitals and clinics around the world through its Global Health Unit.
Anesth, CT Surg, CV Med, Crit-Care, Dent-OMFS,

Derm, ER Med, GI, General, Infect Dis, Logist-Op, MF Med, Medicine, Neonat, Nephro, Nutr, OB-GYN, Ophth-Opt, Ortho, Palliative, Peds, Pod, Psych, Pub Health, Rehab, Rheum, Surg, Urol

📞 +1 800-862-4246
🌐 https://vfapp.org/1723

Global Oncology (GO)
Brings the best in cancer care to underserved patients around the world and collaborates across geographic, professional, and academic borders to improve cancer care, research, and education.
Heme-Onc, Path, Rad-Onc
🌐 https://vfapp.org/fcb8

Global Polio Eradication Initiative
Aims to eradicate polio worldwide.
All-Immu, Logist-Op
📞 +1 847-866-3000
🌐 https://vfapp.org/7e2c

Grassroot Soccer
Leverages the power of soccer to educate, inspire, and mobilize at risk youth in developing countries to overcome their greatest health challenges, live healthier more productive lives, and be agents for change in their communities.
Infect Dis
📞 +1 603-277-9685
🌐 https://vfapp.org/3521

Health Equity Initiative
Aims to build and sustain a global community that engages across sectors and disciplines to advance health equity.
Pub Health
🌐 https://vfapp.org/e2e2

Helen Keller International
Seeks to eliminate preventable vision loss, malnutrition, and diseases of poverty.
Infect Dis, Nutr, OB-GYN, Ophth-Opt, Peds
📞 +1 212-532-0544
🌐 https://vfapp.org/b654

Humanity First
Provides aid and assistance to those in need, offering sustainable development solutions to society while providing and empowering local communities with the resources to help themselves.
ER Med, General, MF Med, Ophth-Opt
📞 +44 20 8417 0082
🌐 https://vfapp.org/13cc

International Agency for the Prevention of Blindness (IAPB), The
Leads international efforts in blindness-prevention activities, works toward a world where no one is needlessly visually impaired, and ensures that everyone has access to the best possible standard of eye health.
Infect Dis, Ophth-Opt, Pub Health
🌐 https://vfapp.org/87a2

International Federation of Gynecology and Obstetrics (FIGO)
Implements global projects on specific women's health issues.
MF Med, Medicine, Neonat, OB-GYN, Surg, Urol
📞 +44 20 7928 1166
🌐 https://vfapp.org/c4b4

International Federation of Red Cross and Red Crescent Societies (IFRC)
Coordinates and directs international assistance following natural and man-made disasters in nonconflict situations through the world's largest humanitarian and development network. Provides disaster-preparedness programs, healthcare activities, and promotes humanitarian values.
ER Med, General, Infect Dis, Nutr
📞 +1 212-338-0161
🌐 https://vfapp.org/b4ee

International Organization for Migration (IOM) – The UN Migration Agency
Promotes evidence-informed policies and holistic, preventive, and curative health programs that are beneficial, accessible, and equitable for vulnerable migrants.
General, Infect Dis, OB-GYN
📞 +27 12 342 2789
🌐 https://vfapp.org/621a

International Planned Parenthood Federation (IPPF)
Leads a locally owned, globally connected civil society movement that provides and enables services and champions sexual and reproductive health and rights for all, especially the underserved.
Infect Dis, MF Med, OB-GYN
📞 +44 20 7939 8200
🌐 https://vfapp.org/dc97

International Trachoma Initiative (iTi)
Works toward a world free from trachoma, a preventable cause of blindness, and provides comprehensive support to national ministries of health and governmental and nongovernmental organizations to implement a comprehensive approach to fight trachoma.
Infect Dis, Ophth-Opt
📞 +1 404-371-0466
🌐 https://vfapp.org/3278

Iris Global
Serves the poor, the destitute, the lost, and the forgotten by providing adoration, outreach, family, education, relief, development, healing, and the arts.
General, Infect Dis, Nutr, Pub Health
📞 +1 530-255-2077
🌐 https://vfapp.org/37f8

Jhpiego
Creates and delivers transformative healthcare solutions that save lives in partnership with national governments, health experts, and local communities.
General, Infect Dis, OB-GYN, Surg
📞 +1 410-537-1800
🌐 https://vfapp.org/45b8

John Snow, Inc. (JSI)
Aims to improve the health and well-being of underserved and vulnerable people and communities throughout the world.
General, Infect Dis, Logist-Op, MF Med, OB-GYN, Peds, Psych, Pub Health
📞 +1 617-482-9485
🌐 https://vfapp.org/ba78

Johns Hopkins Center for Communication Programs
Believes in the power of communication to save lives, by empowering people to adopt healthy behaviors for themselves, their families, and their communities.
General, Infect Dis, Logist-Op, OB-GYN, Pub Health
+1 410-659-6300
https://vfapp.org/1bf9

Joint United Nations Programme on HIV/AIDS (UNAIDS)
Aims to place people living with HIV and people affected by the virus at the decision-making table and at the center of designing, delivering, and monitoring the AIDS response.
Infect Dis
+41 22 791 36 66
https://vfapp.org/464a

Lay Volunteers International Association (LVIA)
Fosters local and global change to help overcome extreme poverty, reinforce equitable and sustainable development, and enhance dialogue between Italian and African communities.
ER Med, Logist-Op, MF Med, Neonat, Nutr, OB-GYN, Peds
+39 0171 696975
https://vfapp.org/ecd4

Lifebox
Seeks to provide safer surgery and anesthesia in low-resource countries by investing in tools, training, and partnerships for safe surgery.
Anesth, Crit-Care, Surg
+44 20 3286 0402
https://vfapp.org/2d4d

Light for the World
Contributes to a world in which persons with disabilities fully exercise their rights and assists persons with disabilities living in poverty.
Ophth-Opt, Rehab
+43 1 8101300
https://vfapp.org/3ff6

Lions Clubs International
Empowers volunteers to serve their communities, meet humanitarian needs, encourage peace, and promote international understanding through Lions clubs.
Heme-Onc, Medicine, Nutr, Ophth-Opt
+1 630-571-5466
https://vfapp.org/7b12

London School of Hygiene & Tropical Medicine: Health in Humanitarian Crises Centre
Advances health and health equity in crisis-affected countries through research, education, and translation of knowledge into policy and practice.
ER Med, Infect Dis, Pub Health
+44 20 7636 8636
https://vfapp.org/96ad

Management Sciences for Health (MSH)
Works with countries and communities to save lives and improve the health of the world's poorest and most vulnerable people by building strong, resilient, sustainable health systems.
Infect Dis, Logist-Op, Pub Health
+1 617-250-9500
https://vfapp.org/6aa2

MAP International
Provides medicines and health supplies to those in need around the world so they might experience life to the fullest.
Logist-Op
+1 800-225-8550
https://vfapp.org/deed

Medical Care Development International (MCD International)
Works to strengthen health systems through innovative, sustainable interventions.
Infect Dis, Logist-Op, OB-GYN, Pub Health
+1 301-562-1920
https://vfapp.org/dc5c

MedShare
Aims to improve the quality of life of people, communities, and the planet by sourcing and directly delivering surplus medical supplies and equipment to communities in need around the world.
Logist-Op
+1 770-323-5858
https://vfapp.org/c8bc

MENTOR Initiative
Saves lives in emergencies through tropical disease control, and helps people recover from crisis with dignity, working side by side with communities, health workers, and health authorities to leave a lasting impact.
ER Med, Infect Dis
+44 1444 412171
https://vfapp.org/3bd5

Mercy Ships
Operates hospital ships staffed by volunteers to bring hope, healing, and healthcare to underserved communities worldwide.
Anesth, Dent-OMFS, Logist-Op, Neonat, OB-GYN, Ophth-Opt, Ortho, Palliative, Plast, Psych, Surg
+1 903-939-7000
https://vfapp.org/2e99

Mérieux Foundation
Committed to fighting infectious diseases that affect developing countries by capacity building, particularly in clinical laboratories, and focusing on diagnosis.
Logist-Op, Path
+33 4 72 40 79 79
https://vfapp.org/a23a

MiracleFeet
Brings low-cost treatment to every child on the planet born with clubfoot, a leading cause of physical disability.
Ortho, Peds, Rehab
+1 919-240-5572
https://vfapp.org/bda8

Neglected Tropical Disease NGO Network
Works to create a global forum for non-governmental organizations working to control onchocerciasis, lymphatic filariasis, schistosomiasis, soil transmitted helminths, and trachoma.
Infect Dis, Logist-Op
+1 929-272-6227
https://vfapp.org/c511

Operation Fistula
Exists to end obstetric fistula by building models of care that serve every woman, everywhere.

MF Med, OB-GYN, Surg

+1 512-687-3479

https://vfapp.org/ce8e

Pact
Works on the ground to improve the lives of those who are challenged by poverty and marginalization, striving for a world where all people are heard, capable, and vibrant.

Infect Dis, Logist-Op, MF Med, Pub Health

+1 202-466-5666

https://vfapp.org/9a6c

RestoringVision
Empowers lives by restoring vision for millions of people in need.

Ophth-Opt

+1 209-980-7323

https://vfapp.org/e121

Rockefeller Foundation, The
Works to promote the well-being of humanity.

Logist-Op, Nutr, Pub Health

+1 212-869-8500

https://vfapp.org/5424

Rotary International
Provides service to others, improves lives, and advances world understanding, goodwill, and peace through its fellowship of business, professional, and community leaders.

ER Med, General, Infect Dis, MF Med, OB-GYN

https://vfapp.org/8fb5

ROW Foundation
Works to improve the quality of training for healthcare providers, and the diagnosis and treatment available to people with epilepsy and associated psychiatric disorders in under-resourced areas of the world.

Neuro, Psych

+1 630-791-0247

https://vfapp.org/25eb

Sanofi Espoir Foundation
Contributes to reducing health inequalities among populations that need it most by applying a socially responsible approach focused on fighting childhood cancers in low-income countries, improving maternal and newborn health, and improving access to care.

ER Med, OB-GYN, Peds

+33 1 53 77 91 38

https://vfapp.org/943b

Save the Children
Gives children around the world a healthy start in life, the opportunity to learn, and protection from harm.

All-Immu, Crit-Care, ER Med, General, Infect Dis, MF Med, Medicine, Neonat, OB-GYN, Peds, Psych, Pub Health

+1 800-728-3843

https://vfapp.org/2e73

Sightsavers
Prevents avoidable blindness in some of the poorest parts of the world by treating debilitating eye diseases.

Infect Dis, Ophth-Opt, Surg

+1 800-707-9746

https://vfapp.org/aa52

SIGN Fracture Care International
Builds orthopedic capacity around the world and provides the injured poor access to fracture surgery by donating orthopedic education and implant systems to surgeons in developing countries.

Ortho, Rehab, Surg

+1 509-371-1107

https://vfapp.org/123d

Smile Train
Seeks to give every child with a cleft the opportunity for a healthy, productive life by providing free cleft repair surgery and comprehensive cleft care in their own communities.

Dent-OMFS, ENT, Plast

+1 800-932-9541

https://vfapp.org/f21d

Solthis
Improves disease prevention and access to quality care by strengthening the health systems and services of the countries served.

General, Infect Dis, Logist-Op, MF Med, Neonat, Path

+33 1 81 70 17 90

https://vfapp.org/a71d

Swiss Tropical and Public Health Institute
Contributes to the improvement of the health of populations internationally, nationally, and locally through excellence in research, education, and services.

Infect Dis, Pub Health

+41 61 284 81 11

https://vfapp.org/2ee4

Task Force for Global Health, The
Consists of programs and focus areas that cover a range of global health issues including neglected tropical diseases, infectious diseases, vaccines, field epidemiology, public health informatics, health workforce development, and global health ethics.

Infect Dis, Logist-Op, Medicine, Ophth-Opt, Peds

+1 404-371-0466

https://vfapp.org/714c

Terre Des Hommes
Works to improve the conditions of the most vulnerable children worldwide by improving the health of children under the age of 3, protecting migrant children, providing humanitarian aid to children and their families in times of crisis, and preventing child exploitation.

ER Med, MF Med, Neonat, OB-GYN, Ped Surg, Peds

+41 58 611 06 66

https://vfapp.org/2689

U.S. President's Malaria Initiative (PMI)
Supports low-income countries to help control and eliminate malaria through cost-effective, lifesaving malaria interventions.

Infect Dis, MF Med, OB-GYN

+1 202-712-0000

https://vfapp.org/dc8b

Union for International Cancer Control (UICC)
Unites and supports the cancer community to reduce the global cancer burden, promote greater equity, and ensure that cancer control continues to be a priority in the world health and development agenda.
Heme-Onc, Pub Health
+41 22 809 18 11
https://vfapp.org/88b1

United Nations Children's Fund (UNICEF)
Works in over 190 countries and territories to save children's lives, to defend their rights, and to help them fulfill their potential, from early childhood through adolescence.
All-Immu, Infect Dis, MF Med, Neonat, Nutr, OB-GYN, Ped Surg, Peds, Pub Health
https://vfapp.org/42d7

United Nations Development Programme (UNDP)
Helps countries achieve the simultaneous eradication of extreme poverty and significant reduction of inequalities and exclusion using a sustainable human development approach.
Infect Dis, Logist-Op, Pub Health
https://vfapp.org/935c

United Nations High Commissioner for Refugees (UNHCR)
Safeguards the rights and well-being of people who have been forced to flee, ensuring that everybody has the right to seek asylum and find safe refuge in another country, with the goal of seeking lasting solutions.
General, MF Med, Medicine, OB-GYN, Peds, Psych, Pub Health
https://vfapp.org/6636

United Nations Population Fund (UNFPA)
Supports reproductive healthcare for women and youth in more than 150 countries, focusing on delivering a world where every pregnancy is wanted, every childbirth is safe, and every young person's potential is fulfilled.
Infect Dis, MF Med, Neonat, OB-GYN, Peds, Pub Health
+1 212-963-6008
https://vfapp.org/c969

United Surgeons for Children (USFC)
Pursues greater health and opportunity for children in the most neglected pockets of the world, with a specific focus and expertise in surgery.
Anesth, CT Surg, Neonat, Neurosurg, OB-GYN, Peds, Radiol, Surg
https://vfapp.org/3b4c

USAID: Maternal and Child Survival Program
Works to prevent child and maternal deaths.
Infect Dis, MF Med, Neonat, OB-GYN, Peds
https://vfapp.org/6fcf

USAID: A2Z The Micronutrient and Child Blindness Project
Aims to increase the use of key micronutrient and blindness interventions to improve child and maternal health.
MF Med, Neonat, Nutr, Ophth-Opt, Surg
+1 202-884-8785
https://vfapp.org/c5f1

USAID: Deliver Project
Builds a global supply chain to deliver lifesaving health products to people in order to enable countries to provide family planning, protect against malaria, and limit the spread of pandemic threats.
Infect Dis, Logist-Op, MF Med
+1 202-712-0000
https://vfapp.org/374e

USAID: Health Finance and Governance Project
Uses research to implement strategies to help countries develop robust governance systems, increase their domestic resources for health, manage those resources more effectively, and make wise purchasing decisions.
Logist-Op
+1 202-712-0000
https://vfapp.org/8652

USAID: Human Resources for Health 2030 (HRH2030)
Helps low- and middle-income countries develop the health workforce needed to prevent maternal and child deaths, support the goals of Family Planning 2020, control the HIV/AIDS epidemic, and protect communities from infectious diseases.
Logist-Op
+1 202-955-3300
https://vfapp.org/9ea8

USAID: Maternal and Child Health Integrated Program
Works to improve the health of women and their families, including programs for maternal, newborn, and child health, immunization, family planning, nutrition, malaria, and HIV/AIDS.
All-Immu, General, Infect Dis, MF Med
+1 202-835-3136
https://vfapp.org/4415

Vitamin Angels
Helps at-risk populations in need—specifically pregnant women, new mothers, and children under age five—to gain access to life-changing vitamins and minerals.
General, Nutr
+1 805-564-8400
https://vfapp.org/7da1

Willing and Abel
Seeks to provide connections between children in developing nations and specialist centers, helping with visas, passports, transportation, and finances.
Anesth, Dent-OMFS, Ped Surg
https://vfapp.org/9dc7

World Health Organization, The (WHO)
The United Nations' agency for health provides leadership on global health matters, shapes the health research agenda, setting norms and standards, articulates evidence-based policy options, provides technical support and monitoring to countries, and assesses health trends.
ER Med, General, Infect Dis, Logist-Op, MF Med, OB-GYN, Peds, Psych, Pub Health
+41 22 791 21 11
https://vfapp.org/c476

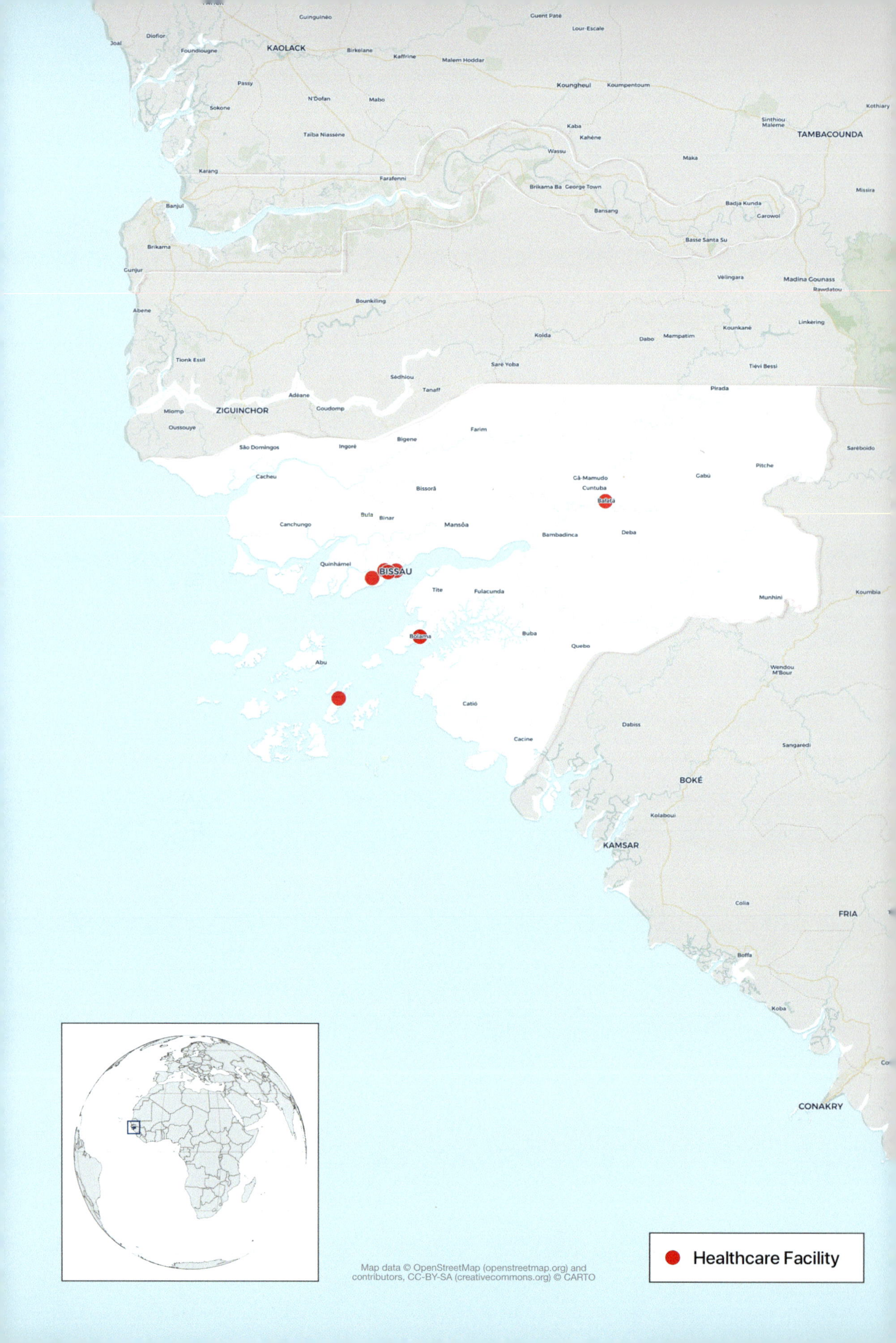

KAOLACK
Guinguinéo
Guent Paté
Lour-Escale
Joal
Diofior
Foundiougne
Birkelane
Kaffrine
Malem Hoddar
Passy
N'Dofan
Mabo
Koungheul
Koumpentoum
Sokone
Kothiary
Taïba Niassène
Kaba
Kahène
Sinthiou Maleme
TAMBACOUNDA
Wassu
Maka
Karang
Farafenni
Brikama Ba
George Town
Missira
Banjul
Badja Kunda
Bansang
Garowol
Brikama
Basse Santa Su
Gunjur
Vélingara
Madina Gounass
Rawdatou
Bounkiling
Abene
Linkéring
Kounkané
Kolda
Dabo
Mampatim
Tionk Essil
Saré Yoba
Tiévi Bessi
Sédhiou
Tanaff
Pirada
Adéane
Mlomp
ZIGUINCHOR
Goudomp
Farim
Oussouye
Bigene
São Domingos
Ingoré
Saréboido
Pitche
Cacheu
Gã-Mamudo
Gabú
Bissorã
Cuntuba
Bafatá
Bula
Binar
Canchungo
Mansôa
Bambadinca
Deba
Quinhámel
BISSAU
Tite
Fulacunda
Koumbia
Munhini
Bolama
Buba
Quebo
Abu
Wendou M'Bour
Catió
Dabiss
Cacine
Sangaredi
BOKÉ
Kolaboui
KAMSAR
Colia
FRIA
Boffa
Koba
CONAKRY
Map data © OpenStreetMap (openstreetmap.org) and contributors, CC-BY-SA (creativecommons.org) © CARTO
Healthcare Facility

Guinea-Bissau

Located on the coast of West Africa, the Republic of Guinea-Bissau has a small, young population of 1.9 million people, two-thirds of whom are under age 30. About one-fifth of the population lives in the capital of Bissau and along the coast. As a coastal country, Guinea-Bissau has countless islands dotting the shoreline, with unique natural features and wildlife. Predominantly Muslim and Christian, Guinea-Bissau's population comprises several ethnic groups such as Fulani, Balanta, Mandinga, Papel, and Manjaco. Crioulo is the lingua franca, while Portuguese is the official language.

Guinea-Bissau was ruled by Portugal until 1974, and since independence, the country has experienced decades of political instability marked by a civil war and several coups. The result is a fragile country with high levels of unemployment, a weak economy, widespread corruption, and endemic poverty. Several public institutions are challenged, including an underdeveloped education infrastructure.

Despite its many economic and political challenges, Guinea-Bissau has seen improvements in recent decades; the under-five mortality rate has declined significantly since 1990, from over 200 deaths per 1,000 live births to under 80. Similarly, life expectancy continues to improve—but it still ranks among the lowest in the world. Despite some improvements in overall population health, top causes of death include neonatal disorders, diarrheal diseases, lower respiratory infections, HIV/AIDS, ischemic heart disease, stroke, tuberculosis, malaria, road injuries, and meningitis. Additionally, cases of measles have been increasing annually, posing a significant public health challenge.

1.9M
Population

$698
GDP Per Capita

58 years
Life Expectancy
↑ Improving

12.7
Doctors/100k
Physician Density

100
Beds/100k
Hospital Bed Density

667
Deaths/100k
Maternal Mortality

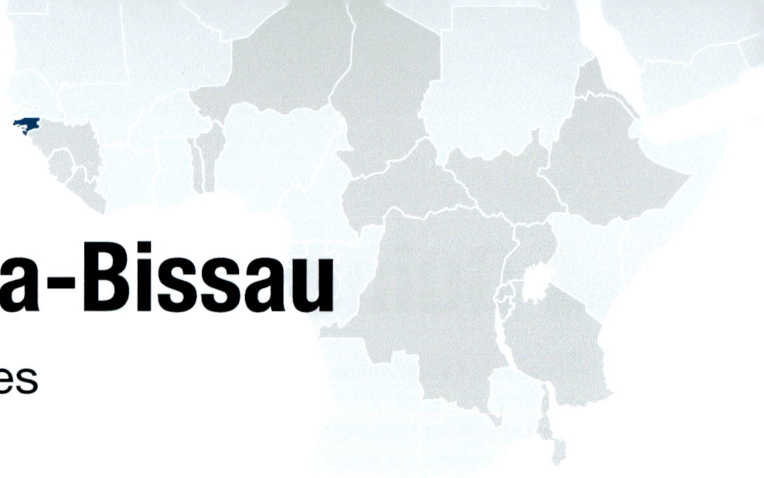

Guinea-Bissau

Healthcare Facilities

Bafatá Hospital
Avenida Principal, Bafatá,
Região de Bafatá,
Guinea-Bissau
https://vfapp.org/ce8c

Hospital 3 de Agosto
Avenida dos Combatentes da Liberdade da Pátria, Bissau,
Sector autónomo de Bissau,
Guinea-Bissau
https://vfapp.org/325b

Hospital Marcelino Banca
Bubaque, Região de Bolama,
Guinea-Bissau
https://vfapp.org/d439

Hospital Militar de Bissau
Avenida dos Combatentes da Liberdade da Pátria, Bissau,
Sector Autónomo de Bissau,
Guinea-Bissau
https://vfapp.org/aad4

Hospital Militar e Civil
Avenida Amílcar Cabral,
Bolama, Região de Bolama,
Guinea-Bissau
https://vfapp.org/7c9f

Hospital Nacional Simão Mendes
Bissau, Guinea-Bissau
https://vfapp.org/bffc

Hospital Raoul Follereau
Bissau, Guinea-Bissau
https://vfapp.org/e9d5

Hospital Solidariedade de Bolama
Bolama, Guinea-Bissau
https://vfapp.org/369d

Hôpital de Cumura
Prábis, Guinea-Bissau
https://vfapp.org/28a6

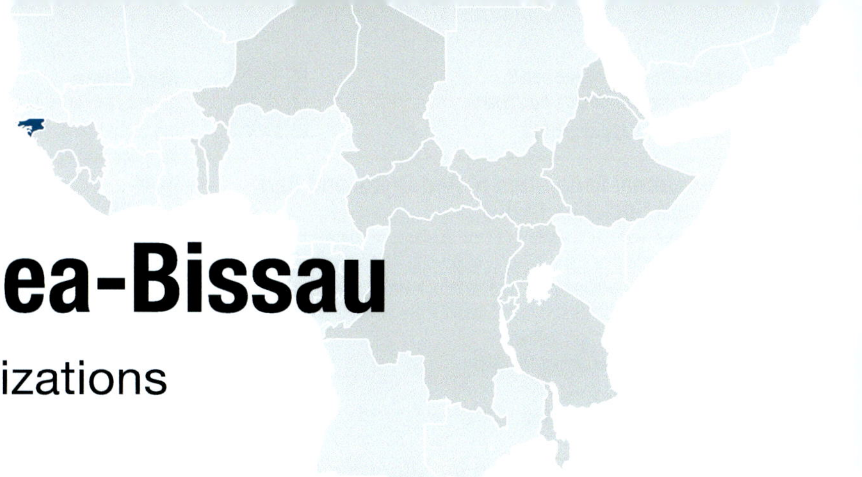

Guinea-Bissau

Nonprofit Organizations

Africa CDC
Aims to strengthen the capacity and capability of Africa's public health institutions as well as partnerships to detect and respond quickly and effectively to disease threats and outbreaks, based on data-driven interventions and programs.
Infect Dis, Logist-Op, Pub Health
☎ +251 11 551 7700
🌐 https://vfapp.org/339c

African Health Now
Promotes and provides information and access to sustainable primary healthcare to women, children, and families living across Sub-Saharan Africa.
Dent-OMFS, Endo, General, Infect Dis, MF Med, OB-GYN
🌐 https://vfapp.org/c766

African Field Epidemiology Network (AFENET)
Strengthens field epidemiology and public health laboratory capacity to contribute effectively to addressing epidemics and other major public health problems in Africa.
All-Immu, Infect Dis, Path, Pub Health
🌐 https://vfapp.org/df2e

BroadReach
Collaborates with governments, multinational health organizations, donors, and private sector companies to affect healthcare reform and solve the world's biggest health challenges.
Logist-Op
☎ +27 21 514 8300
🌐 https://vfapp.org/7812

Center for Strategic and International Studies (CSIS) Commission on Strengthening America's Health Security
Brings together a distinguished and diverse group of high-level opinion leaders bridging security and health, with the core aim to chart a bold vision for the future of U.S. leadership in global health.
ER Med, Infect Dis, MF Med, Pub Health
☎ +1 202-887-0200
🌐 https://vfapp.org/6d7f

Developing Country NGO Delegation: Global Fund to Fight AIDS, TB & Malaria
Works to strengthen the engagement of civil society actors and organizations in developing countries to contribute toward achieving a world in which AIDS, TB, and Malaria are no longer global, public health, and human rights threats.
Infect Dis, Pub Health
☎ +254 20 2515790
🌐 https://vfapp.org/3149

Doctors Without Borders/Médecins Sans Frontières (MSF)
Responds to emergencies and provides lifesaving medical care where needed most, including during disasters, conflicts, and epidemics.
Anesth, Crit-Care, ER Med, General, Infect Dis, Nutr, OB-GYN, Ped Surg, Peds, Psych, Pub Health, Surg
☎ +1 212-679-6800
🌐 https://vfapp.org/f363

Global Oncology (GO)
Brings the best in cancer care to underserved patients around the world and collaborates across geographic, professional, and academic borders to improve cancer care, research, and education.
Heme-Onc, Path, Rad-Onc
🌐 https://vfapp.org/fcb8

Humanity & Inclusion
Works alongside people with disabilities and vulnerable populations, taking action and bearing witness in order to respond to their essential needs, improve their living conditions and health, and promote respect for their dignity and fundamental rights.
General, Infect Dis, MF Med, Medicine, Ortho, Peds, Psych, Pub Health, Rehab
☎ +1 301-891-2138
🌐 https://vfapp.org/16b7

Humanity First
Provides aid and assistance to those in need, offering sustainable development solutions to society while providing and empowering local communities with the resources to help themselves.
ER Med, General, MF Med, Ophth-Opt
☎ +44 20 8417 0082
🌐 https://vfapp.org/13cc

International Agency for the Prevention of Blindness (IAPB), The
Leads international efforts in blindness-prevention activities, works toward a world where no one is needlessly visually impaired, and ensures that everyone has access to the best

possible standard of eye health.
Infect Dis, Ophth-Opt, Pub Health
https://vfapp.org/87a2

International Federation of Red Cross and Red Crescent Societies (IFRC)
Coordinates and directs international assistance following natural and man-made disasters in nonconflict situations through the world's largest humanitarian and development network. Provides disaster-preparedness programs, healthcare activities, and promotes humanitarian values.
ER Med, General, Infect Dis, Nutr
+1 212-338-0161
https://vfapp.org/b4ee

International Organization for Migration (IOM) – The UN Migration Agency
Promotes evidence-informed policies and holistic, preventive, and curative health programs that are beneficial, accessible, and equitable for vulnerable migrants.
General, Infect Dis, OB-GYN
+27 12 342 2789
https://vfapp.org/621a

International Trachoma Initiative (iTi)
Works toward a world free from trachoma, a preventable cause of blindness, and provides comprehensive support to national ministries of health and governmental and nongovernmental organizations to implement a comprehensive approach to fight trachoma.
Infect Dis, Ophth-Opt
+1 404-371-0466
https://vfapp.org/3278

Johns Hopkins Center for Communication Programs
Believes in the power of communication to save lives, by empowering people to adopt healthy behaviors for themselves, their families, and their communities.
General, Infect Dis, Logist-Op, OB-GYN, Pub Health
+1 410-659-6300
https://vfapp.org/1bf9

Joint United Nations Programme on HIV/AIDS (UNAIDS)
Aims to place people living with HIV and people affected by the virus at the decision-making table and at the center of designing, delivering, and monitoring the AIDS response.
Infect Dis
+41 22 791 36 66
https://vfapp.org/464a

Lay Volunteers International Association (LVIA)
Fosters local and global change to help overcome extreme poverty, reinforce equitable and sustainable development, and enhance dialogue between Italian and African communities.
ER Med, Logist-Op, MF Med, Neonat, Nutr, OB-GYN, Peds
+39 0171 696975
https://vfapp.org/ecd4

Lions Clubs International
Empowers volunteers to serve their communities, meet humanitarian needs, encourage peace, and promote international understanding through Lions clubs.
Heme-Onc, Medicine, Nutr, Ophth-Opt
+1 630-571-5466
https://vfapp.org/7b12

MedShare
Aims to improve the quality of life of people, communities, and the planet by sourcing and directly delivering surplus medical supplies and equipment to communities in need around the world.
Logist-Op
+1 770-323-5858
https://vfapp.org/c8bc

Mercy Ships
Operates hospital ships staffed by volunteers to bring hope, healing, and healthcare to underserved communities worldwide.
Anesth, Dent-OMFS, Logist-Op, Neonat, OB-GYN, Ophth-Opt, Ortho, Palliative, Plast, Psych, Surg
+1 903-939-7000
https://vfapp.org/2e99

Mission Bambini
Helps to support children living in poverty, sickness, and without education, giving them the opportunity and hope of a better life.
CT Surg, CV Med, Crit-Care, ER Med, Ped Surg, Peds
+39 02 210 0241
https://vfapp.org/dc1a

Rockefeller Foundation, The
Works to promote the well-being of humanity.
Logist-Op, Nutr, Pub Health
+1 212-869-8500
https://vfapp.org/5424

Rotary International
Provides service to others, improves lives, and advances world understanding, goodwill, and peace through its fellowship of business, professional, and community leaders.
ER Med, General, Infect Dis, MF Med, OB-GYN
https://vfapp.org/8fb5

Sightsavers
Prevents avoidable blindness in some of the poorest parts of the world by treating debilitating eye diseases.
Infect Dis, Ophth-Opt, Surg
+1 800-707-9746
https://vfapp.org/aa52

Sustainable Cardiovascular Health Equity Development Alliance
Fights cardiovascular disease in underserved populations globally via education, training, and increasing interventional capacity.
CV Med, Pub Health, Radiol
+1 608-338-3357
https://vfapp.org/799c

Swiss Tropical and Public Health Institute
Contributes to the improvement of the health of populations internationally, nationally, and locally through excellence in research, education, and services.
Infect Dis, Pub Health
+41 61 284 81 11
https://vfapp.org/2ee4

Task Force for Global Health, The
Consists of programs and focus areas that cover a range of global health issues including neglected tropical diseases,

infectious diseases, vaccines, field epidemiology, public health informatics, health workforce development, and global health ethics.

Infect Dis, Logist-Op, Medicine, Ophth-Opt, Peds

+1 404-371-0466

https://vfapp.org/714c

United Nations Children's Fund (UNICEF)

Works in over 190 countries and territories to save children's lives, to defend their rights, and to help them fulfill their potential, from early childhood through adolescence.

All-Immu, Infect Dis, MF Med, Neonat, Nutr, OB-GYN, Ped Surg, Peds, Pub Health

https://vfapp.org/42d7

United Nations Development Programme (UNDP)

Helps countries achieve the simultaneous eradication of extreme poverty and significant reduction of inequalities and exclusion using a sustainable human development approach.

Infect Dis, Logist-Op, Pub Health

https://vfapp.org/935c

United Nations High Commissioner for Refugees (UNHCR)

Safeguards the rights and well-being of people who have been forced to flee, ensuring that everybody has the right to seek asylum and find safe refuge in another country, with the goal of seeking lasting solutions.

General, MF Med, Medicine, OB-GYN, Peds, Psych, Pub Health

https://vfapp.org/6636

United Nations Population Fund (UNFPA)

Supports reproductive healthcare for women and youth in more than 150 countries, focusing on delivering a world where every pregnancy is wanted, every childbirth is safe, and every young person's potential is fulfilled.

Infect Dis, MF Med, Neonat, OB-GYN, Peds, Pub Health

+1 212-963-6008

https://vfapp.org/c969

World Health Organization, The (WHO)

The United Nations' agency for health provides leadership on global health matters, shapes the health research agenda, setting norms and standards, articulates evidence-based policy options, provides technical support and monitoring to countries, and assesses health trends.

ER Med, General, Infect Dis, Logist-Op, MF Med, OB-GYN, Peds, Psych, Pub Health

+41 22 791 21 11

https://vfapp.org/c476

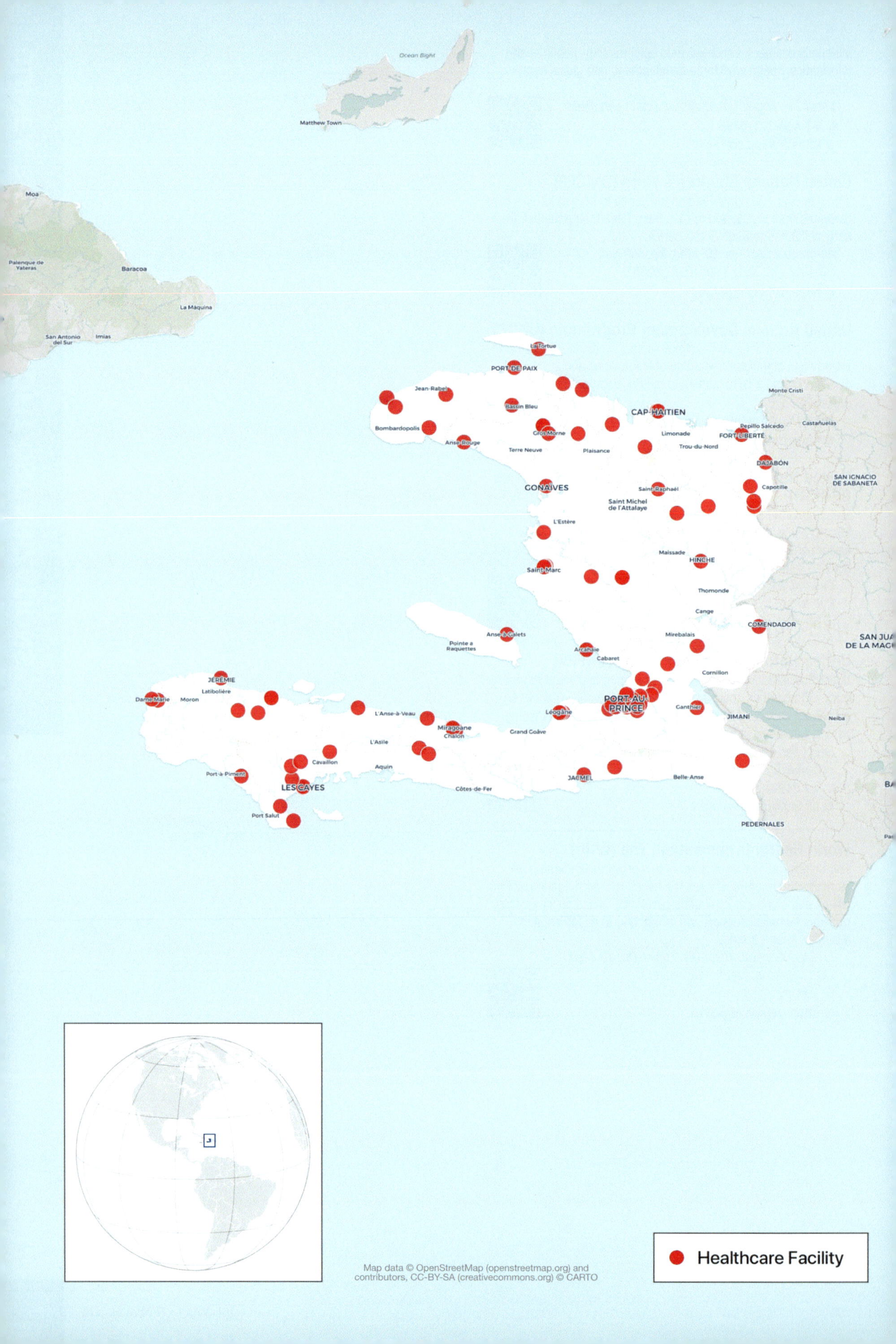
Ocean Bight
Matthew Town
Moa
Palenque de Yateras
Baracoa
La Máquina
San Antonio del Sur
Imías
La Tortue
PORT-DE-PAIX
Jean-Rabel
Bassin Bleu
CAP-HAITIEN
Bombardopolis
Gros Morne
Limonade
Anse-Rouge
Terre Neuve
Plaisance
Trou-du-Nord
Monte Cristi
Pepillo Salcedo
Castañuelas
FORT-LIBERTÉ
DAJABÓN
SAN IGNACIO DE SABANETA
GONAÏVES
Saint-Raphaël
Capotille
Saint Michel de l'Attalaye
L'Estère
Maïssade
HINCHE
Saint-Marc
Thomonde
Cange
COMENDADOR
Anse-à-Galets
Pointe a Raquettes
Mirebalais
Arcahaie
Cabaret
Cornillon
JERÉMIE
Latibolière
Dame-Marie
Moron
PORT-AU-PRINCE
Ganthier
Léogâne
JIMANÍ
Neiba
L'Anse-à-Veau
Miragoâne
Chalon
Grand Goâve
L'Asile
Cavaillon
Aquin
Port-à-Piment
LES CAYES
Côtes-de-Fer
JACMEL
Belle-Anse
Port Salut
PEDERNALES
Map data © OpenStreetMap (openstreetmap.org) and contributors, CC-BY-SA (creativecommons.org) © CARTO
Healthcare Facility

Haiti

The Republic of Haiti is a tropical Caribbean country located south of Cuba and west of the Dominican Republic. The most mountainous country in the Caribbean, Haiti has stunning landscapes and views, along with natural coasts and beaches. The population is young, with 50 percent of Haiti's 11.1 million people under the age of 23. Haitians predominantly speak French and Creole, and are largely Roman Catholic and Protestant while practicing some elements of locally recognized Vodou.

Known for its revolutionary spirit, Haiti won independence from France in a slave-led revolution in 1804. Today, Haiti is the poorest country in the Western Hemisphere and grapples with ongoing political instability and natural disasters. In 2010, an earthquake hit Haiti, devastating its economy and killing more than 300,000 people. In 2016, Hurricane Matthew struck the country, causing losses totaling 32 percent of its GDP. Haiti remains particularly vulnerable to natural disasters, with 96 percent of the population at risk.

With about 65 percent of the population living in poverty, one-quarter of Haitians are unable to cover basic food requirements, and more than 40 percent lack access to clean water. Non-communicable diseases such as ischemic heart disease, stroke, diabetes, congenital defects, and chronic kidney disease have notably increased in recent years as the cause of most deaths in Haiti. While some communicable diseases have decreased on average, lower respiratory infections, HIV/AIDS, neonatal disorders, and diarrheal diseases continue to be significant contributors to deaths in the country.

11.1M
Population

$755
GDP Per Capita

64 years
Life Expectancy
↑ Improving

23.4
Doctors/100k
Physician Density

71
Beds/100k
Hospital Bed Density

480
Deaths/100k
Maternal Mortality

Haiti

Healthcare Facilities

Alma Mater
Rue Balmir, Commune Gros Morne, Département de l'Artibonite, Haiti
https://vfapp.org/4644

Anse Rouge Hospital Anse Rouge (AFME)
Rue St. Joseph, Commune Anse Rouge, Département de l'Artibonite, Haiti
https://vfapp.org/eb93

Arcahaie Hospital Saint Joseph de Galilée
Rue Michel Lafrague, Commune Arcahaie, Département de l'Ouest, Haiti
https://vfapp.org/dd8f

AVSI
Boulevard des Americains, Port-au-Prince, Haiti
https://vfapp.org/f4f8

Baie de Henne
RD 102, Commune Bombardopolis, Département du Nord-Ouest, Haiti
https://vfapp.org/a2cb

Bishop Joseph M. Sullivan Hospital
Plaine Marion, Haiti
https://vfapp.org/32e3

Bon Samaritain des Roseaux
Commune Roseaux, Département de la Grande-Anse, Haiti
https://vfapp.org/5981

Cal de Madian
RD 201, Commune Petite Rivière de Nippes, Département des Nippes, Haiti
https://vfapp.org/48ec

CAL de Mont Organise
RD 602, Commune Mont Organisé, Département du Nord-Est, Haiti
https://vfapp.org/c982

Care SOS France
Rue du Calvaire, Commune Môle-Saint-Nicolas, Département du Nord-Ouest, Haiti
https://vfapp.org/6267

Carrefour Joute
RC 205C, Commune Saint-Jean-du-Sud, Département du Sud, Haiti
https://vfapp.org/f445

CBP St. Raphael
RD 103, Commune Saint-Raphaël, Département du Nord, Haiti
https://vfapp.org/39e4

Centre Ambulancier National
Delmas, Haiti
https://vfapp.org/4cb7

Centre Hospitalier Christian Martinez
1 Rue Beaudrouin, Commune Jacmel, Département du Sud-Est, Haiti
https://vfapp.org/5967

Centre Hospitalier de Lamardelle
RD 111, Commune Ganthier, Département de l'Ouest, Haiti
https://vfapp.org/f15f

Centre Hospitalier Fontaine
Cité Soleil, Port-au-Prince, Haiti
https://vfapp.org/ac3c

Com. Bonne Fin
RD 204, Commune Cavaillon, Département du Sud, Haiti
https://vfapp.org/79d5

Corail Hospital
Route Départementale # 703, Commune Corail, Département de la Grande-Anse, Haiti
https://vfapp.org/1e65

Croix Rouge Haitienne
Impasse Saint Joseph, Commune Arcahaie, Département de l'Ouest, Haiti
https://vfapp.org/ec89

Croix-Rouge at Fort-Liberté
Rue Sainte-Anne, Commune Fort-Liberté, Département du Nord-Est, Haiti
https://vfapp.org/eed6

Fonfred
Route la Fresiliere, Commune Torbeck, Département du Sud, Haiti
https://vfapp.org/ff54

French Hospital/Hôpital Français d'Haiti
Ruelle Nemour, Pòtoprens, Département de l'Ouest, Haiti
https://vfapp.org/7ba8

German Red Cross Basic Care Unit
Delmas 52, Commune de Delmas, Département de l'Ouest, Haiti
https://vfapp.org/343a

Gheskio
33 Boulevard Harry Truman, Pòtoprens, Département de l'Ouest, Haiti
https://vfapp.org/c282

Grace Children's Hospital
Delmas 31, Port-au-Prince, Haiti
https://vfapp.org/4e9f

Help Hospital
Rue Saint Laurent, Commune Léogâne, Département de l'Ouest, Haiti
https://vfapp.org/4aeb

Hospital Bethel Fonds-des-Nègres / Armée du Salut
RN 2, Commune Fonds-des-Nègres, Département des Nippes, Haiti
https://vfapp.org/4f73

Hospital Bonneau St. Joseph
Duval 37, Commune Croix-des-Bouquets, Département de l'Ouest, Haiti
https://vfapp.org/9188

Hospital Finca
Rue Simone Duvalier, Les Cayes, Haiti
https://vfapp.org/45aa

Hospital Fosref/Lakay Saint Marc
Saint-Marc, Haiti
https://vfapp.org/8c95

Hospital La Sainte Famille
Jedo, Jacmel, Département du Sud-Est, Haiti
https://vfapp.org/6583

Hospital Raboteau
16 Rue Frères Simmonds, Cité Militaire, Port-au-Prince, Haiti
https://vfapp.org/1912

Hôpital Adventiste d'Haïti
Diquini 63, Route de la Mairie de Carrefour, Kafou, Port-au-Prince Département de l'Ouest, Haiti
https://vfapp.org/13b5

Hôpital Albert Schweitzer (HAS)
Desjardines, Haiti
https://vfapp.org/be8a

Hôpital Alma Mater
RN 5, Commune Gros Morne, Département de l'Artibonite, Haiti
https://vfapp.org/d47b

Hôpital Beraca la Pointe
Rue Monfort, Commune de Port-de-Paix, Département du Nord-Ouest, Haiti
https://vfapp.org/7fe4

Hôpital Bienfaisance de Pignon
Rue Hôpital de Bienfaisance, Commune Pignon, Département du Nord, Haiti
https://vfapp.org/1c97

Hôpital Borgne
Rue des Pecheurs, Commune Borgne, Département du Nord, Haiti
https://vfapp.org/93e7

Hôpital Charles Colimon
Petite Rivière de l'Artibonite, Haiti
https://vfapp.org/5ce8

Hôpital Christ du Nord
Rues K et 17, Cap Haïtien, Haiti
https://vfapp.org/ac93

Hôpital Communautaire Autrichien-Haïtien
RC 102A, Commune Jean Rabel, Département du Nord-Ouest, Haiti
https://vfapp.org/bc11

Hôpital Communautaire de Référence Dr. Raoul Pierre-Louis
Carrefour, Haiti
https://vfapp.org/e348

Hôpital de Beudet
Rue Rigaud, Commune Croix-des-Bouquets, Département de l'Ouest, Haiti
https://vfapp.org/cfe7

Hôpital de la Communauté Dame-Marienne
220, Commune Dame-Marie, Département de la Grande-Anse, Haiti
https://vfapp.org/5f89

Hôpital de la Nativite
Grand Rue, Commune Belladère, Département du Centre, Haiti
https://vfapp.org/efc8

Hôpital de Petit Trou de Nippes
Boulevard de la Liberté, Commune Petit Trou de Nippes, Département des Nippes, Haiti
https://vfapp.org/72cd

Hôpital de Port-À-Piment
Port-À-Piment, Haiti
https://vfapp.org/435f

Hôpital de Robillard
Road to Citadelle, Commune de Milot, Département du Nord, Haiti
https://vfapp.org/9de6

Hôpital Dessalines Claire Heureuse
La Colline, Commune d'Aquin, Département du Sud, Haiti
https://vfapp.org/a65b

Hôpital Département de l'Ouest
Rue Haut Timo, Commune Léogâne, Département de l'Ouest, Haiti
https://vfapp.org/8975

Hôpital Espoir
Avenue Fragneauville, Commune de Delmas, Département de l'Ouest, Haiti
https://vfapp.org/eb3e

Hôpital Espérance
Route Grande-Savane, Commune Pilate, Département du Nord, Haiti
https://vfapp.org/9c82

Hôpital Français
378 Rue du Centre, Pòtoprens, Département de l'Ouest, Haiti
https://vfapp.org/66cd

Hôpital Glacis Courreaux
Château, Haiti
https://vfapp.org/6fb6

Hôpital Immaculée Conception
Rue Monseigneur Maurice, Commune Les Cayes, Département du Sud, Haiti
https://vfapp.org/ed4a

Hôpital Justinien
Rue 17 Q, Cap Haitien, Haiti
https://vfapp.org/f5cf

Hôpital La Providence des Gonaives
Gonaives, Haiti
https://vfapp.org/3566

Hôpital L'Eglise de Dieu Réformé
Saintard, Haiti
https://vfapp.org/ae26

Hôpital Notre Dame
32 RN 2, Arrondissement des Cayes, Haiti
https://vfapp.org/9e31

Hôpital Notre Dame de La Paix de Jean-Rabel
15, Rue Notre Dame, Jean-Rabel, Nord-Ouest, Haiti
https://vfapp.org/775f

Hôpital Notre Dame des Palmistes
Île de La Tortue, Département du Nord-Ouest, Haiti
https://vfapp.org/8873

Hôpital Saint Antoine
RC 205C, Commune Saint-Jean-du-Sud, Département du Sud, Haiti
https://vfapp.org/7131

Hôpital Saint Boniface
Fond-des-Blancs, Haiti
https://vfapp.org/5fcb

Hôpital Saint Landy
Rue Aubrant, Pétion-Ville, Haiti
https://vfapp.org/b889

Hôpital Saint Nicolas
Rue Savannah, Saint-Marc, Haiti
https://vfapp.org/835d

Hôpital Saint-Jean de Limbé
RN 1, Commune Limbé, Département du Nord, Haiti
https://vfapp.org/a676

Hôpital Saint-Pierre
RD 703, Commune Corail, Département de la Grande-Anse, Haiti
https://vfapp.org/5ca3

Hôpital Sainte Catherine
Avenue Soleil, Cité Soleil, Département de l'Ouest, Haiti
https://vfapp.org/48a2

Hôpital Sainte Croix
1 Rue La Croix, Commune Léogâne, Département de l'Ouest, Haiti
https://vfapp.org/e6b9

Hôpital Sainte Marie Etoile de Mer
Cite Soleil, Ojapon Bas Ti Ayiti, Haiti
https://vfapp.org/8422

Hôpital Sainte Thérèse de Hinche
Rue Paul Eugene Magloire, Commune Hinche, Département du Centre, Haiti
https://vfapp.org/5855

Hôpital Sainte Thérèse de Miragoâne
RD 201, Commune Miragoane, Département des Nippes, Haiti
https://vfapp.org/d96c

Hôpital Sainte-Anne
HT-7, Camp Perrin, Haiti
https://vfapp.org/a125

Hôpital Universitaire de la Paix
Delmas 33, Delmas, Haiti
https://vfapp.org/887c

Hôpital Universitaire de Mirebalais
RD 11, Arrondissement de Mirebalais, Haiti
https://vfapp.org/71b2

Institut Fame Pereo
Pòtoprens, Département de l'Ouest, Haiti
https://vfapp.org/e873

Jeremie Hôpital la Source
Rue Source Dommage, Commune de Jérémie, Département de la Grande-Anse, Haiti
https://vfapp.org/ee83

Kay Sante Pa' W
Rue Jean Baptiste Point du Sable, Commune de Saint-Marc, Département de l'Artibonite, Haiti
https://vfapp.org/3bbb

King's Hospital
Route Petite Place Cazeau, Caradeux, Haiti
https://vfapp.org/3d4d

Medimax Hospital
Avenue Christophe, Pòtoprens, Département de l'Ouest, Haiti
https://vfapp.org/3f19

Miragoane District Hospital
RN 2, Commune Miragoane, Département des Nippes, Haiti
https://vfapp.org/bec1

Miragoane Hospital Paillant
RD 201, Commune Miragoane, Département des Nippes, Haiti
https://vfapp.org/fb63

Mombin Crochu Hospital
Rue Salomon, Commune La Victoire, Département du Nord, Haiti
https://vfapp.org/fa75

Mont Organisé Hospital
RD 602, Commune Mont Organisé, Département du Nord-Est, Haiti
🌐 https://vfapp.org/e174

Notre Dame des Pins d'Orianie
RD 112, Commune Fonds-Verettes, Département du Sud-Est, Haiti
🌐 https://vfapp.org/3498

Ouanaminthe Hospital
RN 6, Commune Ouanaminthe, Département du Nord-Est, Haiti
🌐 https://vfapp.org/b95c

Port Au Prince Hospital Minustah
Boulevard Toussaint Louverture, Commune de Tabarre, Département de l'Ouest, Haiti
🌐 https://vfapp.org/a546

Presidente Néstor C Kirchner Hospital
Corail, Haiti
🌐 https://vfapp.org/e47f

Saint Luke Hospital Croix de Bouquets
Croix-des-Bouquets, Haiti
🌐 https://vfapp.org/dbad

Sainte Claire de Corail
RN 7, Commune Beaumont, Département de la Grande-Anse, Haiti
🌐 https://vfapp.org/da44

Santé Pour Tous
Impasse Colas, Kafou, Département de l'Ouest, Haiti
🌐 https://vfapp.org/f347

Savanne à Roche
Commune Petite Rivière de l'Artibonite, Département de l'Artibonite, Haiti
🌐 https://vfapp.org/4f79

SKS Petite Rivière de Dame Marie
RD 702, Commune Dame-Marie, Département de la Grande-Anse, Haiti
🌐 https://vfapp.org/5d4a

St. Damien's Pediatric Hospital
Port-au-Prince, Haiti
🌐 https://vfapp.org/6eb2

State University of Haiti Hospital
Avenue Monseigneur Guilloux, Pòtoprens, Département de l'Ouest, Haiti
🌐 https://vfapp.org/3182

Wesleyan Hospital
Anse-à-Galets, La Gonave, Haiti
🌐 https://vfapp.org/5549

Haiti

Nonprofit Organizations

100X Development Foundation
Empowers children and families for a more hopeful and productive future through the support and care of orphaned children, education and job training for those in need, help for vulnerable youth to escape trafficking, and healthy nutrition and medical care for mothers to enable a safe birth.

ER Med, Infect Dis, OB-GYN, Peds, Psych
📞 +1 334-387-1178
🌐 https://vfapp.org/b629

Abt Associates
Seeks to improve the quality of life and economic well-being of people worldwide, while striving to meet and exceed the highest professional standards.

General, Logist-Op, MF Med, OB-GYN, Peds
📞 +1 212-779-7700
🌐 https://vfapp.org/cec2

Action Against Hunger
Aims to end life-threatening hunger for good through treating and preventing malnutrition across more than forty-five countries.

📞 +1 212-967-7800
🌐 https://vfapp.org/2dbc

Adventist Health International
Focuses on upgrading and managing mission hospitals by providing governance, consultation, and technical assistance to a number of affiliated Seventh-Day Adventist hospitals throughout Africa, Asia, and the Americas.

Dent-OMFS, General, Pub Health
📞 +1 909-558-5610
🌐 https://vfapp.org/16aa

Agape Global Health for Haiti
Seeks to provide direct medical care, public health education, water filtration kits, and prenatal care to people in La Gonave, Haiti, by utilizing a team of volunteers who are dedicated, knowledgeable, caring professionals with diverse experiences.

General, MF Med, OB-GYN, Peds, Pub Health
📞 +1 401-423-3550
🌐 https://vfapp.org/5139

Aid for Haiti
Seeks to share Christian faith with the people of Haiti through compassionate healthcare, spiritual ministry, and training for service.

ER Med, General, Nutr, OB-GYN, Pub Health
📞 +1 931-635-3531
🌐 https://vfapp.org/96f3

AIDS Healthcare Foundation
Provides cutting-edge HIV/AIDS medical care and advocacy to over one million people in forty-three countries.

Infect Dis
📞 +1 323-860-5200
🌐 https://vfapp.org/b27c

Albert Schweitzer Hospital
Seeks to collaborate with the people of the Artibonite Valley as they strive to improve their health and quality of life. Operates a 131-bed hospital with 24/7 full service; provides access to healthcare for people living in remote areas.

Anesth, Crit-Care, ER Med, Infect Dis, MF Med, Medicine, OB-GYN, Path, Ped Surg, Peds, Radiol, Rehab, Surg
📞 +1 412-361-5200
🌐 https://vfapp.org/c554

Alliance for Children Foundation
Seeks to improve the lives of orphaned and at-risk children and their families where the need is greatest worldwide by working with local partners to provide food, shelter, medical care, and educational programs to the most vulnerable children and families.

General, Nutr, Ped Surg, Peds
📞 +1 781-444-7148
🌐 https://vfapp.org/7acb

American Academy of Ophthalmology
Protects sight and empowers lives by serving as an advocate for patients and the public, leading ophthalmic education, and advancing the profession of ophthalmology.

Ophth-Opt
📞 +1 415-561-8500
🌐 https://vfapp.org/89a2

American Academy of Pediatrics
Seeks to attain optimal physical, mental, and social health and well-being for all infants, children, adolescents, and young adults.

Anesth, Crit-Care, Neonat, Ped Surg
📞 +1 800-433-9016
🌐 https://vfapp.org/9633

Americares

Saves lives and improves health for people affected by poverty or disaster and responds with life-changing medicine, medical supplies, and health programs including domestic and global medical clinics.

All-Immu, ER Med, General, Infect Dis, MF Med, Nutr

+1 203-658-9500

https://vfapp.org/e567

Angel Wings International

Provides compassionate and comprehensive medical care to the underserved people of Haiti by developing the local medical professions and the skill sets of the local population.

ER Med, General, OB-GYN, Peds

+1 954-417-5868

https://vfapp.org/f6c7

Association Haïtienne de Développement Humain (AHDH)

Promotes the welfare of Haitians by contributing to or instituting humanitarian programs in health, education, culture, and development in Haiti and Louisiana.

ENT, General, MF Med, OB-GYN, Ophth-Opt, Peds, Pub Health, Surg

+1 504-957-6233

https://vfapp.org/e462

Association of Haitian Physicians Abroad (AMHE)

Provides professional members a conduit to address the medical needs and concerns of the Haitian community at home and abroad.

General, Medicine, OB-GYN, Ophth-Opt, Peds, Surg

+1 718-245-1015

https://vfapp.org/4599

Association of Medical Doctors of Asia (AMDA)

Strives to support people affected by disasters and economic distress on their road to recovery, establishing a true partnership with special emphasis on local initiative.

ER Med, Logist-Op, Pub Health

+81 86-252-6051

https://vfapp.org/e3d4

Barco's Nightingales Foundation

Aims to honor the women and men who embrace the profession of nursing for their selfless contributions, dedication, and professionalism by focusing its philanthropic efforts on helping children.

General, Heme-Onc, Peds, Plast

+1 310-719-2108

https://vfapp.org/a82d

Basic Foundations

Supports local projects and organizations that seek to meet the basic human needs of others in their community.

ER Med, General, Peds, Rehab, Surg

https://vfapp.org/c4be

Basic Health International

Seeks to eliminate cervical cancer by conducting cutting-edge research on early prevention and treatment as well as implementing sustainable strategies that can be scaled in limited resource settings.

Infect Dis, OB-GYN

+1 646-593-8694

https://vfapp.org/24c9

Batey Relief Alliance

Addresses socio-economic and health needs of children and their families severely affected by poverty, disease, and hunger in the Caribbean, through health, agricultural/cooperative, and development programs.

General

https://vfapp.org/773b

Benjamin H. Josephson, MD Fund

Provides healthcare professionals with the financial resources necessary to deliver medical services for those in need throughout the world.

General, OB-GYN

+1 908-522-2853

https://vfapp.org/6acc

Bethesda Evangelical Mission (BEM)

Provides essential medicines, lifesaving baby formula, training, and education for women and children, prevention and eradication of disease, and promotes better health in some of the most neglected areas of southern Haiti.

General, MF Med, OB-GYN, Peds

https://vfapp.org/45a7

Bicol Clinic Foundation Inc.

Treats patients primarily in the Philippines, Nepal, Haiti, and locally in the USA, while constructing a permanent outpatient clinic in the Bicol region of the Philippines and establishing a disaster-relief fund.

Crit-Care, Derm, ENT, ER Med, Endo, General, Infect Dis, MF Med, Medicine, Nutr, OB-GYN, Ophth-Opt, Pub Health, Surg, Urol

+1 561-864-0298

https://vfapp.org/3f9e

Boston Children's Hospital: Global Health Program

Helps solve pediatric global health care challenges by transferring expertise through long-term partnerships with scalable impact, while working in the field to strengthen healthcare systems, advocate, research and provide care delivery or education as a way of sustainably improving the health of children worldwide.

Anesth, CV Med, Crit-Care, ER Med, Heme-Onc, Infect Dis, Medicine, Nutr, Palliative, Ped Surg, Peds

+1 617-919-6438

https://vfapp.org/f9f8

Bridge of Life

Aims to strengthen healthcare globally through sustainable programs that prevent and treat chronic disease.

Logist-Op, Nephro, OB-GYN, Peds, Surg

+1 888-374-8185

https://vfapp.org/5b68

Brigham and Women's Center for Surgery and Public Health

Advances the science of surgical care delivery by studying effectiveness, quality, equity, and value at the population level, and develops surgeon-scientists committed to excellence in these areas.

Anesth, ER Med, Infect Dis, Pub Health, Surg

+1 617-525-7300

https://vfapp.org/5d64

Brigham and Women's Hospital Global Health Hub

Cares for patients in underserved settings, provides education to staff who work in those areas to create sustainable change, and conducts research designed to improve health in such settings.

General, Infect Dis

https://vfapp.org/a8a3

Brothers Keepers of Haiti

Cultivates empathy and compassion, serves the less fortunate, and cares for the tridimensional well-being of people (mind, body, and spirit) in rural Southeast Haiti (specifically in Jacmel, Cayes-Jacmel, and Orangers), inspired by the Christian faith.

General, Nutr

+1 321-593-3380

https://vfapp.org/6345

Buddhist Tzu Chi Medical Foundation

Provides healthcare to the poor, operates six hospitals in Taiwan and mobile medical and dental clinics in the U.S., manages a bone marrow bank, and organizes over 8,600 physicians who provide free medical services to more than 2 million people globally.

Crit-Care, Dent-OMFS, ER Med, General

+1 626-427-9598

https://vfapp.org/ff61

Burn Advocates

Supports burn survivors as they face the challenges of recovery, rehabilitation, and reintegration.

Anesth, Crit-Care, Derm, Ped Surg, Plast, Rehab, Rehab

+1 844-287-6411

https://vfapp.org/9327

Canadian Medical Assistance Teams (CMAT)

Provides relief and medical aid to the victims of natural and man-made disasters around the world.

Anesth, ER Med, Medicine, OB-GYN, Peds, Psych, Rehab, Surg

+1 855-637-9111

https://vfapp.org/5232

Cap Haitien Dental Institute

Provides oral healthcare in Haiti, serves as a base clinic for outreach mobile dentistry, and provides service opportunities for visiting dentists and non-healthcare workers.

Dent-OMFS

+1 440-541-6889

https://vfapp.org/2b9c

CapraCare

Provides access to medical care, preventive healthcare, mental health services, and health and nutrition education regardless of ability to pay for women, children, families, and the community to combat the physical, psychosocial, and environmental needs from living in Fronfrede, Haiti.

ER Med, General, Medicine, OB-GYN, Peds, Psych

https://vfapp.org/6c94

CardioStart International

Provides free heart surgery and associated medical care to children and adults living in underserved regions of the world, irrespective of political or religious affiliation, through the collective skills of healthcare experts.

Anesth, CT Surg, CV Med, Crit-Care, Pub Health, Pulm-Critic

+1 813-304-2163

https://vfapp.org/85ef

CARE

Works around the globe to save lives, defeat poverty, and achieve social justice.

ER Med, General

+1 800-422-7385

https://vfapp.org/7232

Care 2 Communities (C2C)

Provides vulnerable families access to sustainable, high-quality healthcare services.

General, Logist-Op, MF Med, Neonat

+1 617-559-1032

https://vfapp.org/cb1d

Carter Center, The

Seeks to prevent and resolve conflicts, enhance freedom and democracy, and improve health, while remaining committed to human rights and the alleviation of human suffering.

Infect Dis, MF Med, Ophth-Opt

+1 800-550-3560

https://vfapp.org/6556

Catholic Medical Mission Board (CMMB)

Works in partnership globally to deliver locally sustainable, quality health solutions to women, children, and their communities.

General, MF Med, Peds

+1 800-678-5659

https://vfapp.org/9498

Catholic World Mission

Works to rebuild communities worldwide by helping to alleviate poverty and empower underserved areas, while spreading the message of the Catholic Church.

ER Med, General, Nutr, Peds

+1 770-828-4966

https://vfapp.org/7b5f

Centre Médical Béraca (CMB)

Provides compassionate and quality care, inspired by the Christian faith.

Anesth, CV Med, Endo, Infect Dis, Logist-Op, Medicine, Nephro, Neuro, OB-GYN, Ortho, Path, Ped Surg, Peds, Pub Health, Pulm-Critic, Radiol, Surg

+509 36 12 1867

https://vfapp.org/dc1c

Chain of Hope

Provides lifesaving heart operations for children around the world and supports the development of cardiac services in numerous developing and war-torn countries.

Anesth, CT Surg, CV Med, Crit-Care, Ped Surg, Peds, Pulm-Critic, Surg

+44 20 7351 1978

https://vfapp.org/1b1b

Chain of Hope (La Chaîne de l'Espoir)

Helps underprivileged children around the world by providing them with access to healthcare.

Anesth, CT Surg, Crit-Care, ER Med, Neurosurg, Ortho, Ped Surg, Surg, Vasc Surg

+33 1 44 12 66 66

https://vfapp.org/e871

Chances for Children

Aims to return children to good health through medical attention and good nutrition in a supportive, faith-based environment that is conducive to their emotional and physical development.

Dent-OMFS, General, Path, Peds

+1 480-659-7625

https://vfapp.org/4f75

CharityVision International

Focuses on restoring curable sight impairment worldwide by empowering local physicians and creating sustainable solutions.

Logist-Op, Ophth-Opt, Surg

+1 435-200-4910

https://vfapp.org/6231

Cheerful Heart Mission

Aims to improve the lives of the underprivileged people living on the border of the Dominican Republic and Haiti by funding and managing programs focused on health, education, and economic development.

Dent-OMFS, General, Infect Dis, Peds

+1 973-632-9912

https://vfapp.org/ff1e

Children & Charity International

Puts people first by providing education, leadership, and nutrition programs along with mentoring and healthcare support services to children, youth, and families.

Nutr, Peds

+1 202-234-0488

https://vfapp.org/6538

Children of the Nations

Aims to raise children out of poverty and hopelessness so they can become leaders who transform their nations. Emphasizes caring for the whole child–physically, mentally, socially, and spiritually.

Anesth, Dent-OMFS, General, Surg

+1 360-698-7227

https://vfapp.org/cc52

Children's Health Ministries

Fights to eliminate preventable infant and child deaths due to malnutrition, prematurity, and treatable diseases.

Crit-Care, General, MF Med, Neonat, Nutr, OB-GYN, Peds

+509 42 11 5356

https://vfapp.org/8d86

Children's Surgery International

Provides free medical and surgical services to children in need around the world, and instruction and training to local surgeons and other medical providers such as doctors, anesthesiologists, nurses, and technicians.

Anesth, Dent-OMFS, Ortho, Ped Surg, Peds, Plast, Surg

+1 612-746-4082

https://vfapp.org/26d3

Christian Aid Ministries

Strives to be a trustworthy and efficient channel for Amish, Mennonite, and other conservative Anabaptist groups and individuals to minister to physical and spiritual needs around the world.

CT Surg, ER Med, Logist-Op, Ortho, Pub Health

+1 330-893-2428

https://vfapp.org/7b33

Christian Blind Mission (CBM)

Aims to improve the quality of life of persons with disabilities in the poorest countries, addressing poverty as a cause, and a consequence, of disability, and working in partnership to create a society for all.

ENT, General, Infect Dis, OB-GYN, Ophth-Opt, Ortho, Peds, Psych, Rehab, Surg

+49 6251 131131

https://vfapp.org/3824

Christian Health Service Corps

Brings Christian doctors, health professionals, and health educators who are committed to serving the poor to places that have little or no access to healthcare.

Anesth, Dent-OMFS, General, Medicine, Peds, Surg

+1 903-962-4000

https://vfapp.org/da57

Christie's Heart Samaritan Care Foundation

Addresses the negative impacts of a lack of available outreach services for the underserved populations of Haiti, Dominican Republic, and the United States through medical services and basic needs support.

All-Immu, General, Nutr, Ophth-Opt, Peds

+1 407-442-9845

https://vfapp.org/522e

Circle of Health International (COHI)

Aligns with local, community-based organizations led and powered by women to help respond to the needs of the women and children that they serve. Helps with the provision of professional volunteers, capacity training, and procurement of requested and appropriate supplies and equipment. Raises funds for the organizations to provide the services required.

ER Med, Logist-Op, MF Med, Neonat, OB-GYN, Psych

+1 512-210-7710

https://vfapp.org/8b63

Clinton Health Access Initiative (CHAI)

Aims to save lives and reduce the burden of disease in low- and middle-income countries. Works with partners to strengthen the capabilities of governments and the private sector to create and sustain high-quality health systems.

General, Heme-Onc, Infect Dis, Logist-Op, MF Med, Medicine, Neonat, Nutr, OB-GYN, Path, Peds, Rad-Onc

+1 617-774-0110

https://vfapp.org/9ed7

Cloud Foundation

Provides access to healthcare for medically underserved communities in the Haitian countryside.

ER Med, General, Logist-Op, Peds

+1 240-475-1253

https://vfapp.org/a467

Columbia University: Columbia Office of Global Surgery (COGS)

Helps to increase access to safe and affordable surgical care, as a means to reduce health disparities and the global burden of disease.

Anesth, CT Surg, Crit-Care, Dent-OMFS, ENT, ER Med, Infect Dis, MF Med, Neurosurg, OB-GYN, Ophth-Opt, Ortho, Ped Surg, Plast, Plast, Pub Health, Surg, Urol

https://vfapp.org/4349

Columbia University: Global Mental Health Programs
Pioneers research initiatives, promotes mental health, and aims to reduce the burden of mental illness worldwide.
Psych
+1 646-774-5308
https://vfapp.org/c5cd

Combat Blindness International
Works to eliminate preventable blindness worldwide by providing sustainable, equitable solutions for sight through partnerships and innovation.
Ophth-Opt
+1 608-238-7777
https://vfapp.org/28ad

Community Coalition for Haiti (CCH)
Transforms lives through long-term and community-driven solutions in healthcare, education, and community development.
Anesth, General, Surg
+1 571-250-6554
https://vfapp.org/96dc

Community Health Initiative Haiti
Works to create healthy, empowered, and self-directed communities in Haiti.
General, Logist-Op, Nutr, Peds, Surg
+1 319-313-6619
https://vfapp.org/418a

Community Organized Relief Effort (CORE)
Saves lives and strengthens communities impacted by or vulnerable to crisis.
ER Med
+1 323-934-4400
https://vfapp.org/36dd

Concern Worldwide
Provides education, healthcare, and clothing to children on the northern coast of Haiti.
Logist-Op, MF Med, Nutr, OB-GYN
+353 1 417 7700
https://vfapp.org/77e9

Concerned Haitian Americans of Illinois – C.H.A.I.
Makes an impactful difference in the Haitian community by providing education, healthcare, and clothing to children on the northern coast of Haiti.
General, Logist-Op, Nutr
+1 773-242-9007
https://vfapp.org/684c

Consider Haiti
Works to support grassroot efforts to create sustainable nutrition and medical support.
General, Nutr, Peds
+1 828-209-8780
https://vfapp.org/52c8

Core Group
Aims to improve and expand community health practices for underserved populations, especially women and children, through collaborative action and learning.
General, Infect Dis, MF Med, Medicine, OB-GYN, Peds, Pub Health
+1 202-380-3400
https://vfapp.org/9de3

Critical Care Disaster Foundation
Seeks to educate in-country healthcare providers from developing countries in disaster and crisis medical management and to develop an infrastructure of critical care services.
Anesth, Crit-Care, ER Med, Logist-Op, Pulm-Critic
https://vfapp.org/a445

CRUDEM Foundation, The
Provides quality healthcare to the sick and the poor in the Haitian community.
All-Immu, General, Heme-Onc, Infect Dis, Nutr, Peds
+1 413-642-0450
https://vfapp.org/8c93

Curamericas Global
Partners with communities abroad to save the lives of mothers and children by providing health services and education.
General, Infect Dis, MF Med, OB-GYN, Peds, Pub Health
+1 919-510-8787
https://vfapp.org/286b

CureCervicalCancer
Focuses on the early detection and prevention of cervical cancer around the globe for the women who need it most.
Heme-Onc, OB-GYN
+1 310-601-3002
https://vfapp.org/ace1

Danita's Children
Strives to care for orphans and impoverished children in Haiti by providing education, nutrition, medical, and dental care as well as a nurturing environment to the children and families served.
Dent-OMFS, Peds, Surg
+1 615-721-8433
https://vfapp.org/e889

Direct Relief
Improves the health and lives of people affected by poverty or emergency situations by mobilizing and providing essential medical resources needed for their care.
ER Med, Logist-Op
+1 805-964-4767
https://vfapp.org/58e5

Doctors Without Borders/Médecins Sans Frontières (MSF)
Responds to emergencies and provides lifesaving medical care where needed most, including during disasters, conflicts, and epidemics.
Anesth, Crit-Care, ER Med, General, Infect Dis, Nutr, OB-GYN, Ped Surg, Peds, Psych, Pub Health, Surg
+1 212-679-6800
https://vfapp.org/f363

Dorsainvil Foundation
Provides free medical treatment and healthcare education at the Complexe Medical Sainte Philomene De L'Arcahaie, Haiti.
General, Pub Health
+1 561-843-0578
https://vfapp.org/799f

Douleurs Sans Frontières (Pain Without Borders)
Supports local actors in taking charge of the assessment and treatment of pain and suffering, in an integrated manner and adapted to the realities of each country.
Anesth, Palliative, Psych, Rehab
+33 1 48 78 38 42
https://vfapp.org/324c

Duke University: Global Health Institute
Sparks innovation in global health research and education, and brings together knowledge and resources to address the most important global health issues of our time.
All-Immu, Infect Dis, MF Med, OB-GYN, Pub Health
+1 919-681-7760
https://vfapp.org/c4cd

Edwards Lifesciences
Provides innovative solutions for people fighting cardiovascular disease, as a global leader in patient-focused medical innovations for structural heart disease, as well as critical care and surgical monitoring.
Anesth, CT Surg, CV Med, Crit-Care, Ped Surg, Peds, Pulm-Critic, Surg, Vasc Surg
+1 949-250-5176
https://vfapp.org/d671

Emory Haiti Alliance
Provides essential surgical services to improve patient quality of life, engages in collaborative educational efforts with local healthcare staff, and assists in local healthcare infrastructure
in the town of Pignon within the Central Plateau of Haiti.
Anesth, General, Surg, Urol
+1 404-727-9110
https://vfapp.org/8c8f

Emory University School of Medicine
Aims to provide residents/fellows from clinical departments with knowledge and practical experience in global health by building ongoing collaborations between Emory University and academic instituions abroad.
Anesth, CV Med, General, Infect Dis, Pulm-Critic, Rheum, Surg
+1 404-778-7777
https://vfapp.org/a6f7

Emory University School of Medicine: Global Surgery Program
A leading institution with the highest standards in education, biomedical research, and patient care.
Anesth, Dent-OMFS, ER Med, Pub Health, Surg, Urol
+1 404-727-5660
https://vfapp.org/2b26

Episcopal Relief & Development
Provides relief in times of disaster and promotes sustainable development by identifying and addressing the root causes of suffering.
Infect Dis, MF Med, Neonat, Nutr, Peds
+1 855-312-4325
https://vfapp.org/7cfa

eRanger
Provides sustainable solutions to transportation and medical provision such as ambulances and mobile clinics in developing countries.
ER Med, General, Logist-Op
+27 40 654 3207
https://vfapp.org/4c18

Espwa Foundation, The
Develops projects that empower the people of Haiti, alleviate poverty, build relationships, and ultimately encourage hope, inspired by the Christian faith.
General, Infect Dis, Nutr, Peds
+1 571-234-1643
https://vfapp.org/3252

Evidence Project, The
Improves family-planning policies, programs, and practices through the strategic generation, translation, and use of evidence.
General, MF Med
+1 202-237-9400
https://vfapp.org/f9e7

Eye Foundation of America
Works toward a world without childhood blindness.
Ophth-Opt
+1 304-599-0705
https://vfapp.org/a7eb

F-M Haiti Medical Mission
Aims to provide surgery and improve the healthcare and lives of people in the village of Pignon, Haiti.
General, Ped Surg, Surg
+1 701-412-5643
https://vfapp.org/5fef

Fondation Hôpital Bon Samaritain (HBS)
Provides healthcare services and outreach for the greater population of Haiti's Limbé Valley located in the Département du Nord.
General, MF Med, OB-GYN, Peds
+1 561-246-3360
https://vfapp.org/258e

Forward in Health
Provides medical aid to the people of Fonfred, Haiti, by bringing quality healthcare to the region, one patient at a time.
General, Infect Dis, MF Med, Ortho
+1 978-808-5234
https://vfapp.org/ed32

Foundation for Hope and Health in Haiti (FHHH), The
Provides access to quality medical care to underserved areas in Haiti.
General, MF Med, OB-GYN, Peds
+1 516-489-3681
https://vfapp.org/c8c6

Foundation for Peace
Works with local communities to build schools, medical clinics, water purification facilities, churches, and more.
General, Infect Dis
+1 973-988-1484
https://vfapp.org/e9f7

Friends for Health in Haiti
Aims to improve the health of the people of Haiti in a caring, compassionate manner and seeks to develop a medical facility that

will provide primary healthcare to people of all ages.
ER Med, General
+1 262-227-9581
https://vfapp.org/c7ed

Friends of Haiti
Combines mutual efforts to improve health, education, and economic development in four sections of Thomazeau, Haiti.
Anesth, Dent-OMFS, Ophth-Opt, Surg
https://vfapp.org/eb17

Friends of the Children Medical Mission
Provides medical care and education to the people of LaMontagne, Haiti, during mission trips throughout the year.
General, MF Med, Medicine, Peds, Psych, Rehab
+1 815-540-6976
https://vfapp.org/2377

Friends of the Children of Haiti (FOTCOH)
Provides healthcare and hope to the children of Haiti.
Dent-OMFS, General, Nutr, OB-GYN, Surg
+1 815-310-5872
https://vfapp.org/9424

Friends of UNFPA
Promotes the health, dignity, and rights of women and girls around the world by supporting the lifesaving work of UNFPA, the United Nations reproductive health and rights agency, through education, advocacy, and fundraising.
MF Med, OB-GYN
+1 646-649-9100
https://vfapp.org/2a3a

Functional Literacy Ministry of Haiti: Educational & Medical Mission
Provides healthcare, education, trade skills, and employment to improve the quality of life in Haitian communities.
Dent-OMFS, MF Med, Nutr, OB-GYN, Ophth-Opt, Peds
+1 412-784-0342
https://vfapp.org/f44c

Gaskov Clergé Foundation (GCF)
Promotes health, sports, education, and sciences in both the United States and Haiti through scholarship programs for students.
CV Med, Dent-OMFS, Neuro, OB-GYN, Peds, Psych
+1 561-510-1113
https://vfapp.org/a75e

Gift of Life International
Provides lifesaving cardiac treatment to children in developing countries while developing sustainable pediatric cardiac programs by implementing screening, surgical, and training missions.
Anesth, CT Surg, CV Med, Crit-Care, Ped Surg, Peds, Pulm-Critic
+1 855-734-3278
https://vfapp.org/f2f9

Gift of Sight
Works to eradicate preventable blindness by fostering sustainable healthcare delivery in underserved, global communities.
Ophth-Opt
https://vfapp.org/fdd7

Global Alliance to Prevent Prematurity and Stillbirth (GAPPS)
Seeks to improve birth outcomes worldwide by reducing the burden of premature birth and stillbirth.
All-Immu, Infect Dis, MF Med, Neonat, Neonat, OB-GYN
+1 206-413-7954
https://vfapp.org/3f74

Global Eye Project
Empowers local communities by building locally managed, sustainable eye clinics through education initiatives and volunteer-run professional training services.
Anesth, Ophth-Opt, Surg
https://vfapp.org/cdba

Global First Responder (GFR)
Acts as a centralized network for individuals and agencies involved in relief work worldwide and organizes and executes mission trips to areas in need, focusing not only on healthcare delivery but also health education and improvements.
ER Med
+1 573-424-8370
https://vfapp.org/a3e1

Global Force for Healing
Works to end preventable maternal and newborn deaths by supporting the scaling of effective grassroots. community-led, culturally respectful care and education in underserved areas around the globe using the midwifery model of care.
Neonat, OB-GYN
https://vfapp.org/deb2

Global Healing
Improves access to high-quality healthcare in underserved countries by training medical professionals across the globe to improve pediatric healthcare utilizing sustainable resources.
ER Med, General, Heme-Onc, Path
+1 510-898-1859
https://vfapp.org/a787

Global Health Teams
Provides quality medical care and services to people in great need, supporting medical clinics in rural Southwestern Haiti and providing critical medical services in impoverished, remote areas.
General, Infect Dis, MF Med, Medicine, OB-GYN, Peds
+1 619-905-7157
https://vfapp.org/1f33

Global Health Volunteers
Serves together with in-country partners to provide a transforming healing presence to the poor and underserved within communities in the developing world.
ER Med, General, Ophth-Opt, Rehab
+1 610-355-2003
https://vfapp.org/a3f1

Global Medical Missions Alliance
Brings and promotes Christian-centered missional life to the body

of healthcare professionals and its partners.
Dent-OMFS, ER Med, Pub Health, Rehab, Surg
+1 714-444-3032
https://vfapp.org/29c7

Global Ministries – The United Methodist Church
As the worldwide mission and development agency of The United Methodist Church, Global Ministries works with more than 300 hospitals and clinics around the world through its Global Health Unit.
Anesth, CT Surg, CV Med, Crit-Care, Dent-OMFS, Derm, ER Med, GI, General, Infect Dis, Logist-Op, MF Med, Medicine, Neonat, Nephro, Nutr, OB-GYN, Ophth-Opt, Ortho, Palliative, Peds, Pod, Psych, Pub Health, Rehab, Rheum, Surg, Urol
+1 800-862-4246
https://vfapp.org/1723

Global Offsite Care
Aims to be a catalyst for increasing access to specialized healthcare for all, and provides technology platforms to doctors and clinics around the world through rotary club–sponsored telemedicine projects.
Crit-Care, ER Med, General, Pulm-Critic
+1 707-827-1524
https://vfapp.org/61b5

Global Oncology (GO)
Brings the best in cancer care to underserved patients around the world and collaborates across geographic, professional, and academic borders to improve cancer care, research, and education.
Heme-Onc, Path, Rad-Onc
https://vfapp.org/fcb8

Global Surgical Access Foundation
Partners with underserved communities to provide competent, safe, and sustainable surgical care.
Anesth, Surg
+1 786-223-5046
https://vfapp.org/ea5f

Global Therapy Group
Strives to provide rehabilitation services and sustainable therapy to the people of Haiti.
ER Med, General, Ortho, Rehab
https://vfapp.org/6bcb

GOAL
Works with the most vulnerable communities to help them respond to and recover from humanitarian crises, and to assist them in building transcendent solutions to mitigate poverty and vulnerability.
ER Med, General, Pub Health
+353 1 280 9779
https://vfapp.org/bbea

God's Littlest Angels (GLA)
Provides exceptional neonatal care and a safe haven to the smallest, sickest, and most vulnerable children of Haiti.
MF Med, Neonat, OB-GYN, Peds
+1 719-638-4348
https://vfapp.org/a49e

Grand Anse Surgery Project
Works to holistically and passionately fulfill society's obligation to provide quality surgical care for all by providing surgical care for the residents of Jeremie, Haiti.
Anesth, CT Surg, Endo, Ortho, Plast, Surg
+1 860-573-9287
https://vfapp.org/bcf3

Grassroot Soccer
Leverages the power of soccer to educate, inspire, and mobilize at risk youth in developing countries to overcome their greatest health challenges, live healthier more productive lives, and be agents for change in their communities.
Infect Dis
+1 603-277-9685
https://vfapp.org/3521

Haiti Cardiac Alliance
Works with partners to scale up the availability of lifesaving cardiac surgery to all Haitian children who need it.
Anesth, CT Surg, CV Med, Crit-Care, Peds
+1 617-447-7288
https://vfapp.org/ee78

Haiti Clinic
Works to improve healthcare and health education in the impoverished nation of Haiti.
Dent-OMFS, General, Infect Dis, MF Med
+1 772-226-0403
https://vfapp.org/183c

Haiti Companions
Provides medical, dental, and eye care to three communities in Gressier, Haiti. Except for occasional visits by American providers, all of the medical providers are Haitian and honored to be serving members of their own community.
Dent-OMFS, General, Ophth-Opt
https://vfapp.org/85ea

Haiti Eye Mission
Seeks to provide eye care in Pignon, one of Haiti's most severely impoverished commmunities, to fight preventable and curable blindness through annual medical mission trips, and to build awareness and support networks.
Anesth, Ophth-Opt
+1 701-235-5200
https://vfapp.org/a1d1

Haiti Health & Rehabilitation
Seeks to improve the quality of life in Haiti through healthcare, education, rehabilitation, and nutrition, and aims to improve the health and well-being of the sick and the disabled.
Nutr, Peds, Pub Health
+1 321-536-1986
https://vfapp.org/d8d2

Haiti Health Initiative
Aims to improve the overall health and well-being of rural Haitians, one community at a time, by providing education and services in primary healthcare, dental care, public health, and nutrition.
Dent-OMFS, General, Infect Dis, Nutr, Ophth-Opt
+1 801-830-3043
https://vfapp.org/2f29

Haiti Health Ministries
Provides medical care and ministry through an outpatient medical clinic in Gressier, Haiti.
General, Infect Dis, MF Med, Peds, Radiol, Surg

+1 620-446-9797
https://vfapp.org/11e2

Haiti Health Trust, The
Provides high-quality health and disability care to the most vulnerable in Haiti.
General, Infect Dis, MF Med, Peds, Rehab
https://vfapp.org/e346

Haiti Medical Mission of Wisconsin
Serves the people of rural and remote southeast Haiti by improving access to healthcare through a partnership with Centre de Santé Sacré-Cœur de Thiotte.
Crit-Care, Dent-OMFS, ER Med, General, Ophth-Opt, Ped Surg, Surg
+1 608-556-9775
https://vfapp.org/fdee

Haiti Mobile Medical Mission
Works with Haitian health officials to set up medical clinics in the most underserved communities of Leogane Haiti.
Dent-OMFS, General
https://vfapp.org/24ae

Haiti Neurosurgery Initiative (HNI)
Strives to develop and support a sustainable model of clinical neurosurgical coverage in Haiti.
Neurosurg
https://vfapp.org/955c

Haiti Now
Works to improve the lives of more than 700 impoverished children in Haiti, with a goal of empowering former Restavek girls to achieve a lifetime of emotional and economic self-reliance.
General, Genetics, OB-GYN, Psych
+1 786-664-7747
https://vfapp.org/a7ce

Haiti Outreach Ministries
Provides education and healthcare based in Christian ministry in partnership with the Haitian-led Mission Communautaire de l'Eglise Chretienne des Cites (MICECC).
Dent-OMFS, General, Peds
+1 704-269-8149
https://vfapp.org/2e58

Haiti Outreach Program
Strengthens the spirit, mind, and body of the Haitian community by sending three to four medical teams to Haiti each year, with a focus on providing accessible healthcare and support for construction of a hospital and clinic.
General, Peds
https://vfapp.org/3e2b

Haitian Global Health Alliance
Provides financial support for Les Centres GHESKIO in Port-au-Prince and its network of clinics throughout Haiti that provide clinical service, training, and research in HIV/AIDS and related diseases.
Crit-Care, Heme-Onc, Infect Dis, MF Med, MF Med, OB-GYN, Path, Pulm-Critic
https://vfapp.org/f513

Haitian Health Foundation
Strives to improve the health and well-being of women, children, families, and communities living in the greater Jérémie region of Haiti, serving over 225,000 people in over 100 rural mountain villages, through healthcare, education, and community development.
Dent-OMFS, Endo, General, Infect Dis, OB-GYN, Path, Peds, Radiol
+1 860-886-4357
https://vfapp.org/7fb3

Hands Up for Haiti
Seeks to deliver lifesaving healthcare to the underserved people of northern Haiti through Sante Kominote (community -based healthcare).
ER Med, Nutr, OB-GYN, Ophth-Opt, Peds, Pub Health
https://vfapp.org/ab83

Harvard Medical School: Blavatnik Institute Global Health & Social Medicine
Applies social science and humanities research to constantly improve the practice of medicine, the delivery of treatment, and the development of health care policies locally and worldwide.
General, Infect Dis, Logist-Op, MF Med, Medicine, Neonat, Palliative, Psych, Surg
+1 617-432-1707
https://vfapp.org/9bf1

Headwaters Relief Organization
Addresses public health issues for the most underserved populations in the world, providing psychosocial and medical support as well as disaster debris cleanup and rebuilding in partnership with other organizations.
ER Med, Infect Dis, Logist-Op, Psych, Pub Health
+1 763-233-7655
https://vfapp.org/e511

Healing Art Missions
Aims to provide resources and funding to rural communities in Haiti that lack access to basic resources, such as healthcare, education, employment, and clean drinking water.
Anesth, General, Nutr, OB-GYN, Ophth-Opt, Path, Peds, Surg
+1 740-587-2472
https://vfapp.org/6f58

Healing the Children Northeast
Helps underserved children around the world secure the medical care they need to lead more fulfilling lives.
Anesth, Dent-OMFS, ENT, General, Medicine, Ophth-Opt, Ped Surg, Peds, Plast
+1 860-355-1828
https://vfapp.org/16ba

Health and Education for Haiti
Works collaboratively with the Haitian people to address their critical needs, especially those related to health and education, in four program areas: medical missions, education, infrastructure, and basic needs.
Anesth, ER Med, General, Heme-Onc, OB-GYN, Ophth-Opt, Ortho, Ped Surg, Peds
+1 719-309-6965
https://vfapp.org/f9dc

Health Corps Haiti: Medical Student Missions
Fosters professional and academic medical education

opportunities in Haiti with a "Learning Through Service" model. Designed for medical students, field operations also involve physicians, nurses, paramedics, and lay volunteers to care for the citizens of Artibonite, Haiti.

Dent-OMFS, ER Med, General, Infect Dis, Medicine, OB-GYN, Ophth-Opt, Peds, Surg

📞 +1 877-274-1544

🌐 https://vfapp.org/77c8

Health Equity Initiative

Aims to build and sustain a global community that engages across sectors and disciplines to advance health equity.

Pub Health

🌐 https://vfapp.org/e2e2

Health Equity International

Provides essential health services to the most vulnerable people of southern Haiti, while building a comprehensive, efficient, and resilient health system that provides high-quality care.

Anesth, Dent-OMFS, ER Med, General, Geri, Infect Dis, Logist-Op, MF Med, Medicine, Neonat, OB-GYN, Ped Surg, Peds, Plast, Pub Health, Rehab, Surg, Vasc Surg

📞 +1 617-244-9800

🌐 https://vfapp.org/9bd7

Health Volunteers Overseas (HVO)

Improves the availability and quality of healthcare through the education, training, and professional development of the health workforce in resource-scarce countries.

All-Immu, Anesth, CV Med, Dent-OMFS, Derm, ENT, ER Med, Endo, GI, Heme-Onc, Infect Dis, Medicine, Medicine, Nephro, Neuro, OB-GYN, Ophth-Opt, Ortho, Peds, Plast, Psych, Pulm-Critic, Rehab, Rheum, Surg

📞 +1 202-296-0928

🌐 https://vfapp.org/42b2

Heart Fund, The

Aims to save the lives of children suffering from heart disease by developing innovative solutions that revolutionize access to cardiac care in developing countries.

Anesth, CV Med, Ped Surg, Peds, Surg

🌐 https://vfapp.org/7e67

Heart to Heart International

Strengthens communities through improving health access, providing humanitarian development, and administering crisis relief worldwide. Engages volunteers, collaborates with partners, and deploys resources to achieve this mission.

Anesth, ER Med, General, Logist-Op, Medicine, Path, Path, Peds, Psych, Pub Health, Surg

📞 +1 913-764-5200

🌐 https://vfapp.org/aacb

Heineman Medical Outreach

Provides medical and educational assistance globally to promote sustainable healthcare and enhanced living standards in underserved communities through the International Medical Outreach (IMO) program, a collaborative partnership between Heineman Medical Outreach and Atrium Health.

Anesth, CT Surg, CV Med, ER Med, General, Heme-Onc, Logist-Op, Medicine, Neonat, OB-GYN, Ped Surg, Peds, Surg, Vasc Surg

📞 +1 704-374-0505

🌐 https://vfapp.org/389b

HelpAge International

Works to ensure that people everywhere understand how much older people contribute to society and that they must enjoy their right to healthcare, social services, economic, and physical security.

General, Geri, Infect Dis, Medicine, Pub Health

📞 +44 20 7148 7623

🌐 https://vfapp.org/5d91

Hernia Help

Provides free hernia surgery to underserved children and adults in the Western Hemisphere, practicing the preferential option for the poor. Trains, mentors, develops, and supports local general surgeons who will serve as trainers and future leaders to create self-sustaining teams.

Anesth, Surg

🌐 https://vfapp.org/6319

HERO Foundation USA

Matches veterans, EMS, and civilian medical volunteers with a permanent EMS program in Haiti.

ER Med, Pub Health

📞 +509 42 24 7156

🌐 https://vfapp.org/f54c

Higgins Brothers Surgicenter for Hope

Aims to address the critical shortage of surgical facilities and trained surgeons in Haiti through the volunteer efforts of surgeons and others, and by raising financial resources to develop a long-term solution serving all Haitians in Fonds-Parisien.

Anesth, Dent-OMFS, Heme-Onc, Medicine, OB-GYN, Path, Peds, Pod, Radiol, Surg, Urol, Vasc Surg

📞 +1 816-603-0001

🌐 https://vfapp.org/a959

Hope for Haiti

Improves the quality of life for the Haitian people, particularly children, by taking an integrated approach to sustainability that focuses on education, healthcare, water, infrastructure, and economy.

Dent-OMFS, General, Logist-Op, Medicine, Nutr

📞 +1 239-434-7183

🌐 https://vfapp.org/92a7

Hope for Haiti (The Catholic Church of Saint Monica)

Provides medical, dental, and financial assistance to the poor and underserved of Haiti.

Dent-OMFS, General

🌐 https://vfapp.org/edb2

Hope for Haitians

Provides housing, reliable food sources, clean water, medical care, education, and economic opportunity as part of a comprehensive approach to aid development in Haiti.

General

📞 +1 815-847-0656

🌐 https://vfapp.org/318b

Hope for the Children of Haiti

Seeks to empower Haitian children with the tools they need to succeed, including healthcare, and gives them the opportunity to become well-rounded, self-sufficient adults with a foundation in Christianity.

General, Peds

+1 781-937-8338
https://vfapp.org/fe73

HOPE Haiti Outreach
Aims to help the Borgne, Haiti, community create a safe place where every child can count on food, clean water, healthcare, learning, and livelihood.

General, Infect Dis, Surg
+1 585-262-3370
https://vfapp.org/df32

Hope Health Action
Facilitates sustainable, lifesaving health, and disability care for the world's most vulnerable, without any discrimination.

ER Med, MF Med, Neonat, Nutr, OB-GYN, Peds, Rehab
+44 20 8462 5256
https://vfapp.org/86f7

Hope Smiles
Develops and empowers healthcare leaders to restore hope and transform lives by mobilizing and equipping sustainable dental teams in unreached communities.

Dent-OMFS, Pub Health, Surg
+1 615-324-3904
https://vfapp.org/8a76

Hope Walks
Frees children, families, and communities from the burden of clubfoot, inspired by the Christian faith.

Ortho, Ped Surg, Peds, Rehab
+1 717-502-4400
https://vfapp.org/f6d4

Hope Worldwide
Changes lives through the compassion and commitment of dedicated staff and volunteers delivering sustainable, high-impact, community-based services to the poor and underserved.

Dent-OMFS, General, OB-GYN, Ophth-Opt, Peds
+1 833-446-7399
https://vfapp.org/89b3

HumaniTerra
Helps countries and populations emerging from economic and human crisis to rebuild their healthcare system in a sustainable way. Committed to three fundamental and complementary actions: operating, training, and rebuilding.

Anesth, ENT, ER Med, MF Med, OB-GYN, Ortho, Plast, Surg
+33 4 91 42 10 00
https://vfapp.org/b371

Humanity & Inclusion
Works alongside people with disabilities and vulnerable populations, taking action and bearing witness in order to respond to their essential needs, improve their living conditions and health, and promote respect for their dignity and fundamental rights.

General, Infect Dis, MF Med, Medicine, Ortho, Peds, Psych, Pub Health, Rehab
+1 301-891-2138
https://vfapp.org/16b7

Hôpital Alma Mater
Provides quality preventive and curative care 24 hours a day to patients in Gros Morne, a rural region in northwest Haiti.

Dent-OMFS, General, Infect Dis, MF Med, Medicine, OB-GYN, Path, Peds, Radiol
+509 34 33 6910
https://vfapp.org/65d4

ICAP at Columbia University
Serves as global leader in supporting the scale-up of multidisciplinary HIV/AIDS prevention, care, and treatment programs based on a family-focused approach.

General, Infect Dis, MF Med, Medicine, OB-GYN, Pub Health
+1 212-342-0505
https://vfapp.org/a8ef

IMA World Health
Works to build healthier communities by collaborating with key partners to serve vulnerable people with a focus on health, healing, and well-being for all.

Infect Dis, MF Med, Nutr, OB-GYN, Pub Health
+1 202-888-6200
https://vfapp.org/8316

Innovating Health International (IHI)
Treats chronic diseases and addresses women's health issues in Haiti, Somaliland, and Malawi.

ER Med, Heme-Onc, Medicine, OB-GYN, Path, Plast, Pub Health
+509 48 95 6148
https://vfapp.org/e712

International Allied Missions (IAM), Haiti
Envisions a dynamic healthcare community that will aid the growth of Haitian doctors and nurses, as well as provide year-round support for medical professionals from around the world to care for, teach, and help facilitate a sustainable healthcare system in Haiti.

Anesth, Dent-OMFS, General, Peds, Surg
+1 901-734-7204
https://vfapp.org/edcf

International Children's Heart Foundation
Provides free surgical care, medical training, and technology to save the lives of children with congenital heart disease in developing countries.

Anesth, CT Surg, CV Med, Crit-Care, Ped Surg, Peds, Pulm-Critic
+1 901-869-4243
https://vfapp.org/86c1

International Children's Heart Fund
Aims to promote the international growth and quality of cardiac surgery, particularly in children and young adults.

CT Surg, Ped Surg
https://vfapp.org/33fb

International Council of Ophthalmology
Works with ophthalmologic societies and others to enhance ophthalmic education and improve access to the highest quality eye care in order to preserve and restore vision for the people of the world.

Ophth-Opt

⊕ https://vfapp.org/ffd2

International Eye Foundation (IEF)

Eliminates preventable and treatable blindness by making quality sustainable eye care services accessible and affordable worldwide.

Infect Dis, Logist-Op, Ophth-Opt

📞 +1 240-290-0263

⊕ https://vfapp.org/e839

International Federation of Gynecology and Obstetrics (FIGO)

Implements global projects on specific women's health issues.

MF Med, Medicine, Neonat, OB-GYN, Surg, Urol

📞 +44 20 7928 1166

⊕ https://vfapp.org/c4b4

International Federation of Red Cross and Red Crescent Societies (IFRC)

Coordinates and directs international assistance following natural and man-made disasters in nonconflict situations through the world's largest humanitarian and development network. Provides disaster-preparedness programs, healthcare activities, and promotes humanitarian values.

ER Med, General, Infect Dis, Nutr

📞 +1 212-338-0161

⊕ https://vfapp.org/b4ee

International Learning Movement (ILM UK)

Supports some of the world's poorest people in developing countries with core projects in education, safe drinking water, and healthcare.

General, Ophth-Opt

📞 +44 1254 265451

⊕ https://vfapp.org/b974

International Medical Alliance

Provides access to medical, vision, and dental care in underserved and vulnerable communities around the world, to improve health, wellness, and the quality of life for those populations most in need.

Dent-OMFS, General, Infect Dis, OB-GYN, Ophth-Opt, Peds, Surg

📞 +1 865-325-9063

⊕ https://vfapp.org/2e7d

International Medical Relief

Provides sustainable education, training, medical and dental care, and disaster relief and response in vulnerable communities worldwide.

Dent-OMFS, General, Infect Dis, Medicine, OB-GYN

📞 +1 970-635-0110

⊕ https://vfapp.org/b3ed

International Medical Response

Supplements, supports, and enhances healthcare systems in communities across the world that have been incapacitated by natural disaster, extreme poverty, and/or regional conflict by sending a multidisciplinary team of healthcare professionals.

Anesth, General, OB-GYN, Surg

📞 +1 917-324-8348

⊕ https://vfapp.org/9ccd

International Missionary Fellowship

Serves a Northwestern community in Haiti by meeting basic needs such as medical care, education, and water, inspired by the Christian faith.

Dent-OMFS, General, OB-GYN, Ophth-Opt

📞 +1 813-358-8864

⊕ https://vfapp.org/f62c

International Organization for Migration (IOM) – The UN Migration Agency

Promotes evidence-informed policies and holistic, preventive, and curative health programs that are beneficial, accessible, and equitable for vulnerable migrants.

General, Infect Dis, OB-GYN

📞 +27 12 342 2789

⊕ https://vfapp.org/621a

International Outreach Program of St. Joseph's Health System

Works to save lives in developing countries by training doctors through partnerships with universities, medical schools, and teaching hospitals in countries that need more doctors.

Logist-Op

📞 +1 905-522-1155

⊕ https://vfapp.org/a751

International Planned Parenthood Federation (IPPF)

Leads a locally owned, globally connected civil society movement that provides and enables services and champions sexual and reproductive health and rights for all, especially the underserved.

Infect Dis, MF Med, OB-GYN

📞 +44 20 7939 8200

⊕ https://vfapp.org/dc97

International Smile Power

Partners with people to improve and sustain dental health and build bridges of friendship around the world.

Dent-OMFS

⊕ https://vfapp.org/ba69

International Women & Infant Sustainable Healthcare (IWISH Foundation)

Provides training to local medical care providers in Haiti to sustain quality care for women and children in local communities.

Logist-Op, MF Med, Neonat, OB-GYN, Peds

⊕ https://vfapp.org/db52

Iris Global

Serves the poor, the destitute, the lost, and the forgotten by providing adoration, outreach, family, education, relief, development, healing, and the arts.

General, Infect Dis, Nutr, Pub Health

📞 +1 530-255-2077

⊕ https://vfapp.org/37f8

Islamic Medical Association of North America

Fosters health promotion, disease prevention, and health maintenance in communities around the world through direct patient care and health programs.

Anesth, Dent-OMFS, ER Med, General, Logist-Op, Ophth-Opt, Peds, Plast, Surg

📞 +1 630-932-0000

⊕ https://vfapp.org/a157

IsraAID
Supports people affected by humanitarian crisis and partners with local communities around the world to provide urgent aid, assist recovery, and reduce the risk of future disasters.
ER Med, Infect Dis, Psych, Rehab
+972 3-947-7766
https://vfapp.org/de96

IVUmed
Aims to make quality urological care available worldwide by providing medical and surgical education for physicians and nurses and treatment for thousands of children and adults.
Anesth, OB-GYN, Ped Surg, Surg, Urol
+1 801-524-0201
https://vfapp.org/e619

John Snow, Inc. (JSI)
Aims to improve the health and well-being of underserved and vulnerable people and communities throughout the world.
General, Infect Dis, Logist-Op, MF Med, OB-GYN, Peds, Psych, Pub Health
+1 617-482-9485
https://vfapp.org/ba78

Joint United Nations Programme on HIV/AIDS (UNAIDS)
Aims to place people living with HIV and people affected by the virus at the decision-making table and at the center of designing, delivering, and monitoring the AIDS response.
Infect Dis
+41 22 791 36 66
https://vfapp.org/464a

Kay Mackenson Clinic for Children with Chronic Diseases
Works to improve the health of Haitian children suffering from chronic illnesses by providing high-quality, compassionate, family-centered care, in addition to education and solidarity.
General, Medicine, Peds
+509 36 97 0747
https://vfapp.org/84e5

Kletjian Foundation
Works toward a world in which all people have access to safe, sustainable, and high-quality medical care, building collaborative networks and supporting entrepreneurial leaders that promote global health equity.
CT Surg, ENT, General, Ortho, Surg
https://vfapp.org/12c2

Konbit Sante Cap-Haitien Health Partnership
Supports the development of a sustainable health system to meet the needs of the Cap-Haitien community with maximum local direction and support.
General, OB-GYN, Peds, Pub Health
+1 207-347-6733
https://vfapp.org/16f2

Labakcare
Aims to improve the health of underserved communities by providing no-cost preventive healthcare services.
General, MF Med, Ophth-Opt
+1 856-244-8013
https://vfapp.org/1e61

Lamp for Haiti
Works with and for the people of Haiti to improve the lives of some of the most marginalized persons in Haitian society.
ER Med, General, Infect Dis, Nutr, OB-GYN, Peds
+1 267-499-0516
https://vfapp.org/8788

Last Mile Health
Links community health workers with frontline health workers—nurses, doctors, and midwives at community clinics—and supports them to bring lifesaving services to the doorsteps of people living far from care.
General, Logist-Op, OB-GYN, Pub Health
+1 617-880-6163
https://vfapp.org/37da

Lavi Project
Provides medical care in Haiti by mobilizing medical missions/volunteers and collecting monetary donations and supplies to support clinics and programs.
General
+1 978-855-6494
https://vfapp.org/e1aa

LEAP Global Missions
Provides specialized surgical services to underserved populations around the world.
Anesth, Dent-OMFS, ENT, Ped Surg, Peds, Plast, Surg
+1 972-566-6550
https://vfapp.org/b447

Lespwa Lavi
Supports the community of Verrettes, Haiti, with a school and other programs such as healthcare and nutrition, based in Christian ministry.
ER Med, General, Nutr
https://vfapp.org/dad3

Life for a Child
Supports the provision of the best possible health care, given local circumstances, to all children and youth with diabetes in less-resourced countries, through the strengthening of existing diabetes services.
Endo, Medicine, Peds
https://vfapp.org/d712

Lions Clubs International
Empowers volunteers to serve their communities, meet humanitarian needs, encourage peace, and promote international understanding through Lions clubs.
Heme-Onc, Medicine, Nutr, Ophth-Opt
+1 630-571-5466
https://vfapp.org/7b12

MAGNA International
Helps those who are suffering or recovering from conflicts and disasters by reducing the risks of diseases and treating them immediately.
ER Med, General, Infect Dis, Peds, Surg
+421 2/381 046 69
https://vfapp.org/58f4

Maison de Naissance: Global Birthing Home Foundation
Aims to significantly reduce maternal and infant mortality rates in impoverished communities by sponsoring Maison de Naissance

("Home of Birth"), a modern maternal health center supporting healthy mothers and healthy babies in Haiti.

General, MF Med, Neonat, OB-GYN

+1 913-402-6800

https://vfapp.org/e959

Management Sciences for Health (MSH)

Works with countries and communities to save lives and improve the health of the world's poorest and most vulnerable people by building strong, resilient, sustainable health systems.

Infect Dis, Logist-Op, Pub Health

+1 617-250-9500

https://vfapp.org/6aa2

Massachusetts General Hospital Global Surgery Initiative

Aims to improve surgical education and access to advanced surgical care in resource-limited settings around the world by performing surgical operations as visitors, training local surgeons, and sharing medical technology through international partnerships across disciplines.

Anesth, Crit-Care, ER Med, Heme-Onc, Peds, Surg

+1 617-724-4093

https://vfapp.org/31b1

Maternity Foundation

Works to ensure safer childbirth for women and newborns everywhere through innovative mobile health solutions such as the Safe Delivery App, a mobile training tool for skilled birth attendants.

MF Med, OB-GYN, Pub Health

https://vfapp.org/ff4f

Maternity Worldwide

Works with communities and partners to identify and develop appropriate and effective ways to reduce maternal and newborn mortality and morbidity, facilitate communities to access quality skilled maternity care, and support the provision of quality skilled care.

MF Med, OB-GYN

+44 1273 234033

https://vfapp.org/822b

Maverick Collective

Aims to build a global community of strategic philanthropists and informed advocates who use their intellectual and financial resources to create change.

Infect Dis, MF Med, OB-GYN

+1 202-785-0072

https://vfapp.org/ea49

McGill University Health Centre: Centre for Global Surgery

Works to reduce the impact of injury by advancing surgical care through research and education in resource-limited settings.

ER Med, Logist-Op, Ped Surg, Surg

+1 514-934-1934

https://vfapp.org/7246

Médecins du Monde/Doctors of the World

Provides care, bears witness, and supports social change worldwide with innovative medical programs and evidence-based advocacy initiatives.

ER Med, General, Infect Dis, MF Med, Neonat, OB-GYN, Peds, Pub Health

+33 1 44 92 15 15

https://vfapp.org/a43d

Medical Aid to Haiti (MATH)

Sponsors medical missions to Haiti and sponsors a Haitian-staffed mobile medical clinic in the Port-au-Prince area.

Anesth, MF Med, OB-GYN, Surg

+1 860-760-7009

https://vfapp.org/e3f4

Medical Benevolence Foundation (MBF)

Works with partners in developing countries to build sustainable healthcare for those most in need through faith-based global medical missions.

General, Logist-Op, MF Med, OB-GYN, Surg

+1 800-547-7627

https://vfapp.org/c3e8

Medical Ministry International

Provides compassionate healthcare in areas of need, inspired by the Christian faith.

CT Surg, Dent-OMFS, ENT, General, OB-GYN, Ophth-Opt, Ortho, Plast, Rehab, Surg, Urol, Vasc Surg

+1 905-545-4400

https://vfapp.org/5da6

Medical Mission Exchange (MMEX)

Gives medical mission organizations a way to share information among one another so they can capitalize on each other's strengths, and better serve their patients.

All-Immu, Anesth, CT Surg, CV Med, Dent-OMFS, Derm, ER Med, General, OB-GYN, Ophth-Opt, Ortho, Path, Ped Surg, Plast, Psych, Radiol, Rehab, Surg, Urol

https://vfapp.org/bc8c

Medical Missionaries

Provides medical care, medicine, medical supplies, medical equipment, clothing, food, and other supplies to the poorest of the poor throughout the world.

ER Med, Logist-Op

+1 703-335-1800

https://vfapp.org/5f15

Medical Relief International

Exists to provide dental, medical, humanitarian aid, and other services deemed necessary for the benefit of people in need.

Dent-OMFS, General

+1 206-819-2551

https://vfapp.org/192b

Medical Teams International

Seeks to restore health as the first step to restoring hope, working to bring basic but lifesaving medical care to those in need.

Dent-OMFS, ER Med, General, MF Med, Pub Health

+1 503-624-1000

https://vfapp.org/8d1c

Medicines for Humanity

Aims to save the lives of vulnerable children by strengthening systems of maternal and child health in the communities served.

Infect Dis, MF Med, OB-GYN

+1 781-982-0274

https://vfapp.org/8d13

MedShare
Aims to improve the quality of life of people, communities, and the planet by sourcing and directly delivering surplus medical supplies and equipment to communities in need around the world.
Logist-Op
+1 770-323-5858
https://vfapp.org/c8bc

Mérieux Foundation
Committed to fighting infectious diseases that affect developing countries by capacity building, particularly in clinical laboratories, and focusing on diagnosis.
Logist-Op, Path
+33 4 72 40 79 79
https://vfapp.org/a23a

Middle Ground
Works to fight against malnutrition in Haiti.
Nutr, Peds
+509 33 37 7117
https://vfapp.org/e687

Midwives for Haiti
Increases access to skilled maternity care in Haiti by direct healthcare intervention and training programs through partnerships with Haiti's Ministry of Public Health and Population and other organizations.
MF Med, Neonat, OB-GYN
+1 804-545-6882
https://vfapp.org/2c57

Mission of Hope
Partners with local churches to transform lives through church advancement, nutrition, education, and medical care to bring life transformation to every man, woman, and child.
General
+1 512-256-0835
https://vfapp.org/d3c5

Mission Vision
Seeks to decrease blindness and other eye-related disabilities, as well as to increase academic performance and general quality of life.
Ophth-Opt
+1 724-553-3114
https://vfapp.org/83d8

Mission: Haiti
Serves Jesus Christ by providing medical, educational, and child-focused programs to communities in need.
General, Geri
+1 605-940-7020
https://vfapp.org/4a6a

Mission: Restore
Trains medical professionals abroad in complex reconstructive surgery in order to create a sustainable infrastructure where long-term relationships are forged and permanent change is made.
Plast, Surg
+1 855-777-1350
https://vfapp.org/3f5f

MIVO Foundation
Operates an orthopedic clinic in L'estere, Haiti, and brings orthopedic care and services to underserved communities through medical missions, based in Christian ministry.
Anesth, Ortho, Rehab
+1 717-873-7237
https://vfapp.org/85a1

Mobility Outreach International
Enables mobility for children and adults in under-resourced areas of the world, and creates a sustainable orthopedic surgery model using local resources.
Ortho, Rehab
+1 206-726-1636
https://vfapp.org/9376

More Than Medicine
Provides ENT head/neck care while supporting local doctors to grow the quality of medicine abroad.
Anesth, ENT, Heme-Onc, Surg
+1 501-268-9511
https://vfapp.org/c4e8

MPACT for Mankind
Transforms communities by improving health outcomes, enhancing knowledge, and providing hope while promoting sustainable growth.
ER Med, General
+1 469-998-1381
https://vfapp.org/1c61

MSD for Mothers
Designs scalable solutions that help end preventable maternal deaths.
MF Med, OB-GYN, Pub Health
https://vfapp.org/9f99

Northeast Hope for Haiti
Works to improve the health of the people living in the greater Petite Rivière de l'Artibonite region of Haiti.
General, Surg
https://vfapp.org/d145

Northwest Haiti Christian Mission (NWHCM)
Faciilitates engagement in NWHCM's efforts based in Christian ministry in fostering diverse programs that include primary and secondary schools, nutrition programs, medical clinics, orphanages, and the empowerment of indigenous churches.
Dent-OMFS, ER Med, General, MF Med, Nutr, Ophth-Opt, Surg
+1 317-228-8770
https://vfapp.org/2438

Nuestros Pequeños Hermanos (NPH)
Strives to create a loving and safe family environment for vulnerable children living in extreme conditions.
Psych, Rehab
+52 777 245 6350
https://vfapp.org/57c4

NYC Medics
Deploys mobile medical teams to remote areas of disaster zones and humanitarian emergencies, providing the highest level of medical care to those who otherwise would not have access to aid and relief efforts.
All-Immu, ER Med, Infect Dis, Surg
+1 888-600-1648
https://vfapp.org/aeee

One Spirit Medical Missions
Seeks to encourage and facilitate self-sufficiency in community health by training and supporting local community health workers, based in Christian ministry.

ER Med, General, Medicine

☏ +1 360-739-1345

⊕ https://vfapp.org/d271

Operation Endeavor M99+
Provides direct support for public health and safety, EMS system development, and disaster response in developing and underserved regions, both domestic and abroad, while providing training in rescue, emergency medicine, and trauma care.

Dent-OMFS, ER Med, Infect Dis, Logist-Op, OB-GYN, Peds, Surg

☏ +1 910-849-1140

⊕ https://vfapp.org/d83a

Operation International
Offers medical aid to adults and children suffering from lack of quality healthcare in impoverished countries.

Dent-OMFS, ER Med, Heme-Onc, OB-GYN, Ophth-Opt, Ortho, Ped Surg, Plast, Surg

☏ +1 631-287-6202

⊕ https://vfapp.org/b52a

Operation Medical
Commits efforts to promoting and providing high-quality medical care and education to communities that do not have adequate access.

Anesth, ENT, Logist-Op, OB-GYN, Ped Surg, Plast, Surg, Urol

☏ +1 717-685-9199

⊕ https://vfapp.org/7e1b

Operation Rainbow
Performs free orthopedic surgery for children and young adults in developing countries who do not have access to related medical procedures or equipment.

Anesth, Ortho, Ped Surg, Peds, Rehab, Surg

☏ +1 510-273-2485

⊕ https://vfapp.org/5dad

Operation Smile
Treats patients with cleft lip and cleft palate, and creates solutions that deliver safe surgery to people where it's needed most.

Anesth, Dent-OMFS, ENT, Ped Surg, Plast

☏ +1 757-321-7645

⊕ https://vfapp.org/5c29

OPTIVEST Foundation
Funds strategic opportunities that are holistic and collaborative, inspired by the Christian faith.

General, Nutr

⊕ https://vfapp.org/f1e6

Optometry Giving Sight
Delivers eye exams and low or no-cost glasses, provides training for local eye care professionals, and establishes optometry schools, vision centers and optical labs.

Ophth-Opt

☏ +1 303-526-0430

⊕ https://vfapp.org/33ea

Organization for Renal Care in Haiti, The (TORCH)
Brings lifesaving medical care to patients with kidney disease in Haiti that is not available to them, while providing education, medical equipment, training, and resources to medical professionals and facilities in Haiti.

Medicine, Nephro

☏ +1 617-969-1972

⊕ https://vfapp.org/bda4

Orthopaedic Relief Services International
Provides increased clinical, educational, and infrastructural support for Hopital de l'Universite d'Etat d'Haiti orthopedic surgical services and its residency program.

ER Med, General, Ortho

⊕ https://vfapp.org/e9b3

Partners in Health
Responds to the moral imperative to provide high-quality healthcare globally to those who need it most, while striving to ease suffering by providing a comprehensive model of care that includes access to food, transportation, housing, and other key components of healing.

CT Surg, General, Heme-Onc, Infect Dis, MF Med, Neurosurg, OB-GYN, Ortho, Plast, Psych, Urol

☏ +1 857-880-5600

⊕ https://vfapp.org/dc9c

Pediatric Universal Life-Saving Effort, Inc. (PULSE)
Aims to increase access to acute- and intensive-care services for children, recognizing that a significant amount of childhood mortality is preventable. Utilizes time, talents, and resources and seeks to persuade others to share their gifts to enrich the lives of children worldwide.

Crit-Care, Logist-Op, Neonat, Ped Surg, Peds

☏ +1 347-599-0792

⊕ https://vfapp.org/f6b9

Pharmacists Without Borders Canada
Provides pharmaceutical and technical assistance in the implementation or improvement of community and hospital pharmacies internationally.

☏ +1 514-842-8923

⊕ https://vfapp.org/7658

Phoenix Rising for Haiti
Creates networks of sustainable rehabilitation clinics throughout rural Haiti run by Haitian professionals and locally trained staff.

ER Med, General, OB-GYN, Ortho, Rehab

☏ +1 602-363-0058

⊕ https://vfapp.org/67ee

Picture of Health Foundation
Provides communities with health education and empowers people to alter unhealthy lifestyles, thus increasing both life expectancy and quality.

General, Pub Health

☏ +1 770-807-7813

⊕ https://vfapp.org/83e3

Project Concern International (PCI)
Drives innovation from the ground up to enhance health, end hunger, overcome hardship, and advance women and girls—resulting in meaningful and measurable change in people's lives.

Infect Dis, MF Med, Nutr, OB-GYN, Peds

☏ +1 858-279-9690

⊕ https://vfapp.org/5ed7

Project Haiti
Provides medical care and education in Haiti.
Anesth, General, Medicine, Radiol, Surg, Urol
https://vfapp.org/f95b

Project Medishare for Haiti
Empowers Haitians to provide and receive access to quality healthcare, improves health infrastructure, and strengthen the skills of medical professionals.
General, MF Med, Nutr, OB-GYN, Peds
+1 786-483-8870
https://vfapp.org/5f59

Project SOAR
Conducts HIV operations research around the world to identify practical solutions to improve HIV prevention, care, and treatment services.
ER Med, General, MF Med, OB-GYN, Psych
+1 202-237-9400
https://vfapp.org/1a77

Promise for Haiti
Provides healthcare, education, evangelism, economic development, and safe water in Pignon, Haiti.
Dent-OMFS, General, Infect Dis, MF Med, OB-GYN, Ophth-Opt, Rehab
+1 615-864-0818
https://vfapp.org/79b2

PSI – Population Services International
Dedicates efforts to improving the health of people in the developing world by focusing on challenges such as a lack of family planning, HIV/AIDS, barriers to maternal health, and the greatest threats to children under the age of 5, including malaria, diarrhea, pneumonia, and malnutrition.
Infect Dis, MF Med, OB-GYN, Peds
+1 202-785-0072
https://vfapp.org/ffe3

Queensland Foundation for Children, Health and Education (QFCHE)
Works for children, higher education and scientific research, health, education, environment, public hygiene, population, and development, contributing to the development of the Haitian community.
General
+509 32 22 7685
https://vfapp.org/8e4f

RAD-AID International
Improves and optimizes access to medical imaging and radiology in low-resource regions of the world.
Rad-Onc, Radiol
https://vfapp.org/537f

Real Love Ministries International
Supports the people of Haiti by ministering to the needs of the total person—physical, emotional, and spiritual—based in Christian ministry.
General, MF Med, Nutr, Peds
+1 828-312-9527
https://vfapp.org/c7d2

Real Medicine Foundation (RMF)
Provides humanitarian support to people living in disaster and poverty-stricken areas, focusing on the person as a whole by providing medical/physical, emotional, economic, and social support.
ER Med, General, Infect Dis, Nutr, Peds, Psych
+44 20 8638 0637
https://vfapp.org/d45a

Reconstructing Women International
Treats patients in their local communities through groups of international volunteers made up of female plastic surgeons using local medical facilities, in cooperation with local medical professionals.
Anesth, Plast, Rehab, Surg
https://vfapp.org/924a

Remote Area Medical Volunteer Corps
Brings free high-quality medical, vision, dental, and veterinary care to those in need.
Dent-OMFS, ER Med, General, Heme-Onc, MF Med, OB-GYN, Ophth-Opt
+1 865-579-1530
https://vfapp.org/7669

RestoringVision
Empowers lives by restoring vision for millions of people in need.
Ophth-Opt
+1 209-980-7323
https://vfapp.org/e121

Rose Charities International
Aims to support communities to improve quality of life and reduce the effects of poverty through innovative, self-sustaining projects and partnerships.
ENT, ER Med, General, Infect Dis, Neonat, OB-GYN, Ophth-Opt, Ped Surg, Peds, Rehab, Urol
+1 604-733-0442
https://vfapp.org/53df

Rotary International
Provides service to others, improves lives, and advances world understanding, goodwill, and peace through its fellowship of business, professional, and community leaders.
ER Med, General, Infect Dis, MF Med, OB-GYN
https://vfapp.org/8fb5

ROW Foundation
Works to improve the quality of training for healthcare providers, and the diagnosis and treatment available to people with epilepsy and associated psychiatric disorders in under-resourced areas of the world.
Neuro, Psych
+1 630-791-0247
https://vfapp.org/25eb

Rutgers New Jersey Medical School
Seeks to support and promote the global health efforts of the faculty, staff, and learners in the areas of education, research, and service through The Rutgers New Jersey Medical School's Office of Global Health.
Anesth, CV Med, Crit-Care, Neurosurg, OB-GYN, Psych
+1 732-445-4636
https://vfapp.org/8e67

Saint Rock Haiti Foundation
Provides quality primary healthcare, helps children and young

adults access valuable education opportunities, institutes community outreach programs that support economic sustainability, and invests in infrastructure to support overall health.

Dent-OMFS, General, Infect Dis, MF Med, Nutr, OB-GYN, Path, Peds

+1 617-698-0006

https://vfapp.org/5aa8

Salvation Army International, The

Seeks to meet human needs through services in education, healthcare, community support, emergency response, and ministry development, inspired by the Christian faith.

Dent-OMFS, Derm, ER Med, Infect Dis, MF Med, Medicine, Nutr, OB-GYN, Ophth-Opt, Palliative, Psych, Rehab, Surg

+44 20 7332 0101

https://vfapp.org/8eb3

SAMU Foundation

Provides medical first response and reconstruction when severe international emergencies occur.

ER Med, Infect Dis, Logist-Op, Psych, Pub Health

+1 202-808-0999

https://vfapp.org/3196

Sante Haiti

Ensures that the men, women, and children of Haiti are able to enjoy health as a human right, by providing services in education and empowerment.

General, Pub Health

+1 816-431-6396

https://vfapp.org/c6e7

Save the Children

Gives children around the world a healthy start in life, the opportunity to learn, and protection from harm.

All-Immu, Crit-Care, ER Med, General, Infect Dis, MF Med, Medicine, Neonat, OB-GYN, Peds, Psych, Pub Health

+1 800-728-3843

https://vfapp.org/2e73

Second Chance Haiti

Aims to empower families and leave a legacy through child sponsorship, family empowerment, and medical care programs.

Dent-OMFS, ER Med, General, Ophth-Opt, Psych

+1 336-539-1815

https://vfapp.org/35d9

SEE International

Provides sustainable medical, surgical, and educational services through volunteer ophthalmic surgeons, with the objectives of restoring sight and preventing blindness to disadvantaged individuals worldwide.

Ophth-Opt, Surg

+1 805-963-3303

https://vfapp.org/6e1b

ServeHAITI

Fosters health and development opportunities for the people of Grand-Bois, Haiti.

General, Neonat, OB-GYN, Peds

+1 888-641-0900

https://vfapp.org/1193

SEVA

Delivers vital eye care services to the world's most vulnerable, including women, children, and Indigenous peoples.

Ophth-Opt, Surg

+1 510-845-7382

https://vfapp.org/1e87

SIGN Fracture Care International

Builds orthopedic capacity around the world and provides the injured poor access to fracture surgery by donating orthopedic education and implant systems to surgeons in developing countries.

Ortho, Rehab, Surg

+1 509-371-1107

https://vfapp.org/123d

Soaring Unlimited

Works in partnership with the people of the greater Cap Haitien community to enhance quality of life in the areas of medical services, education, and community development.

General, MF Med, OB-GYN

+1 517-712-3999

https://vfapp.org/c5ac

Spine Care International

Extends spine care to the underprivileged and provides life-changing treatment to those who may otherwise be constrained to living with chronic pain.

Neurosurg, Ortho, Rehab, Surg

+1 720-985-9378

https://vfapp.org/a867

St. Luke Foundation for Haiti

Provides comprehensive medical, educational, and social support services to some of the most marginalized groups in Haiti.

ER Med, Infect Dis, Logist-Op, MF Med, Nutr, OB-GYN, Peds, Peds, Pub Health

+1 703-580-8850

https://vfapp.org/f6c5

Surgical Friends Foundation

Provides reconstructive surgery and post-operative care to individuals living with physical deformities who do not have access to quality medical care.

Dent-OMFS, ENT, Plast, Surg

+1 310-562-3631

https://vfapp.org/8286

Sustainable Kidney Care Foundation (SKCF)

Works to provide treatment for kidney injury where none exists, and aims to reduce mortality from treatable acute kidney injury (AKI).

Infect Dis, Medicine, Nephro

https://vfapp.org/1926

Sustainable Therapy and New Development (STAND): The Haiti Project

Works to establish permanent access to orthopedic rehabilitative services in the country of Haiti through direct patient care and clinical training of Haitian citizens.

General, Ortho, Rehab

https://vfapp.org/8bea

Task Force for Global Health, The

Consists of programs and focus areas that cover a range of global health issues including neglected tropical diseases, infectious diseases, vaccines, field epidemiology, public health informatics, health workforce development, and global health ethics.

Infect Dis, Logist-Op, Medicine, Ophth-Opt, Peds

+1 404-371-0466

https://vfapp.org/714c

Team Broken Earth

Brings medical relief and education to those who need it most by sending volunteer teams of healthcare professionals to areas of wide-ranging relief response.

Medicine, OB-GYN, Ophth-Opt, Rehab, Surg

https://vfapp.org/bfcd

Team Canada Healing Hands

Provides and develops interdisciplinary rehabilitation treatment, education, and training in areas of need.

ENT, Neuro, Psych, Rehab

+1 506-363-3836

https://vfapp.org/2eaf

Tearfund

Responds to crisis and partners with local churches to bring restoration to those living in poverty, inspired by the Christian faith.

ER Med, Logist-Op

+44 20 3906 3906

https://vfapp.org/f6cf

Terre Des Hommes

Works to improve the conditions of the most vulnerable children worldwide by improving the health of children under the age of 3, protecting migrant children, providing humanitarian aid to children and their families in times of crisis, and preventing child exploitation.

ER Med, MF Med, Neonat, OB-GYN, Ped Surg, Peds

+41 58 611 06 66

https://vfapp.org/2689

Union for International Cancer Control (UICC)

Unites and supports the cancer community to reduce the global cancer burden, promote greater equity, and ensure that cancer control continues to be a priority in the world health and development agenda.

Heme-Onc, Pub Health

+41 22 809 18 11

https://vfapp.org/88b1

United Nations Children's Fund (UNICEF)

Works in over 190 countries and territories to save children's lives, to defend their rights, and to help them fulfill their potential, from early childhood through adolescence.

All-Immu, Infect Dis, MF Med, Neonat, Nutr, OB-GYN, Ped Surg, Peds, Pub Health

https://vfapp.org/42d7

United Nations Development Programme (UNDP)

Helps countries achieve the simultaneous eradication of extreme poverty and significant reduction of inequalities and exclusion using a sustainable human development approach.

Infect Dis, Logist-Op, Pub Health

https://vfapp.org/935c

United Nations High Commissioner for Refugees (UNHCR)

Safeguards the rights and well-being of people who have been forced to flee, ensuring that everybody has the right to seek asylum and find safe refuge in another country, with the goal of seeking lasting solutions.

General, MF Med, Medicine, OB-GYN, Peds, Psych, Pub Health

https://vfapp.org/6636

United Nations Office for the Coordination of Humanitarian Affairs (OCHA)

Contributes to principled and effective humanitarian response through coordination, advocacy, policy, information management, and humanitarian financing tools and services, by leveraging functional expertise throughout the organization.

Logist-Op

https://vfapp.org/22b8

United Nations Population Fund (UNFPA)

Supports reproductive healthcare for women and youth in more than 150 countries, focusing on delivering a world where every pregnancy is wanted, every childbirth is safe, and every young person's potential is fulfilled.

Infect Dis, MF Med, Neonat, OB-GYN, Peds, Pub Health

+1 212-963-6008

https://vfapp.org/c969

United States Agency for International Development (USAID)

Promotes and demonstrates democratic values abroad and advances a free, peaceful, and prosperous world. Leads the U.S. government's international development and disaster assistance through partnerships and investments that save lives.

ER Med, Infect Dis, MF Med, OB-GYN, Peds

+1 202-712-0000

https://vfapp.org/9a99

United States President's Emergency Plan for AIDS Relief (PEPFAR)

The U.S. global HIV/AIDS response works to prevent new HIV infections and accelerate progress to control the global epidemic in more than 50 countries, by partnering with governments to support sustainable, integrated, and country-led responses to HIV/AIDS.

Infect Dis, Pub Health

https://vfapp.org/a57c

University of Illinois at Chicago: Center for Global Health

Aims to improve the health of populations around the world and reduce health disparities by collaboratively conducting trans-disciplinary research, training the next generations of global health leaders, and building the capacities of global and local partners.

Pub Health

+1 312-355-4116

https://vfapp.org/b749

University of Chicago: Center for Global Health

Collaborates with communities locally and globally to democratize education, increase service learning opportunities, and advance sustainable solutions to improve health and well-being while reducing global health inequities.

Genetics, MF Med, Peds, Pub Health

+1 773-702-5959

https://vfapp.org/4f8f

University of Massachusetts Medical School: Department of Surgery Global Scholars

Provides state-of-the-art surgical care to patients and serves communities worldwide through education, research, and public service.

Anesth, ER Med, Surg

+1 508-856-3744

https://vfapp.org/3e8e

University of Notre Dame – Haiti Program Neglected Tropical Diseases Initiative

Supports efforts by Hopital Sainte Croix (HSCC) in Leogane, Haiti, to eliminate lymphatic filariasis (LF) through mass drug administration and ease the suffering of Haitians afflicted with the disease through clinical therapies.

Infect Dis, Logist-Op, Pub Health

+1 574-631-3273

https://vfapp.org/3cb8

University of Pennsylvania Perelman School of Medicine Center for Global Health

Aims to improve health equity worldwide – through enhanced public health awareness and access to care, discovery and outcomes based research, and comprehensive educational programs grounded in partnership.

Heme-Onc, Infect Dis, OB-GYN

+1 215-898-0848

https://vfapp.org/cb57

University of Washington: The International Training and Education Center for Health (I-TECH)

Works with local partners to develop skilled healthcare workers and strong national health systems in resource-limited countries.

Infect Dis, Pub Health

+1 206-744-8493

https://vfapp.org/642f

University of Virginia: Anesthesiology Department Global Health Initiatives

Educates and trains physicians, to help people achieve healthy productive lives, and advances knowledge in the medical sciences.

Anesth, Pub Health

+1 434-924-2283

https://vfapp.org/1b8b

USAID: Maternal and Child Survival Program

Works to prevent child and maternal deaths.

Infect Dis, MF Med, Neonat, OB-GYN, Peds

https://vfapp.org/6fcf

USAID: EQUIP Health

Exists as an effective, efficient response mechanism to achieving global HIV epidemic control by delivering the right intervention at the right place and in the right way.

Infect Dis

+27 11 276 8850

https://vfapp.org/d76a

USAID: Health Finance and Governance Project

Uses research to implement strategies to help countries develop robust governance systems, increase their domestic resources for health, manage those resources more effectively, and make wise purchasing decisions.

Logist-Op

+1 202-712-0000

https://vfapp.org/8652

USAID: Health Policy Initiative

Provides field-level programming in health policy development and implementation.

General, Infect Dis, MF Med, OB-GYN, Peds

https://vfapp.org/8f84

USAID: Leadership, Management and Governance Project

Improves leadership, management, and governance practices to strengthen health systems and improve health for all, including vulnerable populations worldwide.

Logist-Op

https://vfapp.org/d35e

Vanderbilt University Medical Center: Global Surgery

Aims to improve the healthcare of individuals and communities regionally, nationally and internationally, combining transformative learning programs and compelling discoveries to provide distinctive personalized care.

CT Surg, CV Med, Neurosurg, Ophth-Opt, Ortho, Ped Surg, Surg, Urol

+1 615-322-5000

https://vfapp.org/ee28

Vision Care

Restores sight and helps patients get regular treatment at short-term eye camps and long-term base clinics by having doctors, missionaries, volunteers, and sponsors work together.

Ophth-Opt

+1 212-769-3056

https://vfapp.org/9d7c

Vision for the Poor

Reduces human suffering and improves quality of life through the recovery of sight by building sustainable eye hospitals in developing countries, empowering local eye specialists, funding essential ophthalmic infrastructure, and partnering with like-minded agencies.

Ophth-Opt

+1 814-823-4486

https://vfapp.org/528e

Vision Outreach International

Advocates for helping the blind in underserved regions of the world and empowers the poor through sight restoration.

Ophth-Opt

+1 269-428-3300

https://vfapp.org/9721

Visitation Hospital Foundation

Provides competent and compassionate healthcare to the people of southwest Haiti by empowering them with resources to pursue their basic right to health and health education.

All-Immu, General, Infect Dis, MF Med

+1 615-673-3501

https://vfapp.org/aa2b

Vitamin Angels

Helps at-risk populations in need—specifically pregnant women, new mothers, and children under age five—to gain access to life-changing vitamins and minerals.

General, Nutr
📞 +1 805-564-8400
🌐 https://vfapp.org/7da1

VOSH (Volunteer Optometric Services to Humanity) International
Facilitates the provision and the sustainability of vision care worldwide for people who can neither afford nor obtain such care.
Ophth-Opt
🌐 https://vfapp.org/a149

Watsi
Uses technology to make healthcare a reality for those who might not otherwise be able to afford it.
Pub Health, Surg
📞 +1 256-792-8747
🌐 https://vfapp.org/41a3

Weill Cornell Medicine: Center for Global Health
Collaborates with international partners to improve the health of people in resource-poor countries through research, training, and service.
General, Infect Dis, OB-GYN
📞 +1 646-962-8140
🌐 https://vfapp.org/1813

Women's Refugee Commission
Seeks to improve lives by protecting the rights of women, children, and youth displaced by conflict and crisis through researching their needs, identifying solutions, and advocating for programs and policies to strengthen their resilience.
General, MF Med, Neonat, OB-GYN, Peds, Psych
📞 +1 212-551-3115
🌐 https://vfapp.org/3d8f

World Compassion Fellowship (WCF)
Serves the global poor and persecuted through relief, medical care, development, and training.
CV Med, ER Med, Endo, GI, General, Infect Dis, Medicine, Nutr, OB-GYN, Ortho, Peds, Psych, Pub Health, Rehab
📞 +1 646-535-2344
🌐 https://vfapp.org/7b97

World Gospel Mission
Mobilizes volunteers to help transform communities through healthcare and education, based in Christian ministry.
ER Med, General
📞 +1 765-664-7331
🌐 https://vfapp.org/efa4

World Health Organization, The (WHO)
The United Nations' agency for health provides leadership on global health matters, shapes the health research agenda, setting norms and standards, articulates evidence-based policy options, provides technical support and monitoring to countries, and assesses health trends.
ER Med, General, Infect Dis, Logist-Op, MF Med, OB-GYN, Peds, Psych, Pub Health
📞 +41 22 791 21 11
🌐 https://vfapp.org/c476

World Health Partnerships
Provides medical care and mental health education to allow people in underserved countries the foundation for improved physical, mental, and spiritual lives.
Anesth, OB-GYN, Psych, Surg
📞 +1 559-903-5664
🌐 https://vfapp.org/5d34

World Hope International
Empowers the poorest individuals around the world so they can become agents of change within their communities, by offering resources and knowledge.
Infect Dis, Logist-Op, MF Med, OB-GYN, Peds
📞 +1 703-923-9414
🌐 https://vfapp.org/a4b8

World Medical Relief
Facilitates the distribution of surplus medical resources where they are needed.
Logist-Op
📞 +1 313-866-5333
🌐 https://vfapp.org/72dc

World Rehabilitation Fund
Enables individuals around the world with functional limitations and participation restrictions to achieve community and social integration through physical and socio-economic rehabilitation and advocacy.
Ortho, Rehab
📞 +1 212-532-6000
🌐 https://vfapp.org/a5bc

World Relief
Brings sustainable solutions to the world's greatest problems: disasters, extreme poverty, violence, oppression, and mass displacement.
ER Med, Nutr, Psych, Pub Health
📞 +1 800-535-5433
🌐 https://vfapp.org/fbcd

World Surgical Foundation
Provides charitable surgical healthcare to the world's poor and underserved in developing nations.
Ped Surg, Surg
📞 +1 717-232-1404
🌐 https://vfapp.org/c162

World Telehealth Initiative
Provides medical expertise to the world's most vulnerable communities to build local capacity and deliver core health services through a network of volunteer healthcare professionals supported with state-of-the-art technology.
Derm, Infect Dis, MF Med, Medicine, Neuro, OB-GYN, Peds, Pulm-Critic
🌐 https://vfapp.org/fa91

World Vision International
Works with vulnerable communities around the world to overcome poverty and injustice with child-focused programs.
ER Med, General, Infect Dis, MF Med, Nutr, OB-GYN, Peds
📞 +1 626-303-8811
🌐 https://vfapp.org/2642

Worldwide Healing Hands
Works to improve the quality of healthcare for women and children in the most underserved areas of the world and to stop the preventable deaths of mothers.
General, MF Med, Neonat, OB-GYN
📞 +1 707-279-8733
🌐 https://vfapp.org/b331

Yale School of Medicine: Global Surgery Division
Addresses the rising worldwide surgical disease burden in low-resource settings both domestically and internationally by mobilizing a community of surgical leaders to engage in international partnerships, implement quality improvement and training protocols.

ER Med, Infect Dis, Medicine, Peds

+1 203-785-2844

https://vfapp.org/2bf7

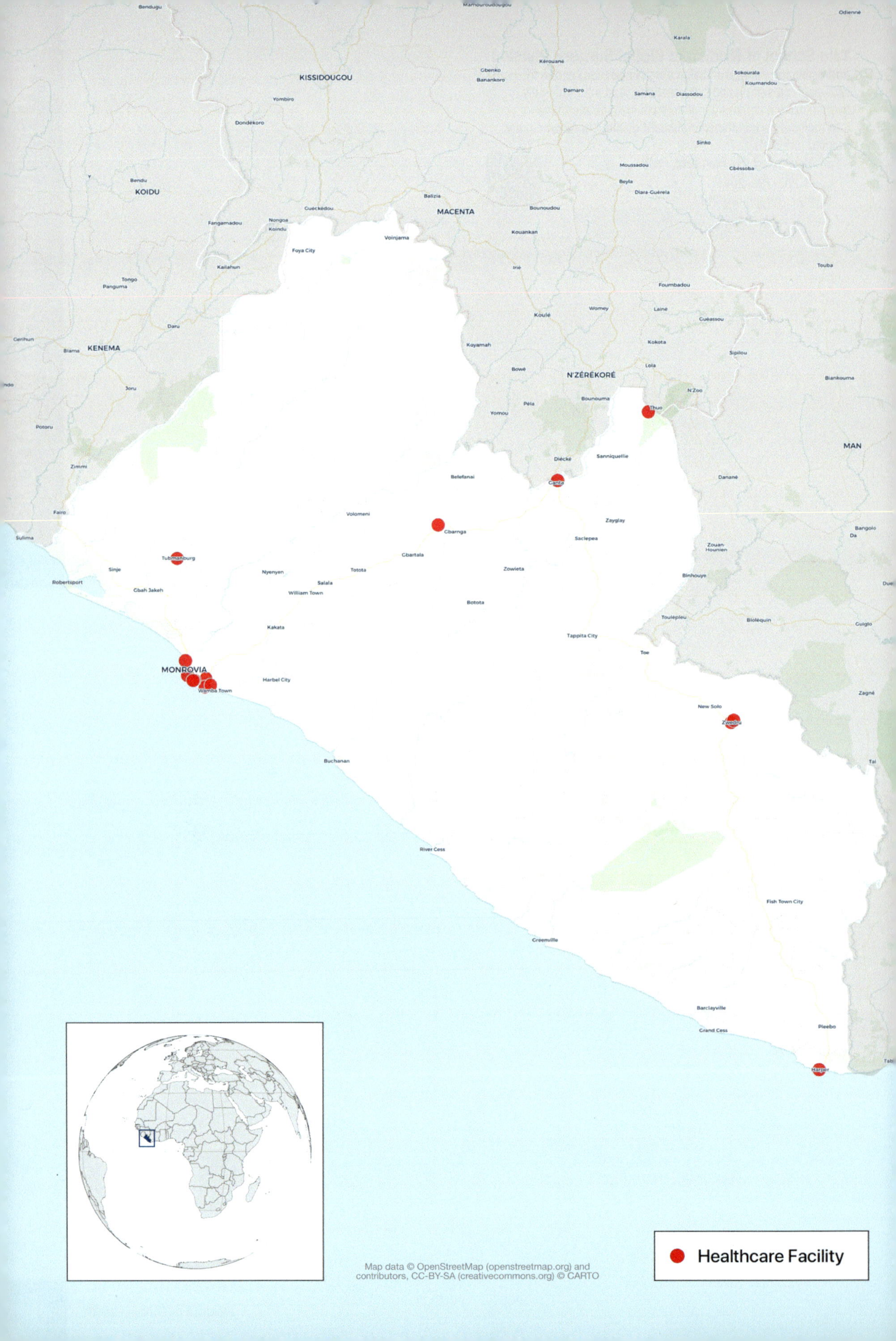
Bendugu
Mamouroudougou
Odienné
Karala
KISSIDOUGOU
Gbenko
Banankoro
Kérouané
Sokourala
Koumandou
Yombiro
Damaro
Samana
Diassodou
Dondékoro
Sinko
Moussadou
Gbéssoba
Bendu
Beyla
KOIDU
Diara-Guérela
Balizia
Guéckédou
MACENTA
Bounoudou
Fangamadou
Nongoa
Koindu
Kouankan
Voinjama
Foya City
Kailahun
Irié
Touba
Tongo
Panguma
Foumbadou
Womey
Lainé
Koulé
Guéassou
Daru
Cerihun
Blama
KENEMA
Koyamah
Kokota
Sipilou
Lola
Bowé
N'ZÉRÉKORÉ
Joru
N'Zoo
Biankouma
Bounouma
Péla
Yomou
Thuo
Potoru
MAN
Diécké
Sanniquellie
Zimmi
Belefanai
Danané
Ganta
Fairo
Volomeni
Zayglay
Bangolo
Gbarnga
Sulima
Saclepea
Tubmanburg
Gbartala
Zouan-Hounien
Sinje
Nyenyen
Totota
Zowieta
Binhouye
Robertsport
Salala
Gbah Jakeh
William Town
Botota
Kakata
Toulépleu
Bloléquin
Guiglo
Tappita City
Toe
MONROVIA
Harbel City
Wamba Town
Zagné
New Solo
Zwedru
Buchanan
River Cess
Fish Town City
Greenville
Barclayville
Pleebo
Grand Cess
Harper
Healthcare Facility
Map data © OpenStreetMap (openstreetmap.org) and contributors, CC-BY-SA (creativecommons.org) © CARTO

Liberia

The Republic of Liberia sits on the West African coast, bordered by Sierra Leone, Guinea, and Cote D'Ivoire. The nation has a small majority Christian population of about 5.1 million people, more than half of whom live in or around urban areas and in close proximity to the capital of Monrovia. The ethnically diverse population comprises groups including Kpelle, Bassa, Grebo, Gio, Mano, Kru, Morma, Kissi, Gola, Krahn, Vai, Mandingo, Gbandi, Mednde, and Sapo. As a result, Liberia offers great linguistic diversity, with as many as 30 different languages spoken in addition to English. The history of Liberia is unique; the country was founded by free people of color emigrating from the United States. As a result, Liberia is a country where both traditional and Western-influenced customs coexist.

Liberia is Africa's oldest republic and has never been ruled by a colonial power. The nation has a history of political instability, which has slowly improved over the decades. However, both unemployment and illiteracy are widespread, and around 50 percent of Liberians live below the poverty line.

Liberians face a variety of health challenges. In 2014, a large Ebola outbreak occurred in Guinea and spread to neighboring Sierra Leone and Liberia. The virus infected more than 10,000 and killed nearly 5,000 Liberians. Despite the turmoil caused by Ebola, life expectancy in Liberia continues to improve significantly, having increased from 46 years in 1990 to almost 64 years in 2018. While overall health may be improving, most deaths in Liberia are caused by malaria, diarrheal disease, neonatal disorders, lower respiratory infections, ischemic heart disease, HIV/AIDS, stroke, tuberculosis, cirrhosis, and maternal disorders.

5.1M
Population

$622
GDP Per Capita

64 years
Life Expectancy
↑ Improving

3.8
Doctors/100k
Physician Density

80
Beds/100k
Hospital Bed Density

661
Deaths/100k
Maternal Mortality

Liberia

Healthcare Facilities

Arcelor Mittal Yekepa Hospital
Yekepa, Liberia
https://vfapp.org/4e41

Benson Hospital
Tubman Boulevard, Monrovia, Montserrado County, Liberia
https://vfapp.org/e8c8

Bomi Tubmanburg ETU
Tubmanburg, Bomi County, Liberia
https://vfapp.org/8183

Catherine Mills Hospital
Dillion Avenue, Monrovia, Montserrado County, Liberia
https://vfapp.org/8a86

Eternal Love Winning Africa Hospital
Monrovia, Liberia
https://vfapp.org/cd26

Ganta Methodist Hospital
Ganta, Liberia
https://vfapp.org/ee41

J.J. Dossen Hospital
Green Street, Harper, Maryland County, Liberia
https://vfapp.org/9b2f

Martha Tubman Memorial Hospital
Breeze Street, Zone 5, Grand Gedeh County, Liberia
https://vfapp.org/4bf9

Phebe Hospital & School of Nursing
Phebe, Liberia
https://vfapp.org/e4b1

Redemption Hospital
New Kru Town, Liberia
https://vfapp.org/ba2e

SDA Cooper Hospital
12th St, Monrovia, Liberia
https://vfapp.org/6363

SOS Hospital
Tubman Boulevard, Monrovia, Montserrado County, Liberia
https://vfapp.org/fb2c

St. Joseph's Catholic Hospital
Tubman Boulevard, Monrovia, Montserrado County, Liberia
https://vfapp.org/c7fb

UN Chinese Hospital and UNMIL Base
Towah Street, Zone 2, Grand Gedeh County, Liberia
https://vfapp.org/fde5

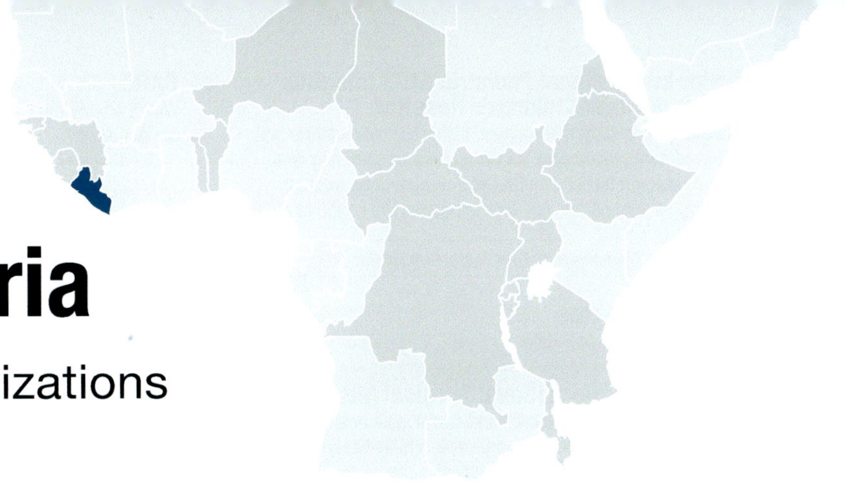

Liberia

Nonprofit Organizations

Abt Associates
Seeks to improve the quality of life and economic well-being of people worldwide, while striving to meet and exceed the highest professional standards.

General, Logist-Op, MF Med, OB-GYN, Peds

+1 212-779-7700

https://vfapp.org/cec2

Aceso Global
Provides strategic healthcare advisory services in low- and middle-income countries to design and deliver highly customized, evidence-based solutions that address the complex nature of healthcare systems, with a goal to strengthen and provide affordable, high-quality care to all.

Logist-Op, Pub Health

+1 202-758-2636

https://vfapp.org/b3b7

Action Against Hunger
Aims to end life-threatening hunger for good through treating and preventing malnutrition across more than forty-five countries.

+1 212-967-7800

https://vfapp.org/2dbc

Adventist Health International
Focuses on upgrading and managing mission hospitals by providing governance, consultation, and technical assistance to a number of affiliated Seventh-Day Adventist hospitals throughout Africa, Asia, and the Americas.

Dent-OMFS, General, Pub Health

+1 909-558-5610

https://vfapp.org/16aa

Africa CDC
Aims to strengthen the capacity and capability of Africa's public health institutions as well as partnerships to detect and respond quickly and effectively to disease threats and outbreaks, based on data-driven interventions and programs.

Infect Dis, Logist-Op, Pub Health

+251 11 551 7700

https://vfapp.org/339c

Africa Humanitarian Action (AHA)
Responds to crises, conflicts, and disasters in Africa, while informing and advising the international community, governments, civil society, and the private sector on humanitarian issues of concern to Africa. Supports institutional and organizational development efforts.

General, Infect Dis, MF Med, Nutr, OB-GYN

+251 11 660 4800

https://vfapp.org/3ca2

Africa Indoor Residual Spraying Project (AIRS)
Aims to protect millions of people in Africa from malaria by spraying insecticide on the walls, ceilings, and other indoor resting places of mosquitoes that transmit malaria.

Infect Dis

+1 301-347-5000

https://vfapp.org/9bd1

African Field Epidemiology Network (AFENET)
Strengthens field epidemiology and public health laboratory capacity to contribute effectively to addressing epidemics and other major public health problems in Africa.

All-Immu, Infect Dis, Path, Pub Health

https://vfapp.org/df2e

American International Health Alliance (AIHA)
Strengthens health systems and workforce capacity worldwide through locally-driven, peer-to-peer institutional partnerships.

CV Med, ER Med, Infect Dis, Medicine, OB-GYN

+1 202-789-1136

https://vfapp.org/69fd

Americares
Saves lives and improves health for people affected by poverty or disaster and responds with life-changing medicine, medical supplies, and health programs including domestic and global medical clinics.

All-Immu, ER Med, General, Infect Dis, MF Med, Nutr

+1 203-658-9500

https://vfapp.org/e567

Amref Health Africa
Serves millions of people across thirty-five countries in Sub-Saharan Africa, strengthening health systems, and training African health workers to respond to the continent's most critical health issues.

All-Immu, General, Infect Dis, Logist-Op, MF Med, OB-GYN, Path, Pub Health, Surg

+254 20 6993000

https://vfapp.org/6985

Baylor International Pediatric AIDS Initiative (BIPAI) at Texas Children's Hospital
Provides high-quality, high-impact, highly ethical pediatric and family-centered healthcare, health professional training, and clinical research focused on HIV/AIDS, tuberculosis, malaria, malnutrition, and other conditions impacting the health of children worldwide.

Infect Dis, Medicine, OB-GYN, Peds, Pub Health, Surg

+1 832-822-1038

https://vfapp.org/e6ba

Bethel SOZO International Surgical Missions
Provides mobile medical clinics and sustainable health education to underserved communities worldwide. A faith-based organization with volunteer opportunities for medical, surgical, and dental professionals and others to provide healthcare.

General

+1 609-656-9228

https://vfapp.org/9d88

Boston Children's Hospital: Global Health Program
Helps solve pediatric global health care challenges by transferring expertise through long-term partnerships with scalable impact, while working in the field to strengthen healthcare systems, advocate, research and provide care delivery or education as a way of sustainably improving the health of children worldwide.

Anesth, CV Med, Crit-Care, ER Med, Heme-Onc, Infect Dis, Medicine, Nutr, Palliative, Ped Surg, Peds

+1 617-919-6438

https://vfapp.org/f9f8

BRAC USA
Seeks to empower people and communities in situations of poverty, illiteracy, disease, and social injustice. Interventions aim to achieve large-scale, positive changes through economic and social programs that enable everyone to realize their potential.

ER Med, General, Infect Dis, Logist-Op, MF Med, OB-GYN

+1 212-808-5615

https://vfapp.org/9d9e

Brigham and Women's Hospital Global Health Hub
Cares for patients in underserved settings, provides education to staff who work in those areas to create sustainable change, and conducts research designed to improve health in such settings.

General, Infect Dis

https://vfapp.org/a8a3

BroadReach
Collaborates with governments, multinational health organizations, donors, and private sector companies to affect healthcare reform and solve the world's biggest health challenges.

Logist-Op

+27 21 514 8300

https://vfapp.org/7812

Brooks Community Health Center, The (TBCHC)
Delivers high-quality, low-cost, ethical, and sustainable healthcare and healthcare-related educational services to underserved communities in Liberia.

Dent-OMFS, General, Geri, Infect Dis, MF Med, Ophth-Opt

+1 401-648-7525

https://vfapp.org/7a89

CARE
Works around the globe to save lives, defeat poverty, and achieve social justice.

ER Med, General

+1 800-422-7385

https://vfapp.org/7232

Carter Center, The
Seeks to prevent and resolve conflicts, enhance freedom and democracy, and improve health, while remaining committed to human rights and the alleviation of human suffering.

Infect Dis, MF Med, Ophth-Opt

+1 800-550-3560

https://vfapp.org/6556

Catholic World Mission
Works to rebuild communities worldwide by helping to alleviate poverty and empower underserved areas, while spreading the message of the Catholic Church.

ER Med, General, Nutr, Peds

+1 770-828-4966

https://vfapp.org/7b5f

CAUSE Canada
Strives to be a catalyst for global justice as a faith-based organization that aims to provide sustainable, integrated community development in rural West Africa and Central America through authentic, collaborative long-term relationships.

General, MF Med, Neonat, OB-GYN, Peds

+1 403-678-3332

https://vfapp.org/6fc1

Center for Epilepsy and Neurologic Diseases Liberia (CEND-LIB)
Provides neurologic care to the people and residents of Liberia, West Africa.

Infect Dis, Neuro

+1 443-956-8962

https://vfapp.org/c4e9

ChildFund Australia
Works to reduce poverty for children in many of the world's most disadvantaged communities.

ER Med, General, Peds

+1 800023600

https://vfapp.org/13df

Children & Charity International
Puts people first by providing education, leadership, and nutrition programs along with mentoring and healthcare support services to children, youth, and families.

Nutr, Peds

+1 202-234-0488

https://vfapp.org/6538

Children of the Nations
Aims to raise children out of poverty and hopelessness so they can become leaders who transform their nations. Emphasizes caring for the whole child–physically, mentally, socially, and spiritually.

Anesth, Dent-OMFS, General, Surg

+1 360-698-7227

https://vfapp.org/cc52

Children's Surgery International
Provides free medical and surgical services to children in need

around the world, and instruction and training to local surgeons and other medical providers such as doctors, anesthesiologists, nurses, and technicians.

Anesth, Dent-OMFS, Ortho, Ped Surg, Peds, Plast, Surg

+1 612-746-4082

https://vfapp.org/26d3

Christian Aid Ministries

Strives to be a trustworthy and efficient channel for Amish, Mennonite, and other conservative Anabaptist groups and individuals to minister to physical and spiritual needs around the world.

CT Surg, ER Med, Logist-Op, Ortho, Pub Health

+1 330-893-2428

https://vfapp.org/7b33

Christian Connections for International Health (CCIH)

Promotes global health and wholeness from a Christian perspective.

All-Immu, General, Infect Dis, MF Med, Neonat, OB-GYN, Psych

+1 703-923-8960

https://vfapp.org/fa5d

Clinton Health Access Initiative (CHAI)

Aims to save lives and reduce the burden of disease in low- and middle-income countries. Works with partners to strengthen the capabilities of governments and the private sector to create and sustain high-quality health systems.

General, Heme-Onc, Infect Dis, Logist-Op, MF Med, Medicine, Neonat, Nutr, OB-GYN, Path, Peds, Rad-Onc

+1 617-774-0110

https://vfapp.org/9ed7

Concern Worldwide

Seeks to permanently transform the lives of people living in extreme poverty, tackling its root causes, and building resilience.

Logist-Op, MF Med, Nutr, OB-GYN

+353 1 417 7700

https://vfapp.org/77e9

CT Medical Mission

Seeks to minister to the physical needs of the sick and suffering with the help of volunteer Christian physicians, dentists, nurses, and other medical personnel. Also aims to educate and provide healthy foods to people while sharing the Christian faith.

Dent-OMFS, ER Med, General, Infect Dis, Surg

+1 610-522-2239

https://vfapp.org/39de

Curamericas Global

Partners with communities abroad to save the lives of mothers and children by providing health services and education.

General, Infect Dis, MF Med, OB-GYN, Peds, Pub Health

+1 919-510-8787

https://vfapp.org/286b

Dignity: Liberia

Aims to bring restoration and hope to women with fistula and their communities through healing, education, and prevention.

MF Med, OB-GYN, Surg

https://vfapp.org/3732

Direct Relief

Improves the health and lives of people affected by poverty or emergency situations by mobilizing and providing essential medical resources needed for their care.

ER Med, Logist-Op

+1 805-964-4767

https://vfapp.org/58e5

Doctors Without Borders/Médecins Sans Frontières (MSF)

Responds to emergencies and provides lifesaving medical care where needed most, including during disasters, conflicts, and epidemics.

Anesth, Crit-Care, ER Med, General, Infect Dis, Nutr, OB-GYN, Ped Surg, Peds, Psych, Pub Health, Surg

+1 212-679-6800

https://vfapp.org/f363

Effect: Hope (The Leprosy Mission Canada)

Connects like-minded Canadians to people suffering in isolation from debilitating neglected tropical diseases like leprosy, lymphatic filariasis, Buruli ulcer, and STH.

General, Infect Dis

+1 888-537-7679

https://vfapp.org/f12a

eHealth Africa

Builds stronger health systems in Africa through the design and implementation of data-driven solutions, responding to local needs and providing underserved communities with the necessary tools to lead healthier lives.

Logist-Op, Path

https://vfapp.org/db6a

Episcopal Relief & Development

Provides relief in times of disaster and promotes sustainable development by identifying and addressing the root causes of suffering.

Infect Dis, MF Med, Neonat, Nutr, Peds

+1 855-312-4325

https://vfapp.org/7cfa

eRanger

Provides sustainable solutions to transportation and medical provision such as ambulances and mobile clinics in developing countries.

ER Med, General, Logist-Op

+27 40 654 3207

https://vfapp.org/4c18

Finn Church Aid

Supports people in the most vulnerable situations within fragile and disaster-affected regions in three thematic priority areas: right to peace, livelihood, and education.

ER Med, Psych, Pub Health

+358 20 7871201

https://vfapp.org/9623

For Hearts and Souls

Provides medical outreach and care for children through heart-related work, such as diagnosing heart problems and performing heart-saving surgeries.

Anesth, CT Surg, CV Med, Crit-Care, Peds, Pulm-Critic
+1 210-289-4753
https://vfapp.org/a162

Foundation for Special Surgery
Provides high-quality, complex surgical care by increasing surgical expertise in Africa through the participation of surgeons across various specialties to provide premium care and skills transfer/education to benefit patients.
Anesth, CT Surg, ENT, Endo, Neurosurg, Plast, Surg, Urol
+1 301-787-8914
https://vfapp.org/53db

Friends of UNFPA
Promotes the health, dignity, and rights of women and girls around the world by supporting the lifesaving work of UNFPA, the United Nations reproductive health and rights agency, through education, advocacy, and fundraising.
MF Med, OB-GYN
+1 646-649-9100
https://vfapp.org/2a3a

Global Alliance to Prevent Prematurity and Stillbirth (GAPPS)
Seeks to improve birth outcomes worldwide by reducing the burden of premature birth and stillbirth.
All-Immu, Infect Dis, MF Med, Neonat, Neonat, OB-GYN
+1 206-413-7954
https://vfapp.org/3f74

Global First Responder (GFR)
Acts as a centralized network for individuals and agencies involved in relief work worldwide and organizes and executes mission trips to areas in need, focusing not only on healthcare delivery but also health education and improvements.
ER Med
+1 573-424-8370
https://vfapp.org/a3e1

Global Ministries – The United Methodist Church
As the worldwide mission and development agency of The United Methodist Church, Global Ministries works with more than 300 hospitals and clinics around the world through its Global Health Unit.
Anesth, CT Surg, CV Med, Crit-Care, Dent-OMFS, Derm, ER Med, GI, General, Infect Dis, Logist-Op, MF Med, Medicine, Neonat, Nephro, Nutr, OB-GYN, Ophth-Opt, Ortho, Palliative, Peds, Pod, Psych, Pub Health, Rehab, Rheum, Surg, Urol
+1 800-862-4246
https://vfapp.org/1723

Global Oncology (GO)
Brings the best in cancer care to underserved patients around the world and collaborates across geographic, professional, and academic borders to improve cancer care, research, and education.
Heme-Onc, Path, Rad-Onc
https://vfapp.org/fcb8

Global Polio Eradication Initiative
Aims to eradicate polio worldwide.
All-Immu, Logist-Op
+1 847-866-3000
https://vfapp.org/7e2c

Global Strategies
Empowers communities in the most neglected areas of the world to improve the lives of women and children through healthcare.
MF Med, Neonat, OB-GYN, Peds
+1 415-451-1814
https://vfapp.org/ef92

GOAL
Works with the most vulnerable communities to help them respond to and recover from humanitarian crises, and to assist them in building transcendent solutions to mitigate poverty and vulnerability.
ER Med, General, Pub Health
+353 1 280 9779
https://vfapp.org/bbea

Grassroot Soccer
Leverages the power of soccer to educate, inspire, and mobilize at risk youth in developing countries to overcome their greatest health challenges, live healthier more productive lives, and be agents for change in their communities.
Infect Dis
+1 603-277-9685
https://vfapp.org/3521

Headwaters Relief Organization
Addresses public health issues for the most underserved populations in the world, providing psychosocial and medical support as well as disaster debris cleanup and rebuilding in partnership with other organizations.
ER Med, Infect Dis, Logist-Op, Psych, Pub Health
+1 763-233-7655
https://vfapp.org/e511

Healing the Children
Helps underserved children around the world secure the medical care they need to lead more fulfilling lives.
Anesth, Dent-OMFS, ENT, General, Medicine, Ophth-Opt, Ped Surg, Peds, Plast, Surg
+1 509-327-4281
https://vfapp.org/d4ee

Health Africa Foundation (HAF)
Provides essential medical equipment and supplies to under-resourced healthcare facilities and builds the capacity of Liberian health workers to enhance the delivery of high quality healthcare services in Liberia. Promotes accountability and demonstrated impact of donations.
Anesth, CV Med, Crit-Care, ER Med, Endo, General, Heme-Onc, Infect Dis, MF Med, Medicine, OB-GYN, Path, Peds, Radiol
+1 267-262-3564
https://vfapp.org/fe3b

Health Education and Relief Through Teaching Foundation (HEARTT Foundation)
Educates and assists local healthcare providers in developing and/or improving the healthcare system and infrastructure.
ER Med, Medicine, OB-GYN, Peds, Psych, Surg
https://vfapp.org/ecc3

Health Equity Initiative
Aims to build and sustain a global community that engages across sectors and disciplines to advance health equity.

Pub Health
https://vfapp.org/e2e2

Heart to Heart International
Strengthens communities through improving health access, providing humanitarian development, and administering crisis relief worldwide. Engages volunteers, collaborates with partners, and deploys resources to achieve this mission.
Anesth, ER Med, General, Logist-Op, Medicine, Path, Path, Peds, Psych, Pub Health, Surg
+1 913-764-5200
https://vfapp.org/aacb

Heineman Medical Outreach
Provides medical and educational assistance globally to promote sustainable healthcare and enhanced living standards in underserved communities through the International Medical Outreach (IMO) program, a collaborative partnership between Heineman Medical Outreach and Atrium Health.
Anesth, CT Surg, CV Med, ER Med, General, Heme-Onc, Logist-Op, Medicine, Neonat, OB-GYN, Ped Surg, Peds, Surg, Vasc Surg
+1 704-374-0505
https://vfapp.org/389b

HOPE2
Renews hope in the Liberian people through safe water, medical care, education, and training.
ER Med, General, Peds
+1 765-729-2695
https://vfapp.org/bf5f

Humanity & Inclusion
Works alongside people with disabilities and vulnerable populations, taking action and bearing witness in order to respond to their essential needs, improve their living conditions and health, and promote respect for their dignity and fundamental rights.
General, Infect Dis, MF Med, Medicine, Ortho, Peds, Psych, Pub Health, Rehab
+1 301-891-2138
https://vfapp.org/16b7

Humanity First
Provides aid and assistance to those in need, offering sustainable development solutions to society while providing and empowering local communities with the resources to help themselves.
ER Med, General, MF Med, Ophth-Opt
+44 20 8417 0082
https://vfapp.org/13cc

HVK Children's Foundation
Works to meet the needs of women, children, and families in Sub-Saharan Africa and Liberia by educating, supporting, and training Liberians to achieve economic self-sufficiency.
All-Immu, Dent-OMFS, Nutr, Ophth-Opt, Peds
+1 508-502-0907
https://vfapp.org/beb5

ICAP at Columbia University
Serves as global leader in supporting the scale-up of multidisciplinary HIV/AIDS prevention, care, and treatment programs based on a family-focused approach.
General, Infect Dis, MF Med, Medicine, OB-GYN, Pub Health
+1 212-342-0505
https://vfapp.org/a8ef

International Agency for the Prevention of Blindness (IAPB), The
Leads international efforts in blindness-prevention activities, works toward a world where no one is needlessly visually impaired, and ensures that everyone has access to the best possible standard of eye health.
Infect Dis, Ophth-Opt, Pub Health
https://vfapp.org/87a2

International Children's Heart Fund
Aims to promote the international growth and quality of cardiac surgery, particularly in children and young adults.
CT Surg, Ped Surg
https://vfapp.org/33fb

International Federation of Red Cross and Red Crescent Societies (IFRC)
Coordinates and directs international assistance following natural and man-made disasters in nonconflict situations through the world's largest humanitarian and development network. Provides disaster-preparedness programs, healthcare activities, and promotes humanitarian values.
ER Med, General, Infect Dis, Nutr
+1 212-338-0161
https://vfapp.org/b4ee

International Medical Response
Supplements, supports, and enhances healthcare systems in communities across the world that have been incapacitated by natural disaster, extreme poverty, and/or regional conflict by sending a multidisciplinary team of healthcare professionals.
Anesth, General, OB-GYN, Surg
+1 917-324-8348
https://vfapp.org/9ccd

International Organization for Migration (IOM) – The UN Migration Agency
Promotes evidence-informed policies and holistic, preventive, and curative health programs that are beneficial, accessible, and equitable for vulnerable migrants.
General, Infect Dis, OB-GYN
+27 12 342 2789
https://vfapp.org/621a

International Planned Parenthood Federation (IPPF)
Leads a locally owned, globally connected civil society movement that provides and enables services and champions sexual and reproductive health and rights for all, especially the underserved.
Infect Dis, MF Med, OB-GYN
+44 20 7939 8200
https://vfapp.org/dc97

International Rescue Committee (IRC)
Responds to the world's worst humanitarian crises and helps people whose lives and livelihoods are shattered by conflict and disaster to survive, recover, and gain control of their future.
ER Med, General, Infect Dis, MF Med, Peds
+1 212-551-3000
https://vfapp.org/5d24

IntraHealth International
Improves the performance of health workers and strengthens the systems in which they work.

CV Med, Endo, General, Infect Dis, MF Med, Neonat, Nutr, OB-GYN

+1 919-313-3554

https://vfapp.org/ddc8

Jhpiego
Creates and delivers transformative healthcare solutions that save lives in partnership with national governments, health experts, and local communities.

General, Infect Dis, OB-GYN, Surg

+1 410-537-1800

https://vfapp.org/45b8

John Snow, Inc. (JSI)
Aims to improve the health and well-being of underserved and vulnerable people and communities throughout the world.

General, Infect Dis, Logist-Op, MF Med, OB-GYN, Peds, Psych, Pub Health

+1 617-482-9485

https://vfapp.org/ba78

Johns Hopkins Center for Communication Programs
Believes in the power of communication to save lives, by empowering people to adopt healthy behaviors for themselves, their families, and their communities.

General, Infect Dis, Logist-Op, OB-GYN, Pub Health

+1 410-659-6300

https://vfapp.org/1bf9

Joint United Nations Programme on HIV/AIDS (UNAIDS)
Aims to place people living with HIV and people affected by the virus at the decision-making table and at the center of designing, delivering, and monitoring the AIDS response.

Infect Dis

+41 22 791 36 66

https://vfapp.org/464a

Korle-Bu Neuroscience Foundation
Committed to providing medical support for brain and spinal injuries and disease to the people of Ghana and West Africa.

Anesth, Logist-Op, Neuro, Neurosurg, Rehab

+1 604-513-0029

https://vfapp.org/6695

Last Mile Health
Links community health workers with frontline health workers—nurses, doctors, and midwives at community clinics—and supports them to bring lifesaving services to the doorsteps of people living far from care.

General, Logist-Op, OB-GYN, Pub Health

+1 617-880-6163

https://vfapp.org/37da

Liberia Medical Mission
Provides free medical, ophthalmic, and mental health services through mission trips to underserved communities in Liberia and other West African countries.

General, Infect Dis, OB-GYN, Ophth-Opt, Ophth-Opt, Palliative, Peds, Psych, Urol

+1 215-901-4731

https://vfapp.org/8193

Life for a Child
Supports the provision of the best possible health care, given local circumstances, to all children and youth with diabetes in less-resourced countries, through the strengthening of existing diabetes services.

Endo, Medicine, Peds

https://vfapp.org/d712

Life for African Mothers
Aims to save the lives of pregnant women in Sub-Saharan Africa.

MF Med, Neonat, OB-GYN

+44 29 2034 3774

https://vfapp.org/fce2

Lions Clubs International
Empowers volunteers to serve their communities, meet humanitarian needs, encourage peace, and promote international understanding through Lions clubs.

Heme-Onc, Medicine, Nutr, Ophth-Opt

+1 630-571-5466

https://vfapp.org/7b12

London School of Hygiene & Tropical Medicine: Health in Humanitarian Crises Centre
Advances health and health equity in crisis-affected countries through research, education, and translation of knowledge into policy and practice.

ER Med, Infect Dis, Pub Health

+44 20 7636 8636

https://vfapp.org/96ad

Management Sciences for Health (MSH)
Works with countries and communities to save lives and improve the health of the world's poorest and most vulnerable people by building strong, resilient, sustainable health systems.

Infect Dis, Logist-Op, Pub Health

+1 617-250-9500

https://vfapp.org/6aa2

MAP International
Provides medicines and health supplies to those in need around the world so they might experience life to the fullest.

Logist-Op

+1 800-225-8550

https://vfapp.org/deed

Massachusetts General Hospital Global Surgery Initiative
Aims to improve surgical education and access to advanced surgical care in resource-limited settings around the world by performing surgical operations as visitors, training local surgeons, and sharing medical technology through international partnerships across disciplines.

Anesth, Crit-Care, ER Med, Heme-Onc, Peds, Surg

+1 617-724-4093

https://vfapp.org/31b1

Maternal & Childhealth Advocacy International
Seeks to save and improve the lives of babies, children, and pregnant women in areas of extreme poverty by empowering and enabling in-country partners to strengthen emergency healthcare.

MF Med, Neonat, OB-GYN, Peds

+44 1445 781354

https://vfapp.org/ea67

Medical Missions for Global Health
Seeks to reduce health disparities by providing surgical, medical, and health care services and education to underserved communities and developing communities throughout Africa, the Caribbean, Central and South America, and the U.S.

Dent-OMFS, General, Surg

+1 212-951-1431

https://vfapp.org/cf52

Medical Teams International
Seeks to restore health as the first step to restoring hope, working to bring basic but lifesaving medical care to those in need.

Dent-OMFS, ER Med, General, MF Med, Pub Health

+1 503-624-1000

https://vfapp.org/8d1c

MedShare
Aims to improve the quality of life of people, communities, and the planet by sourcing and directly delivering surplus medical supplies and equipment to communities in need around the world.

Logist-Op

+1 770-323-5858

https://vfapp.org/c8bc

MENTOR Initiative
Saves lives in emergencies through tropical disease control, and helps people recover from crisis with dignity, working side by side with communities, health workers, and health authorities to leave a lasting impact.

ER Med, Infect Dis

+44 1444 412171

https://vfapp.org/3bd5

Mercy Ships
Operates hospital ships staffed by volunteers to bring hope, healing, and healthcare to underserved communities worldwide.

Anesth, Dent-OMFS, Logist-Op, Neonat, OB-GYN, Ophth-Opt, Ortho, Palliative, Plast, Psych, Surg

+1 903-939-7000

https://vfapp.org/2e99

MiracleFeet
Brings low-cost treatment to every child on the planet born with clubfoot, a leading cause of physical disability.

Ortho, Peds, Rehab

+1 919-240-5572

https://vfapp.org/bda8

Nazarene Compassionate Ministries
Partners with local churches around the world to clothe, shelter, feed, heal, educate, and live in solidarity with those in need.

General, Infect Dis, OB-GYN

+1 800-310-6362

https://vfapp.org/6b4d

Newborn, Infant, and Child Health International (NICHE)
Aims to make outstanding care of newborn babies commonplace in poorly resourced areas of the world.

Crit-Care, General, Neonat, Peds

https://vfapp.org/8817

One Heart Worldwide
Aims to end preventable deaths related to pregnancy and childbirth worldwide.

MF Med, Neonat, OB-GYN, Pub Health

+1 415-379-4762

https://vfapp.org/a865

OneSight
Brings eye exams and glasses to the people who lack access to vision care.

Ophth-Opt

+1 888-935-4589

https://vfapp.org/3ecc

Operation Fistula
Exists to end obstetric fistula by building models of care that serve every woman, everywhere.

MF Med, OB-GYN, Surg

+1 512-687-3479

https://vfapp.org/ce8e

Options
Believes in a world where women and children can access the high-quality health services they need, without financial burden.

Logist-Op, MF Med, Neonat, OB-GYN

+44 20 7430 1900

https://vfapp.org/3a48

Pact
Works on the ground to improve the lives of those who are challenged by poverty and marginalization, striving for a world where all people are heard, capable, and vibrant.

Infect Dis, Logist-Op, MF Med, Pub Health

+1 202-466-5666

https://vfapp.org/9a6c

Partners for Development (PfD)
Works to improve quality of life for vulnerable people in underserved communities through local and international partnerships.

Infect Dis, MF Med, Neonat, Peds

+1 301-608-0426

https://vfapp.org/d2f6

Partners in Health
Responds to the moral imperative to provide high-quality healthcare globally to those who need it most, while striving to ease suffering by providing a comprehensive model of care that includes access to food, transportation, housing, and other key components of healing.

CT Surg, General, Heme-Onc, Infect Dis, MF Med, Neurosurg, OB-GYN, Ortho, Plast, Psych, Urol

+1 857-880-5600

https://vfapp.org/dc9c

Picture of Health Foundation
Provides communities with health education and empowers people to alter unhealthy lifestyles, thus increasing both life expectancy and quality.

General, Pub Health

+1 770-807-7813

https://vfapp.org/83e3

Project Concern International (PCI)
Drives innovation from the ground up to enhance health, end hunger, overcome hardship, and advance women and girls—resulting in meaningful and measurable change in people's lives.

Infect Dis, MF Med, Nutr, OB-GYN, Peds

+1 858-279-9690
https://vfapp.org/5ed7

PSI – Population Services International
Dedicates efforts to improving the health of people in the developing world by focusing on challenges such as a lack of family planning, HIV/AIDS, barriers to maternal health, and the greatest threats to children under the age of 5, including malaria, diarrhea, pneumonia, and malnutrition.
Infect Dis, MF Med, OB-GYN, Peds
+1 202-785-0072
https://vfapp.org/ffe3

RAD-AID International
Improves and optimizes access to medical imaging and radiology in low-resource regions of the world.
Rad-Onc, Radiol
https://vfapp.org/537f

RestoringVision
Empowers lives by restoring vision for millions of people in need.
Ophth-Opt
+1 209-980-7323
https://vfapp.org/e121

Riders for Health International
Aids in the last mile of healthcare delivery, by ensuring that healthcare reaches everyone, everywhere.
ER Med, Infect Dis, Logist-Op, Pub Health
+231 77 704 4287
https://vfapp.org/85aa

Rockefeller Foundation, The
Works to promote the well-being of humanity.
Logist-Op, Nutr, Pub Health
+1 212-869-8500
https://vfapp.org/5424

Rotary International
Provides service to others, improves lives, and advances world understanding, goodwill, and peace through its fellowship of business, professional, and community leaders.
ER Med, General, Infect Dis, MF Med, OB-GYN
https://vfapp.org/8fb5

Rotaplast International
Helps children and families worldwide by eliminating the burden of cleft lip and/or palate, burn scarring, and other deformities by sending medical teams to provide free reconstructive surgery, ancillary treatment, and training.
Anesth, Dent-OMFS, ENT, Ped Surg, Plast, Surg
+1 415-252-1111
https://vfapp.org/78b3

ROW Foundation
Works to improve the quality of training for healthcare providers, and the diagnosis and treatment available to people with epilepsy and associated psychiatric disorders in under-resourced areas of the world.
Neuro, Psych
+1 630-791-0247
https://vfapp.org/25eb

Saint Joseph's Catholic Hospital
Provides healthcare services to all people who need care without any form of discrimination.
Medicine, OB-GYN, Ortho, Peds, Surg
+231 88 673 6888
https://vfapp.org/34d2

Salvation Army International, The
Seeks to meet human needs through services in education, healthcare, community support, emergency response, and ministry development, inspired by the Christian faith.
Dent-OMFS, Derm, ER Med, Infect Dis, MF Med, Medicine, Nutr, OB-GYN, Ophth-Opt, Palliative, Psych, Rehab, Surg
+44 20 7332 0101
https://vfapp.org/8eb3

Save the Children
Gives children around the world a healthy start in life, the opportunity to learn, and protection from harm.
All-Immu, Crit-Care, ER Med, General, Infect Dis, MF Med, Medicine, Neonat, OB-GYN, Peds, Psych, Pub Health
+1 800-728-3843
https://vfapp.org/2e73

SEE International
Provides sustainable medical, surgical, and educational services through volunteer ophthalmic surgeons, with the objectives of restoring sight and preventing blindness to disadvantaged individuals worldwide.
Ophth-Opt, Surg
+1 805-963-3303
https://vfapp.org/6e1b

Seed Global Health
Focuses on human resources for health capacity building at the individual, institutional, and national level through sustained collaborative engagement with partners.
Logist-Op
+1 617-366-1650
https://vfapp.org/d12e

Set Free Alliance
Works with in-country partners to rescue children, provide clean water, host medical clinics, and plant churches, based in Christian ministry.
General, Peds
+1 864-469-9500
https://vfapp.org/bdb8

Sightsavers
Prevents avoidable blindness in some of the poorest parts of the world by treating debilitating eye diseases.
Infect Dis, Ophth-Opt, Surg
+1 800-707-9746
https://vfapp.org/aa52

SIGN Fracture Care International
Builds orthopedic capacity around the world and provides the injured poor access to fracture surgery by donating orthopedic education and implant systems to surgeons in developing countries.
Ortho, Rehab, Surg
+1 509-371-1107
https://vfapp.org/123d

Smile Train

Seeks to give every child with a cleft the opportunity for a healthy, productive life by providing free cleft repair surgery and comprehensive cleft care in their own communities.

Dent-OMFS, ENT, Plast

+1 800-932-9541

https://vfapp.org/f21d

Sustainable Cardiovascular Health Equity Development Alliance

Fights cardiovascular disease in underserved populations globally via education, training, and increasing interventional capacity.

CV Med, Pub Health, Radiol

+1 608-338-3357

https://vfapp.org/799c

Swiss Tropical and Public Health Institute

Contributes to the improvement of the health of populations internationally, nationally, and locally through excellence in research, education, and services.

Infect Dis, Pub Health

+41 61 284 81 11

https://vfapp.org/2ee4

Task Force for Global Health, The

Consists of programs and focus areas that cover a range of global health issues including neglected tropical diseases, infectious diseases, vaccines, field epidemiology, public health informatics, health workforce development, and global health ethics.

Infect Dis, Logist-Op, Medicine, Ophth-Opt, Peds

+1 404-371-0466

https://vfapp.org/714c

Tearfund

Responds to crisis and partners with local churches to bring restoration to those living in poverty, inspired by the Christian faith.

ER Med, Logist-Op

+44 20 3906 3906

https://vfapp.org/f6cf

Turing Foundation

Aims to contribute toward a better world and a better society by focusing on efforts such as health, art, education, and nature.

Infect Dis

+31 20 520 0010

https://vfapp.org/6bcc

U.S. President's Malaria Initiative (PMI)

Supports low-income countries to help control and eliminate malaria through cost-effective, lifesaving malaria interventions.

Infect Dis, MF Med, OB-GYN

+1 202-712-0000

https://vfapp.org/dc8b

United Methodist Volunteers in Mission (UMVIM)

Engages in short-term missions each year in ministries as varied as disaster response, community development, pastor training, microenterprise, agriculture, Vacation Bible School, building repair and construction, and medical/dental services.

Dent-OMFS, ER Med, General

https://vfapp.org/1ee6

United Nations Children's Fund (UNICEF)

Works in over 190 countries and territories to save children's lives, to defend their rights, and to help them fulfill their potential, from early childhood through adolescence.

All-Immu, Infect Dis, MF Med, Neonat, Nutr, OB-GYN, Ped Surg, Peds, Pub Health

https://vfapp.org/42d7

United Nations Development Programme (UNDP)

Helps countries achieve the simultaneous eradication of extreme poverty and significant reduction of inequalities and exclusion using a sustainable human development approach.

Infect Dis, Logist-Op, Pub Health

https://vfapp.org/935c

United Nations High Commissioner for Refugees (UNHCR)

Safeguards the rights and well-being of people who have been forced to flee, ensuring that everybody has the right to seek asylum and find safe refuge in another country, with the goal of seeking lasting solutions.

General, MF Med, Medicine, OB-GYN, Peds, Psych, Pub Health

https://vfapp.org/6636

United Nations Population Fund (UNFPA)

Supports reproductive healthcare for women and youth in more than 150 countries, focusing on delivering a world where every pregnancy is wanted, every childbirth is safe, and every young person's potential is fulfilled.

Infect Dis, MF Med, Neonat, OB-GYN, Peds, Pub Health

+1 212-963-6008

https://vfapp.org/c969

United Surgeons for Children (USFC)

Pursues greater health and opportunity for children in the most neglected pockets of the world, with a specific focus and expertise in surgery.

Anesth, CT Surg, Neonat, Neurosurg, OB-GYN, Peds, Radiol, Surg

https://vfapp.org/3b4c

University of California Los Angeles: David Geffen School of Medicine Global Health Program

Catalyzes opportunities to improve health globally by engaging in multi-disciplinary and innovative education programs, research initiatives, and bilateral partnerships that provide opportunities for trainees, faculty, and staff to contribute to sustainable health initiatives and to address health inequities facing the world today.

All-Immu, Infect Dis, Logist-Op, MF Med, Medicine, Neonat, OB-GYN, Ortho, Ped Surg, Peds, Radiol

+1 310-312-0531

https://vfapp.org/f1a4

University of North Carolina: Institute for Global Health and Infectious Diseases

Harnesses the full resources of UNC and its partners to solve global health problems, reduce the burden of disease, and cultivate the next generation of global health leaders.

Infect Dis, MF Med, OB-GYN, Psych, Surg

+1 919-966-2537

https://vfapp.org/ed5e

USAID: Maternal and Child Survival Program

Works to prevent child and maternal deaths.

Infect Dis, MF Med, Neonat, OB-GYN, Peds

https://vfapp.org/6fcf

USAID: Deliver Project

Builds a global supply chain to deliver lifesaving health products to people in order to enable countries to provide family planning, protect against malaria, and limit the spread of pandemic threats.

Infect Dis, Logist-Op, MF Med

+1 202-712-0000

https://vfapp.org/374e

USAID: Leadership, Management and Governance Project

Improves leadership, management, and governance practices to strengthen health systems and improve health for all, including vulnerable populations worldwide.

Logist-Op

https://vfapp.org/d35e

USAID: Maternal and Child Health Integrated Program

Works to improve the health of women and their families, including programs for maternal, newborn, and child health, immunization, family planning, nutrition, malaria, and HIV/AIDS.

All-Immu, General, Infect Dis, MF Med

+1 202-835-3136

https://vfapp.org/4415

Vitamin Angels

Helps at-risk populations in need—specifically pregnant women, new mothers, and children under age five—to gain access to life-changing vitamins and minerals.

General, Nutr

+1 805-564-8400

https://vfapp.org/7da1

Voices for a Malaria-Free Future

Seeks to expand national movements of private and public sector leaders to mobilize political and popular support for malaria control.

Infect Dis, Path

https://vfapp.org/4213

Women's Refugee Commission

Seeks to improve lives by protecting the rights of women, children, and youth displaced by conflict and crisis through researching their needs, identifying solutions, and advocating for programs and policies to strengthen their resilience.

General, MF Med, Neonat, OB-GYN, Peds, Psych

+1 212-551-3115

https://vfapp.org/3d8f

World Health Organization, The (WHO)

The United Nations' agency for health provides leadership on global health matters, shapes the health research agenda, setting norms and standards, articulates evidence-based policy options, provides technical support and monitoring to countries, and assesses health trends.

ER Med, General, Infect Dis, Logist-Op, MF Med, OB-GYN, Peds, Psych, Pub Health

+41 22 791 21 11

https://vfapp.org/c476

World Hope International

Empowers the poorest individuals around the world so they can become agents of change within their communities, by offering resources and knowledge.

Infect Dis, Logist-Op, MF Med, OB-GYN, Peds

+1 703-923-9414

https://vfapp.org/a4b8

World Medical Relief

Facilitates the distribution of surplus medical resources where they are needed.

Logist-Op

+1 313-866-5333

https://vfapp.org/72dc

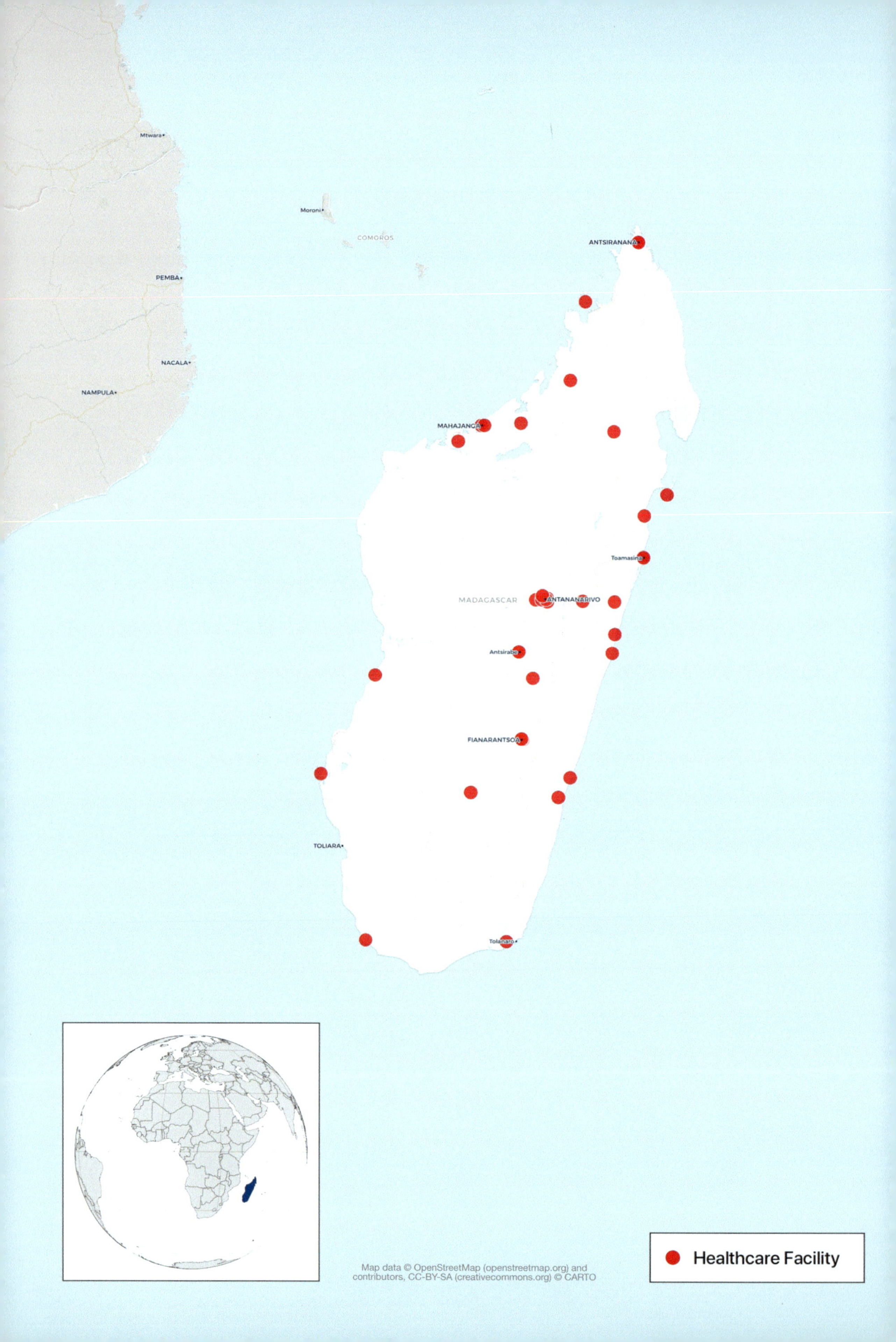
Mtwara
Moroni
COMOROS
ANTSIRANANA
PEMBA
NACALA
NAMPULA
MAHAJANGA
Toamasina
MADAGASCAR
ANTANANARIVO
Antsirabe
FIANARANTSOA
TOLIARA
Tolanaro
Healthcare Facility
Map data © OpenStreetMap (openstreetmap.org) and contributors, CC-BY-SA (creativecommons.org) © CARTO

Madagascar

The Republic of Madagascar is a large island country located about 400 kilometers off the coast of East Africa, in the Indian Ocean. The population of 27 million lives in predominantly rural areas and is made up of various ethnic groups, including Malayo-Indonesian, Cotiers, French, Indian, Creole, and Comoran. Malagasy, French, and English are all spoken, as are local languages; the people practice various forms of Christianity, Islam, and local indigenous religions. The country has diverse animal life, most notably 40 species of indigenous lemurs unique to Madagascar.

Madagascar gained independence from France in 1960 and has since experienced several bouts of political turmoil and instability. A coup in 2009 resulted in a five-year political deadlock; in 2019 the election of a new president ended a decade of political uncertainty. Despite political issues, the country as a whole has made positive economic progress, and the agriculture sector, with crops such as rice, coffee, and vanilla, is the nation's leading employer. Over 70 percent of the young Malagasy population lives in poverty.

Health challenges include chronic malnutrition; nearly half of children under five years of age suffer from stunting. The country also experienced a measles outbreak in 2018 that infected tens of thousands of people. The leading causes of death include diarrheal diseases, lower respiratory infections, neonatal disorders, tuberculosis, malaria, and protein-energy malnutrition. Non-communicable diseases such as stroke, ischemic heart disease, hypertensive heart disease, and cirrhosis have notably increased and are increasingly among the top causes of death in Madagascar.

27M
Population

$522
GDP Per Capita

67 years
Life Expectancy
↑ Improving

18.1 Doctors/100k	**20** Beds/100k	**335** Deaths/100k
Physician Density	Hospital Bed Density	Maternal Mortality

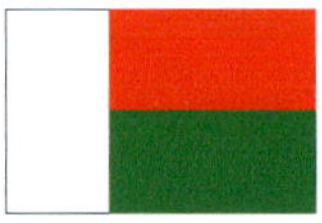

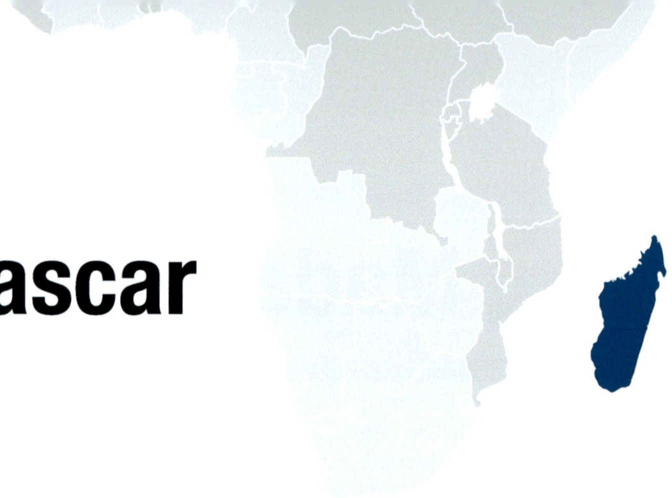

Madagascar

Healthcare Facilities

Andranomadio Hospital
N 34, Antsirabe,
Vakinankaratra, Madagascar
https://vfapp.org/b1b1

Centre Hospitalier de Reference Regional (CHRR) Antsohihy
Antsohihy, Madagascar
https://vfapp.org/83b6

Centre Hospitalier de Référence Régional de Morondava
Morondava, Madagascar
https://vfapp.org/eb4d

Centre Hospitalier de Référence Régionale Ihosy
Ihosy, Madagascar
https://vfapp.org/182d

Centre Hospitalier de Soavinandriana
6 bis, Rue du Dr Moss
Antananarivo, Madagascar
https://vfapp.org/ef5a

Centre Hospitalier Universitaire Zafisaona Gabriel
Rue Marius Barriquand,
Mahajanga, Boeny,
Madagascar
https://vfapp.org/884f

Centre Hosptialier Universitaire Tambohobe
Tambohobe, Fianarantsoa,
Madagascar
https://vfapp.org/9664

CHD I Mahanoro
Mahanoro, Madagascar
https://vfapp.org/2352

CHD II Moramanga
N 2, Moramanga,
Alaotra-Mangoro,
Madagascar
https://vfapp.org/626e

CHRR Manakara
Manakara, Madagascar
https://vfapp.org/32c3

CHU Morafeno Toamasina
Route d'Ivoloina, Toamasina,
Madagascar
https://vfapp.org/3618

Clinique des Soeurs Ankadifotsy
Clinique des Soeurs
Ankadifotsy, Antananarivo,
Madagascar
https://vfapp.org/d12d

CMA
Làlana Nanisana, Antananarivo,
Analamanga, Madagascar
https://vfapp.org/591f

CSB Farafangana
Farafangana,
Madagascar
https://vfapp.org/f232

Espace Medical
Antisiranana,
Madagascar
https://vfapp.org/a947

Hell-Ville Hospital
Avenue Victor Augagneur,
Andoany, Diana, Madagascar
https://vfapp.org/1a61

Hopitaly Atsimo
Rue Daniel Rakotondrainibe,
Antsirabe, Vakinankaratra,
Madagascar
https://vfapp.org/cc83

Hopitaly Kely
Boulevard de la Libération,
Toamasina, Atsinanana,
Madagascar
https://vfapp.org/b99d

Hopitaly Manarapenitra
Avenue Pasteur, Antsiranana,
Diana, Madagascar
https://vfapp.org/c82d

Hospital at Ranomafana
Brickaville, Madagascar
https://vfapp.org/9c4c

Hospital Chrd Ii Atu
N21, Sainte Marie, Madagascar
https://vfapp.org/5fa9

Hospital CSB Ejeda
Ejeda, Madagascar
https://vfapp.org/c462

Hospital Loterana Manambaro
Manambaro, Madagascar
https://vfapp.org/b986

Hospital Mahajanga
Mahajanga,
Madagascar
https://vfapp.org/4c5b

Hôpital de Fénérive-Est
N 5, Fenoarivo Atsinanana,
Analanjirofo, Madagascar
https://vfapp.org/1f67

Hôpital des Enfants
Làlana Andriantsilavo,
Antananarivo, Analamanga,
Madagascar
https://vfapp.org/f664

Hôpital Général de Befelatanana
Làlana Dokotera Ravloud
Jacques, Antananarivo,
Analamanga, Madagascar
https://vfapp.org/b481

Hôpital Itaosy
N 1, Antananarivo,
Analamanga, Madagascar
https://vfapp.org/83d1

Hôpital Jean Paul II
Mahajanga, Madagascar
https://vfapp.org/9c81

Hôpital Joseph Ravoahangy-Andrianavalona
Rue Ravoahangy
Andrianavalona, Antananarivo,
Analamanga, Madagascar
https://vfapp.org/cbd8

Hôpital Luthérien des 67ha
Làlana Agosthino Neto,
Antananarivo, Analamanga,
Madagascar
https://vfapp.org/4a49

Hôpital Mpitsabo Mikambana
Rue Jeneraly Charles
de Gaulle, Antananarivo,
Madagascar
https://vfapp.org/4fc2

Hôpital Municipal de Sandrandahy
Sandrandahy, Madagascar
https://vfapp.org/8bde

Hôpital Universitaire Andrainjato
Route de Mahasoabe,
Fianarantsoa, Matsiatra
Ambony, Madagascar
https://vfapp.org/2946

Hôpital Vaovao Mahafaly – The Good News Hospital
Mandritsara, Madagascar
https://vfapp.org/5197

Hôpital Vezo
Andavadoaka, Madagascar
https://vfapp.org/6952

Joseph Ravoahangy Andrianavalona Hospital
RN 1, Antananarivo 101,
Madagascar
https://vfapp.org/d266

Lutheran Hospital at Ambohibao
Tobim-pitsaboana Loterana
Ambohibao 4 Antananarivo,
105, Madagascar
https://vfapp.org/c754

Orthodoxe
Route d'Alasora, Alasora,
Analamanga, Madagascar
https://vfapp.org/3bf5

OSTIE Anosivavaka
Rue Docteur Joseph
Raseta, Antananarivo,
Madagascar
https://vfapp.org/a5ae

Sampan'asa Loterana Momba ny Fahasalamana Ivory Atsimo
Làlana Pasitera Jessé
Rainihifina, Fianarantsoa,
Matsiatra Ambony, Madagascar
https://vfapp.org/aaa4

Service de Santé de District Mitsinjo
N 19, Antanambao, Boeny,
Madagascar
https://vfapp.org/2193

Smids
Boulevard Duplex,Antsiranana,
Diana, Madagascar
https://vfapp.org/352c

Vatomandry
Vatomandry, Madagascar
https://vfapp.org/b658

Madagascar

Nonprofit Organizations

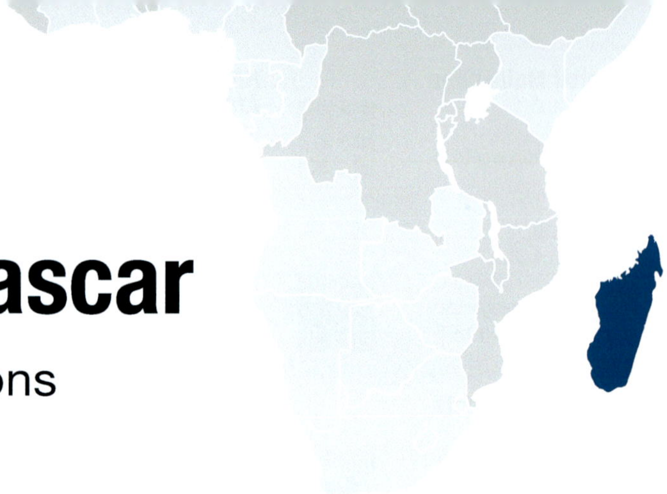

Abt Associates
Seeks to improve the quality of life and economic well-being of people worldwide, while striving to meet and exceed the highest professional standards.

General, Logist-Op, MF Med, OB-GYN, Peds
+1 212-779-7700
https://vfapp.org/cec2

Action Against Hunger
Aims to end life-threatening hunger for good through treating and preventing malnutrition across more than forty-five countries.

+1 212-967-7800
https://vfapp.org/2dbc

Advance Family Planning
Aims to achieve global expansion and access to quality contraceptive information, services, and supplies through financial investment and political commitment.

General, MF Med, Pub Health
+1 410-502-8715
https://vfapp.org/7478

Adventist Health International
Focuses on upgrading and managing mission hospitals by providing governance, consultation, and technical assistance to a number of affiliated Seventh-Day Adventist hospitals throughout Africa, Asia, and the Americas.

Dent-OMFS, General, Pub Health
+1 909-558-5610
https://vfapp.org/16aa

Africa CDC
Aims to strengthen the capacity and capability of Africa's public health institutions as well as partnerships to detect and respond quickly and effectively to disease threats and outbreaks, based on data-driven interventions and programs.

Infect Dis, Logist-Op, Pub Health
+251 11 551 7700
https://vfapp.org/339c

Africa Indoor Residual Spraying Project (AIRS)
Aims to protect millions of people in Africa from malaria by spraying insecticide on the walls, ceilings, and other indoor resting places of mosquitoes that transmit malaria.

Infect Dis
+1 301-347-5000
https://vfapp.org/9bd1

Africa Inland Mission International
Seeks to establish churches and community development programs including health care projects, based in Christian ministry.

Anesth, Dent-OMFS, ER Med, General, MF Med, Medicine, OB-GYN, OB-GYN, Ophth-Opt, Ped Surg, Peds, Rehab
https://vfapp.org/f2f6

Against Malaria Foundation
Helps protect people from malaria. Funds anti-malaria nets, specifically long-lasting insecticidal nets (LLINs), and works with distribution partners to ensure they are used. Tracks and reports on net use and malaria case data.

Infect Dis
+44 20 7371 8735
https://vfapp.org/337d

AISPO
Implements international initiatives in the healthcare sector and remains involved in a variety of projects to combat poverty, social injustice, and disease in the world.

All-Immu, ER Med, GI, General, Infect Dis, Logist-Op, MF Med, Neonat, OB-GYN, Peds, Psych, Pub Health, Radiol
+39 02 2643 4481
https://vfapp.org/c9e6

American Academy of Pediatrics
Seeks to attain optimal physical, mental, and social health and well-being for all infants, children, adolescents, and young adults.

Anesth, Crit-Care, Neonat, Ped Surg
+1 800-433-9016
https://vfapp.org/9633

Amref Health Africa
Serves millions of people across thirty-five countries in Sub-Saharan Africa, strengthening health systems, and training African health workers to respond to the continent's most critical health issues.

All-Immu, General, Infect Dis, Logist-Op, MF Med, OB-GYN, Path, Pub Health, Surg
+254 20 6993000
https://vfapp.org/6985

Australian Doctors for Africa
Develops healthier environments and builds capacity through

the provision of voluntary medical assistance, while training and teaching doctors, nurses, and allied health workers and improving infrastructure and providing medical equipment.

Anesth, ENT, GI, Logist-Op, MF Med, OB-GYN, Ortho, Ped Surg, Peds, Urol

+61 8 6478 8951

https://vfapp.org/f769

Basic Foundations

Supports local projects and organizations that seek to meet the basic human needs of others in their community.

ER Med, General, Peds, Rehab, Surg

https://vfapp.org/c4be

Beta Humanitarian Help

Provides plastic surgery in underserved areas of the world.

Anesth, Plast

+49 228 909075778

https://vfapp.org/7221

BethanyKids

Transforms the lives of African children with surgical conditions and disabilities through pediatric surgery, rehabilitation, public education, spiritual ministry, and training health professionals.

Neurosurg, Nutr, Ortho, Ped Surg, Peds, Rehab, Surg

https://vfapp.org/db4e

CARE

Works around the globe to save lives, defeat poverty, and achieve social justice.

ER Med, General

+1 800-422-7385

https://vfapp.org/7232

Carter Center, The

Seeks to prevent and resolve conflicts, enhance freedom and democracy, and improve health, while remaining committed to human rights and the alleviation of human suffering.

Infect Dis, MF Med, Ophth-Opt

+1 800-550-3560

https://vfapp.org/6556

Chain of Hope (La Chaîne de l'Espoir)

Helps underprivileged children around the world by providing them with access to healthcare.

Anesth, CT Surg, Crit-Care, ER Med, Neurosurg, Ortho, Ped Surg, Surg, Vasc Surg

+33 1 44 12 66 66

https://vfapp.org/e871

CharityVision International

Focuses on restoring curable sight impairment worldwide by empowering local physicians and creating sustainable solutions.

Logist-Op, Ophth-Opt, Surg

+1 435-200-4910

https://vfapp.org/6231

Christian Blind Mission (CBM)

Aims to improve the quality of life of persons with disabilities in the poorest countries, addressing poverty as a cause, and a consequence, of disability, and working in partnership to create a society for all.

ENT, General, Infect Dis, OB-GYN, Ophth-Opt, Ortho, Peds, Psych, Rehab, Surg

+49 6251 131131

https://vfapp.org/3824

Core Group

Aims to improve and expand community health practices for underserved populations, especially women and children, through collaborative action and learning.

General, Infect Dis, MF Med, Medicine, OB-GYN, Peds, Pub Health

+1 202-380-3400

https://vfapp.org/9de3

Direct Relief

Improves the health and lives of people affected by poverty or emergency situations by mobilizing and providing essential medical resources needed for their care.

ER Med, Logist-Op

+1 805-964-4767

https://vfapp.org/58e5

Direct Relief of Poverty & Sickness Foundation (DROPS)

Volunteer led organization that utilizes all donations toward direct relief of poverty and illness through initiatives in healthcare education, improving healthcare systems and providing essential medical help to children and aged people in need.

Dent-OMFS, General, Ophth-Opt

+49 171 3637659

https://vfapp.org/af95

Doctors for Madagascar

Provides direct medical aid with the goal of improving medical treatment in Madagascar in the long term, focusing particularly on the remote south of the island, one of the poorest regions in the country.

General, Logist-Op, Nutr, OB-GYN

+44 7542 752531

https://vfapp.org/12d8

Douleurs Sans Frontières (Pain Without Borders)

Supports local actors in taking charge of the assessment and treatment of pain and suffering, in an integrated manner and adapted to the realities of each country.

Anesth, Palliative, Psych, Rehab

+33 1 48 78 38 42

https://vfapp.org/324c

Duke University: Global Health Institute

Sparks innovation in global health research and education, and brings together knowledge and resources to address the most important global health issues of our time.

All-Immu, Infect Dis, MF Med, OB-GYN, Pub Health

+1 919-681-7760

https://vfapp.org/c4cd

END Fund, The

Aims to control and eliminate the most prevalent neglected diseases among the world's poorest and most vulnerable people.

Infect Dis

+1 646-690-9775

https://vfapp.org/2614

Fistula Foundation
Aims to engage the support of people worldwide who are eager to see the day when no woman suffers from obstetric fistula. Raises and directs funds to doctors and hospitals providing life-transforming surgery to women in need.

OB-GYN

+1 408-249-9596

https://vfapp.org/e958

Fondation Follereau
Promotes the quality of life of the most vulnerable African communities. Alongside trusted partners, the foundation supports local initiatives in healthcare and education.

General, Infect Dis, OB-GYN

+352 44 66 06 34

https://vfapp.org/bcc7

Freedom From Fistula
Helps women and girls who are injured and left incontinent following prolonged, obstructed childbirth by providing free surgical repairs for patients already suffering with fistula, as well as maternity care to prevent fistulas from happening at all.

MF Med, OB-GYN, Peds

+1 646-867-0994

https://vfapp.org/6e11

Friends of Mandritsara Trust
Supports the work of the Good News Hospital in and around the district of Mandritsara in Northern Madagascar. Based in Christian ministry, aims to meet both the medical and spiritual needs of local communities through medical and surgical services as well as church planting.

General, MF Med, OB-GYN, Ophth-Opt, Peds, Pub Health, Surg

https://vfapp.org/279f

Global Alliance to Prevent Prematurity and Stillbirth (GAPPS)
Seeks to improve birth outcomes worldwide by reducing the burden of premature birth and stillbirth.

All-Immu, Infect Dis, MF Med, Neonat, Neonat, OB-GYN

+1 206-413-7954

https://vfapp.org/3f74

Global Ministries – The United Methodist Church
As the worldwide mission and development agency of The United Methodist Church, Global Ministries works with more than 300 hospitals and clinics around the world through its Global Health Unit.

Anesth, CT Surg, CV Med, Crit-Care, Dent-OMFS, Derm, ER Med, GI, General, Infect Dis, Logist-Op, MF Med, Medicine, Neonat, Nephro, Nutr, OB-GYN, Ophth-Opt, Ortho, Palliative, Peds, Pod, Psych, Pub Health, Rehab, Rheum, Surg, Urol

+1 800-862-4246

https://vfapp.org/1723

Global Oncology (GO)
Brings the best in cancer care to underserved patients around the world and collaborates across geographic, professional, and academic borders to improve cancer care, research, and education.

Heme-Onc, Path, Rad-Onc

https://vfapp.org/fcb8

Global Polio Eradication Initiative
Aims to eradicate polio worldwide.

All-Immu, Logist-Op

+1 847-866-3000

https://vfapp.org/7e2c

Grace for Impact
Provides high-quality healthcare and education to the rural poor, where it is needed most, in Sub-Saharan Africa and Southeast Asia.

Dent-OMFS, General, Ophth-Opt

+1 214-646-8055

https://vfapp.org/3ed1

Grassroot Soccer
Leverages the power of soccer to educate, inspire, and mobilize at risk youth in developing countries to overcome their greatest health challenges, live healthier more productive lives, and be agents for change in their communities.

Infect Dis

+1 603-277-9685

https://vfapp.org/3521

Healing the Children Northeast
Helps underserved children around the world secure the medical care they need to lead more fulfilling lives.

Anesth, Dent-OMFS, ENT, General, Medicine, Ophth-Opt, Ped Surg, Peds, Plast

+1 860-355-1828

https://vfapp.org/16ba

Health Equity Initiative
Aims to build and sustain a global community that engages across sectors and disciplines to advance health equity.

Pub Health

https://vfapp.org/e2e2

HelpMeSee
Trains local cataract specialists in Manual Small Incision Cataract Surgery (MSICS) in significant numbers, to meet the increasing demand for surgical services in the communities most impacted by cataract blindness.

Anesth, Ophth-Opt, Surg

+1 844-435-7638

https://vfapp.org/973c

HIS Foundation (Holistic Integrated Services Foundation)
Provides free medical services for patients in underserved communities, such as services in orthopedic surgery, plastic surgery, internal medicine, rehabilitation, and ophthalmology, formed by Christian medical professionals.

Dent-OMFS, Geri, Medicine, Ophth-Opt, Ortho, Plast, Rehab

https://vfapp.org/a24b

Humanity & Inclusion
Works alongside people with disabilities and vulnerable populations, taking action and bearing witness in order to respond to their essential needs, improve their living conditions and health, and promote respect for their dignity and fundamental rights.

General, Infect Dis, MF Med, Medicine, Ortho, Peds, Psych, Pub Health, Rehab

+1 301-891-2138

https://vfapp.org/16b7

International Agency for the Prevention of Blindness (IAPB), The
Leads international efforts in blindness-prevention activities, works toward a world where no one is needlessly visually impaired, and ensures that everyone has access to the best possible standard of eye health.
Infect Dis, Ophth-Opt, Pub Health
🌐 https://vfapp.org/87a2

International Council of Ophthalmology
Works with ophthalmologic societies and others to enhance ophthalmic education and improve access to the highest quality eye care in order to preserve and restore vision for the people of the world.
Ophth-Opt
🌐 https://vfapp.org/ffd2

International Medical and Surgical Aid (IMSA)
Aims to save lives and alleviate suffering through education, healthcare, surgical camps, and quality medical programs.
Anesth, General, Ped Surg, Surg
📞 +44 7598 088806
🌐 https://vfapp.org/2561

International Medical Relief
Provides sustainable education, training, medical and dental care, and disaster relief and response in vulnerable communities worldwide.
Dent-OMFS, General, Infect Dis, Medicine, OB-GYN
📞 +1 970-635-0110
🌐 https://vfapp.org/b3ed

International Organization for Migration (IOM) – The UN Migration Agency
Promotes evidence-informed policies and holistic, preventive, and curative health programs that are beneficial, accessible, and equitable for vulnerable migrants.
General, Infect Dis, OB-GYN
📞 +27 12 342 2789
🌐 https://vfapp.org/621a

International Planned Parenthood Federation (IPPF)
Leads a locally owned, globally connected civil society movement that provides and enables services and champions sexual and reproductive health and rights for all, especially the underserved.
Infect Dis, MF Med, OB-GYN
📞 +44 20 7939 8200
🌐 https://vfapp.org/dc97

InterSurgeon
Fosters collaborative partnerships in the field of global surgery that will advance clinical care, teaching, training, research, and the provision and maintenance of medical equipment.
ENT, Neurosurg, Ortho, Ped Surg, Plast, Surg, Urol
🌐 https://vfapp.org/6f8a

IntraHealth International
Improves the performance of health workers and strengthens the systems in which they work.
CV Med, Endo, General, Infect Dis, MF Med, Neonat, Nutr, OB-GYN
📞 +1 919-313-3554
🌐 https://vfapp.org/ddc8

Iris Global
Serves the poor, the destitute, the lost, and the forgotten by providing adoration, outreach, family, education, relief, development, healing, and the arts.
General, Infect Dis, Nutr, Pub Health
📞 +1 530-255-2077
🌐 https://vfapp.org/37f8

Jhpiego
Creates and delivers transformative healthcare solutions that save lives in partnership with national governments, health experts, and local communities.
General, Infect Dis, OB-GYN, Surg
📞 +1 410-537-1800
🌐 https://vfapp.org/45b8

John Snow, Inc. (JSI)
Aims to improve the health and well-being of underserved and vulnerable people and communities throughout the world.
General, Infect Dis, Logist-Op, MF Med, OB-GYN, Peds, Psych, Pub Health
📞 +1 617-482-9485
🌐 https://vfapp.org/ba78

Johns Hopkins Center for Communication Programs
Believes in the power of communication to save lives, by empowering people to adopt healthy behaviors for themselves, their families, and their communities.
General, Infect Dis, Logist-Op, OB-GYN, Pub Health
📞 +1 410-659-6300
🌐 https://vfapp.org/1bf9

Johns Hopkins Center for Global Health
Facilitates and focuses the extensive expertise and resources of the Johns Hopkins institutions together with global collaborators to effectively address and ameliorate the world's most pressing health issues.
General, Genetics, Logist-Op, MF Med, Peds, Psych, Pub Health, Pulm-Critic
📞 +1 410-502-9872
🌐 https://vfapp.org/54ce

Joint United Nations Programme on HIV/AIDS (UNAIDS)
Aims to place people living with HIV and people affected by the virus at the decision-making table and at the center of designing, delivering, and monitoring the AIDS response.
Infect Dis
📞 +41 22 791 36 66
🌐 https://vfapp.org/464a

Lions Clubs International
Empowers volunteers to serve their communities, meet humanitarian needs, encourage peace, and promote international understanding through Lions clubs.
Heme-Onc, Medicine, Nutr, Ophth-Opt
📞 +1 630-571-5466
🌐 https://vfapp.org/7b12

Management Sciences for Health (MSH)
Works with countries and communities to save lives and improve the health of the world's poorest and most vulnerable people by building strong, resilient, sustainable health systems.
Infect Dis, Logist-Op, Pub Health
📞 +1 617-250-9500
🌐 https://vfapp.org/6aa2

MAP International

Provides medicines and health supplies to those in need around the world so they might experience life to the fullest.

Logist-Op

+1 800-225-8550

https://vfapp.org/deed

Marie Stopes International

Provides the contraception and safe abortion services that enable women all over the world to choose their own futures.

Infect Dis, MF Med, Neonat, OB-GYN, Pub Health

+44 20 7636 6200

https://vfapp.org/9525

Medair

Works to relieve human suffering in some of the world's most remote and devasted places, saving lives in emergencies and helping people in crises survive and recover, inspired by the Christian faith.

ER Med, General, Logist-Op, MF Med, Pub Health

+41 21 694 35 35

https://vfapp.org/5b33

Médecins du Monde/Doctors of the World

Provides care, bears witness, and supports social change worldwide with innovative medical programs and evidence-based advocacy initiatives.

ER Med, General, Infect Dis, MF Med, Neonat, OB-GYN, Peds, Pub Health

+33 1 44 92 15 15

https://vfapp.org/a43d

Medical Care Development International (MCD International)

Works to strengthen health systems through innovative, sustainable interventions.

Infect Dis, Logist-Op, OB-GYN, Pub Health

+1 301-562-1920

https://vfapp.org/dc5c

MedShare

Aims to improve the quality of life of people, communities, and the planet by sourcing and directly delivering surplus medical supplies and equipment to communities in need around the world.

Logist-Op

+1 770-323-5858

https://vfapp.org/c8bc

Mercy Ships

Operates hospital ships staffed by volunteers to bring hope, healing, and healthcare to underserved communities worldwide.

Anesth, Dent-OMFS, Logist-Op, Neonat, OB-GYN, Ophth-Opt, Ortho, Palliative, Plast, Psych, Surg

+1 903-939-7000

https://vfapp.org/2e99

Mérieux Foundation

Committed to fighting infectious diseases that affect developing countries by capacity building, particularly in clinical laboratories, and focusing on diagnosis.

Logist-Op, Path

+33 4 72 40 79 79

https://vfapp.org/a23a

MiracleFeet

Brings low-cost treatment to every child on the planet born with clubfoot, a leading cause of physical disability.

Ortho, Peds, Rehab

+1 919-240-5572

https://vfapp.org/bda8

Mission Bambini

Helps to support children living in poverty, sickness, and without education, giving them the opportunity and hope of a better life.

CT Surg, CV Med, Crit-Care, ER Med, Ped Surg, Peds

+39 02 210 0241

https://vfapp.org/dc1a

Mission Vision

Seeks to decrease blindness and other eye-related disabilities, as well as to increase academic performance and general quality of life.

Ophth-Opt

+1 724-553-3114

https://vfapp.org/83d8

Modern Dental Care Foundation (MDCF)

Works to give the poorest people of Madagascar access to dental care and prevention in a sustainable and effective manner.

Dent-OMFS

+31 172 653 300

https://vfapp.org/5e96

Money for Madagascar

Enables Malagasy people to reduce poverty and protect the environment through sustainable, community-led initiatives.

General

+44 7956 147316

https://vfapp.org/3c86

NCD Alliance

Unites and strengthens civil society to stimulate collaborative advocacy, action, and accountability for NCD (noncommunicable disease) prevention and control.

All-Immu, CV Med, General, Heme-Onc, Medicine, Peds, Psych

+41 22 809 18 11

https://vfapp.org/abdd

Operation Fistula

Exists to end obstetric fistula by building models of care that serve every woman, everywhere.

MF Med, OB-GYN, Surg

+1 512-687-3479

https://vfapp.org/ce8e

Operation Smile

Treats patients with cleft lip and cleft palate, and creates solutions that deliver safe surgery to people where it's needed most.

Anesth, Dent-OMFS, ENT, Ped Surg, Plast

+1 757-321-7645

https://vfapp.org/5c29

Options

Believes in a world where women and children can access the high-quality health services they need, without financial burden.

Logist-Op, MF Med, Neonat, OB-GYN
+44 20 7430 1900
https://vfapp.org/3a48

OPTIVEST Foundation
Funds strategic opportunities that are holistic and collaborative, inspired by the Christian faith.
General, Nutr
https://vfapp.org/f1e6

Pact
Works on the ground to improve the lives of those who are challenged by poverty and marginalization, striving for a world where all people are heard, capable, and vibrant.
Infect Dis, Logist-Op, MF Med, Pub Health
+1 202-466-5666
https://vfapp.org/9a6c

Partners in Health
Responds to the moral imperative to provide high-quality healthcare globally to those who need it most, while striving to ease suffering by providing a comprehensive model of care that includes access to food, transportation, housing, and other key components of healing.
CT Surg, General, Heme-Onc, Infect Dis, MF Med, Neurosurg, OB-GYN, Ortho, Plast, Psych, Urol
+1 857-880-5600
https://vfapp.org/dc9c

Philips Foundation
Aims to reduce healthcare inequality by providing access to quality healthcare for disadvantaged communities.
CV Med, OB-GYN, Ped Surg, Peds, Surg, Urol
https://vfapp.org/bacb

PIVOT
Collaborates with the Ministry of Public Health of Madagascar to strengthen the public health system in order to offer quality care to the population of Ifanadiana district.
ER Med, General, Infect Dis, Logist-Op, MF Med, Nutr, OB-GYN, Path, Peds, Pub Health
https://vfapp.org/84f2

Project Concern International (PCI)
Drives innovation from the ground up to enhance health, end hunger, overcome hardship, and advance women and girls—resulting in meaningful and measurable change in people's lives.
Infect Dis, MF Med, Nutr, OB-GYN, Peds
+1 858-279-9690
https://vfapp.org/5ed7

PSI – Population Services International
Dedicates efforts to improving the health of people in the developing world by focusing on challenges such as a lack of family planning, HIV/AIDS, barriers to maternal health, and the greatest threats to children under the age of 5, including malaria, diarrhea, pneumonia, and malnutrition.
Infect Dis, MF Med, OB-GYN, Peds
+1 202-785-0072
https://vfapp.org/ffe3

RAD-AID International
Improves and optimizes access to medical imaging and radiology in low-resource regions of the world.
Rad-Onc, Radiol
https://vfapp.org/537f

RestoringVision
Empowers lives by restoring vision for millions of people in need.
Ophth-Opt
+1 209-980-7323
https://vfapp.org/e121

Rockefeller Foundation, The
Works to promote the well-being of humanity.
Logist-Op, Nutr, Pub Health
+1 212-869-8500
https://vfapp.org/5424

Rose Charities International
Aims to support communities to improve quality of life and reduce the effects of poverty through innovative, self-sustaining projects and partnerships.
ENT, ER Med, General, Infect Dis, Neonat, OB-GYN, Ophth-Opt, Ped Surg, Peds, Rehab, Urol
+1 604-733-0442
https://vfapp.org/53df

Rotary International
Provides service to others, improves lives, and advances world understanding, goodwill, and peace through its fellowship of business, professional, and community leaders.
ER Med, General, Infect Dis, MF Med, OB-GYN
https://vfapp.org/8fb5

Salvation Army International, The
Seeks to meet human needs through services in education, healthcare, community support, emergency response, and ministry development, inspired by the Christian faith.
Dent-OMFS, Derm, ER Med, Infect Dis, MF Med, Medicine, Nutr, OB-GYN, Ophth-Opt, Palliative, Psych, Rehab, Surg
+44 20 7332 0101
https://vfapp.org/8eb3

Sanofi Espoir Foundation
Contributes to reducing health inequalities among populations that need it most by applying a socially responsible approach focused on fighting childhood cancers in low-income countries, improving maternal and newborn health, and improving access to care.
ER Med, OB-GYN, Peds
+33 1 53 77 91 38
https://vfapp.org/943b

SEVA
Delivers vital eye care services to the world's most vulnerable, including women, children, and Indigenous peoples.
Ophth-Opt, Surg
+1 510-845-7382
https://vfapp.org/1e87

SIGN Fracture Care International
Builds orthopedic capacity around the world and provides the injured poor access to fracture surgery by donating orthopedic education and implant systems to surgeons in developing countries.
Ortho, Rehab, Surg
+1 509-371-1107
https://vfapp.org/123d

Solthis
Improves disease prevention and access to quality care by strengthening the health systems and services of the countries served.

General, Infect Dis, Logist-Op, MF Med, Neonat, Path

+33 1 81 70 17 90

https://vfapp.org/a71d

SOS Children's Villages International
Supports children through alternative care and family strengthening.

ER Med, Peds

+43 1 36824570

https://vfapp.org/aca1

Swiss Tropical and Public Health Institute
Contributes to the improvement of the health of populations internationally, nationally, and locally through excellence in research, education, and services.

Infect Dis, Pub Health

+41 61 284 81 11

https://vfapp.org/2ee4

Task Force for Global Health, The
Consists of programs and focus areas that cover a range of global health issues including neglected tropical diseases, infectious diseases, vaccines, field epidemiology, public health informatics, health workforce development, and global health ethics.

Infect Dis, Logist-Op, Medicine, Ophth-Opt, Peds

+1 404-371-0466

https://vfapp.org/714c

U.S. President's Malaria Initiative (PMI)
Supports low-income countries to help control and eliminate malaria through cost-effective, lifesaving malaria interventions.

Infect Dis, MF Med, OB-GYN

+1 202-712-0000

https://vfapp.org/dc8b

Union for International Cancer Control (UICC)
Unites and supports the cancer community to reduce the global cancer burden, promote greater equity, and ensure that cancer control continues to be a priority in the world health and development agenda.

Heme-Onc, Pub Health

+41 22 809 18 11

https://vfapp.org/88b1

United Nations Children's Fund (UNICEF)
Works in over 190 countries and territories to save children's lives, to defend their rights, and to help them fulfill their potential, from early childhood through adolescence.

All-Immu, Infect Dis, MF Med, Neonat, Nutr, OB-GYN, Ped Surg, Peds, Pub Health

https://vfapp.org/42d7

United Nations Development Programme (UNDP)
Helps countries achieve the simultaneous eradication of extreme poverty and significant reduction of inequalities and exclusion using a sustainable human development approach.

Infect Dis, Logist-Op, Pub Health

https://vfapp.org/935c

United Nations High Commissioner for Refugees (UNHCR)
Safeguards the rights and well-being of people who have been forced to flee, ensuring that everybody has the right to seek asylum and find safe refuge in another country, with the goal of seeking lasting solutions.

General, MF Med, Medicine, OB-GYN, Peds, Psych, Pub Health

https://vfapp.org/6636

United Nations Population Fund (UNFPA)
Supports reproductive healthcare for women and youth in more than 150 countries, focusing on delivering a world where every pregnancy is wanted, every childbirth is safe, and every young person's potential is fulfilled.

Infect Dis, MF Med, Neonat, OB-GYN, Peds, Pub Health

+1 212-963-6008

https://vfapp.org/c969

United States Agency for International Development (USAID)
Promotes and demonstrates democratic values abroad and advances a free, peaceful, and prosperous world. Leads the U.S. government's international development and disaster assistance through partnerships and investments that save lives.

ER Med, Infect Dis, MF Med, OB-GYN, Peds

+1 202-712-0000

https://vfapp.org/9a99

United Surgeons for Children (USFC)
Pursues greater health and opportunity for children in the most neglected pockets of the world, with a specific focus and expertise in surgery.

Anesth, CT Surg, Neonat, Neurosurg, OB-GYN, Peds, Radiol, Surg

https://vfapp.org/3b4c

University of California San Francisco: Institute for Global Health Sciences
Dedicates its efforts to improving health and reducing the burden of disease in the world's most vulnerable populations by integrating expertise in the health, social, and biological sciences to train global health leaders and develop solutions to the most pressing health challenges.

Infect Dis, OB-GYN, Pub Health

+1 415-476-5494

https://vfapp.org/6587

University of Virginia: Anesthesiology Department Global Health Initiatives
Educates and trains physicians, to help people achieve healthy productive lives, and advances knowledge in the medical sciences.

Anesth, Pub Health

+1 434-924-2283

https://vfapp.org/1b8b

USAID: Maternal and Child Survival Program
Works to prevent child and maternal deaths.

Infect Dis, MF Med, Neonat, OB-GYN, Peds

https://vfapp.org/6fcf

USAID: African Strategies for Health
Identifies and advocates for best practices, enhancing technical

capacity of African regional institutions and engaging African stakeholders to address health issues in a sustainable manner.

All-Immu, Infect Dis, OB-GYN, Peds

https://vfapp.org/c272

USAID: Deliver Project

Builds a global supply chain to deliver lifesaving health products to people in order to enable countries to provide family planning, protect against malaria, and limit the spread of pandemic threats.

Infect Dis, Logist-Op, MF Med

+1 202-712-0000

https://vfapp.org/374e

USAID: Health Policy Initiative

Provides field-level programming in health policy development and implementation.

General, Infect Dis, MF Med, OB-GYN, Peds

https://vfapp.org/8f84

USAID: Human Resources for Health 2030 (HRH2030)

Helps low- and middle-income countries develop the health workforce needed to prevent maternal and child deaths, support the goals of Family Planning 2020, control the HIV/AIDS epidemic, and protect communities from infectious diseases.

Logist-Op

+1 202-955-3300

https://vfapp.org/9ea8

USAID: Leadership, Management and Governance Project

Improves leadership, management, and governance practices to strengthen health systems and improve health for all, including vulnerable populations worldwide.

Logist-Op

https://vfapp.org/d35e

USAID: Maternal and Child Health Integrated Program

Works to improve the health of women and their families, including programs for maternal, newborn, and child health, immunization, family planning, nutrition, malaria, and HIV/AIDS.

All-Immu, General, Infect Dis, MF Med

+1 202-835-3136

https://vfapp.org/4415

Vital Strategies

Helps governments strengthen their public health systems to contend with the most important and difficult health challenges, while accelerating progress on the world's most pressing health problems.

CV Med, Infect Dis, Peds

+1 212-500-5720

https://vfapp.org/fe25

Vitamin Angels

Helps at-risk populations in need—specifically pregnant women, new mothers, and children under age five—to gain access to life-changing vitamins and minerals.

General, Nutr

+1 805-564-8400

https://vfapp.org/7da1

VOSH (Volunteer Optometric Services to Humanity) International

Facilitates the provision and the sustainability of vision care worldwide for people who can neither afford nor obtain such care.

Ophth-Opt

https://vfapp.org/a149

World Children's Initiative (WCI)

Aims to improve and rebuild the healthcare and educational infrastructure for children in developing areas, both domestically and worldwide.

CV Med, Ped Surg, Surg

+1 408-554-4188

https://vfapp.org/9ca7

World Health Organization, The (WHO)

The United Nations' agency for health provides leadership on global health matters, shapes the health research agenda, setting norms and standards, articulates evidence-based policy options, provides technical support and monitoring to countries, and assesses health trends.

ER Med, General, Infect Dis, Logist-Op, MF Med, OB-GYN, Peds, Psych, Pub Health

+41 22 791 21 11

https://vfapp.org/c476

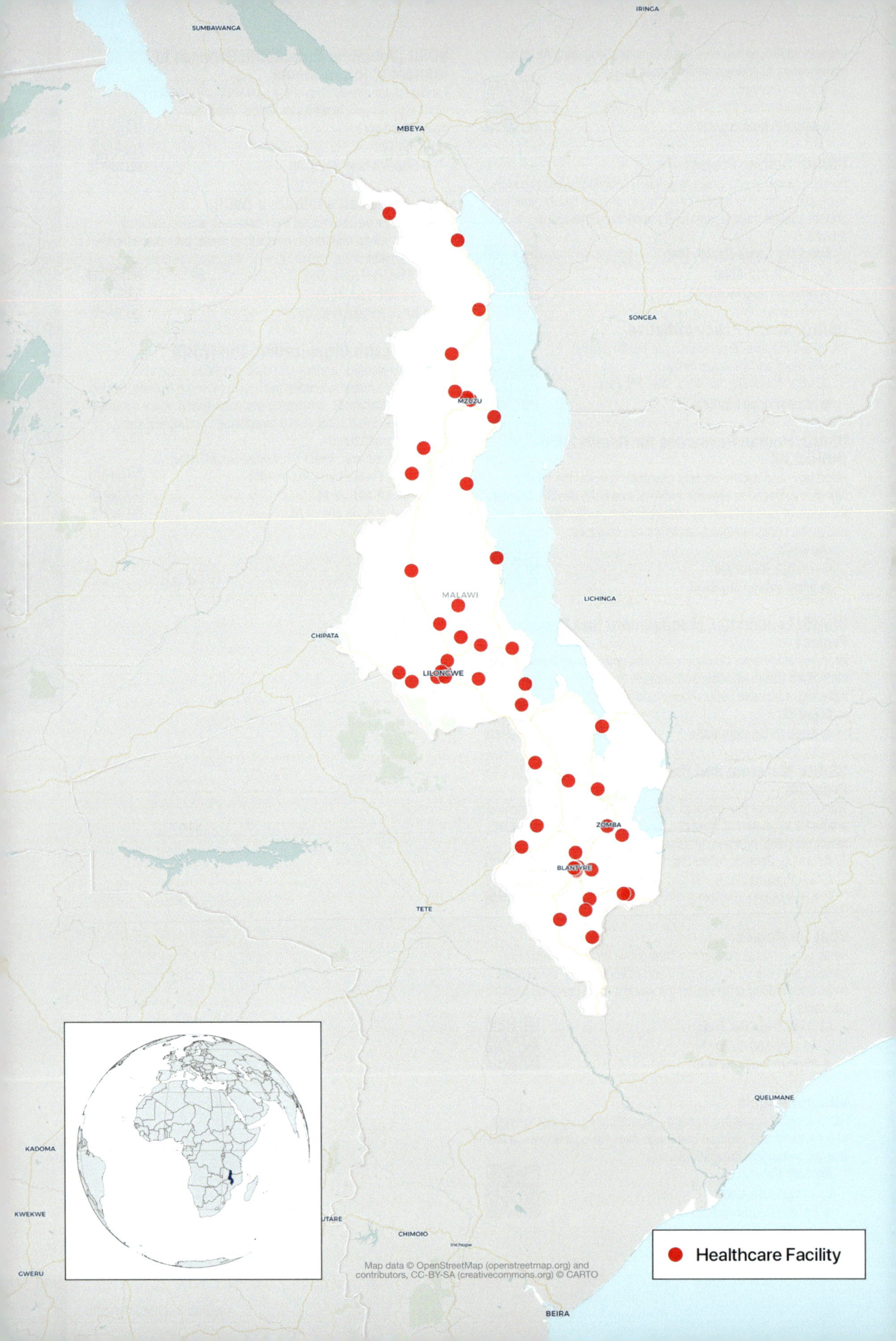
SUMBAWANGA
IRINGA
MBEYA
SONGEA
MZUZU
MALAWI
LICHINGA
CHIPATA
LILONGWE
ZOMBA
BLANTYRE
TETE
QUELIMANE
KADOMA
KWEKWE
CHIMOIO
Inchope
GWERU
BEIRA
Healthcare Facility
Map data © OpenStreetMap (openstreetmap.org) and contributors, CC-BY-SA (creativecommons.org) © CARTO

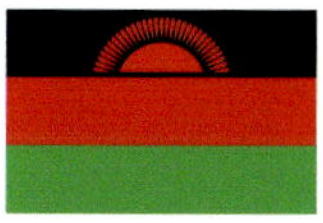

Malawi

The Republic of Malawi, a landlocked country in Southern Africa, shares a border with Tanzania, Mozambique, and Zambia. Lake Nyasa, also known as Lake Malawi, takes up about a third of Malawi's area, and is a UNESCO World Heritage Site. The country has a population of 21.2 million people, many of whom live in the highest-density, southern, rural parts of the country and close to Lake Nyasa. Most of the population is Christian and speak the Bantu languages of Chichewa, Chitumbuka, and Chiyao. English is the official language of Malawi.

Formerly a colony of Britain, Malawi is politically stable and has implemented structural and economic reforms to sustain growth. Agriculture is the primary employer for 80 percent of Malawi's people, with tobacco, sugar cane, tea, and corn among the biggest cash crops. Free primary education was made available in the mid-1990s, leading to increased school enrollment. As much as half of the population lives in poverty.

Despite the challenges that poverty presents, there has been an increase in life expectancy, from 40 years to around 64 years between 2000 and 2018. The diseases causing the most deaths in Malawi include HIV/AIDS, neonatal disorders, lower respiratory infections, tuberculosis, diarrheal diseases, and meningitis. Non-communicable diseases have notably increased to cause significant deaths as well, with marked increases in stroke, ischemic heart disease, and cirrhosis. Malawi's healthcare system might not be equipped to face some of these health challenges, as it is susceptible to shortages of supplies, drugs, and health workers. While Malawi initiated the Drug Revolving Funds to supply communities with medications at a discounted cost and has expanded training of health workers, the country is still in need of assistance.

21.2M
Population

$412
GDP Per Capita

64 years
Life Expectancy
↑ Improving

3.6
Doctors/100k
Physician Density

130
Beds/100k
Hospital Bed Density

349
Deaths/100k
Maternal Mortality

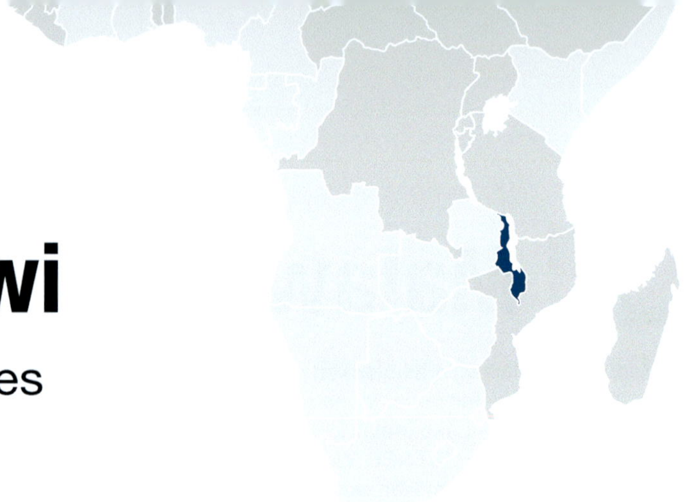

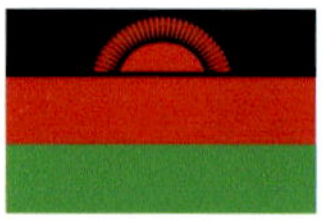

Malawi

Healthcare Facilities

Balaka District Hospital
Balaka, Malawi
https://vfapp.org/9f65

Baylor College of Medicine Children's Foundation Malawi
Mzimba Street, Lilongwe, Lilongwe, Malawi
https://vfapp.org/5aab

Beit CURE International Hospital
Chipatala, Blantyre, Malawi
https://vfapp.org/e8d9

Blantyre Malaria Project
Ndirande Ring Road, Blantyre, Blantyre, Malawi
https://vfapp.org/3d45

Bwaila Hospital
M1, Lilongwe, Lilongwe, Malawi
https://vfapp.org/b184

CCAP Embangweni Mission Hospital
S112, Loudon, Malawi
https://vfapp.org/f8e1

Child Legacy Hospital
T345, Lilongwe, Lilongwe, Malawi
https://vfapp.org/6cbb

Chitawira Private Hospital
Chitawira Road, Limbe, Blantyre, Malawi
https://vfapp.org/6718

Chitipa District Hospital
M9, Chitipa, Chitipa, Malawi
https://vfapp.org/48f3

Daeyang Luke Hospital
Lilongwe, Malawi
https://vfapp.org/86d4

David Gordon Memorial – Livingstonia Hospital
Golodi Road, Livingstonia, Rumphi, Malawi
https://vfapp.org/a8dd

District Hospital Mangochi
M3, Mangochi, Mangochi, Malawi
https://vfapp.org/b9d2

Dowa District Hospital
M16, Dowa, Dowa, Malawi
https://vfapp.org/a85d

Dwambazi Rural Hospital
M5, Dwambazi, Nkhotakota, Malawi
https://vfapp.org/f8dd

Ekwendeni Mission Hospital
M1, Ekwendeni, Malawi
https://vfapp.org/611d

Kamuzu Central Hospital
Lilongwe, Malawi
https://vfapp.org/5efd

Karonga District Hospital
M1, Karonga, Karonga, Malawi
https://vfapp.org/43f5

Kasungu District Hospital
M18, Kasungu, Malawi
https://vfapp.org/f39c

Lifeline
Salima, Malawi
https://vfapp.org/8ff9

Likuni Hospital
S124, Likuni, Lilongwe, Malawi
https://vfapp.org/f9b3

Machinga District Hospital
Machinga, Liwonde, Malawi
https://vfapp.org/2cb2

Malamulo Rural Hospital
S151, Mangwalala, Thyolo, Malawi
https://vfapp.org/e576

Mlambe Hospital
M1, Lunzu, Blantyre, Malawi
https://vfapp.org/2123

Mponela Hospital
Mponela, Malawi
https://vfapp.org/d8c1

Mua Mission Hospital
M5, Mua, Dedza, Malawi
https://vfapp.org/addb

Mulanje District Hospital
M2, Mulanje, Malawi
https://vfapp.org/384c

Mulanje Mission Hospital
Mulanje Mission Road, Nkhonya, Mulanje, Malawi
https://vfapp.org/5cc1

Mvera Mission Hospital
M14, Mvera Mission, Dowa, Malawi
https://vfapp.org/3831

Mwaiwathu Private Hospital
Chileka Road, Blantyre, Blantyre, Malawi
https://vfapp.org/a316

Mwanza Hospital
S135, Mwanza, Mwanza, Malawi
https://vfapp.org/88cc

Mzimba South District Hospital
M9, Mzimba, Mzimba, Malawi
https://vfapp.org/aaad

Mzuzu Central Hospital
M1, Mzuzu, Mzimba, Malawi
https://vfapp.org/21ce

Nchalo Baptist Church
M1, Nchalo, Chikwawa, Malawi
https://vfapp.org/9972

Neno District Hospital
T397, Neno, Malawi
https://vfapp.org/4671

Nguludi Mission Hospital
T411, Nguludi, Chiradzulu, Malawi
https://vfapp.org/1d63

Nkhata District Hospital
M5, Nkhata Bay, Nkhata Bay, Malawi
https://vfapp.org/187e

Nkhoma Hospital
T374, Gwenembe, Lilongwe, Malawi
https://vfapp.org/dee3

Nkhotakota District Hospital
Kasungo Road, Kachuma, Nkhotakota, Malawi
https://vfapp.org/c557

Ntcheu District Hospital
M1, Mtandizi, Ntcheu, Malawi
https://vfapp.org/32b2

Ntchisi Hospital
T350, Ntchisi, Ntchisi, Malawi
https://vfapp.org/276e

Partners in Hope
M1, Lilongwe, Lilongwe, Malawi
https://vfapp.org/cfc5

Pirimiti Community Hospital
S144, Thondwe, Zomba, Malawi
https://vfapp.org/58fe

Queen Elizabeth Central Hospital
Chipatala Avenue, Blantyre, Blantyre, Malawi
https://vfapp.org/d2e7

Rumphi District Hospital
M24, Mputa, Rumphi, Malawi
https://vfapp.org/4d77

Salima District Hospital
M5, Salima, Salima, Malawi
https://vfapp.org/bdf2

Shifa Hospital
Haile Selassie Avenue, Blantyre, Blantyre, Malawi
https://vfapp.org/829b

St. Gabriel Mission Hospital
M12, Namitete, Lilongwe, Malawi
https://vfapp.org/3798

St. John's Hospital
Chimaliro Road, Mzuzu, Mzimba, Malawi
https://vfapp.org/5955

Surgery Hospital at Blantyre
Sharpe Road, Blantyre, Blantyre, Malawi
https://vfapp.org/515e

Thyolo District Hospital
Thyolo Road, Ndalama, Thyolo, Malawi
https://vfapp.org/8fbe

Trinity Hospital
S152, Malothi, Nsanje, Malawi
https://vfapp.org/c9f5

ZMK Hospital
Queens Road, Lilongwe, Lilongwe, Malawi
https://vfapp.org/28c9

Zomba Central Hospital
M3, Matawale, Zomba, Malawi
https://vfapp.org/33fc

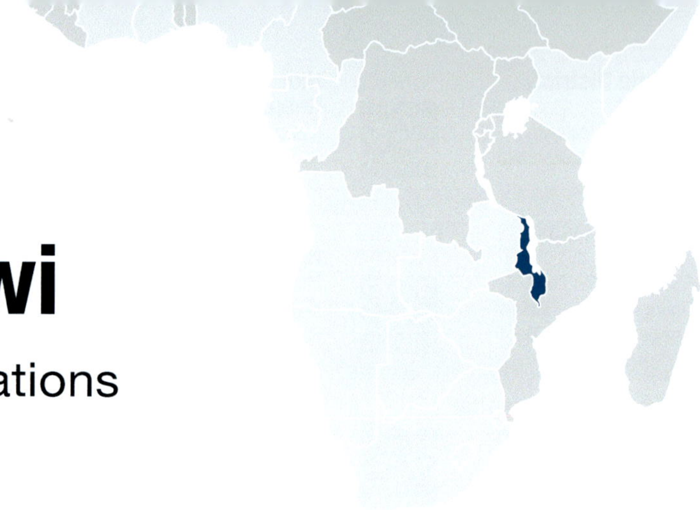

Malawi

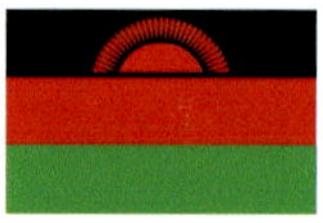

Nonprofit Organizations

100X Development Foundation
Empowers children and families for a more hopeful and productive future through the support and care of orphaned children, education and job training for those in need, help for vulnerable youth to escape trafficking, and healthy nutrition and medical care for mothers to enable a safe birth.

ER Med, Infect Dis, OB-GYN, Peds, Psych
- +1 334-387-1178
- https://vfapp.org/b629

A Broader View Volunteers
Provides developing countries around the world with significant volunteer programs that both aid the neediest communities and forge a lasting bond between those volunteering and those they have helped.

Dent-OMFS, ER Med, Infect Dis, MF Med
- +1 215-780-1845
- https://vfapp.org/3bec

Access Health Africa
Provides surgical services to Malawi, operating on those who otherwise may not have access to surgical services.

CV Med, Dent-OMFS, Infect Dis, Ped Surg, Pulm-Critic, Surg
- +1 828-263-6877
- https://vfapp.org/1b57

Accomplish Children's Trust
Provides education and medical care to children with disabilities. Also addresses the financial implications of caring for a child with disabilities by helping families to earn an income.

Neuro, Peds, Rehab
- https://vfapp.org/de84

Adventist Health International
Focuses on upgrading and managing mission hospitals by providing governance, consultation, and technical assistance to a number of affiliated Seventh-Day Adventist hospitals throughout Africa, Asia, and the Americas.

Dent-OMFS, General, Pub Health
- +1 909-558-5610
- https://vfapp.org/16aa

Africa CDC
Aims to strengthen the capacity and capability of Africa's public health institutions as well as partnerships to detect and respond quickly and effectively to disease threats and outbreaks, based on data-driven interventions and programs.

Infect Dis, Logist-Op, Pub Health
- +251 11 551 7700
- https://vfapp.org/339c

Africa Indoor Residual Spraying Project (AIRS)
Aims to protect millions of people in Africa from malaria by spraying insecticide on the walls, ceilings, and other indoor resting places of mosquitoes that transmit malaria.

Infect Dis
- +1 301-347-5000
- https://vfapp.org/9bd1

African Field Epidemiology Network (AFENET)
Strengthens field epidemiology and public health laboratory capacity to contribute effectively to addressing epidemics and other major public health problems in Africa.

All-Immu, Infect Dis, Path, Pub Health
- https://vfapp.org/df2e

African Vision
Strives to help children and vulnerable people in Malawi with the goal of creating a healthy, educated, and self-sufficient community.

Infect Dis, MF Med, Nutr, OB-GYN
- +44 82878169
- https://vfapp.org/be7f

Against Malaria Foundation
Helps protect people from malaria. Funds anti-malaria nets, specifically long-lasting insecticidal nets (LLINs), and works with distribution partners to ensure they are used. Tracks and reports on net use and malaria case data.

Infect Dis
- +44 20 7371 8735
- https://vfapp.org/337d

Aid Africa's Children
Aims to empower impoverished African children and communities with healthcare, food, clean water, educational, and entrepreneurial opportunities.

ER Med, General, Infect Dis, Nutr, OB-GYN, Palliative, Peds, Pub Health
- +1 708-269-1139
- https://vfapp.org/5e2e

AIDS Healthcare Foundation
Provides cutting-edge HIV/AIDS medical care and advocacy to over one million people in forty-three countries.

Infect Dis

+1 323-860-5200

https://vfapp.org/b27c

AMARI (African Mental Health Research Initiative)
Seeks to build an Africa-led network of future leaders in mental, neurological, and substance use (MNS) research in Ethiopia, Malawi, South Africa, and Zimbabwe.

Neuro, Psych

+263 24 2708020

https://vfapp.org/5e9d

Americares
Saves lives and improves health for people affected by poverty or disaster and responds with life-changing medicine, medical supplies, and health programs including domestic and global medical clinics.

All-Immu, ER Med, General, Infect Dis, MF Med, Nutr

+1 203-658-9500

https://vfapp.org/e567

AMOR (Aide Mondiale Orphelins Reconfort)
Aims to contribute to significant reductions in global infant and maternal mortality rates by providing medical services to at-risk mothers and appropriate care for orphans.

Infect Dis, MF Med, Neonat, OB-GYN, Ophth-Opt, Ped Surg

+33 6 80 86 19 75

https://vfapp.org/98a4

Amref Health Africa
Serves millions of people across thirty-five countries in Sub-Saharan Africa, strengthening health systems, and training African health workers to respond to the continent's most critical health issues.

All-Immu, General, Infect Dis, Logist-Op, MF Med, OB-GYN, Path, Pub Health, Surg

+254 20 6993000

https://vfapp.org/6985

AO Alliance
Builds solutions to lessen the burden of injuries in low- and middle-income countries, while enhancing the care of the injured to reduce human suffering, disability, and poverty.

Ortho, Surg

https://vfapp.org/8cd5

Aspen Management Partnership for Health (AMP Health)
Works to improve health systems and outcomes by collaborating with governments to strengthen leadership and management capabilities through public-private partnership.

Logist-Op

+1 202-736-5800

https://vfapp.org/ea78

Avert
Works to ensure widespread understanding of HIV and AIDS in order to reduce new infections and improve the lives of those affected.

Infect Dis, Path

+44 1273 947749

https://vfapp.org/312d

Baylor College of Medicine: Global Surgery
Trains leaders in academic global surgery and remains dedicated to advancements in the arenas of patient care, biomedical research, and medical education.

ENT, Infect Dis, OB-GYN, Ortho, Ped Surg, Plast, Pub Health, Radiol, Surg, Urol

+1 713-798-6078

https://vfapp.org/21f5

Baylor International Pediatric AIDS Initiative (BIPAI) at Texas Children's Hospital
Provides high-quality, high-impact, highly ethical pediatric and family-centered healthcare, health professional training, and clinical research focused on HIV/AIDS, tuberculosis, malaria, malnutrition, and other conditions impacting the health of children worldwide.

Infect Dis, Medicine, OB-GYN, Peds, Pub Health, Surg

+1 832-822-1038

https://vfapp.org/e6ba

Benjamin H. Josephson, MD Fund
Provides healthcare professionals with the financial resources necessary to deliver medical services for those in need throughout the world.

General, OB-GYN

+1 908-522-2853

https://vfapp.org/6acc

Billy's Malawi Project
Works to improve the overall health status of the village of Cape Maclear (Chembe Village) through the provision of a medical clinic and health center, and also provides educational opportunities and support.

General, OB-GYN, Ophth-Opt, Peds

https://vfapp.org/f787

Boston Children's Hospital: Global Health Program
Helps solve pediatric global health care challenges by transferring expertise through long-term partnerships with scalable impact, while working in the field to strengthen healthcare systems, advocate, research and provide care delivery or education as a way of sustainably improving the health of children worldwide.

Anesth, CV Med, Crit-Care, ER Med, Heme-Onc, Infect Dis, Medicine, Nutr, Palliative, Ped Surg, Peds

+1 617-919-6438

https://vfapp.org/f9f8

Called to Go Chiropractic Missions
Provides chiropractic care and education to people in Malawi.

+1 816-694-9003

https://vfapp.org/afdb

Canadian Foundation for Women's Health
Seeks to advance the health of women in Canada and around the world through research, education, and advocacy in obstetrics and gynecology.

MF Med, OB-GYN

+1 613-730-4192

https://vfapp.org/f41e

Canadian Vision Care

Consists of eye healthcare professionals who donate time and resources to the development of vision care in the developing world.

Ophth-Opt

+1 403-803-5563

https://vfapp.org/3a38

CARE

Works around the globe to save lives, defeat poverty, and achieve social justice.

ER Med, General

+1 800-422-7385

https://vfapp.org/7232

Carter Center, The

Seeks to prevent and resolve conflicts, enhance freedom and democracy, and improve health, while remaining committed to human rights and the alleviation of human suffering.

Infect Dis, MF Med, Ophth-Opt

+1 800-550-3560

https://vfapp.org/6556

Catholic Health Commission

Implements health programs and provides health/nutrition care services in remote areas of the central region of Malawi. Provides equitable, sustainable, and quality healthcare to all targeted communities regardless of faith.

Anesth, Dent-OMFS, General, General, Infect Dis, MF Med, Medicine, Nutr, OB-GYN, Palliative, Peds, Surg

+265 1 766 645

https://vfapp.org/c786

Catholic World Mission

Works to rebuild communities worldwide by helping to alleviate poverty and empower underserved areas, while spreading the message of the Catholic Church.

ER Med, General, Nutr, Peds

+1 770-828-4966

https://vfapp.org/7b5f

Center for Strategic and International Studies (CSIS) Commission on Strengthening America's Health Security

Brings together a distinguished and diverse group of high-level opinion leaders bridging security and health, with the core aim to chart a bold vision for the future of U.S. leadership in global health.

ER Med, Infect Dis, MF Med, Pub Health

+1 202-887-0200

https://vfapp.org/6d7f

Centre for Global Mental Health

Closes the care gap and reduces human rights abuses experienced by people living with mental, neurological, and substance use conditions, particularly in low-resource settings.

Neuro, OB-GYN, Palliative, Peds, Psych

https://vfapp.org/a96d

Chain of Hope

Provides lifesaving heart operations for children around the world and supports the development of cardiac services in numerous developing and war-torn countries.

Anesth, CT Surg, CV Med, Crit-Care, Ped Surg, Peds, Pulm-Critic, Surg

+44 20 7351 1978

https://vfapp.org/1b1b

Chikondi Health Foundation

Promotes spiritual and physical health through medical missions at Blessings Hospital in Lumbadzi, Malawi, and through the support of local churches.

Infect Dis, OB-GYN, Surg

+1 334-315-5225

https://vfapp.org/9125

Child Legacy International

Works in Africa to transform lives by providing opportunities that break the generational cycle of poverty and despair, inspired by the Christian faith.

All-Immu, General, Heme-Onc, Surg

+1 830-331-9428

https://vfapp.org/a2bd

Children of the Nations

Aims to raise children out of poverty and hopelessness so they can become leaders who transform their nations. Emphasizes caring for the whole child–physically, mentally, socially, and spiritually.

Anesth, Dent-OMFS, General, Surg

+1 360-698-7227

https://vfapp.org/cc52

Christian Aid Ministries

Strives to be a trustworthy and efficient channel for Amish, Mennonite, and other conservative Anabaptist groups and individuals to minister to physical and spiritual needs around the world.

CT Surg, ER Med, Logist-Op, Ortho, Pub Health

+1 330-893-2428

https://vfapp.org/7b33

Christian Blind Mission (CBM)

Aims to improve the quality of life of persons with disabilities in the poorest countries, addressing poverty as a cause, and a consequence, of disability, and working in partnership to create a society for all.

ENT, General, Infect Dis, OB-GYN, Ophth-Opt, Ortho, Peds, Psych, Rehab, Surg

+49 6251 131131

https://vfapp.org/3824

Christian Connections for International Health (CCIH)

Promotes global health and wholeness from a Christian perspective.

All-Immu, General, Infect Dis, MF Med, Neonat, OB-GYN, Psych

+1 703-923-8960

https://vfapp.org/fa5d

Christian Health Service Corps

Brings Christian doctors, health professionals, and health educators who are committed to serving the poor to places that have little or no access to healthcare.

Anesth, Dent-OMFS, General, Medicine, Peds, Surg

+1 903-962-4000

https://vfapp.org/da57

Clinton Health Access Initiative (CHAI)

Aims to save lives and reduce the burden of disease in low- and middle-income countries. Works with partners to strengthen the capabilities of governments and the private sector to create and sustain high-quality health systems.

General, Heme-Onc, Infect Dis, Logist-Op, MF Med, Medicine, Neonat, Nutr, OB-GYN, Path, Peds, Rad-Onc

+1 617-774-0110

https://vfapp.org/9ed7

Columbia University: Global Mental Health Programs

Pioneers research initiatives, promotes mental health, and aims to reduce the burden of mental illness worldwide.

Psych

+1 646-774-5308

https://vfapp.org/c5cd

Concern Worldwide

Seeks to permanently transform the lives of people living in extreme poverty, tackling its root causes, and building resilience.

Logist-Op, MF Med, Nutr, OB-GYN

+353 1 417 7700

https://vfapp.org/77e9

Core Group

Aims to improve and expand community health practices for underserved populations, especially women and children, through collaborative action and learning.

General, Infect Dis, MF Med, Medicine, OB-GYN, Peds, Pub Health

+1 202-380-3400

https://vfapp.org/9de3

CURE

Operates charitable hospitals and programs in underserved countries worldwide where patients receive surgical treatment, based in Christian ministry.

Anesth, Neurosurg, Ortho, Ped Surg, Peds, Rehab, Surg

+1 616-512-3105

https://vfapp.org/aa16

D-tree Digital Global Health

Demonstrates and advocates for the potential of digital technology to transform health systems and improve health and wellbeing for all.

Logist-Op, MF Med, OB-GYN, Peds, Pub Health

+1 978-238-9122

https://vfapp.org/1f79

Dentaid

Seeks to treat, equip, train, and educate people in need of dental care.

Dent-OMFS

+44 1794 324249

https://vfapp.org/a183

Development Aid from People to People (DAPP)

Strives to promote social and economic development. Through a variety of development models, DAPP complements the government's effort in implementing the Malawi Growth and Development Strategy to achieve the nation's Vision 2020.

Infect Dis, Nutr, Path

+265 888 86 17 91

https://vfapp.org/f8c8

Direct Relief

Improves the health and lives of people affected by poverty or emergency situations by mobilizing and providing essential medical resources needed for their care.

ER Med, Logist-Op

+1 805-964-4767

https://vfapp.org/58e5

Direct Relief of Poverty & Sickness Foundation (DROPS)

Volunteer led organization that utilizes all donations toward direct relief of poverty and illness through initiatives in healthcare education, improving healthcare systems and providing essential medical help to children and aged people in need.

Dent-OMFS, General, Ophth-Opt

+49 171 3637659

https://vfapp.org/af95

Doctors Without Borders/Médecins Sans Frontières (MSF)

Responds to emergencies and provides lifesaving medical care where needed most, including during disasters, conflicts, and epidemics.

Anesth, Crit-Care, ER Med, General, Infect Dis, Nutr, OB-GYN, Ped Surg, Peds, Psych, Pub Health, Surg

+1 212-679-6800

https://vfapp.org/f363

Doctors Worldwide

Focuses on health access, health improvement, and health emergencies to serve communities in need so they can build healthier and happier futures.

Dent-OMFS, ER Med, General, MF Med, Palliative, Peds

+44 7308 139100

https://vfapp.org/99cd

Dream Sant'Egidio

Seeks to counter HIV/AIDS in Africa by eliminating the transmission of HIV from mother to child, with a focus on women because of the importance of their role in the community.

Infect Dis, MF Med, Neonat, OB-GYN, Path, Peds

+39 06 899 2225

https://vfapp.org/f466

Drugs for Neglected Diseases Initiative

Develops lifesaving medicines for people with neglected diseases around the world, having developed eight treatments for five deadly diseases and saving millions of lives since 2003.

Infect Dis, Pub Health

+41 22 906 92 30

https://vfapp.org/969c

Elizabeth Glaser Pediatric AIDS Foundation

Seeks to end global pediatric HIV/AIDS through prevention and treatment programs, research, and advocacy.

Infect Dis, Nutr, OB-GYN, Peds

+1 888-499-4673

https://vfapp.org/d6ec

Embangweni Mission Hospital

Promotes and provides holistic, accessible, and patient-centered care, inspired by the Christian faith. Serves patients from Malawi and Zambia, offering a broad range of services as the main healthcare provider in the Mzimba region of Malawi.

Anesth, Dent-OMFS, General, MF Med, Neonat, Ophth-Opt, Ortho, Path, Peds, Surg
+265 999 19 18 70
https://vfapp.org/b5ae

Episcopal Relief & Development
Provides relief in times of disaster and promotes sustainable development by identifying and addressing the root causes of suffering.
Infect Dis, MF Med, Neonat, Nutr, Peds
+1 855-312-4325
https://vfapp.org/7cfa

eRanger
Provides sustainable solutions to transportation and medical provision such as ambulances and mobile clinics in developing countries.
ER Med, General, Logist-Op
+27 40 654 3207
https://vfapp.org/4c18

Evidence Action
Aims to be a world leader in scaling evidence-based and cost-effective programs to reduce the burden of poverty.
General, Infect Dis
+1 202-888-9886
https://vfapp.org/94b6

Eye Foundation of America
Works toward a world without childhood blindness.
Ophth-Opt
+1 304-599-0705
https://vfapp.org/a7eb

Feet First Worldwide
Aims to prevent and correct clubfoot in Malawi so that every child is diagnosed at birth and given access to surgical and other treatment. Also provides care for existing neglected cases, with an emphasis on training local staff in basic surgical techniques and clubfoot management.
Anesth, Ortho, Peds, Radiol, Rehab
+44 7565 922609
https://vfapp.org/f119

Freedom From Fistula
Helps women and girls who are injured and left incontinent following prolonged, obstructed childbirth by providing free surgical repairs for patients already suffering with fistula, as well as maternity care to prevent fistulas from happening at all.
MF Med, OB-GYN, Peds
+1 646-867-0994
https://vfapp.org/6e11

Global Alliance to Prevent Prematurity and Stillbirth (GAPPS)
Seeks to improve birth outcomes worldwide by reducing the burden of premature birth and stillbirth.
All-Immu, Infect Dis, MF Med, Neonat, Neonat, OB-GYN
+1 206-413-7954
https://vfapp.org/3f74

Global Health Corps
Mobilizes a diverse community of leaders to build the movement for global health equity, working toward a world where every person lives a healthy life.
ER Med, General, Pub Health
https://vfapp.org/31c6

Global Medical Missions
Organizes medical missions and partners with local medical organizations, usually hospitals or health systems, in fulfilling their mission of reaching their community's health needs in developing countries by providing needed medical care and screening to those underserved.
General
+1 661-865-8120
https://vfapp.org/8d73

Global Ministries – The United Methodist Church
As the worldwide mission and development agency of The United Methodist Church, Global Ministries works with more than 300 hospitals and clinics around the world through its Global Health Unit.
Anesth, CT Surg, CV Med, Crit-Care, Dent-OMFS, Derm, ER Med, GI, General, Infect Dis, Logist-Op, MF Med, Medicine, Neonat, Nephro, Nutr, OB-GYN, Ophth-Opt, Ortho, Palliative, Peds, Pod, Psych, Pub Health, Rehab, Rheum, Surg, Urol
+1 800-862-4246
https://vfapp.org/1723

Global Oncology (GO)
Brings the best in cancer care to underserved patients around the world and collaborates across geographic, professional, and academic borders to improve cancer care, research, and education.
Heme-Onc, Path, Rad-Onc
https://vfapp.org/fcb8

GOAL
Works with the most vulnerable communities to help them respond to and recover from humanitarian crises, and to assist them in building transcendent solutions to mitigate poverty and vulnerability.
ER Med, General, Pub Health
+353 1 280 9779
https://vfapp.org/bbea

Grassroot Soccer
Leverages the power of soccer to educate, inspire, and mobilize at risk youth in developing countries to overcome their greatest health challenges, live healthier more productive lives, and be agents for change in their communities.
Infect Dis
+1 603-277-9685
https://vfapp.org/3521

Health Equity Initiative
Aims to build and sustain a global community that engages across sectors and disciplines to advance health equity.
Pub Health
https://vfapp.org/e2e2

Health Poverty Action
Works in partnership with people around the world who are pursuing change in their own communities to demand health justice and challenge power imbalances.
ER Med, General, Infect Dis, Psych, Pub Health
+44 20 7840 3777
https://vfapp.org/ee58

Health Volunteers Overseas (HVO)
Improves the availability and quality of healthcare through the education, training, and professional development of the health workforce in resource-scarce countries.

All-Immu, Anesth, CV Med, Dent-OMFS, Derm, ENT, ER Med, Endo, GI, Heme-Onc, Infect Dis, Medicine, Medicine, Nephro, Neuro, OB-GYN, Ophth-Opt, Ortho, Peds, Plast, Psych, Pulm-Critic, Rehab, Rheum, Surg

+1 202-296-0928

https://vfapp.org/42b2

Healthy Developments
Provides Germany-supported health and social protection programs around the globe in a collaborative knowledge management process.

All-Immu, General, Infect Dis, Logist-Op, MF Med

https://vfapp.org/dc31

Heart to Heart International
Strengthens communities through improving health access, providing humanitarian development, and administering crisis relief worldwide. Engages volunteers, collaborates with partners, and deploys resources to achieve this mission.

Anesth, ER Med, General, Logist-Op, Medicine, Path, Path, Peds, Psych, Pub Health, Surg

+1 913-764-5200

https://vfapp.org/aacb

Hope and Healing International
Gives hope and healing to children and families trapped by poverty and disability.

General, Nutr, Ophth-Opt, Peds, Rehab

+1 905-640-6464

https://vfapp.org/c638

Hope Walks
Frees children, families, and communities from the burden of clubfoot, inspired by the Christian faith.

Ortho, Ped Surg, Peds, Rehab

+1 717-502-4400

https://vfapp.org/f6d4

Hunger Project, The
Aims to end hunger and poverty by pioneering sustainable, grassroots, women-centered strategies and advocating for their widespread adoption in countries throughout the world.

Infect Dis, Nutr, OB-GYN, Pub Health

+1 212-251-9100

https://vfapp.org/3a49

ICAP at Columbia University
Serves as global leader in supporting the scale-up of multidisciplinary HIV/AIDS prevention, care, and treatment programs based on a family-focused approach.

General, Infect Dis, MF Med, Medicine, OB-GYN, Pub Health

+1 212-342-0505

https://vfapp.org/a8ef

Imaging the World
Develops sustainable models for ultrasound imaging in the world's lowest resource settings and uses a technology-enabled solution to improve healthcare access, integrating lifesaving ultrasound and training programs in rural communities.

Logist-Op, OB-GYN, Radiol

https://vfapp.org/59e4

Innovating Health International (IHI)
Treats chronic diseases and addresses women's health issues in Haiti, Somaliland, and Malawi.

ER Med, Heme-Onc, Medicine, OB-GYN, Path, Plast, Pub Health

+509 48 95 6148

https://vfapp.org/e712

Institute for Healthcare Improvement (IHI)
Aims to improve health and healthcare worldwide by working with health professionals to strengthen systems.

Crit-Care, Infect Dis, MF Med, Medicine, Neonat, OB-GYN, Pub Health

+1 617-301-4800

https://vfapp.org/ecae

International Agency for the Prevention of Blindness (IAPB), The
Leads international efforts in blindness-prevention activities, works toward a world where no one is needlessly visually impaired, and ensures that everyone has access to the best possible standard of eye health.

Infect Dis, Ophth-Opt, Pub Health

https://vfapp.org/87a2

International Campaign for Women's Right to Safe Abortion
Works to build an international network and campaign that brings together organizations with an interest in promoting and providing safe abortion to create a shared platform for advocacy, debate, and dialogue and the sharing of skills and experience.

OB-GYN, Pub Health, Surg

https://vfapp.org/f341

International Council of Ophthalmology
Works with ophthalmologic societies and others to enhance ophthalmic education and improve access to the highest quality eye care in order to preserve and restore vision for the people of the world.

Ophth-Opt

https://vfapp.org/ffd2

International Eye Foundation (IEF)
Eliminates preventable and treatable blindness by making quality sustainable eye care services accessible and affordable worldwide.

Infect Dis, Logist-Op, Ophth-Opt

+1 240-290-0263

https://vfapp.org/e839

International Federation of Gynecology and Obstetrics (FIGO)
Implements global projects on specific women's health issues.

MF Med, Medicine, Neonat, OB-GYN, Surg, Urol

+44 20 7928 1166

https://vfapp.org/c4b4

International Federation of Red Cross and Red Crescent Societies (IFRC)
Coordinates and directs international assistance following natural and man-made disasters in nonconflict situations through the

world's largest humanitarian and development network. Provides disaster-preparedness programs, healthcare activities, and promotes humanitarian values.

ER Med, General, Infect Dis, Nutr

+1 212-338-0161

https://vfapp.org/b4ee

International Learning Movement (ILM UK)

Supports some of the world's poorest people in developing countries with core projects in education, safe drinking water, and healthcare.

General, Ophth-Opt

+44 1254 265451

https://vfapp.org/b974

International Medical Response

Supplements, supports, and enhances healthcare systems in communities across the world that have been incapacitated by natural disaster, extreme poverty, and/or regional conflict by sending a multidisciplinary team of healthcare professionals.

Anesth, General, OB-GYN, Surg

+1 917-324-8348

https://vfapp.org/9ccd

International Organization for Migration (IOM) – The UN Migration Agency

Promotes evidence-informed policies and holistic, preventive, and curative health programs that are beneficial, accessible, and equitable for vulnerable migrants.

General, Infect Dis, OB-GYN

+27 12 342 2789

https://vfapp.org/621a

International Pediatric Nephrology Association (IPNA)

Leads the global efforts to successfully address the care for all children with kidney disease through advocacy, education, and training.

Medicine, Nephro, Peds

https://vfapp.org/b59d

International Planned Parenthood Federation (IPPF)

Leads a locally owned, globally connected civil society movement that provides and enables services and champions sexual and reproductive health and rights for all, especially the underserved.

Infect Dis, MF Med, OB-GYN

+44 20 7939 8200

https://vfapp.org/dc97

International Relief Teams

Helps families survive and recover after a disaster by delivering timely and effective assistance through programs that improve their health and well-being while also providing a hopeful future for underserved communities.

Dent-OMFS, ER Med, General, Nutr, Ophth-Opt

+1 619-284-7979

https://vfapp.org/ffd5

International Society of Nephrology

Aims to advance worldwide kidney health.

Nephro

+32 2 808 04 20

https://vfapp.org/1bae

International Trachoma Initiative (iTi)

Works toward a world free from trachoma, a preventable cause of blindness, and provides comprehensive support to national ministries of health and governmental and nongovernmental organizations to implement a comprehensive approach to fight trachoma.

Infect Dis, Ophth-Opt

+1 404-371-0466

https://vfapp.org/3278

International Union Against Tuberculosis and Lung Disease

Develops, implements, and assesses anti-tuberculosis, lung health, and noncommunicable disease programs.

Infect Dis, Pub Health, Pulm-Critic

+33 1 44 32 03 60

https://vfapp.org/3e82

InterSurgeon

Fosters collaborative partnerships in the field of global surgery that will advance clinical care, teaching, training, research, and the provision and maintenance of medical equipment.

ENT, Neurosurg, Ortho, Ped Surg, Plast, Surg, Urol

https://vfapp.org/6f8a

Ipas

Focuses efforts on women and girls who want contraception or abortion, and builds programs around their needs and how best to support them.

OB-GYN

https://vfapp.org/8e39

Iris Global

Serves the poor, the destitute, the lost, and the forgotten by providing adoration, outreach, family, education, relief, development, healing, and the arts.

General, Infect Dis, Nutr, Pub Health

+1 530-255-2077

https://vfapp.org/37f8

Islamic Medical Association of North America

Fosters health promotion, disease prevention, and health maintenance in communities around the world through direct patient care and health programs.

Anesth, Dent-OMFS, ER Med, General, Logist-Op, Ophth-Opt, Peds, Plast, Surg

+1 630-932-0000

https://vfapp.org/a157

Jacaranda Foundation

Provides orphans and vulnerable children in Malawi with education, comprehensive care, and enrichment programs to enable them to become leaders and change agents in their communities.

Nutr, Peds, Rehab

+265 999 91 90 56

https://vfapp.org/acf4

Jhpiego

Creates and delivers transformative healthcare solutions that save lives in partnership with national governments, health experts, and local communities.

General, Infect Dis, OB-GYN, Surg

+1 410-537-1800

https://vfapp.org/45b8

John Snow, Inc. (JSI)
Aims to improve the health and well-being of underserved and vulnerable people and communities throughout the world.

General, Infect Dis, Logist-Op, MF Med, OB-GYN, Peds, Psych, Pub Health

+1 617-482-9485

https://vfapp.org/ba78

Johns Hopkins Center for Communication Programs
Believes in the power of communication to save lives, by empowering people to adopt healthy behaviors for themselves, their families, and their communities.

General, Infect Dis, Logist-Op, OB-GYN, Pub Health

+1 410-659-6300

https://vfapp.org/1bf9

Joint United Nations Programme on HIV/AIDS (UNAIDS)
Aims to place people living with HIV and people affected by the virus at the decision-making table and at the center of designing, delivering, and monitoring the AIDS response.

Infect Dis

+41 22 791 36 66

https://vfapp.org/464a

Kansas University Medical Center: Global Surgery
Improves the lives and communities in Kansas and beyond through innovation in education, research and health care.

Neurosurg, Ortho, Ped Surg, Surg, Urol

+1 913-588-5000

https://vfapp.org/bc97

Last Mile Health
Links community health workers with frontline health workers—nurses, doctors, and midwives at community clinics—and supports them to bring lifesaving services to the doorsteps of people living far from care.

General, Logist-Op, OB-GYN, Pub Health

+1 617-880-6163

https://vfapp.org/37da

Life Support Foundation
Aims to prevent deaths due to acute, life-threatening conditions in low-income countries through improving the access to, and quality of, basic lifesaving interventions.

Anesth, Crit-Care, ER Med, OB-GYN, Peds

https://vfapp.org/799e

LifeCare Malawi Foundation (LCMF)
Inspired by faith, aims to fight for the survival and personal development of Malawi's most vulnerable and disadvantaged citizens, regardless of their tribal, religious, or political affiliation.

General, Infect Dis, MF Med, Nutr

+265 998 68 59 00

https://vfapp.org/839f

LifeNet International
Transforms African healthcare by equipping and empowering existing local health centers to provide quality, sustainable, and lifesaving care to patients.

General, Infect Dis, MF Med, Neonat, OB-GYN, Pub Health

+1 407-630-9518

https://vfapp.org/e5d2

Lighthouse Trust
Provides improved quality treatment, care, and support services for people living with HIV in Malawi.

General, Infect Dis

+265 1 725 549

https://vfapp.org/fbd1

Lions Clubs International
Empowers volunteers to serve their communities, meet humanitarian needs, encourage peace, and promote international understanding through Lions clubs.

Heme-Onc, Medicine, Nutr, Ophth-Opt

+1 630-571-5466

https://vfapp.org/7b12

London School of Hygiene & Tropical Medicine: International Centre for Eye Health
Works to improve eye health and eliminate avoidable visual impairment and blindness with a focus on low-income populations.

Logist-Op, Ophth-Opt, Pub Health

+44 20 7958 8316

https://vfapp.org/6f5f

Luke International (LIN)
Builds bridges between local and international development partners, creates interfaces between health and technology, and advocates and serves where the greatest needs are.

General, Infect Dis, OB-GYN, Peds, Pub Health

+47 908 92 582

https://vfapp.org/4681

Malawi AIDS Counseling and Resource Organization (MACRO MW)
Provides high-quality HIV and AIDS treatment and other health-related services to the Malawian population.

Infect Dis, Psych, Pub Health

+265 999 37 45 71

https://vfapp.org/6138

Malawi Children's Initiative
Works to improve the lives of Malawian children through better healthcare, education, and nutrition by building bridges between communities in the United States and Malawi.

General, Logist-Op, Nutr, Peds

+1 336-212-5394

https://vfapp.org/e9a9

Malawi Healthcare Support UK (MAHECAS UK)
Aims to provide relief and preserve good health among patients in hospitals, health clinics, and other primary healthcare locations across Malawi.

Dent-OMFS, General

https://vfapp.org/7b2a

Malawi Stroke Unit
Aims to build and run the first integrated stroke pathway in Malawi, based at Queen Elizabeth Central Hospital, Malawi, and demonstrate substantial improvement in stroke-related mortality and long-term disability while reducing stroke care costs.

CV Med, Neuro, Rehab, Vasc Surg

+265 1 876 213

https://vfapp.org/97ba

Malawi Washington Foundation
Aims to improve and strengthen the lives of vulnerable communities through the provision of charitable educational services and supporting sustainable programs for

the poor, especially women and youth.
Logist-Op
https://vfapp.org/7d2a

Maloto
Seeks to transform the lives of vulnerable populations in Malawi living in extreme poverty and provide women and children with the opportunity to reach their full potential in an actively sustainable way.
Nutr
+1 646-576-6485
https://vfapp.org/f56a

Management Sciences for Health (MSH)
Works with countries and communities to save lives and improve the health of the world's poorest and most vulnerable people by building strong, resilient, sustainable health systems.
Infect Dis, Logist-Op, Pub Health
+1 617-250-9500
https://vfapp.org/6aa2

MAP International
Provides medicines and health supplies to those in need around the world so they might experience life to the fullest.
Logist-Op
+1 800-225-8550
https://vfapp.org/deed

Marie Stopes International
Provides the contraception and safe abortion services that enable women all over the world to choose their own futures.
Infect Dis, MF Med, Neonat, OB-GYN, Pub Health
+44 20 7636 6200
https://vfapp.org/9525

Maternity Worldwide
Works with communities and partners to identify and develop appropriate and effective ways to reduce maternal and newborn mortality and morbidity, facilitate communities to access quality skilled maternity care, and support the provision of quality skilled care.
MF Med, OB-GYN
+44 1273 234033
https://vfapp.org/822b

Medic Malawi
Provides quality, accessible, sustainable healthcare through partnership with St. Andrew's Hospital and aims to create a safe, loving, supportive, and sustainable environment for the children in Malawi.
Peds
+44 7990 678676
https://vfapp.org/1c83

Medical Benevolence Foundation (MBF)
Works with partners in developing countries to build sustainable healthcare for those most in need through faith-based global medical missions.
General, Logist-Op, MF Med, OB-GYN, Surg
+1 800-547-7627
https://vfapp.org/c3e8

Medical Ministry International
Provides compassionate healthcare in areas of need, inspired by the Christian faith.
CT Surg, Dent-OMFS, ENT, General, OB-GYN, Ophth-Opt, Ortho, Plast, Rehab, Surg, Urol, Vasc Surg
+1 905-545-4400
https://vfapp.org/5da6

Medical Servants International
Provides medical care, inspired by the Christian faith.
Dent-OMFS, General, OB-GYN, Peds
+1 760-644-4316
https://vfapp.org/6371

MedSend
Funds qualified healthcare professionals to serve the physical and spiritual needs of people around the world, enabling healthcare providers to work where they have been called.
General
+1 203-891-8223
https://vfapp.org/661c

MedShare
Aims to improve the quality of life of people, communities, and the planet by sourcing and directly delivering surplus medical supplies and equipment to communities in need around the world.
Logist-Op
+1 770-323-5858
https://vfapp.org/c8bc

MicroResearch: Africa/Asia
Seeks to improve health outcomes in Africa by training, mentoring, and supporting local multidisciplinary health professional researchers.
Infect Dis, Nutr, OB-GYN, Psych
https://vfapp.org/13e7

Miracle for Africa Foundation
Works to end poverty in Malawi by building programs focused on health, education, and agriculture.
Crit-Care, ER Med, General, MF Med, Path, Radiol, Surg
+265 1 711 398
https://vfapp.org/b1e3

Mission Vision
Seeks to decrease blindness and other eye-related disabilities, as well as to increase academic performance and general quality of life.
Ophth-Opt
+1 724-553-3114
https://vfapp.org/83d8

mothers2mothers (m2m)
Employs and trains local women living with HIV as community health workers called Mentor Mothers to support women, children, and adolescents with vital medical services, education, and support.
Infect Dis, MF Med, OB-GYN, Peds, Pub Health
+27 21 466 9160
https://vfapp.org/6557

MSD for Mothers
Designs scalable solutions that help end preventable maternal deaths.
MF Med, OB-GYN, Pub Health
https://vfapp.org/9f99

Mua Mission Hospital

Works to provide affordable and quality healthcare services to all people in Bwanje Valley and beyond, serving as the principal referral hospital within a poor and remote rural area with a population of more than 130,000 people.

Dent-OMFS, General, Infect Dis, MF Med, Peds, Pub Health, Surg

☎ +265 995 29 32 33

🌐 https://vfapp.org/ae41

Mulanje Mission Hospital

Works with a local government hospital to serve a population of 685,000 people in the Mulanje District of southeast Malawi.

General, Infect Dis, MF Med, OB-GYN, Peds, Pub Health, Surg

☎ +265 999 28 65 03

🌐 https://vfapp.org/9212

NCD Alliance

Unites and strengthens civil society to stimulate collaborative advocacy, action, and accountability for NCD (noncommunicable disease) prevention and control.

All-Immu, CV Med, General, Heme-Onc, Medicine, Peds, Psych

☎ +41 22 809 18 11

🌐 https://vfapp.org/abdd

Ndi Moyo: The Place Giving Life

Provides patient-centered, home-based palliative care for people in Salima, Malawi, who are sick and dying.

General, Heme-Onc, Palliative

☎ +265 1 262 644

🌐 https://vfapp.org/745e

NEST 360

Works to ensure that hospitals in Africa can deliver lifesaving care for small and sick newborns, by developing and distributing high-quality technologies and services.

MF Med, Neonat, Peds, Pub Health

☎ +1 713-348-4174

🌐 https://vfapp.org/cea9

Network for Improving Critical Care Systems and Training (NICST)

Provides critical-care training for staff in developing countries.

Crit-Care, General, Pulm-Critic

☎ +94 114 063 739

🌐 https://vfapp.org/71f8

NYC Medics

Deploys mobile medical teams to remote areas of disaster zones and humanitarian emergencies, providing the highest level of medical care to those who otherwise would not have access to aid and relief efforts.

All-Immu, ER Med, Infect Dis, Surg

☎ +1 888-600-1648

🌐 https://vfapp.org/aeee

OB Foundation

Works in partnership globally to deliver locally sustainable, quality healthcare, health education, and health solutions to medically underserved, rural communities.

General

☎ +1 614-500-7345

🌐 https://vfapp.org/91d7

Operation Medical

Commits efforts to promoting and providing high-quality medical care and education to communities that do not have adequate access.

Anesth, ENT, Logist-Op, OB-GYN, Ped Surg, Plast, Surg, Urol

☎ +1 717-685-9199

🌐 https://vfapp.org/7e1b

Operation Smile

Treats patients with cleft lip and cleft palate, and creates solutions that deliver safe surgery to people where it's needed most.

Anesth, Dent-OMFS, ENT, Ped Surg, Plast

☎ +1 757-321-7645

🌐 https://vfapp.org/5c29

Options

Believes in a world where women and children can access the high-quality health services they need, without financial burden.

Logist-Op, MF Med, Neonat, OB-GYN

☎ +44 20 7430 1900

🌐 https://vfapp.org/3a48

OPTIVEST Foundation

Funds strategic opportunities that are holistic and collaborative, inspired by the Christian faith.

General, Nutr

🌐 https://vfapp.org/f1e6

Optometry Giving Sight

Delivers eye exams and low or no-cost glasses, provides training for local eye care professionals, and establishes optometry schools, vision centers and optical labs.

Ophth-Opt

☎ +1 303-526-0430

🌐 https://vfapp.org/33ea

Orbis International

Works to prevent and treat blindness through hands-on training and improved access to quality eye care.

Anesth, Ophth-Opt, Surg

☎ +1 646-674-5500

🌐 https://vfapp.org/f2b2

Oxford University Global Surgery Group (OUGSG)

Aims to contribute to the provision of high-quality surgical care globally, particularly in low- and middle-income countries (LMICs) while bringing together students, researchers, and clinicians with an interest in global surgery, anaesthesia, and obstetrics and gynecology.

Anesth, MF Med, OB-GYN, Ortho, Surg

☎ +44 1865 737543

🌐 https://vfapp.org/c624

PACHI Trust (Parent and Child Health Initiative)

Promotes high-quality, sustainable, and cost-effective maternal and child care delivery, capacity building, and research that promotes the health of families in Malawi and beyond.

MF Med, Neonat, OB-GYN, Peds, Pub Health

☎ +265 111 75 84 77

🌐 https://vfapp.org/c49c

Pact

Works on the ground to improve the lives of those who are

challenged by poverty and marginalization, striving for a world where all people are heard, capable, and vibrant.

Infect Dis, Logist-Op, MF Med, Pub Health

+1 202-466-5666

https://vfapp.org/9a6c

Pan African Thoracic Society (PATS)

Aims to promote lung health in Africa, the continent most afflicted by morbidity and death from respiratory diseases, by promoting education, research, advocacy, optimal care, and the development of African capacity to address respiratory challenges in the continent.

CV Med, Crit-Care, Pulm-Critic

https://vfapp.org/5457

Pan-African Academy of Christian Surgeons (PAACS)

Exists to train and support African surgeons to provide excellent, compassionate care to those most in need, inspired by the Christian faith.

Anesth, CT Surg, Neurosurg, OB-GYN, Ortho, Ped Surg, Plast, Surg

+1 847-571-9926

https://vfapp.org/85ba

Partners in Health

Responds to the moral imperative to provide high-quality healthcare globally to those who need it most, while striving to ease suffering by providing a comprehensive model of care that includes access to food, transportation, housing, and other key components of healing.

CT Surg, General, Heme-Onc, Infect Dis, MF Med, Neurosurg, OB-GYN, Ortho, Plast, Psych, Urol

+1 857-880-5600

https://vfapp.org/dc9c

Partners in Hope

Aims to strengthen the capacity of Malawi's healthcare system to deliver quality, equitable, and sustainable services.

ER Med, General, Infect Dis, Nutr, Path, Radiol, Rehab, Surg

+265 999 97 17 31

https://vfapp.org/2a75

PATH

Advances health equity through innovation and partnerships so people, communities, and economies can thrive.

All-Immu, CV Med, Endo, Heme-Onc, Infect Dis, MF Med, Neonat, Nutr, OB-GYN, Path, Peds, Pulm-Critic

+1 202-822-0033

https://vfapp.org/b4db

Pediatric Health Initiative

Supports the spread of quality pediatric care and its development and progress in low- and middle-income countries.

ER Med, Infect Dis, Neonat, Palliative, Ped Surg, Peds

https://vfapp.org/614b

Physicians for Peace

Educates and empowers local providers of surgical care to alleviate suffering and transform lives in under-resourced communities around the world.

Crit-Care, Ped Surg, Plast, Psych, Surg, Urol

+1 757-625-7569

https://vfapp.org/6a65

PINCC Preventing Cervical Cancer

Seeks to prevent female-specific diseases in developing countries by utilizing low-cost and low-technology methods to create sustainable programs through patient education, medical personnel training, and facility outfitting.

OB-GYN

+1 830-708-6009

https://vfapp.org/9666

Project Concern International (PCI)

Drives innovation from the ground up to enhance health, end hunger, overcome hardship, and advance women and girls—resulting in meaningful and measurable change in people's lives.

Infect Dis, MF Med, Nutr, OB-GYN, Peds

+1 858-279-9690

https://vfapp.org/5ed7

Project HOPE

Works on the front lines of the world's health challenges, partnering hand-in-hand with communities, healthcare workers, and public health systems to ensure sustainable change.

CV Med, ER Med, Endo, General, Infect Dis, MF Med, Peds

+1 844-349-0188

https://vfapp.org/2bd7

Project SOAR

Conducts HIV operations research around the world to identify practical solutions to improve HIV prevention, care, and treatment services.

ER Med, General, MF Med, OB-GYN, Psych

+1 202-237-9400

https://vfapp.org/1a77

PSI – Population Services International

Dedicates efforts to improving the health of people in the developing world by focusing on challenges such as a lack of family planning, HIV/AIDS, barriers to maternal health, and the greatest threats to children under the age of 5, including malaria, diarrhea, pneumonia, and malnutrition.

Infect Dis, MF Med, OB-GYN, Peds

+1 202-785-0072

https://vfapp.org/ffe3

RAD-AID International

Improves and optimizes access to medical imaging and radiology in low-resource regions of the world.

Rad-Onc, Radiol

https://vfapp.org/537f

Raising Malawi

Supports community-based organizations that provide Malawi's orphans, vulnerable children, and their caregivers with education, medical care, food and shelter, and psycho-social support.

Crit-Care, General, Infect Dis, Ped Surg, Peds, Pub Health, Surg

https://vfapp.org/34c3

RestoringVision

Empowers lives by restoring vision for millions of people in need.

Ophth-Opt

+1 209-980-7323

https://vfapp.org/e121

Rice 360 Institute for Global Health

Brings together an international group of faculty, students, clinicians, and private and public sector partners to design innovative health technologies for low-resource settings, while developing and implementing entrepreneurial approaches that increase access to these technologies around the world.

Crit-Care, Infect Dis, Logist-Op, MF Med, Neonat, Pub Health

+1 713-348-2923

https://vfapp.org/c82b

Riders for Health International

Aids in the last mile of healthcare delivery, by ensuring that healthcare reaches everyone, everywhere.

ER Med, Infect Dis, Logist-Op, Pub Health

+231 77 704 4287

https://vfapp.org/85aa

Right to Care

Responds to public health needs by supporting and delivering innovative, quality healthcare solutions, based on the latest medical research and established best practices, for the prevention, treatment, and management of infectious and chronic diseases.

ER Med, Infect Dis, Logist-Op

+27 11 276 8850

https://vfapp.org/3383

Ripple Africa

Empowers communities to achieve a sustainable future by providing a hand up, not a handout, by developing programs in such areas as the environment, education, and healthcare.

General, Infect Dis, OB-GYN, Ortho, Pub Health, Rehab

+1 941-782-7956

https://vfapp.org/63bb

Rockefeller Foundation, The

Works to promote the well-being of humanity.

Logist-Op, Nutr, Pub Health

+1 212-869-8500

https://vfapp.org/5424

Rotary International

Provides service to others, improves lives, and advances world understanding, goodwill, and peace through its fellowship of business, professional, and community leaders.

ER Med, General, Infect Dis, MF Med, OB-GYN

https://vfapp.org/8fb5

ROW Foundation

Works to improve the quality of training for healthcare providers, and the diagnosis and treatment available to people with epilepsy and associated psychiatric disorders in under-resourced areas of the world.

Neuro, Psych

+1 630-791-0247

https://vfapp.org/25eb

Salvation Army International, The

Seeks to meet human needs through services in education, healthcare, community support, emergency response, and ministry development, inspired by the Christian faith.

Dent-OMFS, Derm, ER Med, Infect Dis, MF Med, Medicine, Nutr, OB-GYN, Ophth-Opt, Palliative, Psych, Rehab, Surg

+44 20 7332 0101

https://vfapp.org/8eb3

Samaritan's Purse International Disaster Relief

Provides spiritual and physical aid to hurting people around the world, such as victims of war, poverty, natural disasters, disease, and famine, based in Christian ministry.

Anesth, CT Surg, Crit-Care, Dent-OMFS, Derm, ENT, ER Med, Endo, GI, General, Heme-Onc, Infect Dis, MF Med, Neonat, Nephro, Neuro, Neurosurg, Nutr, OB-GYN, Ophth-Opt, Ortho, Path, Ped Surg, Peds, Plast, Psych, Pulm-Critic, Radiol, Rehab, Rheum, Surg, Urol, Vasc Surg

+1 800-528-1980

https://vfapp.org/87e3

Sanofi Espoir Foundation

Contributes to reducing health inequalities among populations that need it most by applying a socially responsible approach focused on fighting childhood cancers in low-income countries, improving maternal and newborn health, and improving access to care.

ER Med, OB-GYN, Peds

+33 1 53 77 91 38

https://vfapp.org/943b

Save A Child's Heart

Provides lifesaving cardiac treatment to children in developing countries, and trains healthcare professionals from these countries to deliver quality care in their communities.

CT Surg, CV Med, Crit-Care, Ped Surg, Peds

+1 240-223-3940

https://vfapp.org/1bef

Save the Children

Gives children around the world a healthy start in life, the opportunity to learn, and protection from harm.

All-Immu, Crit-Care, ER Med, General, Infect Dis, MF Med, Medicine, Neonat, OB-GYN, Peds, Psych, Pub Health

+1 800-728-3843

https://vfapp.org/2e73

SEE International

Provides sustainable medical, surgical, and educational services through volunteer ophthalmic surgeons, with the objectives of restoring sight and preventing blindness to disadvantaged individuals worldwide.

Ophth-Opt, Surg

+1 805-963-3303

https://vfapp.org/6e1b

Seed Global Health

Focuses on human resources for health capacity building at the individual, institutional, and national level through sustained collaborative engagement with partners.

Logist-Op

+1 617-366-1650

https://vfapp.org/d12e

Sightsavers

Prevents avoidable blindness in some of the poorest parts of the world by treating debilitating eye diseases.

Infect Dis, Ophth-Opt, Surg

+1 800-707-9746

https://vfapp.org/aa52

SIGN Fracture Care International

Builds orthopedic capacity around the world and provides the injured poor access to fracture surgery by donating orthopedic education and implant systems to surgeons in developing countries.

Ortho, Rehab, Surg
+1 509-371-1107
https://vfapp.org/123d

Simavi

Strives for a world in which all women and girls are socially and economically empowered and pursue their rights to live a healthy life, free from discrimination, coercion, and violence.

MF Med, OB-GYN
+31 88 313 1500
https://vfapp.org/b57b

Smile Train

Seeks to give every child with a cleft the opportunity for a healthy, productive life by providing free cleft repair surgery and comprehensive cleft care in their own communities.

Dent-OMFS, ENT, Plast
+1 800-932-9541
https://vfapp.org/f21d

Sound Seekers

Supports people with hearing loss by enabling access to healthcare and education.

ENT
+44 7305 433250
https://vfapp.org/ef1c

Sponsel Foundation

Provides resources and services to advance the education, screening, research, diagnosis, and treatment of ophthalmic diseases and ocular trauma for medically underserved communities locally and worldwide.

Ophth-Opt, Surg
+1 210-223-9292
https://vfapp.org/d93e

Surgeons OverSeas (SOS)

Works to reduce death and disability from surgically treatable conditions in developing countries.

Anesth, Heme-Onc, Surg
https://vfapp.org/5d16

Surgical Healing of Africa's Youth Foundation, The (S.H.A.Y.)

Provides volunteer reconstructive surgery to children in need, including treating congenital anomalies such as cleft lip/palate and general reconstruction.

Anesth, Dent-OMFS, Peds, Plast
+1 310-860-0646
https://vfapp.org/41a7

Swiss Tropical and Public Health Institute

Contributes to the improvement of the health of populations internationally, nationally, and locally through excellence in research, education, and services.

Infect Dis, Pub Health
+41 61 284 81 11
https://vfapp.org/2ee4

Task Force for Global Health, The

Consists of programs and focus areas that cover a range of global health issues including neglected tropical diseases, infectious diseases, vaccines, field epidemiology, public health informatics, health workforce development, and global health ethics.

Infect Dis, Logist-Op, Medicine, Ophth-Opt, Peds
+1 404-371-0466
https://vfapp.org/714c

Tearfund

Responds to crisis and partners with local churches to bring restoration to those living in poverty, inspired by the Christian faith.

ER Med, Logist-Op
+44 20 3906 3906
https://vfapp.org/f6cf

Texas Children's Global Health

Addresses healthcare needs in resource-limited settings locally and globally by improving maternal and child health through the implementation of innovative, sustainable, in-country programs to train health professionals and build functional healthcare infrastructure.

Anesth, ER Med, Heme-Onc, Infect Dis, MF Med, Nutr, OB-GYN, Peds, Pub Health, Surg
+1 832-824-1141
https://vfapp.org/4a1d

Together! ACT Now

Aims to end the spread of HIV in poor and rural areas of Malawi through theater, education, and access.

Infect Dis, Pub Health
+1 323-300-4929
https://vfapp.org/2fdc

U.S. President's Malaria Initiative (PMI)

Supports low-income countries to help control and eliminate malaria through cost-effective, lifesaving malaria interventions.

Infect Dis, MF Med, OB-GYN
+1 202-712-0000
https://vfapp.org/dc8b

Union for International Cancer Control (UICC)

Unites and supports the cancer community to reduce the global cancer burden, promote greater equity, and ensure that cancer control continues to be a priority in the world health and development agenda.

Heme-Onc, Pub Health
+41 22 809 18 11
https://vfapp.org/88b1

United Nations Children's Fund (UNICEF)

Works in over 190 countries and territories to save children's lives, to defend their rights, and to help them fulfill their potential, from early childhood through adolescence.

All-Immu, Infect Dis, MF Med, Neonat, Nutr, OB-GYN, Ped Surg, Peds, Pub Health
https://vfapp.org/42d7

United Nations Development Programme (UNDP)

Helps countries achieve the simultaneous eradication of extreme poverty and significant reduction of inequalities and exclusion using a sustainable human development approach.

Infect Dis, Logist-Op, Pub Health
https://vfapp.org/935c

United Nations High Commissioner for Refugees (UNHCR)

Safeguards the rights and well-being of people who have been forced to flee, ensuring that everybody has the right to seek asylum and find safe refuge in another country, with the goal of seeking lasting solutions.

General, MF Med, Medicine, OB-GYN, Peds, Psych, Pub Health

https://vfapp.org/6636

United Nations Population Fund (UNFPA)

Supports reproductive healthcare for women and youth in more than 150 countries, focusing on delivering a world where every pregnancy is wanted, every childbirth is safe, and every young person's potential is fulfilled.

Infect Dis, MF Med, Neonat, OB-GYN, Peds, Pub Health

+1 212-963-6008

https://vfapp.org/c969

United States Agency for International Development (USAID)

Promotes and demonstrates democratic values abroad and advances a free, peaceful, and prosperous world. Leads the U.S. government's international development and disaster assistance through partnerships and investments that save lives.

ER Med, Infect Dis, MF Med, OB-GYN, Peds

+1 202-712-0000

https://vfapp.org/9a99

University of California Los Angeles: David Geffen School of Medicine Global Health Program

Catalyzes opportunities to improve health globally by engaging in multi-disciplinary and innovative education programs, research initiatives, and bilateral partnerships that provide opportunities for trainees, faculty, and staff to contribute to sustainable health initiatives and to address health inequities facing the world today.

All-Immu, Infect Dis, Logist-Op, MF Med, Medicine, Neonat, OB-GYN, Ortho, Ped Surg, Peds, Radiol

+1 310-312-0531

https://vfapp.org/f1a4

University of California San Francisco: Institute for Global Health Sciences

Dedicates its efforts to improving health and reducing the burden of disease in the world's most vulnerable populations by integrating expertise in the health, social, and biological sciences to train global health leaders and develop solutions to the most pressing health challenges.

Infect Dis, OB-GYN, Pub Health

+1 415-476-5494

https://vfapp.org/6587

University of Cincinnati: College of Medicine Global Surgery

Aims to inspire a transformative approach to global health by training the next generation of surgeons, scholars, and leaders.

Plast, Surg

+1 513-558-7333

https://vfapp.org/13c9

University of New Mexico School of Medicine: Project Echo

Seeks to improve health outcomes worldwide through the use of a technology called telementoring, a guided-practice model in which the participating clinician retains responsibility for managing the patient.

General, Infect Dis, MF Med, OB-GYN, Path, Peds

+1 505-750-3246

https://vfapp.org/6c9a

University of North Carolina: Institute for Global Health and Infectious Diseases

Leads and supports the efforts to improve global health through research, teaching and service programs.

ENT, Infect Dis, MF Med, Neonat, OB-GYN, Surg

+1 919-966-2536

https://vfapp.org/9519

University of North Carolina: Institute for Global Health and Infectious Diseases

Harnesses the full resources of UNC and its partners to solve global health problems, reduce the burden of disease, and cultivate the next generation of global health leaders.

Infect Dis, MF Med, OB-GYN, Psych, Surg

+1 919-966-2537

https://vfapp.org/ed5e

University of Pennsylvania Perelman School of Medicine Center for Global Health

Aims to improve health equity worldwide – through enhanced public health awareness and access to care, discovery and outcomes based research, and comprehensive educational programs grounded in partnership.

Heme-Onc, Infect Dis, OB-GYN

+1 215-898-0848

https://vfapp.org/cb57

University of Virginia: Anesthesiology Department Global Health Initiatives

Educates and trains physicians, to help people achieve healthy productive lives, and advances knowledge in the medical sciences.

Anesth, Pub Health

+1 434-924-2283

https://vfapp.org/1b8b

University of Washington: The International Training and Education Center for Health (I-TECH)

Works with local partners to develop skilled healthcare workers and strong national health systems in resource-limited countries.

Infect Dis, Pub Health

+1 206-744-8493

https://vfapp.org/642f

USAID: Maternal and Child Survival Program

Works to prevent child and maternal deaths.

Infect Dis, MF Med, Neonat, OB-GYN, Peds

https://vfapp.org/6fcf

USAID: African Strategies for Health

Identifies and advocates for best practices, enhancing technical capacity of African regional institutions and engaging African stakeholders to address health issues in a sustainable manner.

All-Immu, Infect Dis, OB-GYN, Peds

https://vfapp.org/c272

USAID: A2Z The Micronutrient and Child Blindness Project
Aims to increase the use of key micronutrient and blindness interventions to improve child and maternal health.
MF Med, Neonat, Nutr, Ophth-Opt, Surg
+1 202-884-8785
https://vfapp.org/c5f1

USAID: Deliver Project
Builds a global supply chain to deliver lifesaving health products to people in order to enable countries to provide family planning, protect against malaria, and limit the spread of pandemic threats.
Infect Dis, Logist-Op, MF Med
+1 202-712-0000
https://vfapp.org/374e

USAID: EQUIP Health
Exists as an effective, efficient response mechanism to achieving global HIV epidemic control by delivering the right intervention at the right place and in the right way.
Infect Dis
+27 11 276 8850
https://vfapp.org/d76a

USAID: Health Policy Initiative
Provides field-level programming in health policy development and implementation.
General, Infect Dis, MF Med, OB-GYN, Peds
https://vfapp.org/8f84

USAID: Human Resources for Health 2030 (HRH2030)
Helps low- and middle-income countries develop the health workforce needed to prevent maternal and child deaths, support the goals of Family Planning 2020, control the HIV/AIDS epidemic, and protect communities from infectious diseases.
Logist-Op
+1 202-955-3300
https://vfapp.org/9ea8

USAID: Maternal and Child Health Integrated Program
Works to improve the health of women and their families, including programs for maternal, newborn, and child health, immunization, family planning, nutrition, malaria, and HIV/AIDS.
All-Immu, General, Infect Dis, MF Med
+1 202-835-3136
https://vfapp.org/4415

USAID: TB Care II
Focuses on tuberculosis care and treatment.
Infect Dis
+1 301-654-8338
https://vfapp.org/57d4

Virtual Doctors, The
Uses local mobile broadband networks to connect rural clinics with doctors around the world, connecting isolated health centers with volunteer doctors around the world.
Anesth, Derm, ENT, Endo, General, Heme-Onc, Infect Dis, Medicine, Neuro, OB-GYN, Ophth-Opt, Ortho, Palliative, Ped Surg, Peds, Plast, Psych, Surg
+44 1903 203720
https://vfapp.org/3d94

Vision Care
Restores sight and helps patients get regular treatment at short-term eye camps and long-term base clinics by having doctors, missionaries, volunteers, and sponsors work together.
Ophth-Opt
+1 212-769-3056
https://vfapp.org/9d7c

Vitamin Angels
Helps at-risk populations in need—specifically pregnant women, new mothers, and children under age five—to gain access to life-changing vitamins and minerals.
General, Nutr
+1 805-564-8400
https://vfapp.org/7da1

Voluntary Service Overseas (VSO)
Works with health workers, communities, and governments to improve health services and rights for women, babies, youth, people with disabilities, and prisoners.
General, MF Med, OB-GYN
+44 20 8780 7500
https://vfapp.org/213d

Watsi
Uses technology to make healthcare a reality for those who might not otherwise be able to afford it.
Pub Health, Surg
+1 256-792-8747
https://vfapp.org/41a3

White Ribbon Alliance, The
Leads a movement for reproductive, maternal, and newborn health and accelerates progress by putting citizens at the center of global, national, and local health efforts.
MF Med, OB-GYN
+1 202-204-0324
https://vfapp.org/496b

Women and Children First
Pioneers approaches that support communities to solve problems themselves.
MF Med, Neonat, OB-GYN, Peds
+44 20 7700 6309
https://vfapp.org/cdc9

World Blind Union (WBU)
Represents those experiencing blindness, speaking to governments and international bodies on issues concerning visual impairments.
Ophth-Opt
https://vfapp.org/2bd3

World Child Cancer
Works to improve diagnosis, treatment, and support for children with cancer, and their families, in the low- and middle-income world.
Heme-Onc, Ped Surg, Rad-Onc
+1 480-269-7380
https://vfapp.org/fbbc

World Compassion Fellowship (WCF)
Serves the global poor and persecuted through relief, medical care, development, and training.
CV Med, ER Med, Endo, GI, General, Infect Dis,

Medicine, Nutr, OB-GYN, Ortho, Peds, Psych, Pub Health, Rehab
+1 646-535-2344
https://vfapp.org/7b97

World Health Organization, The (WHO)

The United Nations' agency for health provides leadership on global health matters, shapes the health research agenda, setting norms and standards, articulates evidence-based policy options, provides technical support and monitoring to countries, and assesses health trends.

ER Med, General, Infect Dis, Logist-Op, MF Med, OB-GYN, Peds, Psych, Pub Health
+41 22 791 21 11
https://vfapp.org/c476

World Medical Relief

Facilitates the distribution of surplus medical resources where they are needed.

Logist-Op
+1 313-866-5333
https://vfapp.org/72dc

World Relief

Brings sustainable solutions to the world's greatest problems: disasters, extreme poverty, violence, oppression, and mass displacement.

ER Med, Nutr, Psych, Pub Health
+1 800-535-5433
https://vfapp.org/fbcd

World Telehealth Initiative

Provides medical expertise to the world's most vulnerable communities to build local capacity and deliver core health services through a network of volunteer healthcare professionals supported with state-of-the-art technology.

Derm, Infect Dis, MF Med, Medicine, Neuro, OB-GYN, Peds, Pulm-Critic
https://vfapp.org/fa91

World Vision International

Works with vulnerable communities around the world to overcome poverty and injustice with child-focused programs.

ER Med, General, Infect Dis, MF Med, Nutr, OB-GYN, Peds
+1 626-303-8811
https://vfapp.org/2642

Worldwide Radiology

Works to strengthen access to quality diagnostic imaging in underserved areas of low- and middle-income countries, and educates/supports professionals in the use of relevant and appropriate diagnostic imaging equipment and technologies.

Radiol
https://vfapp.org/b35b

Yamba Malawi

Uplifts Malawi's most vulnerable children by building local businesses and by enabling investment in children's care.

Nutr, Peds
+1 646-963-6076
https://vfapp.org/8d5f

Yathu Hospice

Provides hospice palliative care services to individuals with life-limiting conditions and their loved ones, and those who are facing end of life and going through grief and loss.

General, Palliative, Psych
+265 888 47 64 20
https://vfapp.org/ecbb

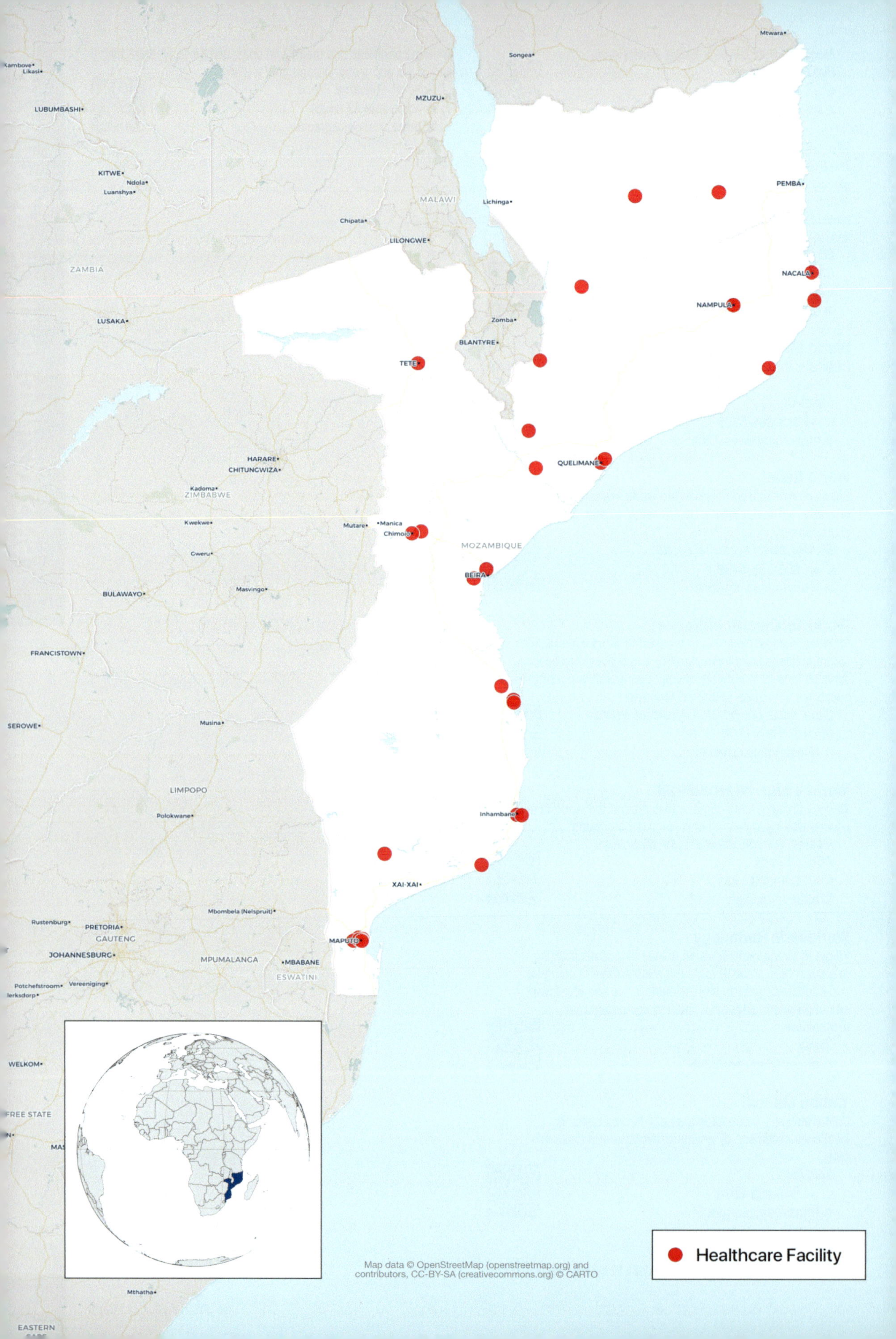

Mtwara
Songea
Kambove
Likasi
LUBUMBASHI
MZUZU
KITWE
Ndola
Luanshya
PEMBA
MALAWI
Lichinga
Chipata
LILONGWE
ZAMBIA
NACALA
NAMPULA
LUSAKA
Zomba
BLANTYRE
TETE
HARARE
CHITUNGWIZA
QUELIMANE
Kadoma
ZIMBABWE
Kwekwe
Mutare
Manica
Chimoio
MOZAMBIQUE
Gweru
BEIRA
Masvingo
BULAWAYO
FRANCISTOWN
SEROWE
Musina
LIMPOPO
Polokwane
Inhambane
XAI-XAI
Mbombela (Nelspruit)
Rustenburg
PRETORIA
GAUTENG
MAPUTO
JOHANNESBURG
MPUMALANGA
MBABANE
ESWATINI
Potchefstroom
Vereeniging
WELKOM
FREE STATE
Mthatha
EASTERN
Map data © OpenStreetMap (openstreetmap.org) and contributors, CC-BY-SA (creativecommons.org) © CARTO
Healthcare Facility

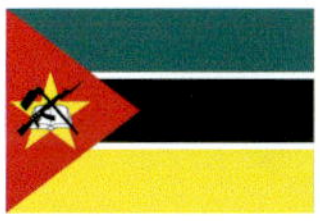

Mozambique

Located on the coast of southwest Africa, the Republic of Mozambique is a large country of about 30.1 million people. As much as two-thirds of the Mozambican population live in rural areas and along its long coastline. Maputo, the capital, is located on the shore and is known for being a vibrant and lively tropical city. Nearly 99 percent of the population falls into a few major ethnic groups, including the Makhuwa, Tsonga, Lomwe, and Sena. Portuguese is the official language, but local languages are used as well. Mozambique is also a religiously diverse country, with a population that includes Roman Catholics, Muslims, Zionist Christians, Evangelicals, and Pentecostals.

Ruled by Portugal in the colonial era, Mozambique experienced violent conflict during the latter half of the 20th century. In 1975, a temporary and controversial Marxist government held power. Over the past three decades, Mozambique has seen its economy grow steadily. Yet despite economic and political progress, Mozambique faces an Islamic rebellion in Cabo Delgado, which has contributed to instability. In addition, much of the country's population is vulnerable to natural disasters such as cyclones and tropical storms. These factors, among others, have resulted in endemic poverty rates countrywide.

Mozambique is challenged by a burden of disease that can be largely attributed to high poverty levels. Only 35 percent of the population is within 30 minutes of a health facility. As a result, diseases that cause the most deaths include HIV/AIDS, neonatal disorders, tuberculosis, malaria, lower respiratory infections, diarrheal diseases, and protein-energy malnutrition. Additionally, stroke and ischemic heart disease have risen over time as the non-communicable diseases that contribute to the most deaths in Mozambique. Road injuries have also increased and pose a significant health challenge, becoming a top cause of death in the country.

30.1M
Population

$492
GDP Per Capita

60 years
Life Expectancy
↑ Improving

8.4
Doctors/100k
Physician Density

70
Beds/100k
Hospital Bed Density

289
Deaths/100k
Maternal Mortality

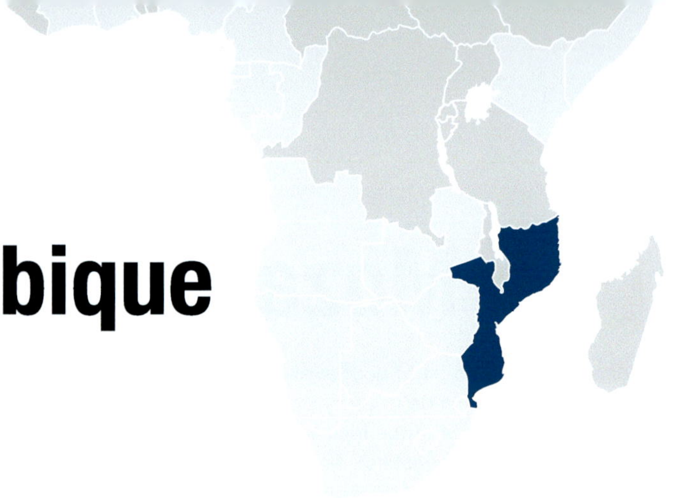

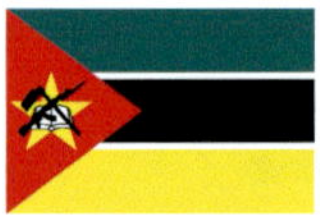

Mozambique

Healthcare Facilities

Central Hospital Nampula
Rua dos Continuadores, Nampula, Nampula, Mozambique
https://vfapp.org/c4b9

Distrital Hospital de Marrupa
N360, Marrupa, Niassa, Mozambique
https://vfapp.org/ec55

Hospital Antiga da Baixa
N12, Nacala, Nampula, Mozambique
https://vfapp.org/3623

Hospital at Inhamizua
Inhamizua, Beira, Mozambique
https://vfapp.org/4659

Hospital Central de Maputo
1653 Avenida Eduardo Mondlane, Maputo, Mozambique
https://vfapp.org/19b8

Hospital Central de Quelimane
Quelimane, Mozambique
https://vfapp.org/5778

Hospital da Ilha
Rua da Solidariedade, Ilha de Mocambique, Nampula, Mozambique
https://vfapp.org/242a

Hospital da Salela
N242, Salela, Inhambane, Mozambique
https://vfapp.org/153b

Hospital Distrital de Gondola
N6, Gondola, Manica, Mozambique
https://vfapp.org/ba9e

Hospital Distrital de Mopeia
R640, Mopeia, Zambézia, Mozambique
https://vfapp.org/e2aa

Hospital Distrital de Quissico
N1, Chissibuca, Inhambane, Mozambique
https://vfapp.org/f722

Hospital Geral da Machava
Matola, Mozambique
https://vfapp.org/e318

Hospital Geral de J. Macamo
Maputo, Mozambique
https://vfapp.org/6a3e

Hospital Militar de Maputo
Rua Pêro d'Anaya, Cidade de Maputo, Mozambique
https://vfapp.org/ba49

Hospital Polana Caniço A
Rua 3.730, Cidade de Maputo, Mozambique
https://vfapp.org/f772

Hospital Privado de Maputo
Rua do Rio Inhamiara, Cidade de Maputo, Mozambique
https://vfapp.org/4662

Hospital Provincial de Quelimane
Avenida 7 de Julho, Quelimane, Zambézia, Mozambique
https://vfapp.org/8355

Hospital Provincial da Matola
N2, Matola, Maputo, Mozambique
https://vfapp.org/d44d

Hospital Provincial de Inhambane
1300 Inhambane, Inhambane, Mozambique
https://vfapp.org/d7bb

Hospital Provincial de Manica
Rua do Hospital, Chimoio, Manica, Mozambique
https://vfapp.org/7af2

Hospital Provincial de Tete
R1051, Tete, Tete, Mozambique
https://vfapp.org/2c1d

Hospital Rural de Angoche
Rua de Parapato, Angoche, Nampula, Mozambique
https://vfapp.org/dab6

Hospital Rural de Buzi
Buzi, Sofala, Mozambique
https://vfapp.org/75af

Hospital Rural de Chokwe
Avenida 7 de Abril, Chókwè, Gaza, Mozambique
https://vfapp.org/32df

Hospital Rural de Cuamba

N13, Cuamba, Niassa, Mozambique
https://vfapp.org/b3cf

Hospital Rural de Montepuez

N14, Montepuez, Cabo Delgado, Mozambique
https://vfapp.org/5827

Hospital Rural de Vilankulo

N240, Vilankulo, Inhambane, Mozambique
https://vfapp.org/f3cc

Hospital Rural do Milange

Rua Joaquim Maquival, Milange, Zambézia, Mozambique
https://vfapp.org/6fb2

Instituto do Coração – ICOR

1111 Avenida Kenneth Kaunda, Cidade de Maputo, Mozambique
https://vfapp.org/558c

Lenmed Hospital Privado de Maputo

Rua do Rio Inhamiara, 1100 Maputo, Maputo City, Mozambique
https://vfapp.org/b34a

Mangungumete Health Home

Maimelane, Mozambique
https://vfapp.org/b4b1

Nampula Military Hospital

N104, Nampula, Nampula, Mozambique
https://vfapp.org/95fb

Netcare Nhamacunda

N240, Vilankulo, Inhambane, Mozambique
https://vfapp.org/e5ac

Rural Hospital of Morrumbala

477, Morrumbala, Zambézia, Mozambique
https://vfapp.org/7559

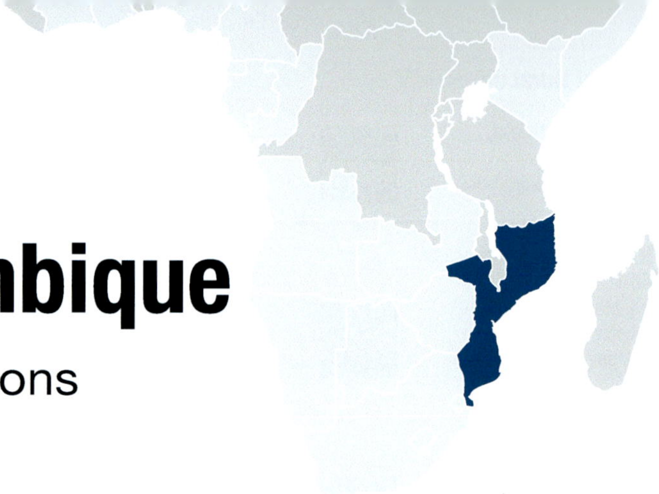

Mozambique

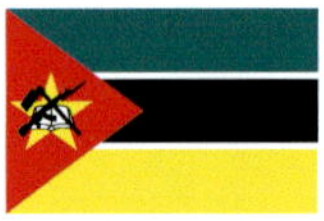

Nonprofit Organizations

Abt Associates
Seeks to improve the quality of life and economic well-being of people worldwide, while striving to meet and exceed the highest professional standards.

General, Logist-Op, MF Med, OB-GYN, Peds

📞 +1 212-779-7700

🌐 https://vfapp.org/cec2

Aceso Global
Provides strategic healthcare advisory services in low- and middle-income countries to design and deliver highly customized, evidence-based solutions that address the complex nature of healthcare systems, with a goal to strengthen and provide affordable, high-quality care to all.

Logist-Op, Pub Health

📞 +1 202-758-2636

🌐 https://vfapp.org/b3b7

Adventist Development and Relief Agency (ADRA) Moçambique
Improves lives through emergency relief, community-based projects that target food security, economic development, primary health, and basic education.

General, Infect Dis, Pub Health

📞 +258 21 304 4223

🌐 https://vfapp.org/1d91

Africa CDC
Aims to strengthen the capacity and capability of Africa's public health institutions as well as partnerships to detect and respond quickly and effectively to disease threats and outbreaks, based on data-driven interventions and programs.

Infect Dis, Logist-Op, Pub Health

📞 +251 11 551 7700

🌐 https://vfapp.org/339c

African Health Now
Promotes and provides information and access to sustainable primary healthcare to women, children, and families living across Sub-Saharan Africa.

Dent-OMFS, Endo, General, Infect Dis, MF Med, OB-GYN

🌐 https://vfapp.org/c766

Africa Indoor Residual Spraying Project (AIRS)
Aims to protect millions of people in Africa from malaria by spraying insecticide on the walls, ceilings, and other indoor resting places of mosquitoes that transmit malaria.

Infect Dis

📞 +1 301-347-5000

🌐 https://vfapp.org/9bd1

African Field Epidemiology Network (AFENET)
Strengthens field epidemiology and public health laboratory capacity to contribute effectively to addressing epidemics and other major public health problems in Africa.

All-Immu, Infect Dis, Path, Pub Health

🌐 https://vfapp.org/df2e

Africa Inland Mission International
Seeks to establish churches and community development programs including health care projects, based in Christian ministry.

Anesth, Dent-OMFS, ER Med, General, MF Med, Medicine, OB-GYN, OB-GYN, Ophth-Opt, Ped Surg, Peds, Rehab

🌐 https://vfapp.org/f2f6

Aid for the Development of People for People (ADPP) Mozambique
Promotes the social and economic development of the most vulnerable people in society with special attention to children, orphans, women, and girls.

Infect Dis, Nutr, Pub Health

📞 +258 82 309 2050

🌐 https://vfapp.org/cf53

AIDS Healthcare Foundation
Provides cutting-edge HIV/AIDS medical care and advocacy to over one million people in forty-three countries.

Infect Dis

📞 +1 323-860-5200

🌐 https://vfapp.org/b27c

AISPO
Implements international initiatives in the healthcare sector and remains involved in a variety of projects to combat poverty, social injustice, and disease in the world.

All-Immu, ER Med, GI, General, Infect Dis, Logist-Op, MF Med, Neonat, OB-GYN, Peds, Psych, Pub Health, Radiol

📞 +39 02 2643 4481

🌐 https://vfapp.org/c9e6

American International Health Alliance (AIHA)
Strengthens health systems and workforce capacity worldwide through locally-driven, peer-to-peer institutional partnerships.
CV Med, ER Med, Infect Dis, Medicine, OB-GYN
+1 202-789-1136
https://vfapp.org/69fd

Americares
Saves lives and improves health for people affected by poverty or disaster and responds with life-changing medicine, medical supplies, and health programs including domestic and global medical clinics.
All-Immu, ER Med, General, Infect Dis, MF Med, Nutr
+1 203-658-9500
https://vfapp.org/e567

AMOR (Aide Mondiale Orphelins Reconfort)
Aims to contribute to significant reductions in global infant and maternal mortality rates by providing medical services to at-risk mothers and appropriate care for orphans.
Infect Dis, MF Med, Neonat, OB-GYN, Ophth-Opt, Ped Surg
+33 6 80 86 19 75
https://vfapp.org/98a4

Amref Health Africa
Serves millions of people across thirty-five countries in Sub-Saharan Africa, strengthening health systems, and training African health workers to respond to the continent's most critical health issues.
All-Immu, General, Infect Dis, Logist-Op, MF Med, OB-GYN, Path, Pub Health, Surg
+254 20 6993000
https://vfapp.org/6985

Amsterdam Institute for Global Health and Development (AIGHD)
Provides sustainable solutions to major health problems across our planet by forging synergies between disciplines, healthcare delivery, research, and education.
Infect Dis
+31 20 210 3960
https://vfapp.org/d73d

Anan Clinica
Focuses on expanding local knowledge on health, while offering basic healthcare, education, agriculture, and water management.
General, Infect Dis, Nutr
https://vfapp.org/8281

Aurum Institute, The
Seeks to impact global health by designing and delivering high-quality care and treatment to people in developing countries.
Infect Dis, Pub Health
+27 10 590 1300
https://vfapp.org/ae2a

Basic Foundations
Supports local projects and organizations that seek to meet the basic human needs of others in their community.
ER Med, General, Peds, Rehab, Surg
https://vfapp.org/c4be

CARE
Works around the globe to save lives, defeat poverty, and achieve social justice.
ER Med, General
+1 800-422-7385
https://vfapp.org/7232

Carter Center, The
Seeks to prevent and resolve conflicts, enhance freedom and democracy, and improve health, while remaining committed to human rights and the alleviation of human suffering.
Infect Dis, MF Med, Ophth-Opt
+1 800-550-3560
https://vfapp.org/6556

Center for Strategic and International Studies (CSIS) Commission on Strengthening America's Health Security
Brings together a distinguished and diverse group of high-level opinion leaders bridging security and health, with the core aim to chart a bold vision for the future of U.S. leadership in global health.
ER Med, Infect Dis, MF Med, Pub Health
+1 202-887-0200
https://vfapp.org/6d7f

Centre for Global Mental Health
Closes the care gap and reduces human rights abuses experienced by people living with mental, neurological, and substance use conditions, particularly in low-resource settings.
Neuro, OB-GYN, Palliative, Peds, Psych
https://vfapp.org/a96d

Centro de Colaboração em Saúde
Seeks to promote health activities, prevent disease, and improve the quality and equity of access to care and treatment of common diseases in Mozambique, focusing on the health of women, children, and other vulnerable groups.
General, Infect Dis, OB-GYN, Path, Peds
+258 84 301 3341
https://vfapp.org/6f6c

Chain of Hope
Provides lifesaving heart operations for children around the world and supports the development of cardiac services in numerous developing and war-torn countries.
Anesth, CT Surg, CV Med, Crit-Care, Ped Surg, Peds, Pulm-Critic, Surg
+44 20 7351 1978
https://vfapp.org/1b1b

Chain of Hope (La Chaîne de l'Espoir)
Helps underprivileged children around the world by providing them with access to healthcare.
Anesth, CT Surg, Crit-Care, ER Med, Neurosurg, Ortho, Ped Surg, Surg, Vasc Surg
+33 1 44 12 66 66
https://vfapp.org/e871

Christian Aid Ministries
Strives to be a trustworthy and efficient channel for Amish, Mennonite, and other conservative Anabaptist groups and individuals to minister to physical and spiritual needs around the world.
CT Surg, ER Med, Logist-Op, Ortho, Pub Health
+1 330-893-2428
https://vfapp.org/7b33

Clinton Health Access Initiative (CHAI)
Aims to save lives and reduce the burden of disease in low- and middle-income countries. Works with partners to strengthen the capabilities of governments and the private sector to create and sustain high-quality health systems.

General, Heme-Onc, Infect Dis, Logist-Op, MF Med, Medicine, Neonat, Nutr, OB-GYN, Path, Peds, Rad-Onc

☎ +1 617-774-0110

🌐 https://vfapp.org/9ed7

Columbia University: Global Mental Health Programs
Pioneers research initiatives, promotes mental health, and aims to reduce the burden of mental illness worldwide.

Psych

☎ +1 646-774-5308

🌐 https://vfapp.org/c5cd

Core Group
Aims to improve and expand community health practices for underserved populations, especially women and children, through collaborative action and learning.

General, Infect Dis, MF Med, Medicine, OB-GYN, Peds, Pub Health

☎ +1 202-380-3400

🌐 https://vfapp.org/9de3

Developing Country NGO Delegation: Global Fund to Fight AIDS, TB & Malaria
Works to strengthen the engagement of civil society actors and organizations in developing countries to contribute toward achieving a world in which AIDS, TB, and Malaria are no longer global, public health, and human rights threats.

Infect Dis, Pub Health

☎ +254 20 2515790

🌐 https://vfapp.org/3149

Direct Relief
Improves the health and lives of people affected by poverty or emergency situations by mobilizing and providing essential medical resources needed for their care.

ER Med, Logist-Op

☎ +1 805-964-4767

🌐 https://vfapp.org/58e5

Doctors with Africa (CUAMM)
Advocates for the universal right to health and promotes the values of international solidarity, justice, and peace. Works to protect and improve the well-being and health of vulnerable communities in Africa with a long-term development perspective.

ER Med, Infect Dis, MF Med, Neonat, OB-GYN, Peds

🌐 https://vfapp.org/d2fb

Doctors Without Borders/Médecins Sans Frontières
Responds to emergencies and provides lifesaving medical care where needed most, including during disasters, conflicts, and epidemics.

Anesth, Crit-Care, ER Med, General, Infect Dis, Nutr, OB-GYN, Ped Surg, Peds, Psych, Pub Health, Surg

☎ +1 212-679-6800

🌐 https://vfapp.org/f363

Douleurs Sans Frontières (Pain Without Borders)
Supports local actors in taking charge of the assessment and treatment of pain and suffering, in an integrated manner and adapted to the realities of each country.

Anesth, Palliative, Psych, Rehab

☎ +33 1 48 78 38 42

🌐 https://vfapp.org/324c

Dream Sant'Egidio
Seeks to counter HIV/AIDS in Africa by eliminating the transmission of HIV from mother to child, with a focus on women because of the importance of their role in the community.

Infect Dis, MF Med, Neonat, OB-GYN, Path, Peds

☎ +39 06 899 2225

🌐 https://vfapp.org/f466

Duke University: Global Health Institute
Sparks innovation in global health research and education, and brings together knowledge and resources to address the most important global health issues of our time.

All-Immu, Infect Dis, MF Med, OB-GYN, Pub Health

☎ +1 919-681-7760

🌐 https://vfapp.org/c4cd

Elizabeth Glaser Pediatric AIDS Foundation
Seeks to end global pediatric HIV/AIDS through prevention and treatment programs, research, and advocacy.

Infect Dis, Nutr, OB-GYN, Peds

☎ +1 888-499-4673

🌐 https://vfapp.org/d6ec

Enabel
As the development agency of the Belgian federal government, charged with implementing Belgium's international development policy, carries out public service assignments in Belgium and abroad pursuant to the 2030 Agenda for Sustainable Development.

General, Infect Dis, Logist-Op, MF Med, OB-GYN, Peds, Pub Health

☎ +32 2 505 37 00

🌐 https://vfapp.org/5af7

EngenderHealth
Works to implement high-quality, gender-equitable programs that advance sexual and reproductive health and rights.

General, MF Med, OB-GYN, Peds

☎ +1 202-902-2000

🌐 https://vfapp.org/1cb2

Episcopal Relief & Development
Provides relief in times of disaster and promotes sustainable development by identifying and addressing the root causes of suffering.

Infect Dis, MF Med, Neonat, Nutr, Peds

☎ +1 855-312-4325

🌐 https://vfapp.org/7cfa

eRanger
Provides sustainable solutions to transportation and medical provision such as ambulances and mobile clinics in developing countries.

ER Med, General, Logist-Op

☎ +27 40 654 3207

🌐 https://vfapp.org/4c18

Esperança
Works to improve health and provide hope through disease prevention, education, and medical/surgical treatment.

Anesth, Dent-OMFS, ENT, General, Neurosurg, Nutr, OB-GYN, Ophth-Opt, Ortho, Ped Surg, Peds, Plast, Pub Health, Surg, Urol, Vasc Surg

📞 +1 602-252-7772

🌐 https://vfapp.org/5cf3

Evangelical Alliance Mission, The (TEAM)

Provides services in the areas of church planting, community development, healthcare, social justice, business as mission, and more.

Dent-OMFS, General, Ophth-Opt

📞 +1 800-343-3144

🌐 https://vfapp.org/9faa

Eye Foundation of America

Works toward a world without childhood blindness.

Ophth-Opt

📞 +1 304-599-0705

🌐 https://vfapp.org/a7eb

USAID: Fistula Care Plus

A fistula repair and prevention project from USAID that builds on, enhances, and expands the work undertaken by the previous Fistula Care project (2007–2013), with attention to new areas of focus so that obstetric fistula can become a rare event for future generations.

MF Med, OB-GYN, Surg

📞 +1 202-902-2000

🌐 https://vfapp.org/a7cd

Friends of UNFPA

Promotes the health, dignity, and rights of women and girls around the world by supporting the lifesaving work of UNFPA, the United Nations reproductive health and rights agency, through education, advocacy, and fundraising.

MF Med, OB-GYN

📞 +1 646-649-9100

🌐 https://vfapp.org/2a3a

Global Alliance to Prevent Prematurity and Stillbirth (GAPPS)

Seeks to improve birth outcomes worldwide by reducing the burden of premature birth and stillbirth.

All-Immu, Infect Dis, MF Med, Neonat, Neonat, OB-GYN

📞 +1 206-413-7954

🌐 https://vfapp.org/3f74

Global Clubfoot Initiative (GCI)

Promotes and resources the treatment of children with clubfoot in developing countries using the Ponseti technique.

Ortho, Ped Surg

🌐 https://vfapp.org/f229

Global Ministries – The United Methodist Church

As the worldwide mission and development agency of The United Methodist Church, Global Ministries works with more than 300 hospitals and clinics around the world through its Global Health Unit.

Anesth, CT Surg, CV Med, Crit-Care, Dent-OMFS, Derm, ER Med, GI, General, Infect Dis, Logist-Op, MF Med, Medicine, Neonat, Nephro, Nutr, OB-GYN, Ophth-Opt, Ortho, Palliative, Peds, Pod, Psych, Pub Health, Rehab, Rheum, Surg, Urol

📞 +1 800-862-4246

🌐 https://vfapp.org/1723

Global Oncology (GO)

Brings the best in cancer care to underserved patients around the world and collaborates across geographic, professional, and academic borders to improve cancer care, research, and education.

Heme-Onc, Path, Rad-Onc

🌐 https://vfapp.org/fcb8

Grassroot Soccer

Leverages the power of soccer to educate, inspire, and mobilize at risk youth in developing countries to overcome their greatest health challenges, live healthier more productive lives, and be agents for change in their communities.

Infect Dis

📞 +1 603-277-9685

🌐 https://vfapp.org/3521

Health Alliance International

Promotes policies and support programs that strengthen government primary healthcare and foster social, economic, and health equity for all.

General, Infect Dis, Logist-Op, MF Med, Neonat, OB-GYN, Psych

📞 +1 206-543-8382

🌐 https://vfapp.org/6f2d

Health Equity Initiative

Aims to build and sustain a global community that engages across sectors and disciplines to advance health equity.

Pub Health

🌐 https://vfapp.org/e2e2

Health Poverty Action

Works in partnership with people around the world who are pursuing change in their own communities to demand health justice and challenge power imbalances.

ER Med, General, Infect Dis, Psych, Pub Health

📞 +44 20 7840 3777

🌐 https://vfapp.org/ee58

HEART (High-Quality Technical Assistance for Results)

Works to support the use of evidence and expert advice in policymaking in the areas of international development, health, nutrition, education, social protection, and water and sanitation (WASH).

General, Infect Dis, Infect Dis, Logist-Op, MF Med, Medicine, Nutr, OB-GYN, Peds, Psych

📞 +44 1865 207333

🌐 https://vfapp.org/c491

Helen Keller International

Seeks to eliminate preventable vision loss, malnutrition, and diseases of poverty.

Infect Dis, Nutr, OB-GYN, Ophth-Opt, Peds

📞 +1 212-532-0544

🌐 https://vfapp.org/b654

HelpAge International

Works to ensure that people everywhere understand how much older people contribute to society and that they must enjoy their right to healthcare, social services, economic, and physical security.

General, Geri, Infect Dis, Medicine, Pub Health

📞 +44 20 7148 7623

🌐 https://vfapp.org/5d91

Hope Walks
Frees children, families, and communities from the burden of clubfoot, inspired by the Christian faith.
Ortho, Ped Surg, Peds, Rehab
+1 717-502-4400
https://vfapp.org/f6d4

Humanity & Inclusion
Works alongside people with disabilities and vulnerable populations, taking action and bearing witness in order to respond to their essential needs, improve their living conditions and health, and promote respect for their dignity and fundamental rights.
General, Infect Dis, MF Med, Medicine, Ortho, Peds, Psych, Pub Health, Rehab
+1 301-891-2138
https://vfapp.org/16b7

Hunger Project, The
Aims to end hunger and poverty by pioneering sustainable, grassroots, women-centered strategies and advocating for their widespread adoption in countries throughout the world.
Infect Dis, Nutr, OB-GYN, Pub Health
+1 212-251-9100
https://vfapp.org/3a49

ICAP at Columbia University
Serves as global leader in supporting the scale-up of multidisciplinary HIV/AIDS prevention, care, and treatment programs based on a family-focused approach.
General, Infect Dis, MF Med, Medicine, OB-GYN, Pub Health
+1 212-342-0505
https://vfapp.org/a8ef

Imaging the World
Develops sustainable models for ultrasound imaging in the world's lowest resource settings and uses a technology-enabled solution to improve healthcare access, integrating lifesaving ultrasound and training programs in rural communities.
Logist-Op, OB-GYN, Radiol
https://vfapp.org/59e4

International Agency for the Prevention of Blindness (IAPB), The
Leads international efforts in blindness-prevention activities, works toward a world where no one is needlessly visually impaired, and ensures that everyone has access to the best possible standard of eye health.
Infect Dis, Ophth-Opt, Pub Health
https://vfapp.org/87a2

International Federation of Gynecology and Obstetrics (FIGO)
Implements global projects on specific women's health issues.
MF Med, Medicine, Neonat, OB-GYN, Surg, Urol
+44 20 7928 1166
https://vfapp.org/c4b4

International Federation of Red Cross and Red Crescent Societies (IFRC)
Coordinates and directs international assistance following natural and man-made disasters in nonconflict situations through the world's largest humanitarian and development network. Provides disaster-preparedness programs, healthcare activities, and promotes humanitarian values.
ER Med, General, Infect Dis, Nutr
+1 212-338-0161
https://vfapp.org/b4ee

International Insulin Foundation
Aims to prolong the life and promote the health of people with diabetes in developing countries by improving the supply of insulin and education in its use.
Endo, Logist-Op
https://vfapp.org/d34f

International Organization for Migration (IOM) – The UN Migration Agency
Promotes evidence-informed policies and holistic, preventive, and curative health programs that are beneficial, accessible, and equitable for vulnerable migrants.
General, Infect Dis, OB-GYN
+27 12 342 2789
https://vfapp.org/621a

International Planned Parenthood Federation (IPPF)
Leads a locally owned, globally connected civil society movement that provides and enables services and champions sexual and reproductive health and rights for all, especially the underserved.
Infect Dis, MF Med, OB-GYN
+44 20 7939 8200
https://vfapp.org/dc97

International Relief Teams
Helps families survive and recover after a disaster by delivering timely and effective assistance through programs that improve their health and well-being while also providing a hopeful future for underserved communities.
Dent-OMFS, ER Med, General, Nutr, Ophth-Opt
+1 619-284-7979
https://vfapp.org/ffd5

International Trachoma Initiative (iTi)
Works toward a world free from trachoma, a preventable cause of blindness, and provides comprehensive support to national ministries of health and governmental and nongovernmental organizations to implement a comprehensive approach to fight trachoma.
Infect Dis, Ophth-Opt
+1 404-371-0466
https://vfapp.org/3278

IntraHealth International
Improves the performance of health workers and strengthens the systems in which they work.
CV Med, Endo, General, Infect Dis, MF Med, Neonat, Nutr, OB-GYN
+1 919-313-3554
https://vfapp.org/ddc8

Ipas
Focuses efforts on women and girls who want contraception or abortion, and builds programs around their needs and how best to support them.
OB-GYN
https://vfapp.org/8e39

Iris Global
Serves the poor, the destitute, the lost, and the forgotten

by providing adoration, outreach, family, education, relief, development, healing, and the arts.

General, Infect Dis, Nutr, Pub Health

+1 530-255-2077

https://vfapp.org/37f8

Islamic Medical Association of North America

Fosters health promotion, disease prevention, and health maintenance in communities around the world through direct patient care and health programs.

Anesth, Dent-OMFS, ER Med, General, Logist-Op, Ophth-Opt, Peds, Plast, Surg

+1 630-932-0000

https://vfapp.org/a157

IsraAID

Supports people affected by humanitarian crisis and partners with local communities around the world to provide urgent aid, assist recovery, and reduce the risk of future disasters.

ER Med, Infect Dis, Psych, Rehab

+972 3-947-7766

https://vfapp.org/de96

IVUmed

Aims to make quality urological care available worldwide by providing medical and surgical education for physicians and nurses and treatment for thousands of children and adults.

Anesth, OB-GYN, Ped Surg, Surg, Urol

+1 801-524-0201

https://vfapp.org/e619

Jhpiego

Creates and delivers transformative healthcare solutions that save lives in partnership with national governments, health experts, and local communities.

General, Infect Dis, OB-GYN, Surg

+1 410-537-1800

https://vfapp.org/45b8

John Snow, Inc. (JSI)

Aims to improve the health and well-being of underserved and vulnerable people and communities throughout the world.

General, Infect Dis, Logist-Op, MF Med, OB-GYN, Peds, Psych, Pub Health

+1 617-482-9485

https://vfapp.org/ba78

Johns Hopkins Center for Communication Programs

Believes in the power of communication to save lives, by empowering people to adopt healthy behaviors for themselves, their families, and their communities.

General, Infect Dis, Logist-Op, OB-GYN, Pub Health

+1 410-659-6300

https://vfapp.org/1bf9

Joint Aid Management (JAM)

Provides food security, nutrition, water, and sanitation to vulnerable communities in Africa in dignified and sustainable ways.

ER Med, Nutr

+27 11 548 3900

https://vfapp.org/dcac

Kaya Responsible Travel

Promotes sustainable social, environmental, and economic development, empowers communities, and cultivates educated, compassionate global citizens through responsible travel.

All-Immu, Crit-Care, Dent-OMFS, ER Med, General, Geri, Infect Dis, MF Med, Medicine, Nutr, OB-GYN, Peds, Psych, Pub Health, Rehab

+1 413-517-0266

https://vfapp.org/b2cf

Lay Volunteers International Association (LVIA)

Fosters local and global change to help overcome extreme poverty, reinforce equitable and sustainable development, and enhance dialogue between Italian and African communities.

ER Med, Logist-Op, MF Med, Neonat, Nutr, OB-GYN, Peds

+39 0171 696975

https://vfapp.org/ecd4

Lepra

Works directly with communities in Bangladesh, India, Mozambique, and Zimbabwe to find, treat, and rehabilitate people affected by leprosy.

Infect Dis, Pub Health, Rehab

+44 1206 216700

https://vfapp.org/5d1c

Leprosy Mission England and Wales, The

Leads the fight against leprosy by supporting people living with leprosy today and serving future generations by working to end the transmission of the disease.

Infect Dis, Pub Health

https://vfapp.org/4c67

Light for the World

Contributes to a world in which persons with disabilities fully exercise their rights and assists persons with disabilities living in poverty.

Ophth-Opt, Rehab

+43 1 8101300

https://vfapp.org/3ff6

Lions Clubs International

Empowers volunteers to serve their communities, meet humanitarian needs, encourage peace, and promote international understanding through Lions clubs.

Heme-Onc, Medicine, Nutr, Ophth-Opt

+1 630-571-5466

https://vfapp.org/7b12

Management Sciences for Health (MSH)

Works with countries and communities to save lives and improve the health of the world's poorest and most vulnerable people by building strong, resilient, sustainable health systems.

Infect Dis, Logist-Op, Pub Health

+1 617-250-9500

https://vfapp.org/6aa2

MAP International

Provides medicines and health supplies to those in need around the world so they might experience life to the fullest.

Logist-Op

+1 800-225-8550

https://vfapp.org/deed

Maverick Collective
Aims to build a global community of strategic philanthropists and informed advocates who use their intellectual and financial resources to create change.

Infect Dis, MF Med, OB-GYN
+1 202-785-0072
https://vfapp.org/ea49

Médecins du Monde/Doctors of the World
Provides care, bears witness, and supports social change worldwide with innovative medical programs and evidence-based advocacy initiatives.

ER Med, General, Infect Dis, MF Med, Neonat, OB-GYN, Peds, Pub Health
+33 1 44 92 15 15
https://vfapp.org/a43d

MedShare
Aims to improve the quality of life of people, communities, and the planet by sourcing and directly delivering surplus medical supplies and equipment to communities in need around the world.

Logist-Op
+1 770-323-5858
https://vfapp.org/c8bc

Mending Kids
Provides free, lifesaving surgical care to sick children worldwide by deploying volunteer medical teams and teaching communities to become medically self-sustaining by educating local medical staff.

Anesth, CT Surg, ENT, Ortho, Ortho, Ped Surg, Plast, Surg
+1 818-843-6363
https://vfapp.org/4d61

MENTOR Initiative
Saves lives in emergencies through tropical disease control, and helps people recover from crisis with dignity, working side by side with communities, health workers, and health authorities to leave a lasting impact.

ER Med, Infect Dis
+44 1444 412171
https://vfapp.org/3bd5

Mercy Ships
Operates hospital ships staffed by volunteers to bring hope, healing, and healthcare to underserved communities worldwide.

Anesth, Dent-OMFS, Logist-Op, Neonat, OB-GYN, Ophth-Opt, Ortho, Palliative, Plast, Psych, Surg
+1 903-939-7000
https://vfapp.org/2e99

mothers2mothers (m2m)
Employs and trains local women living with HIV as community health workers called Mentor Mothers to support women, children, and adolescents with vital medical services, education, and support.

Infect Dis, MF Med, OB-GYN, Peds, Pub Health
+27 21 466 9160
https://vfapp.org/6557

MSD for Mothers
Designs scalable solutions that help end preventable maternal deaths.

MF Med, OB-GYN, Pub Health
https://vfapp.org/9f99

Nazarene Compassionate Ministries
Partners with local churches around the world to clothe, shelter, feed, heal, educate, and live in solidarity with those in need.

General, Infect Dis, OB-GYN
+1 800-310-6362
https://vfapp.org/6b4d

NCD Alliance
Unites and strengthens civil society to stimulate collaborative advocacy, action, and accountability for NCD (noncommunicable disease) prevention and control.

All-Immu, CV Med, General, Heme-Onc, Medicine, Peds, Psych
+41 22 809 18 11
https://vfapp.org/abdd

New Hope in Africa
Aims to reach the people of Africa through healthcare, education, and basic necessities such as food and water.

Dent-OMFS, Infect Dis, MF Med, Nutr, OB-GYN, Pub Health
+1 970-640-5597
https://vfapp.org/b2a8

NLR International
Promotes and supports the prevention and treatment of leprosy, prevention of disabilities, social inclusion, and stigma reduction of people affected by leprosy.

Infect Dis, Pub Health
+31 20 595 0500
https://vfapp.org/d7bd

Norwegian People's Aid
Aims to improve living conditions, to create a democratic, just, and safe society.

ER Med, Logist-Op
+47 22 03 77 00
https://vfapp.org/2d8e

Ohana One International Surgical Aid & Education
Provides surgical care for the global family through technology and training.

Anesth, Logist-Op, Ped Surg, Peds, Plast, Surg
+1 310-529-7824
https://vfapp.org/86b8

Operation Fistula
Exists to end obstetric fistula by building models of care that serve every woman, everywhere.

MF Med, OB-GYN, Surg
+1 512-687-3479
https://vfapp.org/ce8e

Operation Smile
Treats patients with cleft lip and cleft palate, and creates solutions that deliver safe surgery to people where it's needed most.

Anesth, Dent-OMFS, ENT, Ped Surg, Plast
+1 757-321-7645
https://vfapp.org/5c29

Options
Believes in a world where women and children can access the high-quality health services they need, without financial burden.

Logist-Op, MF Med, Neonat, OB-GYN
📞 +44 20 7430 1900
🌐 https://vfapp.org/3a48

Optometry Giving Sight

Delivers eye exams and low or no-cost glasses, provides training for local eye care professionals, and establishes optometry schools, vision centers and optical labs.
Ophth-Opt
📞 +1 303-526-0430
🌐 https://vfapp.org/33ea

PATH

Advances health equity through innovation and partnerships so people, communities, and economies can thrive.
All-Immu, CV Med, Endo, Heme-Onc, Infect Dis, MF Med, Neonat, Nutr, OB-GYN, Path, Peds, Pulm-Critic
📞 +1 202-822-0033
🌐 https://vfapp.org/b4db

Pathfinder International

Champions sexual and reproductive health and rights worldwide, mobilizing communities most in need to break through barriers and forge paths to a healthier future.
OB-GYN
📞 +1 617-924-7200
🌐 https://vfapp.org/a7b3

PINCC Preventing Cervical Cancer

Seeks to prevent female-specific diseases in developing countries by utilizing low-cost and low-technology methods to create sustainable programs through patient education, medical personnel training, and facility outfitting.
OB-GYN
📞 +1 830-708-6009
🌐 https://vfapp.org/9666

PLeDGE Health

Aims to improve emergency medical care around the world through sustainable partnerships, open-source material development and dissemination, and development of the next generation of educational leaders in low-resource areas.
ER Med, General
🌐 https://vfapp.org/3a7d

Project Concern International (PCI)

Drives innovation from the ground up to enhance health, end hunger, overcome hardship, and advance women and girls—resulting in meaningful and measurable change in people's lives.
Infect Dis, MF Med, Nutr, OB-GYN, Peds
📞 +1 858-279-9690
🌐 https://vfapp.org/5ed7

Project SOAR

Conducts HIV operations research around the world to identify practical solutions to improve HIV prevention, care, and treatment services.
ER Med, General, MF Med, OB-GYN, Psych
📞 +1 202-237-9400
🌐 https://vfapp.org/1a77

PSI – Population Services International

Dedicates efforts to improving the health of people in the developing world by focusing on challenges such as a lack of family planning, HIV/AIDS, barriers to maternal health, and the greatest threats to children under the age of 5, including malaria, diarrhea, pneumonia, and malnutrition.
Infect Dis, MF Med, OB-GYN, Peds
📞 +1 202-785-0072
🌐 https://vfapp.org/ffe3

Real Medicine Foundation (RMF)

Provides humanitarian support to people living in disaster and poverty-stricken areas, focusing on the person as a whole by providing medical/physical, emotional, economic, and social support.
ER Med, General, Infect Dis, Nutr, Peds, Psych
📞 +44 20 8638 0637
🌐 https://vfapp.org/d45a

RestoringVision

Empowers lives by restoring vision for millions of people in need.
Ophth-Opt
📞 +1 209-980-7323
🌐 https://vfapp.org/e121

ReSurge International

Provides reconstructive surgical care and builds surgical capacity in developing countries.
Anesth, Dent-OMFS, Ped Surg, Plast, Surg
📞 +1 408-737-8743
🌐 https://vfapp.org/9937

Rockefeller Foundation, The

Works to promote the well-being of humanity.
Logist-Op, Nutr, Pub Health
📞 +1 212-869-8500
🌐 https://vfapp.org/5424

Rotary International

Provides service to others, improves lives, and advances world understanding, goodwill, and peace through its fellowship of business, professional, and community leaders.
ER Med, General, Infect Dis, MF Med, OB-GYN
🌐 https://vfapp.org/8fb5

Salvation Army International, The

Seeks to meet human needs through services in education, healthcare, community support, emergency response, and ministry development, inspired by the Christian faith.
Dent-OMFS, Derm, ER Med, Infect Dis, MF Med, Medicine, Nutr, OB-GYN, Ophth-Opt, Palliative, Psych, Rehab, Surg
📞 +44 20 7332 0101
🌐 https://vfapp.org/8eb3

Samaritan's Purse International Disaster Relief

Provides spiritual and physical aid to hurting people around the world, such as victims of war, poverty, natural disasters, disease, and famine, based in Christian ministry.
Anesth, CT Surg, Crit-Care, Dent-OMFS, Derm, ENT, ER Med, Endo, GI, General, Heme-Onc, Infect Dis, MF Med, Neonat, Nephro, Neuro, Neurosurg, Nutr, OB-GYN, Ophth-Opt, Ortho, Path, Ped Surg, Peds, Plast, Psych, Pulm-Critic, Radiol, Rehab, Rheum, Surg, Urol, Vasc Surg
📞 +1 800-528-1980
🌐 https://vfapp.org/87e3

Save the Children
Gives children around the world a healthy start in life, the opportunity to learn, and protection from harm.
All-Immu, Crit-Care, ER Med, General, Infect Dis, MF Med, Medicine, Neonat, OB-GYN, Peds, Psych, Pub Health
+1 800-728-3843
https://vfapp.org/2e73

SEVA
Delivers vital eye care services to the world's most vulnerable, including women, children, and Indigenous peoples.
Ophth-Opt, Surg
+1 510-845-7382
https://vfapp.org/1e87

Sightsavers
Prevents avoidable blindness in some of the poorest parts of the world by treating debilitating eye diseases.
Infect Dis, Ophth-Opt, Surg
+1 800-707-9746
https://vfapp.org/aa52

Smile Train
Seeks to give every child with a cleft the opportunity for a healthy, productive life by providing free cleft repair surgery and comprehensive cleft care in their own communities.
Dent-OMFS, ENT, Plast
+1 800-932-9541
https://vfapp.org/f21d

SOS Children's Villages International
Supports children through alternative care and family strengthening.
ER Med, Peds
+43 1 36824570
https://vfapp.org/aca1

Swiss Tropical and Public Health Institute
Contributes to the improvement of the health of populations internationally, nationally, and locally through excellence in research, education, and services.
Infect Dis, Pub Health
+41 61 284 81 11
https://vfapp.org/2ee4

Task Force for Global Health, The
Consists of programs and focus areas that cover a range of global health issues including neglected tropical diseases, infectious diseases, vaccines, field epidemiology, public health informatics, health workforce development, and global health ethics.
Infect Dis, Logist-Op, Medicine, Ophth-Opt, Peds
+1 404-371-0466
https://vfapp.org/714c

Tearfund
Responds to crisis and partners with local churches to bring restoration to those living in poverty, inspired by the Christian faith.
ER Med, Logist-Op
+44 20 3906 3906
https://vfapp.org/f6cf

U.S. President's Malaria Initiative (PMI)
Supports low-income countries to help control and eliminate malaria through cost-effective, lifesaving malaria interventions.
Infect Dis, MF Med, OB-GYN
+1 202-712-0000
https://vfapp.org/dc8b

Union for International Cancer Control (UICC)
Unites and supports the cancer community to reduce the global cancer burden, promote greater equity, and ensure that cancer control continues to be a priority in the world health and development agenda.
Heme-Onc, Pub Health
+41 22 809 18 11
https://vfapp.org/88b1

United Methodist Volunteers in Mission (UMVIM)
Engages in short-term missions each year in ministries as varied as disaster response, community development, pastor training, microenterprise, agriculture, Vacation Bible School, building repair and construction, and medical/dental services.
Dent-OMFS, ER Med, General
https://vfapp.org/1ee6

United Nations Children's Fund (UNICEF)
Works in over 190 countries and territories to save children's lives, to defend their rights, and to help them fulfill their potential, from early childhood through adolescence.
All-Immu, Infect Dis, MF Med, Neonat, Nutr, OB-GYN, Ped Surg, Peds, Pub Health
https://vfapp.org/42d7

United Nations Development Programme (UNDP)
Helps countries achieve the simultaneous eradication of extreme poverty and significant reduction of inequalities and exclusion using a sustainable human development approach.
Infect Dis, Logist-Op, Pub Health
https://vfapp.org/935c

United Nations High Commissioner for Refugees (UNHCR)
Safeguards the rights and well-being of people who have been forced to flee, ensuring that everybody has the right to seek asylum and find safe refuge in another country, with the goal of seeking lasting solutions.
General, MF Med, Medicine, OB-GYN, Peds, Psych, Pub Health
https://vfapp.org/6636

United Nations Population Fund (UNFPA)
Supports reproductive healthcare for women and youth in more than 150 countries, focusing on delivering a world where every pregnancy is wanted, every childbirth is safe, and every young person's potential is fulfilled.
Infect Dis, MF Med, Neonat, OB-GYN, Peds, Pub Health
+1 212-963-6008
https://vfapp.org/c969

United States Agency for International Development (USAID)
Promotes and demonstrates democratic values abroad and advances a free, peaceful, and prosperous world. Leads the U.S. government's international development and disaster assistance through partnerships and investments that save lives.
ER Med, Infect Dis, MF Med, OB-GYN, Peds
+1 202-712-0000
https://vfapp.org/9a99

United States President's Emergency Plan for AIDS Relief (PEPFAR)
The U.S. global HIV/AIDS response works to prevent new HIV infections and accelerate progress to control the global epidemic in more than 50 countries, by partnering with governments to support sustainable, integrated, and country-led responses to HIV/AIDS.
Infect Dis, Pub Health
🌐 https://vfapp.org/a57c

United Surgeons for Children (USFC)
Pursues greater health and opportunity for children in the most neglected pockets of the world, with a specific focus and expertise in surgery.
Anesth, CT Surg, Neonat, Neurosurg, OB-GYN, Peds, Radiol, Surg
🌐 https://vfapp.org/3b4c

University of California Los Angeles: David Geffen School of Medicine Global Health Program
Catalyzes opportunities to improve health globally by engaging in multi-disciplinary and innovative education programs, research initiatives, and bilateral partnerships that provide opportunities for trainees, faculty, and staff to contribute to sustainable health initiatives and to address health inequities facing the world today.
All-Immu, Infect Dis, Logist-Op, MF Med, Medicine, Neonat, OB-GYN, Ortho, Ped Surg, Peds, Radiol
📞 +1 310-312-0531
🌐 https://vfapp.org/f1a4

University of California San Francisco: Institute for Global Health Sciences
Dedicates its efforts to improving health and reducing the burden of disease in the world's most vulnerable populations by integrating expertise in the health, social, and biological sciences to train global health leaders and develop solutions to the most pressing health challenges.
Infect Dis, OB-GYN, Pub Health
📞 +1 415-476-5494
🌐 https://vfapp.org/6587

University of Washington: The International Training and Education Center for Health (I-TECH)
Works with local partners to develop skilled healthcare workers and strong national health systems in resource-limited countries.
Infect Dis, Pub Health
📞 +1 206-744-8493
🌐 https://vfapp.org/642f

USAID: Maternal and Child Survival Program
Works to prevent child and maternal deaths.
Infect Dis, MF Med, Neonat, OB-GYN, Peds
🌐 https://vfapp.org/6fcf

USAID: Deliver Project
Builds a global supply chain to deliver lifesaving health products to people in order to enable countries to provide family planning, protect against malaria, and limit the spread of pandemic threats.
Infect Dis, Logist-Op, MF Med
📞 +1 202-712-0000
🌐 https://vfapp.org/374e

USAID: EQUIP Health
Exists as an effective, efficient response mechanism to achieving global HIV epidemic control by delivering the right intervention at the right place and in the right way.
Infect Dis
📞 +27 11 276 8850
🌐 https://vfapp.org/d76a

USAID: Health Finance and Governance Project
Uses research to implement strategies to help countries develop robust governance systems, increase their domestic resources for health, manage those resources more effectively, and make wise purchasing decisions.
Logist-Op
📞 +1 202-712-0000
🌐 https://vfapp.org/8652

USAID: Health Policy Initiative
Provides field-level programming in health policy development and implementation.
General, Infect Dis, MF Med, OB-GYN, Peds
🌐 https://vfapp.org/8f84

USAID: Maternal and Child Health Integrated Program
Works to improve the health of women and their families, including programs for maternal, newborn, and child health, immunization, family planning, nutrition, malaria, and HIV/AIDS.
All-Immu, General, Infect Dis, MF Med
📞 +1 202-835-3136
🌐 https://vfapp.org/4415

Vision Care
Restores sight and helps patients get regular treatment at short-term eye camps and long-term base clinics by having doctors, missionaries, volunteers, and sponsors work together.
Ophth-Opt
📞 +1 212-769-3056
🌐 https://vfapp.org/9d7c

Voluntary Service Overseas (VSO)
Works with health workers, communities, and governments to improve health services and rights for women, babies, youth, people with disabilities, and prisoners.
General, MF Med, OB-GYN
📞 +44 20 8780 7500
🌐 https://vfapp.org/213d

World Blind Union (WBU)
Represents those experiencing blindness, speaking to governments and international bodies on issues concerning visual impairments.
Ophth-Opt
🌐 https://vfapp.org/2bd3

World Health Organization, The (WHO)
The United Nations' agency for health provides leadership on global health matters, shapes the health research agenda, setting norms and standards, articulates evidence-based policy options, provides technical support and monitoring to countries, and assesses health trends.
ER Med, General, Infect Dis, Logist-Op, MF Med, OB-GYN, Peds, Psych, Pub Health
📞 +41 22 791 21 11
🌐 https://vfapp.org/c476

World Hope International
Empowers the poorest individuals around the world so they can become agents of change within their communities, by offering

resources and knowledge.

Infect Dis, Logist-Op, MF Med, OB-GYN, Peds

+1 703-923-9414

https://vfapp.org/a4b8

World Medical Relief

Facilitates the distribution of surplus medical resources where they are needed.

Logist-Op

+1 313-866-5333

https://vfapp.org/72dc

World Vision International

Works with vulnerable communities around the world to overcome poverty and injustice with child-focused programs.

ER Med, General, Infect Dis, MF Med, Nutr, OB-GYN, Peds

+1 626-303-8811

https://vfapp.org/2642

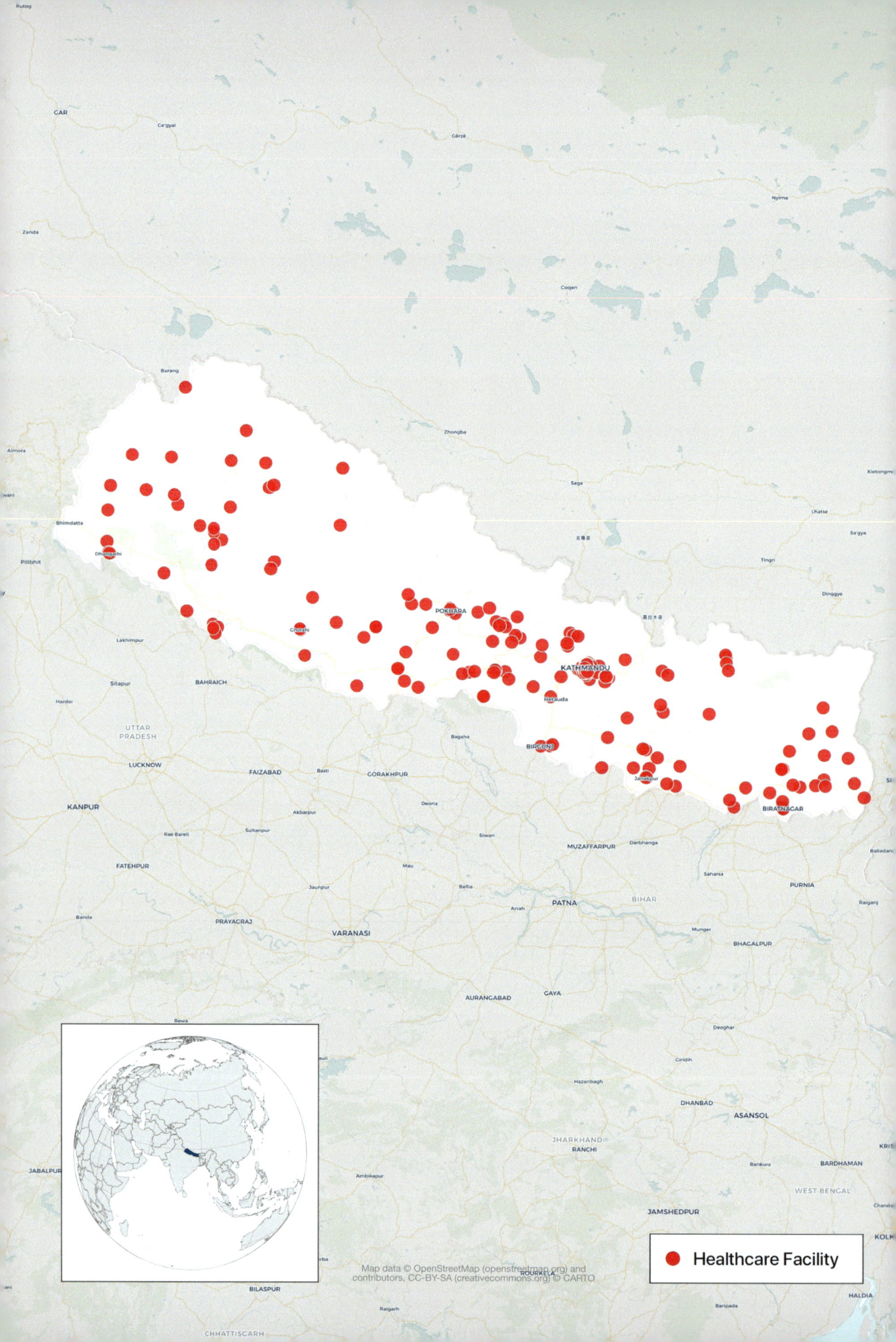
Rutog
GAR
Ce'gyai
Gêrzê
Nyima
Zanda
Coqen
Burang
Zhongba
Almora
Saga
Xietongmen
Lhatse
Bhimdatta
Sa'gya
Dhangarhi
Pilibhit
Tingri
Dinggye
POKHARA
Lakhimpur
Ghorahi
KATHMANDU
Sitapur
BAHRAICH
Hardoi
Hetauda
UTTAR
PRADESH
Bagaha
BIRGUNJ
LUCKNOW
FAIZABAD
Basti
GORAKHPUR
Janakpur
KANPUR
Akbarpur
Deoria
BIRATNAGAR
Rae Bareli
Sultanpur
Siwan
MUZAFFARPUR
Darbhanga
Baliadangi
FATEHPUR
Mau
Saharsa
Jaunpur
Ballia
PURNIA
Arrah
PATNA
BIHAR
Raiganj
Banda
PRAYAGRAJ
VARANASI
Munger
BHAGALPUR
AURANGABAD
GAYA
Rewa
Deoghar
Giridih
Hazaribagh
DHANBAD
ASANSOL
JHARKHAND
RANCHI
JABALPUR
Bankura
BARDHAMAN
Ambikapur
WEST BENGAL
JAMSHEDPUR
Healthcare Facility
Map data © OpenStreetMap (openstreetmap.org) and contributors, CC-BY-SA (creativecommons.org) © CARTO
ROURKELA
BILASPUR
HALDIA
Raigarh
Baripada
CHHATTISGARH

Nepal

The Federal Democratic Republic of Nepal is a landlocked Asian country flanked by China and India. Located in the Himalayas, Nepal is best known for its mountainous terrain, which includes the tallest peak in the world, Mount Everest. The predominantly Hindu nation is home to 30.3 million people, most of whom live in the southern plains region or the hilly central region. Nepal has an incredibly diverse population of 125 different ethnic and caste groups speaking 123 different languages.

For the past several decades, Nepal has experienced periods of turmoil and change, including a Maoist insurgency and the abolition of its monarchy. The creation of a multiparty parliamentary system has resulted in greater political stability as well as opportunities to improve infrastructure and economic conditions. While the poverty rate has largely improved, dropping from 15 percent to 8 percent between 2010 and 2019, around 31 percent of people face significant risk of falling into extreme poverty, and substantial inequities persist in regard to urban-rural areas, gender, and caste.

Free basic health services are available to all citizens, which may have contributed to improving health indicators. The country's life expectancy has increased from 60 years to 70 years since the 1990s. Additionally, Nepal has made significant progress in reducing HIV and TB and is on track to be malaria-free by 2025. Non-communicable diseases increasingly contribute to the most deaths in the country, including COPD, ischemic heart disease, stroke, cirrhosis, asthma, and chronic kidney disease. Ailments such as lower respiratory infections, neonatal disorders, tuberculosis, and diarrheal diseases continue to cause significant deaths, but have decreased over time. Epidemics still occur frequently, leading to high rates of both morbidity and mortality. It should be noted that mental health challenges and depressive disorders also contribute greatly to disability in Nepal, with self-harm being a top cause of death.

30.3M
Population

$1,071
GDP Per Capita

70 years
Life Expectancy
↑ Improving

74.9
Doctors/100k
Physician Density

30
Beds/100k
Hospital Bed Density

186
Deaths/100k
Maternal Mortality

Nepal

Healthcare Facilities

Aama-Baa Hospital Pvt. Ltd.
Abukhaireni-Gorkha Hwy, Gorkha 34000, Nepal
https://vfapp.org/487c

Aarogya Swasthya Sadan
Jawalakhel, Patan, वाग्मती प्रदेश, Nepal
https://vfapp.org/72a9

Achham District Hospital
69DR017, Mangalsen, Mangalsen, Nepal
https://vfapp.org/bb8c

Alive Hospital & Trauma Centre
Bharatpur 44207, Nepal
https://vfapp.org/74b1

Alka Hospital Pvt. Ltd.
Lalitpur 44600, Nepal
https://vfapp.org/d564

All Nepal Hospital Pvt. Ltd.
Kathmandu 44600, Nepal
https://vfapp.org/1e2b

Alpine Medical College Teaching Hospital
Gadhimai 44400, Simara, Nepal
https://vfapp.org/cccf

Araddhya Hospital Pvt. Ltd.
Janakpur, Nepal
https://vfapp.org/93ee

Asia Medicare Hospital Pvt. Ltd.
Birgunj Busspark, Birgunj, प्रदेश नं. २, Nepal
https://vfapp.org/de6f

Ayurveda Hospital
Yogbir Singh Marg, Kathmandu, Bagmati Pradesh, Nepal
https://vfapp.org/62c1

Ayurvedic Hospital
Kirtipur Road, Kirtipur, Vagmati Pradesh, Nepal
https://vfapp.org/cff7

Ayush Hospital
Suruchi Marga, Kathmandu 44600, Nepal
https://vfapp.org/b53d

B.P. Koirala Institute of Health Science
Buddha Road, Dharan 56700, Nepal
https://vfapp.org/6794

B.P. Koirala Memorial Cancer Hospital
Madi Thori, Bharatpur Metro, Vagmati Pradesh, Nepal
https://vfapp.org/33d6

B.P. Smriti Hospital
Srikanti Marg, Kathmandu 44600, Nepal
https://vfapp.org/77e2

Bagmati Health Hub Pvt. Ltd
Sinamangal Marg, Kathmandu, Bagmati Pradesh, Nepal
https://vfapp.org/53bc

Bajhang District Hospital
F49, Jaya Prithvi, JayaPrithvi, Nepal
https://vfapp.org/6634

Bandipur Hospital
Bandipur 33904, Nepal
https://vfapp.org/d9cd

Banepa Hospital and Education Foundation
Banepa 45210, Nepal
https://vfapp.org/382d

Bardiya District Hospital
Hospital Road, Gulariya 21800, Nepal
https://vfapp.org/879e

Bayalpata Hospital
Madhya Pahaadi Rajmaarga, Sanfebagar 10700, Nepal
https://vfapp.org/fe8b

Besisahar Hospital Pvt. Ltd.
Dumre-Besishahar, Besishahar,Gandaki Pradesh, Nepal
https://vfapp.org/322f

Bhaktapur Cancer Hospital
Bhaktapur 44800, Nepal
https://vfapp.org/37a2

Bhaktapur Hospital Emergency Block
Itachhen, Bhaktapur, Vagmati Pradesh, Nepal
https://vfapp.org/54e2

Bharatpur Hospital
Hospital Road, Bharatpur Metro, Vagmati Pradesh, Nepal
https://vfapp.org/54ea

Bharosa Hospital Pvt. Ltd.
Devkota Sadak, Kathmandu 44600, Nepal
https://vfapp.org/951b

Bheri Zonal Hospital
Nepalgunj 21900, Nepal
https://vfapp.org/f2a6

Bijayapur Hospital
Putali line, Dharan 56700, Nepal
https://vfapp.org/74d7

Bir Hospital
Aspatal Marg, Kathmandu, Bagmati Pradesh, Nepal
https://vfapp.org/b269

Birat Medical and Teaching Hospital
Tankisinuwari 56613, Nepal
https://vfapp.org/f2a9

Blue Cross Hospital
Kathmandu, Nepal
https://vfapp.org/c2ae

Blue Lotus Hospital
Tripura Marg, Tripureswor 44601, Nepal
https://vfapp.org/212b

Bungkot Hospital
36DR036, Bunkot,Gandaki Pradesh, Nepal
https://vfapp.org/fcad

Butwal Hospital Pvt. Ltd.
E – W Hwy, Butwal 32907, Nepal
https://vfapp.org/b76c

C.P. Hospital Pvt. Ltd.
Bhimdatta Hwy, Dhangadhi 10900, Nepal
https://vfapp.org/9981

Charak Hospital
Siddhartha St, Pokhara 33700, Nepal
https://vfapp.org/dd2e

Charak Memorial Hospital
New Bazaar, Pokhara, Gandaki Pradesh, Nepal
https://vfapp.org/3832

Chirayu National Hospital & Medical Institute Pvt. Ltd.
रिङ्ग रोड, Kathmandu 44600, Nepal
https://vfapp.org/35d5

Chitwan Hospital
Madi-Thori, Madi, Vagmati Pradesh, Nepal
https://vfapp.org/daae

Chitwan Hospital Pvt. Ltd.
E – W Hwy, Bharatpur 44207, Nepal
https://vfapp.org/26dc

Chitwan Medical College Teaching Hospital
Mahendra Highway, Bharatpur Metro, Vagmati Pradesh,Nepal
https://vfapp.org/5866

Chitwan Valley Model Hospital
Doorsanchar Road, Bharatpur Metro,Vagmati Pradesh, Nepal
https://vfapp.org/7b75

City Hospital
Siddharthanagar 32900, Nepal
https://vfapp.org/198f

Civil Service Hospital
Minbhawan Marg, Kathmandu 44600, Nepal
https://vfapp.org/5443

Dadeldhura District Hospital
Hospital Road, Amargadhi, Amargadhi, Nepal
https://vfapp.org/1311

Dailekh District Hospital
Dailekh Rajmarg, Narayan Municipality, कर्णाली प्रदेश, Nepal
https://vfapp.org/11bb

Dailekh District Hospital
Dailekh Sadak, Narayan Municipality 21600, Nepal
https://vfapp.org/46a2

Devchuli Hospital
AH2, Devachuli 33000, Nepal
https://vfapp.org/b598

Dhading Hospital
Dhading Besi Marga, Dhading Besi, Vagmati Pradesh, Nilkantha 45100, Nepal
https://vfapp.org/33cc

Dhankuta District Hospital
Hulak Tole & Thadobazar Street, Dhankuta 56800, Nepal
https://vfapp.org/65c1

Dhaulagiri Zonal Hospital
Darling 33300, Nepal
https://vfapp.org/1c98

Dhulikhel Hospital
Dhulikhel 45200, Nepal
https://vfapp.org/ef8f

Dullu Hospital
Kal Bhairab Dullu 21600, Nepal
https://vfapp.org/cc3d

Dunai District Hospital
F47, Dunai, Karnali Pradesh, Nepal
https://vfapp.org/1e5b

Era Hospital
Puspalal Path, Kathmandu 44600, Nepal
https://vfapp.org/68a7

Everest Hospital
Madan Bhandari Road, Kathmandu, Nepal
https://vfapp.org/8dfb

Fewa City Hospital
Indrapuri Marg, Pokhara, गण्डकी प्रदेश, Nepal
https://vfapp.org/c16c

Gadhawa Hospital
Gadhawa 22414, Nepal
https://vfapp.org/e147

Gajuri Hospital
Prithvi Rajmarg, Gajuri, Vagmati Pradesh, Nepal
https://vfapp.org/49a6

Gandaki Medical College Teaching Hospital & Research Centre Ltd.
New Bazaar, Pokhara, Gandaki Pradesh, Nayabazar Rd, Pokhara 33700, Nepal
https://vfapp.org/7632

Gauri Shankar Hospital
Charikot – Lamabagar Rd, Bhimeshwor Municipality 45500, Nepal
https://vfapp.org/5f3a

Gautam Buddha Int'l Cardiac Hospital
Bridge, Ring Road Near Balkumari, Kathmandu 44600, Nepal
https://vfapp.org/341f

Ghorahi Hospital Pvt. Ltd.
Tribhuwan Park Road, Ghorahi 22400, Nepal
https://vfapp.org/9333

Global Hospital
Ring Road, Patan, वाग्मती प्रदेश, Nepal
https://vfapp.org/d8e3

Golden Hospital
Rangeli Road, Biratnagar, प्रदेश नं. १, Nepal
https://vfapp.org/86c7

Gorkha District Hospital
Gorkha-Ghyampesal Road, Gorkha, गण्डकी प्रदेश, Nepal
https://vfapp.org/836e

Grande City Hospital
Kanti Path, Kathmandu, Bagmati Pradesh, Nepal
https://vfapp.org/c947

Grande International Hospital
Tokha Rd, Kathmandu 44600, Nepal
https://vfapp.org/99ea

Green City Hospital
Ring Road, Kathmandu, Bagmati Pradesh, Nepal
https://vfapp.org/2dc9

Hamro Sahayatri Hospital and Birthing Centre
Arniko Raj Marga, Lokanthali, वाग्मती प्रदेश, Nepal
https://vfapp.org/33ee

HCH Hospital
Khadichaur – Jiri Highway, Namdu, वाग्मती प्रदेश, Nepal
https://vfapp.org/edeb

HDCS Chaurjahari Mission Hospital
Bijayashwari 22000, Nepal
https://vfapp.org/6fef

Hillary Hospital
Khumjung, Province No. 1, Nepal
https://vfapp.org/997e

Hilsa Hospital
F145, Muchu, Karnali Pradesh, Nepal
https://vfapp.org/d513

Himal Hospital
Thirbom Sadak, Chardobato, Gyaneshwor, Kathmandu, Nepal
https://vfapp.org/baf8

Himalaya Sherpa Hospital
Khumjung 56000, Nepal
https://vfapp.org/853d

Himalayan Healthcare Inc.
Manbhawan Ekta Galli, Patan, Vagmati Pradesh, Nepal
https://vfapp.org/7ce5

Hospital at Bardibas
Bardibas Jaleshwar Highway, Aurahi, प्रदेश नं. २, Nepal
https://vfapp.org/4889

Hospital at Bhijer
Bhijer, Nepal
https://vfapp.org/badb

Hospital at Bhorle
Bhorle 45000, Nepal
https://vfapp.org/d4f8

Hospital at Bidur
Pasang Lhamu Highway, Bidur, वाग्मती प्रदेश, Nepal
https://vfapp.org/52a7

Hospital at Biratchok
महेन्द्र राजमार्ग, Sundar Dulari, प्रदेश नं. १, Nepal
https://vfapp.org/cd3b

Hospital at Chakratirtha
37DR042, Chakratirtha, गण्डकी प्रदेश, Nepal
https://vfapp.org/e97e

Hospital at Gilunng
37DR013, Gilunng, गण्डकी प्रदेश, Nepal
https://vfapp.org/3518

Hospital at Hanspur
36DR012, Hanspur, गण्डकी प्रदेश, Nepal
https://vfapp.org/df47

Hospital at Hirmaniya
Hirmaniya Road, Hirminiya, प्रदेश नं. ५, Nepal
https://vfapp.org/8fb8

Hospital at Kalikathum
60DR005, Mairi Kalikathum, कर्णाली प्रदेश, Nepal
https://vfapp.org/3d6a

Hospital at Khali Puraini Road
Puraini, Nepal
https://vfapp.org/56c9

Hospital at Machijhitkaiya
H17, Marchaijhitakaiya, प्रदेश नं. २, Nepal
https://vfapp.org/ba92

Hospital at Marmaparikanda
Marmaparikanda, Nepal
https://vfapp.org/5c31

Hospital at Nepalgung Gulariya Road
Nepalgung Gulariya Road, Khajura Khurda, प्रदेश नं. ५, Nepal
https://vfapp.org/b8d4

Hospital at Raghunathpur
Raghunathpur, Nepal
https://vfapp.org/a268

Hospital at Ramgram
Ramgram, Nepal
⊕ https://vfapp.org/ea9f

Hospital at Rawatkot
H18, Rawatkot, कर्णाली प्रदेश, Nepal
⊕ https://vfapp.org/3d99

Hospital at Sandhikharka
Gorusinge-Sandhikharka Rajmarga, Sandhikharka, प्रदेश नं. ५, Nepal
⊕ https://vfapp.org/d993

Hospital at Santalla
H18, Dailekh, Santalla, Nepal
⊕ https://vfapp.org/e37b

Hospital at Sukhadhik
Sukhadhik, Nepal
⊕ https://vfapp.org/c55c

Hospital at Thaha
Tribhuvan Highway, Thaha 44100, Nepal
⊕ https://vfapp.org/a282

Hospital at Urthu-Ghodsen Road
Urthu-Ghodsen, Patmara, Karnali Pradesh,Nepal
⊕ https://vfapp.org/f963

Hospital Bakulahat Ratnanagar
35DR012, Ratnanagar, Vagmati Pradesh, Nepal
⊕ https://vfapp.org/f47b

Hospital Mai Manakamana Hospital Pvt. Ltd.
Manakamana, Nepal
⊕ https://vfapp.org/4b33

Hospital of Amppipal
Thalipokhari-Amppipal, Palumtar, Gandaki Pradesh, Nepal
⊕ https://vfapp.org/bc74

Hospital Tamakoshi
Khurkot Manthali Rd, Manthali, वाग्मती प्रदेश, Nepal
⊕ https://vfapp.org/1511

Ilam District Hospital
Ilam, Nepal
⊕ https://vfapp.org/21d6

Inaruwa Hospital
06DR021, Inaruwa, प्रदेश नं. १, Nepal
⊕ https://vfapp.org/198e

International Friendship Children's Hospital
Kathmandu 44600, Nepal
⊕ https://vfapp.org/c7bb

Janaki Medical College and Teaching Hospital
Janaki Medical College-Ramdaiya-Sabaila-paterwa Road, Tarapatti Sirsiya, प्रदेश नं. २, Nepal
⊕ https://vfapp.org/2487

Janakpur Zonal Hospital
Janakpur 45600, Nepal
⊕ https://vfapp.org/49c6

Jeevan Jyoti Hospital & Diagnostic Center Pvt. Ltd.
Samsi Bajar Tengar Road, Mahottari, Janakpur, Nepal
⊕ https://vfapp.org/9854

Jilla Pashusewa Karyalaya Dhangadhi
Main Road, Dhangadi Sub Metropolitan, Dhanhadhi, Nepal
⊕ https://vfapp.org/4c54

Kalaiya Hospital
Barewa Road, Kalaiya, प्रदेश नं. २, Nepal
⊕ https://vfapp.org/23e6

Kalika Community Hospital
Siddartha Rajmarg, Darsing Dahathum 33800, Nepal
⊕ https://vfapp.org/8eff

Kanti Children's Hospital
Kathmandu, Nepal
⊕ https://vfapp.org/2ac6

Kantipur Hospital
Shree Ganesh Marga, काठमाडौं, वाग्मती प्रदेश, Nepal
⊕ https://vfapp.org/cbc5

Kantipur Institute of Health Science
Bhakti Marg, Pokhara, गण्डकी प्रदेश, Nepal
⊕ https://vfapp.org/bc45

Kaski Model Hospital
Pragati Marg, Pokhara, गण्डकी प्रदेश, Nepal
⊕ https://vfapp.org/ea62

Kathmandu Hospital
त्रिपुरेश्वर मार्ग, Kathmandu 44600, Nepal
⊕ https://vfapp.org/47c8

Kathmandu Medical College
Goshwara Marga, काठमाडौं, वाग्मती प्रदेश, Nepal
⊕ https://vfapp.org/362c

Kathmandu Medical College Teaching Hospital
Om Nagar Marg, काठमाडौं, वाग्मती प्रदेश, Nepal
⊕ https://vfapp.org/e4dd

Kathmandu Military Hospital
King Birendra Marg, Kathmandu, Bagmati Pradesh, Nepal
⊕ https://vfapp.org/768b

Kathmandu Model Hospital
Red Cross Marga, काठमाडौं, वाग्मती प्रदेश, Nepal
⊕ https://vfapp.org/82f2

Kawasoti Ayurvedic Hospital
48DR025, Kawaswoti, गण्डकी प्रदेश, Nepal
⊕ https://vfapp.org/3d55

Kirtipur Hospital
Kirtipur Ring Road, Kirtipur, वाग्मती प्रदेश, Nepal
⊕ https://vfapp.org/3aa4

KIST Hospital
Sundar Marga, Patan, वाग्मती प्रदेश, Nepal
⊕ https://vfapp.org/4782

KIST Medical College Teaching Hospital
Gwarko-Lamatar, Imadol, वाग्मती प्रदेश, Nepal
⊕ https://vfapp.org/2443

Koshi Hospital
Rangeli Road, Biratnagar 56700, Nepal
https://vfapp.org/8c77

Koshi Zonal Hospital
Sahid Marg, Biratnagar, प्रदेश नं. १, Nepal
https://vfapp.org/37f5

Krisna Prasad Hospital
Banepa-Panauti-Khopasi Road, Banepa 45210, Nepal
https://vfapp.org/3c39

Lake City Hospital and Critical Care
Parshyang – Bagale Tole Marga, Pokhara 33700, Nepal
https://vfapp.org/fc12

Lalgadh Leprosy Hospital & Services Centre
Ward 10, East – West Highway, Mithila, Dhanusha 45600, Nepal
https://vfapp.org/effe

Lalgadh Model Hospital Pvt. Ltd.
E – W Hwy, Mithila 45600, Nepal
https://vfapp.org/77d9

Laxmimarga-Dangihat Hospital
34 Laxmimarga-Dangihat Road, Dangihat, प्रदेश नं. १, Nepal
https://vfapp.org/1994

Lekhnath City Hospital
Prithvi Highway, Pokhara, गण्डकी प्रदेश, Nepal
https://vfapp.org/ada5

Life Care Hospital at Bharatpur
Mahendra Highway, Bharatpur Metro, वाग्मती प्रदेश, Nepal
https://vfapp.org/d894

Life Care Hospital at Kathmandu
Bagdurbar Marg, काठमाडौं, वाग्मती प्रदेश, Nepal
https://vfapp.org/3f5e

Lifeguard Hospital
Bargachhi Chowk, Biratnagar, Eastern Region, Chandani Marg, Biratnagar 56613, Nepal
https://vfapp.org/889c

Lukla Hospital
Chaurikharka, प्रदेश नं. १, Nepal
https://vfapp.org/6aa4

Lumbini City Hospital
Sarvan Path, Butwal 32907, Nepal
https://vfapp.org/6679

Lumbini Medical College
H 10, Tansen 32500, Nepal
https://vfapp.org/afcc

Madhyapur Hospital
Araniko Highway, Madhyapur Thimi, Nepal
https://vfapp.org/cf2e

Madi Samudayik Hospital Pvt. Ltd.
Madi-Thori, Madi, वाग्मती प्रदेश, Nepal
https://vfapp.org/79a7

Mahendra Narayan Nidhi Memorial Hospital
Shreekanti Marg, Kathmandu 44600, Nepal
https://vfapp.org/fbfd

Makawanpur Sahakari Hospital
Bhintuna Marg, Hetauda 44107, Nepal
https://vfapp.org/8d2f

Manahari Hospital
Manahari 44100, Nepal
https://vfapp.org/fe1b

Mangalbare Hospital Urlabari
Urlabari 56600, Nepal
https://vfapp.org/4f8c

Manmohan Memorial Hospital
Thamel Marg, Kathmandu 44600, Nepal
https://vfapp.org/41b4

Marie Stopes Nepal
Ring Road 44600, Lalitpur 44700, Nepal
https://vfapp.org/f7b8

Maruti Children Hospital
Shree Kanti Marg,Kathmandu, Bagmati Pradesh, Nepal
https://vfapp.org/f6df

Maya Metro Hospital
H14, Dhangadi Sub Metropolitan, Dhanhadhi, Nepal
https://vfapp.org/b572

Mechi Zonal Hospital
Bhadra Purjhapa Mechi Highway, Bhadrapur, Province No. 1, Nepal
https://vfapp.org/d7be

Medical House
Shanischare-Milldanda, Shani-Arjun, Province No. 1, Nepal
https://vfapp.org/c3af

Metro City Hospital
Srijana Chowk, Pokhara 33700, Nepal
https://vfapp.org/4dc3

Mid City Hospital
Arniko Raj Marga, Lokanthali, Vagmati Pradesh, Nepal
https://vfapp.org/2bb6

Mid Western Regional Hospital
Ratna Rajmarg, Birendranagar, Karnali Pradesh, Nepal
https://vfapp.org/a963

Midat Hospital
Thaina-Prayagpokhari Road, Patan, Bagmati Pradesh, Nepal
https://vfapp.org/386f

Mirchaiya Hospital
F52, Mirchaiya, प्रदेश नं. २, Nepal
https://vfapp.org/deeb

Mission Hospital Simikot
Simikot 21000, Nepal
https://vfapp.org/3dc7

Myagdi Hospital
Beni – Jomsom Road,
Arthunge, गण्डकी प्रदेश, Nepal
⊕ https://vfapp.org/aca7

Namaste Public Hospital
E – W Hwy, Damak 57217,
Nepal
⊕ https://vfapp.org/7b9d

National Tuberculosis Control Center
Araniko Highway, Madhyapur
Thimi 44600, Nepal
⊕ https://vfapp.org/9181

Natural Health Hospital
Prayag Marg, काठमाडौं,
वाग्मती प्रदेश, Nepal
⊕ https://vfapp.org/a999

Navajeevan Hospital
Main Road, Dhangadi Sub
Metropolitan, Dhanhadhi, Nepal
⊕ https://vfapp.org/61ef

Nepal Armed Police Force Hospital
Tribhuvan Rajpath, Naya
Naikap, वाग्मती प्रदेश, Nepal
⊕ https://vfapp.org/bd99

Nepal Bharat Maitri Hospital
Ring Road, काठमाडौं, वाग्मती
प्रदेश, Nepal
⊕ https://vfapp.org/e5ea

Nepal Cancer Hospital and Research Centre
सातदोबाटो – गोदावरी रोड,
Lalitpur 44700, Nepal
⊕ https://vfapp.org/72e7

Nepal Korea Friendship Hospital
Purano Thimi- Naya Thimi,
थिमि, वाग्मती प्रदेश, Nepal
⊕ https://vfapp.org/3ed4

Nepal Medical College and Teaching Hospital
Gokarneshwar, Nepal
⊕ https://vfapp.org/d131

Nepal Mediciti Hospital
Bhaisepati Lalitpur, Nepal
⊕ https://vfapp.org/ca1f

Nepal National Hospital
Ring Road, काठमाडौं, वाग्मती
प्रदेश, Nepal
⊕ https://vfapp.org/c367

Nepal Orthopaedic Hospital
Way to Pashupati, Kathmandu,
वाग्मती प्रदेश, Nepal
⊕ https://vfapp.org/9fba

Nepal Skin Hospital
Madan Bhandari Path,
काठमाडौं, वाग्मती प्रदेश, Nepal
⊕ https://vfapp.org/c334

Nepalgunj Medical College
Kasturi Marg, Nepalgunj Sub
Metropolitan City, प्रदेश नं. ५,
Nepal
⊕ https://vfapp.org/47ee

New Amda Hospital
New Amda Road, Damak
57217, Nepal
⊕ https://vfapp.org/2788

New Life Health Care Pvt. Ltd.
Tushal Marga, काठमाडौं,
वाग्मती प्रदेश, Nepal
⊕ https://vfapp.org/e63c

New Padma Hospital
Mahakali Highway, Chhatiwan,
Jorayal, Nepal
⊕ https://vfapp.org/adc3

Nidan Hospital
Pulchowk Marg, Patan, वाग्मती
प्रदेश, Nepal
⊕ https://vfapp.org/66e4

Nobel Hospital
Sinamangal Marg, काठमाडौं,
वाग्मती प्रदेश, Nepal
⊕ https://vfapp.org/49a1

Nobel Medical College Teaching Hospital
Kanchanbari, Biratnagar
Metropolitan City– 5,
Biratnagar 56700, Nepal
⊕ https://vfapp.org/21a7

North Point Hospital
Golfutar Main Road, Tokha,
वाग्मती प्रदेश, Nepal
⊕ https://vfapp.org/a7aa

Okhaldhunga Community Hospital
Siddhicharan 56100, Nepal
⊕ https://vfapp.org/338d

Om Hospital
Hospital Road, Bharatpur
Metro, वाग्मती प्रदेश, Nepal
⊕ https://vfapp.org/67ab

Padma Hospital Private Limited
Attaria Chowk, Attariya 10900,
Nepal
⊕ https://vfapp.org/d832

Panchamukhi Nagarik Hospital Pvt. Ltd.
Yagyabhumi, Dharapani
– Kunaghat marga,
Dhanusadham 33000, Nepal
⊕ https://vfapp.org/75ab

Panchthar Hospital
मेची राजमार्ग, Phidim, प्रदेश नं.
१, Nepal
⊕ https://vfapp.org/939b

Parkland Hospital
Amar Sing Chowk 10, Pokhara
33700, Nepal
⊕ https://vfapp.org/6dca

Patan Hospital
Mahalaxmisthan Road, Patan,
वाग्मती प्रदेश, Nepal
⊕ https://vfapp.org/f435

Pina Hospital
Pina, कर्णाली प्रदेश, Nepal
⊕ https://vfapp.org/89df

Pokhara Regional Hospital, Pvt. Ltd.
Pokhara Baglung Rajmarg,
Pokhara, गण्डकी प्रदेश, Nepal
⊕ https://vfapp.org/14ed

Pulse Health Care & Diagnostics Pvt. Ltd.
Kathmandu 44600, Nepal
⊕ https://vfapp.org/b7ad

Punarjiban Hospital
Ring Road, Patan, वाग्मती
प्रदेश, Nepal
⊕ https://vfapp.org/8c32

Pyuthan Hospital
F14, Pyuthan, प्रदेश नं. ५, Nepal
https://vfapp.org/ad21

Rajhar Ayurved Aushadhalaya
Mahendra Highway, Rajahar, गण्डकी प्रदेश, Nepal
https://vfapp.org/5945

Ramechhap District Hospital
21DR033, Ramechhap, वाग्मती प्रदेश, Nepal
https://vfapp.org/b28d

Rapti Sub-Regional Hospital
F179, घोराही, प्रदेश नं. ५, Nepal
https://vfapp.org/3cf9

Red Cross – Patan
Patan, वाग्मती प्रदेश, Nepal
https://vfapp.org/7998

Red Cross – Panauti
Malpi Road, Panauti, वाग्मती प्रदेश, Nepal
https://vfapp.org/c643

Resunga Hospital
Purano Bazar Road, Tamghas, प्रदेश नं. ५, Nepal
https://vfapp.org/ac83

Rolpa District Hospital
F13, Liwang, प्रदेश नं. ५, Nepal
https://vfapp.org/dde5

Sagarmatha Zonal Hospital
8 Kunauli Road, Rajbiraj, प्रदेश नं. २, Nepal
https://vfapp.org/5423

Sahara Hospital
Pokhara, गण्डकी प्रदेश, Nepal
https://vfapp.org/e51f

Sahodar Hospital
Dhamilikuwa 33600, Nepal
https://vfapp.org/fac2

Sai Archana Hospital
Hospital Marg, Pokhara, गण्डकी प्रदेश, Nepal
https://vfapp.org/787f

Saptari Model Hospital
Kushaha 56400, Nepal
https://vfapp.org/ac1a

Sarbodhaya Sewa Ashram
Tarkughat, Nepal
https://vfapp.org/e39b

Sarvanga Hospital
Kupondol Marg, Patan, वाग्मती प्रदेश, Nepal
https://vfapp.org/62df

Satya Sai Hospital
Araniko Highway, Banepa, वाग्मती प्रदेश, Nepal
https://vfapp.org/adc7

Scheer Memorial Adventist Hospital
Banepa 45210, Nepal
https://vfapp.org/cafb

Seti Zonal Hospital, Dhangadhi
Main Road, Dhangadhi Sub Metropolitan, Dhanhadhi, Nepal
https://vfapp.org/e7bd

Shankarapur Hospital
Jorpati Main Road, Kathmandu, वाग्मती प्रदेश, Nepal
https://vfapp.org/b782

Shanti Sewa Griha
Tilaganga B marga, काठमाडौं, वाग्मती प्रदेश, Nepal
https://vfapp.org/3c71

Shree Birendra Hospital
Chhauni Hospital Rd, Kathmandu 44600, Nepal
https://vfapp.org/3e34

Shree Memorial Hospital
Chandeshwori Marga, Banepa, वाग्मती प्रदेश, Nepal
https://vfapp.org/b13d

Shree Tribhuwan Chandra Sainik Hospital
New Road, काठमाडौं, वाग्मती प्रदेश, Nepal
https://vfapp.org/761f

Shuvatara Hospital
Mahalaxmisthan Road, Patan, Bagmati Pradesh, Nepal
https://vfapp.org/deb7

Siddhi Memorial Hospital
Hanumante, Bhaktapur, Vagmati Pradesh Nepal
https://vfapp.org/7511

Sindhupalchok District Hospital
Chautara-Nawalpur Road , Chautara 45301 Nepal
https://vfapp.org/82e7

Siraha District Hospital
Madar – Siraha – Choharwa, Siraha, State No. 2, Nepal
https://vfapp.org/ca43

Spark B and D Hospital
Jalpa Road, Pokhara,Gandaki Pradesh Nepal
https://vfapp.org/544e

Sri Tribhubana Chandra Military Hospital
New Rd, Kathmandu 44600, Nepal
https://vfapp.org/942f

Star Hospital
Ring Road, Patan, Bagmati Pradesh, Nepal
https://vfapp.org/e99a

Sumeru City Hospital
Patan, Bagmati Pradesh, Nepal
https://vfapp.org/2738

Sumeru Hospital
F102, Dhapakhel, Vagmati Pradesh, Nepal
https://vfapp.org/4b98

Summit Hospital
Tikathali-Lokanthali Road, Lokanthali,Vagmati Pradesh, Nepal
https://vfapp.org/6d8b

Surkhet Hospital Pvt. Ltd.
Birendranagar 21700, Nepal
https://vfapp.org/26e5

Susma Koirala Memorial Hospital
Sankhu Road, Shankharapur, Vagmati Pradesh, Nepal
🌐 https://vfapp.org/e92d

Suvechhya Hospital
F75, Kathmandu, Bagmati Pradesh, Nepal
🌐 https://vfapp.org/8f5c

Swabhiman Hospital Pvt. Ltd.
Hariwon-11, Hariyon, Nepal
🌐 https://vfapp.org/2e38

T. U. Teaching Hospital
Kathepul Parsa Road, Khairahani, Bagmati Pradesh, Nepal
🌐 https://vfapp.org/a9fb

Tamghas Hospital
Resunga 32600, Nepal
🌐 https://vfapp.org/63e7

Taplejung District Hospital
Taplejung 57500, Nepal
🌐 https://vfapp.org/4dcd

Taulihawa District Hospital
Kapilvastu, Nepal
🌐 https://vfapp.org/2d25

Teaching Hospital, Karnali Academy of Health Sciences
Hospital Route, Chandannath 21200, Nepal
🌐 https://vfapp.org/71a8

Terhathum District Hospital
Myanglung 57100, Nepal
🌐 https://vfapp.org/78d7

The Mountain Medical Institute
Namche 56000, Nepal
🌐 https://vfapp.org/8468

The Skin Hospital
Lazimpat Road, Kathmandu, Bagmati Pradesh, Nepal
🌐 https://vfapp.org/d774

Tikapur Hospital
Tikapur Hospital Road, Tikapur, Tikapur, Nepal
🌐 https://vfapp.org/c48d

Tilahar Old Hospital
Tilahar Sadak, Tilahar 33400, Nepal
🌐 https://vfapp.org/7d62

Tilottama Hospital
Butwal 32907, Nepal
🌐 https://vfapp.org/f294

Trishuli Hospital
28DR008, Bidur, Bagmati Pradesh, Nepal
🌐 https://vfapp.org/5899

TU Teaching Hospital
Maharajgunj, Kathmandu, Nepal
🌐 https://vfapp.org/a5c7

United Mission Hospital Tansen
Tansen, Nepal
🌐 https://vfapp.org/f35f

Vayodha Hospital
Ring Road, Kathmadou, Vagmati Pradesh, Nepal
🌐 https://vfapp.org/f81b

Venus International Hospital
Puja Pratisthan Marga,Kathmadou, Vagmati Pradesh, Nepal
🌐 https://vfapp.org/3777

Wellness Hospital Pvt. Ltd.
Bansbari Road, Kathmadou, Vagmati Pradesh, Nepal
🌐 https://vfapp.org/8e52

Western Hospital
Charbahini Rd 10, Nepalgunj 21900, Nepal
🌐 https://vfapp.org/91fe

Western Regional Hospital
Hospital Marg, Pokhara,Gandaki Region, Nepal
🌐 https://vfapp.org/214f

Yeti Hospital
Ring Road, Kathmadou, Vagmati Pradesh, Nepal
🌐 https://vfapp.org/293a

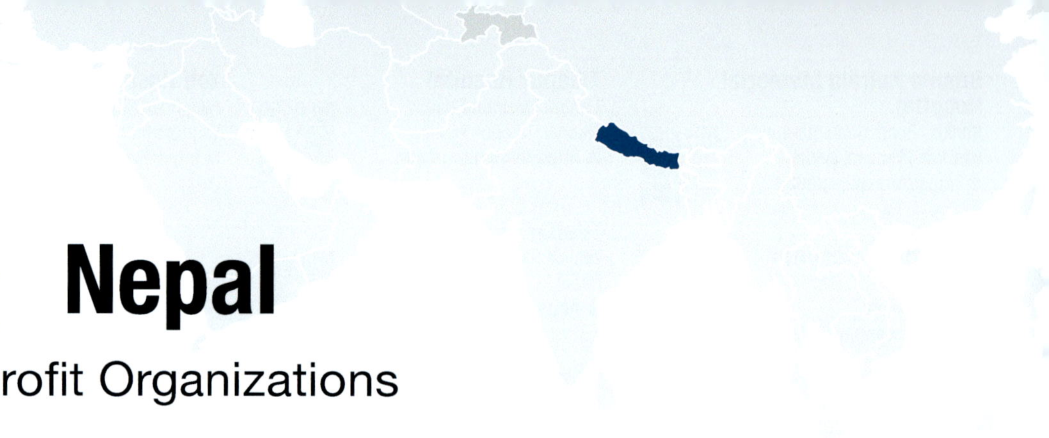

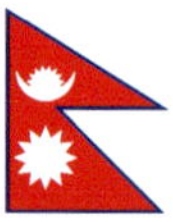

Nepal

Nonprofit Organizations

1789 Fund, The
Promotes gender equality worldwide through investment in the economic empowerment of women and the health of mothers and newborns.
MF Med, Neonat, OB-GYN
+1 215-439-3256
https://vfapp.org/7145

A Broader View Volunteers
Provides developing countries around the world with significant volunteer programs that both aid the neediest communities and forge a lasting bond between those volunteering and those they have helped.
Dent-OMFS, ER Med, Infect Dis, MF Med
+1 215-780-1845
https://vfapp.org/3bec

Abt Associates
Seeks to improve the quality of life and economic well-being of people worldwide, while striving to meet and exceed the highest professional standards.
General, Logist-Op, MF Med, OB-GYN, Peds
+1 212-779-7700
https://vfapp.org/cec2

Action Against Hunger
Aims to end life-threatening hunger for good through treating and preventing malnutrition across more than forty-five countries.
+1 212-967-7800
https://vfapp.org/2dbc

Adara Group
Seeks to bridge the world of business with the people in extreme poverty, and to support vulnerable communities with health, education, and other essential services.
General, MF Med, Neonat, OB-GYN, Ped Surg, Peds
+1 425-967-5115
https://vfapp.org/c8b4

Advance Family Planning
Aims to achieve global expansion and access to quality contraceptive information, services, and supplies through financial investment and political commitment.
General, MF Med, Pub Health
+1 410-502-8715
https://vfapp.org/7478

Adventist Health International
Focuses on upgrading and managing mission hospitals by providing governance, consultation, and technical assistance to a number of affiliated Seventh-Day Adventist hospitals throughout Africa, Asia, and the Americas.
Dent-OMFS, General, Pub Health
+1 909-558-5610
https://vfapp.org/16aa

Against Malaria Foundation
Helps protect people from malaria. Funds anti-malaria nets, specifically long-lasting insecticidal nets (LLINs), and works with distribution partners to ensure they are used. Tracks and reports on net use and malaria case data.
Infect Dis
+44 20 7371 8735
https://vfapp.org/337d

AIDS Healthcare Foundation
Provides cutting-edge HIV/AIDS medical care and advocacy to over one million people in forty-three countries.
Infect Dis
+1 323-860-5200
https://vfapp.org/b27c

Aloha Medical Mission
Bringing hope and changing the lives of the people served overseas and in Hawai‘i.
Anesth, Crit-Care, Dent-OMFS, ENT, ER Med, General, Medicine, OB-GYN, Ophth-Opt, Ortho, Ped Surg, Peds, Plast, Surg, Urol
+1 808-847-3400
https://vfapp.org/72ac

America Nepal Medical Foundation
Promotes the advancement of medical training and practice in Nepal and helps strengthen its existing medical capabilities through fostering academic and professional cooperations.
ER Med, General, Surg
https://vfapp.org/ec64

American Academy of Pediatrics
Seeks to attain optimal physical, mental, and social health and well-being for all infants, children, adolescents, and young adults.
Anesth, Crit-Care, Neonat, Ped Surg
+1 800-433-9016
https://vfapp.org/9633

American Heart Association (AHA)
Fights heart disease and stroke, striving to save and improve lives.
CV Med, Crit-Care, General, Heme-Onc, Medicine, Peds
☎ +1 212-878-5900
⊕ https://vfapp.org/4747

American Stroke Association
Works to prevent, treat, and beat stroke by funding innovative research, fighting for stronger public health policies, and providing lifesaving tools and information.
CV Med, Crit-Care, Heme-Onc, Medicine, Neuro, Pub Health, Pulm-Critic, Vasc Surg
☎ +1 800-242-8721
⊕ https://vfapp.org/746f

Americares
Saves lives and improves health for people affected by poverty or disaster and responds with life-changing medicine, medical supplies, and health programs including domestic and global medical clinics.
All-Immu, ER Med, General, Infect Dis, MF Med, Nutr
☎ +1 203-658-9500
⊕ https://vfapp.org/e567

AO Alliance
Builds solutions to lessen the burden of injuries in low- and middle-income countries, while enhancing the care of the injured to reduce human suffering, disability, and poverty.
Ortho, Surg
⊕ https://vfapp.org/8cd5

Association of Medical Doctors of Asia (AMDA)
Strives to support people affected by disasters and economic distress on their road to recovery, establishing a true partnership with special emphasis on local initiative.
ER Med, Logist-Op, Pub Health
☎ +81 86-252-6051
⊕ https://vfapp.org/e3d4

Australians for Women's Health
Aims to provide sustainable medical treatment and public health interventions for women in developing countries suffering from gynecological or pregnancy-related conditions.
Crit-Care, MF Med, OB-GYN, Surg
☎ +61 2 6584 7210
⊕ https://vfapp.org/b4d4

Australian Himalayan Foundation
Works in partnership with people of the remote Himalaya to improve living standards through better education and training, improved health services, and environmental sustainability.
General, MF Med, OB-GYN, Peds
☎ +61 2 9438 1822
⊕ https://vfapp.org/3428

Autism Care Nepal Society
Empowers people with autism to protect and promote their rights and utilize their skills to have a meaningful and effective participation in the society.
General, Neuro, Peds, Psych
☎ +977 1015251554
⊕ https://vfapp.org/1394

Backpacker Medics
Aims to bring effective medical care to those who need it most through a platform for paramedics and other pre-hospital workers to engage with humanitarian work and travel to remote areas of the world to deliver healthcare, establish healthcare facilities, and provide education.
Crit-Care, ER Med, OB-GYN
⊕ https://vfapp.org/c4e5

Basic Foundations
Supports local projects and organizations that seek to meet the basic human needs of others in their community.
ER Med, General, Peds, Rehab, Surg
⊕ https://vfapp.org/c4be

Benjamin H. Josephson, MD Fund
Provides healthcare professionals with the financial resources necessary to deliver medical services for those in need throughout the world.
General, OB-GYN
☎ +1 908-522-2853
⊕ https://vfapp.org/6acc

Beta Humanitarian Help
Provides plastic surgery in underserved areas of the world.
Anesth, Plast
☎ +49 228 909075778
⊕ https://vfapp.org/7221

Better Vision Foundation Nepal
Aims to provide quality, sustainable, comprehensive, and affordable eye care by identifying and mobilizing resources to eliminate avoidable blindness in Nepal to align with the global initiative of Vision 2020.
Ophth-Opt
☎ +977 98667605333
⊕ https://vfapp.org/61a1

BFIRST – British Foundation for International Reconstructive Surgery & Training
Supports projects across the developing world to train surgeons in their local environment to effectively manage devastating injuries.
Anesth, Plast, Surg
☎ +44 20 7831 5161
⊕ https://vfapp.org/ad4f

Bicol Clinic Foundation Inc.
Treats patients primarily in the Philippines, Nepal, Haiti, and locally in the USA, while constructing a permanent outpatient clinic in the Bicol region of the Philippines and establishing a disaster-relief fund.
Crit-Care, Derm, ENT, ER Med, Endo, General, Infect Dis, MF Med, Medicine, Nutr, OB-GYN, Ophth-Opt, Pub Health, Surg, Urol
☎ +1 561-864-0298
⊕ https://vfapp.org/3f9e

Birat Nepal Medical Trust (BNMT Nepal)
Ensures equitable access to quality healthcare for socially and economically disadvantaged people.
General, Infect Dis, OB-GYN, Psych
☎ +977 1-4436434
⊕ https://vfapp.org/6a41

B.P. Eye Foundation
Empowers people to achieve their full human potential by eliminating barriers of ill health, illiteracy, inequity, and poverty by employing health as an entry point and education as a door opener for poverty reduction, equity, and social inclusion.
ENT, General, Ophth-Opt, Peds, Pub Health, Rehab
+977 1-6631705
https://vfapp.org/c16e

BRAC USA
Seeks to empower people and communities in situations of poverty, illiteracy, disease, and social injustice. Interventions aim to achieve large-scale, positive changes through economic and social programs that enable everyone to realize their potential.
ER Med, General, Infect Dis, Logist-Op, MF Med, OB-GYN
+1 212-808-5615
https://vfapp.org/9d9e

Bridge of Life
Aims to strengthen healthcare globally through sustainable programs that prevent and treat chronic disease.
Logist-Op, Nephro, OB-GYN, Peds, Surg
+1 888-374-8185
https://vfapp.org/5b68

Canadian Medical Assistance Teams (CMAT)
Provides relief and medical aid to the victims of natural and man-made disasters around the world.
Anesth, ER Med, Medicine, OB-GYN, Peds, Psych, Rehab, Surg
+1 855-637-9111
https://vfapp.org/5232

Canadian Reconstructive Surgery Foundation, The
Develops, organizes, and manages, in participation with developing countries, the delivery of reconstructive medical-care programs, technologies, and education to those not able to obtain the care needed.
Anesth, Dent-OMFS, Plast
https://vfapp.org/15f4

CardioStart International
Provides free heart surgery and associated medical care to children and adults living in underserved regions of the world, irrespective of political or religious affiliation, through the collective skills of healthcare experts.
Anesth, CT Surg, CV Med, Crit-Care, Pub Health, Pulm-Critic
+1 813-304-2163
https://vfapp.org/85ef

CARE
Works around the globe to save lives, defeat poverty, and achieve social justice.
ER Med, General
+1 800-422-7385
https://vfapp.org/7232

Care and Development Organization (CDO) Nepal
Works to improve the lives of underprivileged people, children working in brick and carpet factories, internally displaced people, and women in need by providing medical care, health awareness, and training.
General, MF Med, Nutr, Ophth-Opt
+977 1-5560403
https://vfapp.org/4c98

Carter Center, The
Seeks to prevent and resolve conflicts, enhance freedom and democracy, and improve health, while remaining committed to human rights and the alleviation of human suffering.
Infect Dis, MF Med, Ophth-Opt
+1 800-550-3560
https://vfapp.org/6556

Center for Private Sector Health Initiatives
Aims to improve the health and well-being of people in developing countries by facilitating partnerships between the public and private sectors.
Infect Dis, Nutr, Peds
+1 202-884-8334
https://vfapp.org/b198

Chain of Hope (La Chaîne de l'Espoir)
Helps underprivileged children around the world by providing them with access to healthcare.
Anesth, CT Surg, Crit-Care, ER Med, Neurosurg, Ortho, Ped Surg, Surg, Vasc Surg
+33 1 44 12 66 66
https://vfapp.org/e871

Chance for Nepal
Works closely with established and trusted organizations, schools, and hospitals in Nepal to guarantee aid and support to those families in need and to offer education and training opportunities.
Derm, General, Ped Surg, Peds, Plast
https://vfapp.org/f436

CharityVision International
Focuses on restoring curable sight impairment worldwide by empowering local physicians and creating sustainable solutions.
Logist-Op, Ophth-Opt, Surg
+1 435-200-4910
https://vfapp.org/6231

ChildFund Australia
Works to reduce poverty for children in many of the world's most disadvantaged communities.
ER Med, General, Peds
+1 800023600
https://vfapp.org/13df

Christian Aid Ministries
Strives to be a trustworthy and efficient channel for Amish, Mennonite, and other conservative Anabaptist groups and individuals to minister to physical and spiritual needs around the world.
CT Surg, ER Med, Logist-Op, Ortho, Pub Health
+1 330-893-2428
https://vfapp.org/7b33

Christian Blind Mission (CBM)
Aims to improve the quality of life of persons with disabilities in the poorest countries, addressing poverty as a cause, and a consequence, of disability, and working in partnership to create a society for all.
ENT, General, Infect Dis, OB-GYN, Ophth-Opt, Ortho, Peds, Psych, Rehab, Surg
+49 6251 131131
https://vfapp.org/3824

Circle of Health International (COHI)

Aligns with local, community-based organizations led and powered by women to help respond to the needs of the women and children that they serve. Helps with the provision of professional volunteers, capacity training, and procurement of requested and appropriate supplies and equipment. Raises funds for the organizations to provide the services required.

ER Med, Logist-Op, MF Med, Neonat, OB-GYN, Psych

+1 512-210-7710

https://vfapp.org/8b63

Clinic Nepal

Seeks to help the Meghauli and Daldale communities gain access to education, healthcare, and clean water and sanitary facilities.

ER Med, General, Medicine, Peds, Surg

+977 1-4387774

https://vfapp.org/5acd

Columbia University: Global Mental Health Programs

Pioneers research initiatives, promotes mental health, and aims to reduce the burden of mental illness worldwide.

Psych

+1 646-774-5308

https://vfapp.org/c5cd

Community Action Nepal

Focuses on supporting remote mountain communities and strengthening their resilience by improving healthcare and educational services.

ER Med, General, Pub Health

+44 7500 828711

https://vfapp.org/d39a

Concern Worldwide

Seeks to permanently transform the lives of people living in extreme poverty, tackling its root causes, and building resilience.

Logist-Op, MF Med, Nutr, OB-GYN

+353 1 417 7700

https://vfapp.org/77e9

Core Group

Aims to improve and expand community health practices for underserved populations, especially women and children, through collaborative action and learning.

General, Infect Dis, MF Med, Medicine, OB-GYN, Peds, Pub Health

+1 202-380-3400

https://vfapp.org/9de3

Critical Care Disaster Foundation

Seeks to educate in-country healthcare providers from developing countries in disaster and crisis medical management and to develop an infrastructure of critical care services.

Anesth, Crit-Care, ER Med, Logist-Op, Pulm-Critic

https://vfapp.org/a445

Cura for the World

Seeks to heal, nourish, and embrace the neglected by building medical clinics in remote communities in dire need of medical care.

ER Med, General, Peds

https://vfapp.org/c55f

Dentaid

Seeks to treat, equip, train, and educate people in need of dental care.

Dent-OMFS

+44 1794 324249

https://vfapp.org/a183

Direct Relief

Improves the health and lives of people affected by poverty or emergency situations by mobilizing and providing essential medical resources needed for their care.

ER Med, Logist-Op

+1 805-964-4767

https://vfapp.org/58e5

Doctors for Nepal

Aims to improve healthcare in rural Nepal through healthcare projects, continuing education for health workers, and by sponsoring students from poor rural areas to attend medical, nursing, and midwifery schools in Nepal and then work in these communities post-graduation.

General

+44 7768 980960

https://vfapp.org/f9ff

Duke University: Global Health Institute

Sparks innovation in global health research and education, and brings together knowledge and resources to address the most important global health issues of our time.

All-Immu, Infect Dis, MF Med, OB-GYN, Pub Health

+1 919-681-7760

https://vfapp.org/c4cd

Ear Aid Nepal

Promotes good ear health by treating and preventing hearing disability in Nepal.

ENT, Surg

+977 61-431015

https://vfapp.org/ef32

Education and Health Nepal

Aims to make a difference by matching volunteers from the growing volunteer movement with placements that support underserved communities.

General, Geri, Medicine, OB-GYN, Peds, Psych, Radiol, Surg

+977 980-3719037

https://vfapp.org/fb12

Edwards Lifesciences

Provides innovative solutions for people fighting cardiovascular disease, as a global leader in patient-focused medical innovations for structural heart disease, as well as critical care and surgical monitoring.

Anesth, CT Surg, CV Med, Crit-Care, Ped Surg, Peds, Pulm-Critic, Surg, Vasc Surg

+1 949-250-5176

https://vfapp.org/d671

EngenderHealth

Works to implement high-quality, gender-equitable programs that advance sexual and reproductive health and rights.

General, MF Med, OB-GYN, Peds

+1 202-902-2000

https://vfapp.org/1cb2

Eye Care Foundation
Helps prevent and cure avoidable blindness and visual impairment in low-income countries.
Ophth-Opt, Surg
+31 20 647 3879
https://vfapp.org/c8f9

Eye Foundation of America
Works toward a world without childhood blindness.
Ophth-Opt
+1 304-599-0705
https://vfapp.org/a7eb

Eyes4Everest
Provides primary eye care and prescription eyewear for people of the Everest National Park.
Ophth-Opt
https://vfapp.org/436f

Finn Church Aid
Supports people in the most vulnerable situations within fragile and disaster-affected regions in three thematic priority areas: right to peace, livelihood, and education.
ER Med, Psych, Pub Health
+358 20 7871201
https://vfapp.org/9623

Fistula Foundation
Aims to engage the support of people worldwide who are eager to see the day when no woman suffers from obstetric fistula. Raises and directs funds to doctors and hospitals providing life-transforming surgery to women in need.
OB-GYN
+1 408-249-9596
https://vfapp.org/e958

For Hearts and Souls
Provides medical outreach and care for children through heart-related work, such as diagnosing heart problems and performing heart-saving surgeries.
Anesth, CT Surg, CV Med, Crit-Care, Peds, Pulm-Critic
+1 210-289-4753
https://vfapp.org/a162

Foundation for International Development Relief (FIDR)
Implements assistance projects in developing countries to improve the living environment of residents, while promoting regional development centered on the welfare of children.
Pub Health
+81 3-5282-5211
https://vfapp.org/7356

Foundation For International Education In Neurological Surgery (FIENS), The
Provides hands-on training and education to neurosurgeons around the world.
Neuro, Neurosurg, Surg
https://vfapp.org/bab8

Foundation Human Nature (FHN)
Helps marginalized communities by providing technical, human, and financial resources to sustainably strengthen primary healthcare and public health in Ecuador, Ghana, and Nepal.
ER Med, General, Infect Dis, OB-GYN, Peds, Pub Health
https://vfapp.org/6e8c

Fred Hollows Foundation, The
Works toward a world in which no person is needlessly blind or vision impaired.
Ophth-Opt, Pub Health, Surg
+1 646-374-0445
https://vfapp.org/73e5

Friends for Asia Foundation, The
Develops international volunteer projects that assist local communities in overcoming challenges, and provides volunteers with the experience of contributing to those communities as a valued participant.
General
+66 53 232 053
https://vfapp.org/f8a9

Friends of UNFPA
Promotes the health, dignity, and rights of women and girls around the world by supporting the lifesaving work of UNFPA, the United Nations reproductive health and rights agency, through education, advocacy, and fundraising.
MF Med, OB-GYN
+1 646-649-9100
https://vfapp.org/2a3a

Gastro & Liver Foundation Nepal
Seeks to raise public awareness of the prevention of liver and gastrointestinal diseases and works to create facilities providing treatment of liver diseases at an affordable cost or free of cost.
GI, Heme-Onc
+977 980-3529126
https://vfapp.org/5b59

Global Alliance to Prevent Prematurity and Stillbirth (GAPPS)
Seeks to improve birth outcomes worldwide by reducing the burden of premature birth and stillbirth.
All-Immu, Infect Dis, MF Med, Neonat, Neonat, OB-GYN
+1 206-413-7954
https://vfapp.org/3f74

Global Dental Relief
Brings free dental care to impoverished children in partnership with local organizations, and delivers treatment and preventive care in dental clinics that serve children in schools and remote villages.
Dent-OMFS
+1 303-858-8857
https://vfapp.org/29b6

Global Eye Project
Empowers local communities by building locally managed, sustainable eye clinics through education initiatives and volunteer-run professional training services.
Anesth, Ophth-Opt, Surg
https://vfapp.org/cdba

Global First Responder (GFR)
Acts as a centralized network for individuals and agencies involved in relief work worldwide and organizes and executes mission trips to areas in need, focusing not only on healthcare delivery but also health education and improvements.
ER Med
+1 573-424-8370
https://vfapp.org/a3e1

Global Force for Healing
Works to end preventable maternal and newborn deaths by supporting the scaling of effective grassroots. community-led, culturally respectful care and education in underserved areas around the globe using the midwifery model of care.

Neonat, OB-GYN

🌐 https://vfapp.org/deb2

Global Medical Foundation Australia
Provides medical, surgical, dental, and educational welfare to underprivileged communities and gives them access to the basics that are often take for granted.

Dent-OMFS, ER Med, General, OB-GYN, Ortho, Surg

🌐 https://vfapp.org/fa56

Global Ministries – The United Methodist Church
As the worldwide mission and development agency of The United Methodist Church, Global Ministries works with more than 300 hospitals and clinics around the world through its Global Health Unit.

Anesth, CT Surg, CV Med, Crit-Care, Dent-OMFS, Derm, ER Med, GI, General, Infect Dis, Logist-Op, MF Med, Medicine, Neonat, Nephro, Nutr, OB-GYN, Ophth-Opt, Ortho, Palliative, Peds, Pod, Psych, Pub Health, Rehab, Rheum, Surg, Urol

📞 +1 800-862-4246

🌐 https://vfapp.org/1723

Global Mission Partners, Inc.
Provides opportunities for short-term global medical mission opportunities, as well as evangelism and construction missions, to serve persons who have little or no access to healthcare, adequate housing, and community outreach.

Dent-OMFS, General, Geri, Palliative, Psych

📞 +1 405-623-7667

🌐 https://vfapp.org/7db4

Global Offsite Care
Aims to be a catalyst for increasing access to specialized healthcare for all, and provides technology platforms to doctors and clinics around the world through rotary club–sponsored telemedicine projects.

Crit-Care, ER Med, General, Pulm-Critic

📞 +1 707-827-1524

🌐 https://vfapp.org/61b5

Global Oncology (GO)
Brings the best in cancer care to underserved patients around the world and collaborates across geographic, professional, and academic borders to improve cancer care, research, and education.

Heme-Onc, Path, Rad-Onc

🌐 https://vfapp.org/fcb8

Global Outreach Doctors
Provides global health medical services in developing countries affected by famine, infant mortality, and chronic health issues.

All-Immu, Anesth, ER Med, General, Infect Dis, MF Med, Peds, Surg

📞 +1 505-473-9333

🌐 https://vfapp.org/8514

GOAL
Works with the most vulnerable communities to help them respond to and recover from humanitarian crises, and to assist them in building transcendent solutions to mitigate poverty and vulnerability.

ER Med, General, Pub Health

📞 +353 1 280 9779

🌐 https://vfapp.org/bbea

Hands for Health Foundation
Aims to provide healthcare access and medical supplies to people living in the developing world, who are less fortunate.

General, Nutr, Ophth-Opt

📞 +1 720-875-2814

🌐 https://vfapp.org/776e

Headwaters Relief Organization
Addresses public health issues for the most underserved populations in the world, providing psychosocial and medical support as well as disaster debris cleanup and rebuilding in partnership with other organizations.

ER Med, Infect Dis, Logist-Op, Psych, Pub Health

📞 +1 763-233-7655

🌐 https://vfapp.org/e511

Healing the Children
Helps underserved children around the world secure the medical care they need to lead more fulfilling lives.

Anesth, Dent-OMFS, ENT, General, Medicine, Ophth-Opt, Ped Surg, Peds, Plast, Surg

📞 +1 509-327-4281

🌐 https://vfapp.org/d4ee

Health and Development Society Nepal
Aims to provide quality oral health services, integrated general health services, and also engages in development initiatives with a focus on overall health and well-being.

Dent-OMFS, Pub Health

📞 +977 1-5251067

🌐 https://vfapp.org/71da

Health Equity Initiative
Aims to build and sustain a global community that engages across sectors and disciplines to advance health equity.

Pub Health

🌐 https://vfapp.org/e2e2

Health Volunteers Overseas (HVO)
Improves the availability and quality of healthcare through the education, training, and professional development of the health workforce in resource-scarce countries.

All-Immu, Anesth, CV Med, Dent-OMFS, Derm, ENT, ER Med, Endo, GI, Heme-Onc, Infect Dis, Medicine, Medicine, Nephro, Neuro, OB-GYN, Ophth-Opt, Ortho, Peds, Plast, Psych, Pulm-Critic, Rehab, Rheum, Surg

📞 +1 202-296-0928

🌐 https://vfapp.org/42b2

Healthcare Nepal
Works to improve healthcare and education in Nepal.

Anesth, Dent-OMFS, MF Med, Neonat, Peds, Plast, Surg

🌐 https://vfapp.org/3bab

HealthRight International
Leverages global resources to address local health challenges and create sustainable solutions that empower marginalized

communities to live healthy lives.

General, Infect Dis, MF Med, OB-GYN, Psych, Pub Health

+1 212-226-9890

https://vfapp.org/129d

Healthy Developments

Provides Germany-supported health and social protection programs around the globe in a collaborative knowledge management process.

All-Immu, General, Infect Dis, Logist-Op, MF Med

https://vfapp.org/dc31

Heart to Heart International

Strengthens communities through improving health access, providing humanitarian development, and administering crisis relief worldwide. Engages volunteers, collaborates with partners, and deploys resources to achieve this mission.

Anesth, ER Med, General, Logist-Op, Medicine, Path, Path, Peds, Psych, Pub Health, Surg

+1 913-764-5200

https://vfapp.org/aacb

Helen Keller International

Seeks to eliminate preventable vision loss, malnutrition, and diseases of poverty.

Infect Dis, Nutr, OB-GYN, Ophth-Opt, Peds

+1 212-532-0544

https://vfapp.org/b654

HelpAge International

Works to ensure that people everywhere understand how much older people contribute to society and that they must enjoy their right to healthcare, social services, economic, and physical security.

General, Geri, Infect Dis, Medicine, Pub Health

+44 20 7148 7623

https://vfapp.org/5d91

Helping Hands Health Education

Provides sustainable health and education services to children and adults throughout the world.

Dent-OMFS, General, Logist-Op, OB-GYN, Ophth-Opt, Peds

+1 303-448-1811

https://vfapp.org/36da

HelpMeSee

Trains local cataract specialists in Manual Small Incision Cataract Surgery (MSICS) in significant numbers, to meet the increasing demand for surgical services in the communities most impacted by cataract blindness.

Anesth, Ophth-Opt, Surg

+1 844-435-7638

https://vfapp.org/973c

High Elevation Lives Project

Aims to provide children and adults with healthcare and health education, inspired by faith, compassion and caring.

General, MF Med, Neonat, Peds

+1 207-944-7705

https://vfapp.org/91a6

Himalayan Cataract Project

Works to cure needless blindness with the highest quality care at the lowest cost.

Anesth, Ophth-Opt, Surg

+1 888-287-8530

https://vfapp.org/3b3d

Himalayan Development Foundation

Ensures access to education for all children in the remote Kanchenjunga and Indrawati communities of Nepal.

General, OB-GYN

+61 414 804 055

https://vfapp.org/a36b

Himalayan HealthCare

Creates sustainable development programs in remote areas of Nepal that will improve the quality of life for its people by strengthening primary healthcare, community education, and income-generation opportunities.

ER Med, General, Infect Dis, Medicine, OB-GYN, Ophth-Opt, Peds

+1 646-464-0248

https://vfapp.org/e6cd

Hospital & Rehabilitation Centre for Disabled Children (HRCD)

Ensures equitable access to quality of life through appropriate interventions and enabling environments for children with physical disabilities.

Ortho, Ped Surg, Peds, Rehab, Surg

+977 11-661666

https://vfapp.org/ea2c

Human Development and Community Services (HDCS)

Aims to provide access and use of affordable, quality health services for poor and marginalized people.

General, MF Med, Peds

+977 1-5015062

https://vfapp.org/4568

Humanity & Inclusion

Works alongside people with disabilities and vulnerable populations, taking action and bearing witness in order to respond to their essential needs, improve their living conditions and health, and promote respect for their dignity and fundamental rights.

General, Infect Dis, MF Med, Medicine, Ortho, Peds, Psych, Pub Health, Rehab

+1 301-891-2138

https://vfapp.org/16b7

Humla Fund

Seeks to strengthen the Bon culture and traditions in the Humla region of Nepal through access to quality education, healthcare, and sustainable economic development.

General, Infect Dis, MF Med, Neuro, Peds, Peds

+1 518-567-1361

https://vfapp.org/2b74

Icahn School of Medicine at Mt. Sinai Arnhold Institute for Global Health

Specializes in global health systems and implementation research, working toward a world where vulnerable people in every community have access to health care.

CV Med, Endo, General, Infect Dis, Logist-Op, MF Med, Medicine, Neonat, OB-GYN, Ophth-Opt, Peds, Plast, Pub Health

+1 212-824-7950

https://vfapp.org/a327

IMA World Health
Works to build healthier communities by collaborating with key partners to serve vulnerable people with a focus on health, healing, and well-being for all.

Infect Dis, MF Med, Nutr, OB-GYN, Pub Health

+1 202-888-6200

https://vfapp.org/8316

IMPACT Foundation
Works to prevent and alleviate needless disability by restoring sight, mobility, and hearing.

ENT, MF Med, OB-GYN, Ophth-Opt, Ortho, Peds, Surg

+44 1444 457080

https://vfapp.org/ba28

International Agency for the Prevention of Blindness (IAPB), The
Leads international efforts in blindness-prevention activities, works toward a world where no one is needlessly visually impaired, and ensures that everyone has access to the best possible standard of eye health.

Infect Dis, Ophth-Opt, Pub Health

https://vfapp.org/87a2

International Children's Heart Fund
Aims to promote the international growth and quality of cardiac surgery, particularly in children and young adults.

CT Surg, Ped Surg

https://vfapp.org/33fb

International Council of Ophthalmology
Works with ophthalmologic societies and others to enhance ophthalmic education and improve access to the highest quality eye care in order to preserve and restore vision for the people of the world.

Ophth-Opt

https://vfapp.org/ffd2

International Federation of Gynecology and Obstetrics (FIGO)
Implements global projects on specific women's health issues.

MF Med, Medicine, Neonat, OB-GYN, Surg, Urol

+44 20 7928 1166

https://vfapp.org/c4b4

International Federation of Red Cross and Red Crescent Societies (IFRC)
Coordinates and directs international assistance following natural and man-made disasters in nonconflict situations through the world's largest humanitarian and development network. Provides disaster-preparedness programs, healthcare activities, and promotes humanitarian values.

ER Med, General, Infect Dis, Nutr

+1 212-338-0161

https://vfapp.org/b4ee

International Learning Movement (ILM UK)
Supports some of the world's poorest people in developing countries with core projects in education, safe drinking water, and healthcare.

General, Ophth-Opt

+44 1254 265451

https://vfapp.org/b974

International Medical Relief
Provides sustainable education, training, medical and dental care, and disaster relief and response in vulnerable communities worldwide.

Dent-OMFS, General, Infect Dis, Medicine, OB-GYN

+1 970-635-0110

https://vfapp.org/b3ed

International Nepal Fellowship
Helps people affected by leprosy, spinal cord injuries, and other disabilities by facilitating development in some of Nepal's most remote and poorest communities and running medical outreach programs.

ENT, ER Med, MF Med, Nutr, Ortho, Palliative, Rehab, Surg

+977 61-520111

https://vfapp.org/4673

International Nepal Fellowship (INF)
Supports local Nepali communities by providing healthcare services to improve health, reduce poverty, and promote social inclusion.

Derm, ER Med, General, Ortho, Peds, Surg

+44 121 472 2425

https://vfapp.org/d9ca

International Organization for Migration (IOM) – The UN Migration Agency
Promotes evidence-informed policies and holistic, preventive, and curative health programs that are beneficial, accessible, and equitable for vulnerable migrants.

General, Infect Dis, OB-GYN

+27 12 342 2789

https://vfapp.org/621a

International Planned Parenthood Federation (IPPF)
Leads a locally owned, globally connected civil society movement that provides and enables services and champions sexual and reproductive health and rights for all, especially the underserved.

Infect Dis, MF Med, OB-GYN

+44 20 7939 8200

https://vfapp.org/dc97

International Society of Nephrology
Aims to advance worldwide kidney health.

Nephro

+32 2 808 04 20

https://vfapp.org/1bae

International Trachoma Initiative (iTi)
Works toward a world free from trachoma, a preventable cause of blindness, and provides comprehensive support to national ministries of health and governmental and nongovernmental organizations to implement a comprehensive approach to fight trachoma.

Infect Dis, Ophth-Opt

+1 404-371-0466

https://vfapp.org/3278

International Union Against Tuberculosis and Lung Disease
Develops, implements, and assesses anti-tuberculosis, lung health, and noncommunicable disease programs.

Infect Dis, Pub Health, Pulm-Critic

+33 1 44 32 03 60

https://vfapp.org/3e82

InterSurgeon
Fosters collaborative partnerships in the field of global surgery that will advance clinical care, teaching, training, research, and the provision and maintenance of medical equipment.
ENT, Neurosurg, Ortho, Ped Surg, Plast, Surg, Urol
https://vfapp.org/6f8a

IntraHealth International
Improves the performance of health workers and strengthens the systems in which they work.
CV Med, Endo, General, Infect Dis, MF Med, Neonat, Nutr, OB-GYN
+1 919-313-3554
https://vfapp.org/ddc8

Ipas
Focuses efforts on women and girls who want contraception or abortion, and builds programs around their needs and how best to support them.
OB-GYN
https://vfapp.org/8e39

Iris Global
Serves the poor, the destitute, the lost, and the forgotten by providing adoration, outreach, family, education, relief, development, healing, and the arts.
General, Infect Dis, Nutr, Pub Health
+1 530-255-2077
https://vfapp.org/37f8

Islamic Medical Association of North America
Fosters health promotion, disease prevention, and health maintenance in communities around the world through direct patient care and health programs.
Anesth, Dent-OMFS, ER Med, General, Logist-Op, Ophth-Opt, Peds, Plast, Surg
+1 630-932-0000
https://vfapp.org/a157

IsraAID
Supports people affected by humanitarian crisis and partners with local communities around the world to provide urgent aid, assist recovery, and reduce the risk of future disasters.
ER Med, Infect Dis, Psych, Rehab
+972 3-947-7766
https://vfapp.org/de96

Janata Clinic
Aims to improve population health by providing more effective health services, and promotes health as a collaborative service by developing a sustainable model of community-endorsed health programs.
General, OB-GYN, Peds
+977 1-4106287
https://vfapp.org/992f

Jeewasha Foundation
Relieves the suffering of kidney patients in Nepal and helps others to avoid kidney failure in their lives.
Medicine, Nephro
+977 61-526604
https://vfapp.org/bc2a

Jericho Road Community Health Center
Provides holistic healthcare for underserved and marginalized communities around the world, inspired by the Christian faith.
Anesth, General, Heme-Onc, Infect Dis, Medicine, OB-GYN, Ped Surg, Peds, Psych, Surg
+1 716-348-3000
https://vfapp.org/3d6b

Jhpiego
Creates and delivers transformative healthcare solutions that save lives in partnership with national governments, health experts, and local communities.
General, Infect Dis, OB-GYN, Surg
+1 410-537-1800
https://vfapp.org/45b8

John Snow, Inc. (JSI)
Aims to improve the health and well-being of underserved and vulnerable people and communities throughout the world.
General, Infect Dis, Logist-Op, MF Med, OB-GYN, Peds, Psych, Pub Health
+1 617-482-9485
https://vfapp.org/ba78

Johns Hopkins Center for Communication Programs
Believes in the power of communication to save lives, by empowering people to adopt healthy behaviors for themselves, their families, and their communities.
General, Infect Dis, Logist-Op, OB-GYN, Pub Health
+1 410-659-6300
https://vfapp.org/1bf9

Johns Hopkins Center for Global Health
Facilitates and focuses the extensive expertise and resources of the Johns Hopkins institutions together with global collaborators to effectively address and ameliorate the world's most pressing health issues.
General, Genetics, Logist-Op, MF Med, Peds, Psych, Pub Health, Pulm-Critic
+1 410-502-9872
https://vfapp.org/54ce

Joint United Nations Programme on HIV/AIDS (UNAIDS)
Aims to place people living with HIV and people affected by the virus at the decision-making table and at the center of designing, delivering, and monitoring the AIDS response.
Infect Dis
+41 22 791 36 66
https://vfapp.org/464a

Kailash Medical Foundation
Aims to improve the health and well-being of those in need around the world by going on missions to developing countries and providing medical, dental, and vision services to the underprivileged.
Dent-OMFS, General, Ophth-Opt
+1 925-699-4609
https://vfapp.org/db41

Karma Thalo Foundation
Delivers sustainable health programs to the poor in the most remote areas of Nepal, improving quality of life through access to medical care and health education.
Dent-OMFS, General, Geri, MF Med, Ophth-Opt, Peds
+1 314-223-1293
https://vfapp.org/382b

Karuna Foundation Nepal
Improves the lives of children with disabilities, prevents disabilities, empowers communities, and creates a more inclusive society.

Ortho, Ped Surg, Peds, Rehab

☎ +977 1-4410687

🌐 https://vfapp.org/1f5f

Kaya Responsible Travel
Promotes sustainable social, environmental, and economic development, empowers communities, and cultivates educated, compassionate global citizens through responsible travel.

All-Immu, Crit-Care, Dent-OMFS, ER Med, General, Geri, Infect Dis, MF Med, Medicine, Nutr, OB-GYN, Peds, Psych, Pub Health, Rehab

☎ +1 413-517-0266

🌐 https://vfapp.org/b2cf

Kids Care Everywhere
Seeks to empower physicians in under-resourced environments with multimedia, state-of-the-art medical software, and to inspire young professionals to become future global healthcare leaders.

Logist-Op, Ped Surg, Peds

🌐 https://vfapp.org/bc23

Leprosy Mission England and Wales, The
Leads the fight against leprosy by supporting people living with leprosy today and serving future generations by working to end the transmission of the disease.

Infect Dis, Pub Health

🌐 https://vfapp.org/4c67

Leprosy Mission: Northern Ireland, The
Leads the fight against leprosy by supporting people living with leprosy today and serving future generations by working to end the transmission of the disease.

General, Infect Dis

☎ +44 28 9262 9500

🌐 https://vfapp.org/e265

Life for a Child
Supports the provision of the best possible health care, given local circumstances, to all children and youth with diabetes in less-resourced countries, through the strengthening of existing diabetes services.

Endo, Medicine, Peds

🌐 https://vfapp.org/d712

Lifebox
Seeks to provide safer surgery and anesthesia in low-resource countries by investing in tools, training, and partnerships for safe surgery.

Anesth, Crit-Care, Surg

☎ +44 20 3286 0402

🌐 https://vfapp.org/2d4d

Lions Clubs International
Empowers volunteers to serve their communities, meet humanitarian needs, encourage peace, and promote international understanding through Lions clubs.

Heme-Onc, Medicine, Nutr, Ophth-Opt

☎ +1 630-571-5466

🌐 https://vfapp.org/7b12

London School of Hygiene & Tropical Medicine: Health in Humanitarian Crises Centre
Advances health and health equity in crisis-affected countries through research, education, and translation of knowledge into policy and practice.

ER Med, Infect Dis, Pub Health

☎ +44 20 7636 8636

🌐 https://vfapp.org/96ad

MAGNA International
Helps those who are suffering or recovering from conflicts and disasters by reducing the risks of diseases and treating them immediately.

ER Med, General, Infect Dis, Peds, Surg

☎ +421 2/381 046 69

🌐 https://vfapp.org/58f4

Management Sciences for Health (MSH)
Works with countries and communities to save lives and improve the health of the world's poorest and most vulnerable people by building strong, resilient, sustainable health systems.

Infect Dis, Logist-Op, Pub Health

☎ +1 617-250-9500

🌐 https://vfapp.org/6aa2

MAP International
Provides medicines and health supplies to those in need around the world so they might experience life to the fullest.

Logist-Op

☎ +1 800-225-8550

🌐 https://vfapp.org/deed

Marie Stopes International
Provides the contraception and safe abortion services that enable women all over the world to choose their own futures.

Infect Dis, MF Med, Neonat, OB-GYN, Pub Health

☎ +44 20 7636 6200

🌐 https://vfapp.org/9525

Massachusetts General Hospital Global Surgery Initiative
Aims to improve surgical education and access to advanced surgical care in resource-limited settings around the world by performing surgical operations as visitors, training local surgeons, and sharing medical technology through international partnerships across disciplines.

Anesth, Crit-Care, ER Med, Heme-Onc, Peds, Surg

☎ +1 617-724-4093

🌐 https://vfapp.org/31b1

Maverick Collective
Aims to build a global community of strategic philanthropists and informed advocates who use their intellectual and financial resources to create change.

Infect Dis, MF Med, OB-GYN

☎ +1 202-785-0072

🌐 https://vfapp.org/ea49

McGill University Health Centre: Centre for Global Surgery
Works to reduce the impact of injury by advancing surgical care through research and education in resource-limited settings.

ER Med, Logist-Op, Ped Surg, Surg

☎ +1 514-934-1934

🌐 https://vfapp.org/7246

Médecins du Monde/Doctors of the World
Provides care, bears witness, and supports social change worldwide with innovative medical programs and evidence-based advocacy initiatives.

ER Med, General, Infect Dis, MF Med, Neonat, OB-GYN, Peds, Pub Health
+33 1 44 92 15 15
https://vfapp.org/a43d

Medical Mercy Canada
Seeks to improve the quality of life in impoverished areas through humanitarian projects with local participation; provides funding for orphanages, geriatric and childcare centers, remote health clinics, medical aid centers, hospitals, rural schools and health programs.

General
+1 403-717-0933
https://vfapp.org/81dc

Medical Ministry International
Provides compassionate healthcare in areas of need, inspired by the Christian faith.

CT Surg, Dent-OMFS, ENT, General, OB-GYN, Ophth-Opt, Ortho, Plast, Rehab, Surg, Urol, Vasc Surg
+1 905-545-4400
https://vfapp.org/5da6

Medical Teams International
Seeks to restore health as the first step to restoring hope, working to bring basic but lifesaving medical care to those in need.

Dent-OMFS, ER Med, General, MF Med, Pub Health
+1 503-624-1000
https://vfapp.org/8d1c

MedShare
Aims to improve the quality of life of people, communities, and the planet by sourcing and directly delivering surplus medical supplies and equipment to communities in need around the world.

Logist-Op
+1 770-323-5858
https://vfapp.org/c8bc

Milan Foundation Nepal
Provides access to a good education and good health.

General, Ophth-Opt
+977 67-420986
https://vfapp.org/9e11

MiracleFeet
Brings low-cost treatment to every child on the planet born with clubfoot, a leading cause of physical disability.

Ortho, Peds, Rehab
+1 919-240-5572
https://vfapp.org/bda8

Mission Bambini
Helps to support children living in poverty, sickness, and without education, giving them the opportunity and hope of a better life.

CT Surg, CV Med, Crit-Care, ER Med, Ped Surg, Peds
+39 02 210 0241
https://vfapp.org/dc1a

Mission Plasticos
Provides reconstructive plastic surgical care to those in need, and generates sustainable outcomes through training, education, and research.

Plast
+1 714-769-9974
https://vfapp.org/97cb

Mission: Restore
Trains medical professionals abroad in complex reconstructive surgery in order to create a sustainable infrastructure where long-term relationships are forged and permanent change is made.

Plast, Surg
+1 855-777-1350
https://vfapp.org/3f5f

Multi-Agency International Training and Support (MAITS)
Improves the lives of some of the world's poorest people living with disabilities through better access to quality health and education services and support.

Neuro, Psych, Rehab
+44 20 7258 8443
https://vfapp.org/9dcd

Muna Foundation Nepal
Works for the welfare of children, women and girls, and minorities of Nepal to provide shelter, food, clothing, education, and healthcare as well as hope, compassion, and love.

General, Infect Dis, Ophth-Opt
+977 1-6200160
https://vfapp.org/51d3

Namaste Children Nepal
Provides proper shelter, quality education, and healthcare to children without parents.

General, Peds
+977 1-4254987
https://vfapp.org/ee74

NCD Alliance
Unites and strengthens civil society to stimulate collaborative advocacy, action, and accountability for NCD (noncommunicable disease) prevention and control.

All-Immu, CV Med, General, Heme-Onc, Medicine, Peds, Psych
+41 22 809 18 11
https://vfapp.org/abdd

Neglected Tropical Disease NGO Network
Works to create a global forum for non-governmental organizations working to control onchocerciasis, lymphatic filariasis, schistosomiasis, soil transmitted helminths, and trachoma.

Infect Dis, Logist-Op
+1 929-272-6227
https://vfapp.org/c511

Nepal Bharat Maitri Hospital
Delivers high-quality healthcare services that are affordable and accessible for the general public.

Crit-Care, ER Med, General, OB-GYN, Radiol, Surg
+977 1-5241288
https://vfapp.org/adbd

Nepal Eye Hospital
Provides eye care services to the Nepalese community.

Ophth-Opt, Surg

+977 1-4260813

https://vfapp.org/e2e3

Nepal Fertility Care Center (NFCC)
Helps to provide available, accessible, and affordable reproductive health for all.

Infect Dis, MF Med, OB-GYN

+977 1-5904789

https://vfapp.org/e917

Nepal Healthcare Equipment Development Foundation (NHEDF)
Accepts donated biomedical equipment from government hospitals and health clinics, repurposes it, and tailors its use to the specific needs of Nepalese patients.

ER Med, General, Logist-Op, Psych

+977 985-1015746

https://vfapp.org/8399

Nepal Heart Foundation
Promotes awareness among the people to reduce the incidence of heart diseases which have been taking an increased toll of death in the world.

CV Med, Crit-Care, Heme-Onc, Medicine, Peds

+977 1-5009263

https://vfapp.org/2c9e

Nepal Leprosy Trust
Aims for the ultimate elimination of leprosy, improved health, and socio-economic development.

Infect Dis, Pub Health

+977 1-5521622

https://vfapp.org/37d5

Nepal Netra Jyoti Sangh (NNJS)
Provides high-quality, sustainable, comprehensive, and affordable eye care services by identifying and mobilizing local, national, and international resources.

Infect Dis, Ophth-Opt

+977 1-4261921

https://vfapp.org/cddc

Nepal Youth Foundation
Brings freedom, health, shelter, and education to Nepal's most impoverished children.

Infect Dis, Nutr, Psych

+1 415-331-8585

https://vfapp.org/6f8e

Nestling Trust, The (TNT)
Facilitates the construction of village health clinics in collaboration with the Nepal Ministry of Health, equips staff, and ensures sustainability in order to provide basic healthcare in remote areas.

General, OB-GYN, Pub Health

+977 7747062757

https://vfapp.org/498c

NLR International
Promotes and supports the prevention and treatment of leprosy, prevention of disabilities, social inclusion, and stigma reduction of people affected by leprosy.

Infect Dis, Pub Health

+31 20 595 0500

https://vfapp.org/d7bd

NPI Narayani Samudayik Hospital
Delivers patient-centered care to enhance and contribute to health and well-being in Nepal.

Anesth, CV Med, Dent-OMFS, Derm, ENT, ER Med, General, Heme-Onc, Neuro, OB-GYN, Ortho, Path, Peds, Surg

+977 56-525517

https://vfapp.org/4877

Nyaya Health Nepal
Provides free, quality healthcare for underserved communities in Nepal, through a sustainable model. Works in Achham, a remote district in Far West Province that was disinvested during the decade-long civil war, and Dolakha, in Bagmati Province, an epicenter of the 2015 earthquake.

Anesth, CV Med, ER Med, Endo, General, Infect Dis, Logist-Op, Medicine, OB-GYN, Ortho, Ortho, Path, Peds, Radiol, Surg

https://vfapp.org/7825

NYC Medics
Deploys mobile medical teams to remote areas of disaster zones and humanitarian emergencies, providing the highest level of medical care to those who otherwise would not have access to aid and relief efforts.

All-Immu, ER Med, Infect Dis, Surg

+1 888-600-1648

https://vfapp.org/aeee

Oda Foundation
Develops community-led solutions, helping Nepal's most impoverished and remote communities to thrive.

ER Med, General, OB-GYN

+1 954-817-1446

https://vfapp.org/9884

One Heart Worldwide
Aims to end preventable deaths related to pregnancy and childbirth worldwide.

MF Med, Neonat, OB-GYN, Pub Health

+1 415-379-4762

https://vfapp.org/a865

One World – One Heart Foundation
Seeks to help people and improve the lives of those in need in Nepal.

Dent-OMFS, ER Med, General, Medicine, OB-GYN, Ophth-Opt

+1 575-758-9511

https://vfapp.org/c3f2

Open Heart International
Provides surgical interventions and best practices to the most disadvantaged communities on the planet.

CT Surg, MF Med, OB-GYN, Ophth-Opt, Plast, Surg

+61 2 9487 9295

https://vfapp.org/dab2

Operation Eyesight
Works to eliminate blindness in partnership with governments, hospitals, medical professionals, corporations, and community development teams.

Ophth-Opt, Surg
+1 403-283-6323
https://vfapp.org/b95d

Operation International
Offers medical aid to adults and children suffering from lack of quality healthcare in impoverished countries.
Dent-OMFS, ER Med, Heme-Onc, OB-GYN, Ophth-Opt, Ortho, Ped Surg, Plast, Surg
+1 631-287-6202
https://vfapp.org/b52a

Operation Medical
Commits efforts to promoting and providing high-quality medical care and education to communities that do not have adequate access.
Anesth, ENT, Logist-Op, OB-GYN, Ped Surg, Plast, Surg, Urol
+1 717-685-9199
https://vfapp.org/7e1b

Operation Walk
Provides the gift of mobility through life-changing joint replacement surgeries at no cost for those in need in the U.S. and globally.
Anesth, Ortho, Rehab, Surg
+1 310-493-8073
https://vfapp.org/bafe

Operation Walk New York
Provides free surgical treatment for patients who have no access to life-improving care for arthritis or other debilitating bone and joint conditions.
Anesth, Ortho, Rehab, Rheum
+1 315-883-5875
https://vfapp.org/4bf4

Options
Believes in a world where women and children can access the high-quality health services they need, without financial burden.
Logist-Op, MF Med, Neonat, OB-GYN
+44 20 7430 1900
https://vfapp.org/3a48

OPTIVEST Foundation
Funds strategic opportunities that are holistic and collaborative, inspired by the Christian faith.
General, Nutr
https://vfapp.org/f1e6

Optometry Giving Sight
Delivers eye exams and low or no-cost glasses, provides training for local eye care professionals, and establishes optometry schools, vision centers and optical labs.
Ophth-Opt
+1 303-526-0430
https://vfapp.org/33ea

Orbis International
Works to prevent and treat blindness through hands-on training and improved access to quality eye care.
Anesth, Ophth-Opt, Surg
+1 646-674-5500
https://vfapp.org/f2b2

Oxford University Global Surgery Group (OUGSG)
Aims to contribute to the provision of high-quality surgical care globally, particularly in low- and middle-income countries (LMICs) while bringing together students, researchers, and clinicians with an interest in global surgery, anaesthesia, and obstetrics and gynecology.
Anesth, MF Med, OB-GYN, Ortho, Surg
+44 1865 737543
https://vfapp.org/c624

Pact
Works on the ground to improve the lives of those who are challenged by poverty and marginalization, striving for a world where all people are heard capable, and vibrant.
Infect Dis, Logist-Op, MF Med, Pub Health
+1 202-466-5666
https://vfapp.org/9a6c

Partners in Health
Responds to the moral imperative to provide high-quality healthcare globally to those who need it most, while striving to ease suffering by providing a comprehensive model of care that includes access to food, transportation, housing, and other key components of healing.
CT Surg, General, Heme-Onc, Infect Dis, MF Med, Neurosurg, OB-GYN, Ortho, Plast, Psych, Urol
+1 857-880-5600
https://vfapp.org/dc9c

Partnership for Sustainable Development (PSD) Nepal
Builds capacity in the poorest and most vulnerable communities in Nepal.
General, OB-GYN, Ped Surg, Peds, Psych, Surg
+977 1-4411648
https://vfapp.org/1de6

PASHA
Creates opportunities to improve health among vulnerable populations around the world, by bringing together diverse individuals with various areas of expertise and engaging them in solving local and global health challenges.
Derm, Logist-Op, Ophth-Opt, Ortho
+1 310-400-0205
https://vfapp.org/efbc

PATH
Advances health equity through innovation and partnerships so people, communities, and economies can thrive.
All-Immu, CV Med, Endo, Heme-Onc, Infect Dis, MF Med, Neonat, Nutr, OB-GYN, Path, Peds, Pulm-Critic
+1 202-822-0033
https://vfapp.org/b4db

Pediatric Universal Life-Saving Effort, Inc. (PULSE)
Aims to increase access to acute- and intensive-care services for children, recognizing that a significant amount of childhood mortality is preventable. Utilizes time, talents, and resources and seeks to persuade others to share their gifts to enrich the lives of children worldwide.
Crit-Care, Logist-Op, Neonat, Ped Surg, Peds
+1 347-599-0792
https://vfapp.org/f6b9

Phase Worldwide
Empowers isolated communities through integrated and

sustainable programs in health, education, and livelihoods.
General, Heme-Onc, MF Med, Medicine, Nutr, OB-GYN, Peds
+44 117 916 6423
https://vfapp.org/fc74

Philips Foundation
Aims to reduce healthcare inequality by providing access to quality healthcare for disadvantaged communities.
CV Med, OB-GYN, Ped Surg, Peds, Surg, Urol
https://vfapp.org/bacb

PLeDGE Health
Aims to improve emergency medical care around the world through sustainable partnerships, open-source material development and dissemination, and development of the next generation of educational leaders in low-resource areas.
ER Med, General
https://vfapp.org/3a7d

Possible / Nyaya Health
Improves healthcare for underserved communities in Nepal and has piloted an integrated care-delivery model that coordinates care from home to facility, using an electronic health record (EHR) that was optimized for low-resource settings.
General, OB-GYN, Peds
+1 212-344-2100
https://vfapp.org/d949

PSI – Population Services International
Dedicates efforts to improving the health of people in the developing world by focusing on challenges such as a lack of family planning, HIV/AIDS, barriers to maternal health, and the greatest threats to children under the age of 5, including malaria, diarrhea, pneumonia, and malnutrition.
Infect Dis, MF Med, OB-GYN, Peds
+1 202-785-0072
https://vfapp.org/ffe3

Public Health Concern Trust Nepal (phect-Nepal)
Advocates for individual rights to healthcare and strives to provide better and affordable healthcare services to people in both urban as well as rural areas of Nepal.
Crit-Care, Dent-OMFS, ENT, General, MF Med, Medicine, Neurosurg, OB-GYN, Ophth-Opt, Ortho, Ped Surg, Peds, Psych, Pub Health, Radiol, Rehab, Surg
+977 1-4222450
https://vfapp.org/26c5

RAD-AID International
Improves and optimizes access to medical imaging and radiology in low-resource regions of the world.
Rad-Onc, Radiol
https://vfapp.org/537f

Reach Beyond
Aims to reach and impact underserved communities with medical care and community development, based in Christian ministry.
ER Med, General
+1 800-873-4859
https://vfapp.org/cc5c

Real Medicine Foundation (RMF)
Provides humanitarian support to people living in disaster and poverty-stricken areas, focusing on the person as a whole by providing medical/physical, emotional, economic, and social support.
ER Med, General, Infect Dis, Nutr, Peds, Psych
+44 20 8638 0637
https://vfapp.org/d45a

RestoringVision
Empowers lives by restoring vision for millions of people in need.
Ophth-Opt
+1 209-980-7323
https://vfapp.org/e121

ReSurge International
Provides reconstructive surgical care and builds surgical capacity in developing countries.
Anesth, Dent-OMFS, Ped Surg, Plast, Surg
+1 408-737-8743
https://vfapp.org/9937

RHD Action
Seeks to reduce the burden of rheumatic heart disease in vulnerable populations throughout the world.
CV Med, Medicine, Pub Health
https://vfapp.org/f5d9

Rockefeller Foundation, The
Works to promote the well-being of humanity.
Logist-Op, Nutr, Pub Health
+1 212-869-8500
https://vfapp.org/5424

Rose Charities International
Aims to support communities to improve quality of life and reduce the effects of poverty through innovative, self-sustaining projects and partnerships.
ENT, ER Med, General, Infect Dis, Neonat, OB-GYN, Ophth-Opt, Ped Surg, Peds, Rehab, Urol
+1 604-733-0442
https://vfapp.org/53df

Rotary International
Provides service to others, improves lives, and advances world understanding, goodwill, and peace through its fellowship of business, professional, and community leaders.
ER Med, General, Infect Dis, MF Med, OB-GYN
https://vfapp.org/8fb5

Rotaplast International
Helps children and families worldwide by eliminating the burden of cleft lip and/or palate, burn scarring, and other deformities by sending medical teams to provide free reconstructive surgery, ancillary treatment, and training.
Anesth, Dent-OMFS, ENT, Ped Surg, Plast, Surg
+1 415-252-1111
https://vfapp.org/78b3

Safe Anaesthesia Worldwide
Provides anesthesia to those in need in low-income countries to enable lifesaving surgery.

Anesth, Plast
+44 7527 506969
https://vfapp.org/134a

Salvation Army International, The
Seeks to meet human needs through services in education, healthcare, community support, emergency response, and ministry development, inspired by the Christian faith.
Dent-OMFS, Derm, ER Med, Infect Dis, MF Med, Medicine, Nutr, OB-GYN, Ophth-Opt, Palliative, Psych, Rehab, Surg
+44 20 7332 0101
https://vfapp.org/8eb3

SAMU Foundation
Provides medical first response and reconstruction when severe international emergencies occur.
ER Med, Infect Dis, Logist-Op, Psych, Pub Health
+1 202-808-0999
https://vfapp.org/3196

Save A Child's Heart
Provides lifesaving cardiac treatment to children in developing countries, and trains healthcare professionals from these countries to deliver quality care in their communities.
CT Surg, CV Med, Crit-Care, Ped Surg, Peds
+1 240-223-3940
https://vfapp.org/1bef

Save the Children
Gives children around the world a healthy start in life, the opportunity to learn, and protection from harm.
All-Immu, Crit-Care, ER Med, General, Infect Dis, MF Med, Medicine, Neonat, OB-GYN, Peds, Psych, Pub Health
+1 800-728-3843
https://vfapp.org/2e73

Scheer Memorial Adventist Hospital
Provides compassionate, patient-centered care at international standards for all patients.
Anesth, CV Med, Crit-Care, Dent-OMFS, Derm, Endo, OB-GYN, Ortho, Path, Peds, Radiol, Rehab, Surg, Urol
+977 11-661111
https://vfapp.org/fd87

SEE International
Provides sustainable medical, surgical, and educational services through volunteer ophthalmic surgeons, with the objectives of restoring sight and preventing blindness to disadvantaged individuals worldwide.
Ophth-Opt, Surg
+1 805-963-3303
https://vfapp.org/6e1b

SEVA
Delivers vital eye care services to the world's most vulnerable, including women, children, and Indigenous peoples.
Ophth-Opt, Surg
+1 510-845-7382
https://vfapp.org/1e87

Siddhi Memorial Foundation
Seeks to provide quality, accessible healthcare services for women and children through Siddhi Memorial Hospital (SMH) and to serve children, women, and senior citizens in need.
Anesth, Dent-OMFS, ER Med, General, MF Med, Neonat, OB-GYN, Path, Ped Surg, Peds, Surg
+977 1-6619382
https://vfapp.org/a52a

Sight for All
Empowers communities to deliver comprehensive, evidence-based, high-quality eye healthcare through the provision of research, education, and equipment.
Logist-Op, Ophth-Opt, Surg
+66 42 804 9888
https://vfapp.org/e34b

SIGN Fracture Care International
Builds orthopedic capacity around the world and provides the injured poor access to fracture surgery by donating orthopedic education and implant systems to surgeons in developing countries.
Ortho, Rehab, Surg
+1 509-371-1107
https://vfapp.org/123d

Simavi
Strives for a world in which all women and girls are socially and economically empowered and pursue their rights to live a healthy life, free from discrimination, coercion, and violence.
MF Med, OB-GYN
+31 88 313 1500
https://vfapp.org/b57b

Smile Train
Seeks to give every child with a cleft the opportunity for a healthy, productive life by providing free cleft repair surgery and comprehensive cleft care in their own communities.
Dent-OMFS, ENT, Plast
+1 800-932-9541
https://vfapp.org/f21d

SmileOnU
Empowers dental professionals to help and educate those who may not have adequate dental knowledge and access to oral-health services.
Dent-OMFS, Surg
+1 916-538-1466
https://vfapp.org/cb6d

Social Welfare Association of Nepal (SWAN Nepal)
Strives to support disadvantaged and rural communities in Nepal by providing accessible health care and educational opportunities for children, and enabling women to achieve financial independence.
Pub Health
+977 1-4720776
https://vfapp.org/a151

SOS Children's Villages International
Supports children through alternative care and family strengthening.
ER Med, Peds
+43 1 36824570
https://vfapp.org/aca1

Stand By Me
Helps children facing terrible circumstances and provides the care, love, and attention they need to thrive through children's homes and schools.

Peds
+44 1708 442271
https://vfapp.org/a224

Surgeons OverSeas (SOS)
Works to reduce death and disability from surgically treatable conditions in developing countries.
Anesth, Heme-Onc, Surg
https://vfapp.org/5d16

Swiss Tropical and Public Health Institute
Contributes to the improvement of the health of populations internationally, nationally, and locally through excellence in research, education, and services.
Infect Dis, Pub Health
+41 61 284 81 11
https://vfapp.org/2ee4

Task Force for Global Health, The
Consists of programs and focus areas that cover a range of global health issues including neglected tropical diseases, infectious diseases, vaccines, field epidemiology, public health informatics, health workforce development, and global health ethics.
Infect Dis, Logist-Op, Medicine, Ophth-Opt, Peds
+1 404-371-0466
https://vfapp.org/714c

Tearfund
Responds to crisis and partners with local churches to bring restoration to those living in poverty, inspired by the Christian faith.
ER Med, Logist-Op
+44 20 3906 3906
https://vfapp.org/f6cf

Terre Des Hommes
Works to improve the conditions of the most vulnerable children worldwide by improving the health of children under the age of 3, protecting migrant children, providing humanitarian aid to children and their families in times of crisis, and preventing child exploitation.
ER Med, MF Med, Neonat, OB-GYN, Ped Surg, Peds
+41 58 611 06 66
https://vfapp.org/2689

Third World Eye Care Society (TWECS)
Collects old, unused eyeglasses and distributes them in conjunction with eye exams given by properly trained individuals.
Logist-Op, Ophth-Opt
+1 604-874-2733
https://vfapp.org/8618

Training for Health Equity Network (THEnet)
Contributes to health equity through health workforce education, research, and service, based on the principles of social accountability and community engagement.
ER Med, General
https://vfapp.org/38c6

Tsering's Fund
Provides assistance through private donations for deserving underprivileged children, young women, and families in Nepal, helping to change lives with educational scholarships, medical care, and basic living assistance.

Dent-OMFS, General
+1 406-579-2911
https://vfapp.org/39c1

Two Worlds Cancer Collaboration
Collaborates with local care professionals in lesser-resourced countries to help reduce the burden of cancer and other life-limiting illnesses.
Heme-Onc, Palliative, Peds, Pub Health, Rad-Onc
https://vfapp.org/fbdd

Union for International Cancer Control (UICC)
Unites and supports the cancer community to reduce the global cancer burden, promote greater equity, and ensure that cancer control continues to be a priority in the world health and development agenda.
Heme-Onc, Pub Health
+41 22 809 18 11
https://vfapp.org/88b1

United Mission Hospital Tansen
Aims to improve the quality of life of the people of Palpa District by providing high-quality primary healthcare and to provide training in primary healthcare.
All-Immu, Anesth, Dent-OMFS, Infect Dis, MF Med, Neonat, Psych
+977 75-520111
https://vfapp.org/5811

United Mission to Nepal (UMN)
Strives to address root causes of poverty as it serves the people of Nepal.
ER Med, General, Infect Dis, MF Med, Psych
+977 1-4268900
https://vfapp.org/cb26

United Nations Children's Fund (UNICEF)
Works in over 190 countries and territories to save children's lives, to defend their rights, and to help them fulfill their potential, from early childhood through adolescence.
All-Immu, Infect Dis, MF Med, Neonat, Nutr, OB-GYN, Ped Surg, Peds, Pub Health
https://vfapp.org/42d7

United Nations Development Programme (UNDP)
Helps countries achieve the simultaneous eradication of extreme poverty and significant reduction of inequalities and exclusion using a sustainable human development approach.
Infect Dis, Logist-Op, Pub Health
https://vfapp.org/935c

United Nations High Commissioner for Refugees (UNHCR)
Safeguards the rights and well-being of people who have been forced to flee, ensuring that everybody has the right to seek asylum and find safe refuge in another country, with the goal of seeking lasting solutions.
General, MF Med, Medicine, OB-GYN, Peds, Psych, Pub Health
https://vfapp.org/6636

United Nations Population Fund (UNFPA)
Supports reproductive healthcare for women and youth in more than 150 countries, focusing on delivering a world where every pregnancy is wanted, every childbirth is safe, and every young

person's potential is fulfilled.

Infect Dis, MF Med, Neonat, OB-GYN, Peds, Pub Health

+1 212-963-6008

https://vfapp.org/c969

United States Agency for International Development (USAID)

Promotes and demonstrates democratic values abroad and advances a free, peaceful, and prosperous world. Leads the U.S. government's international development and disaster assistance through partnerships and investments that save lives.

ER Med, Infect Dis, MF Med, OB-GYN, Peds

+1 202-712-0000

https://vfapp.org/9a99

United Surgeons for Children (USFC)

Pursues greater health and opportunity for children in the most neglected pockets of the world, with a specific focus and expertise in surgery.

Anesth, CT Surg, Neonat, Neurosurg, OB-GYN, Peds, Radiol, Surg

https://vfapp.org/3b4c

University of Illinois at Chicago: Center for Global Health

Aims to improve the health of populations around the world and reduce health disparities by collaboratively conducting trans-disciplinary research, training the next generations of global health leaders, and building the capacities of global and local partners.

Pub Health

+1 312-355-4116

https://vfapp.org/b749

University of California Los Angeles: David Geffen School of Medicine Global Health Program

Catalyzes opportunities to improve health globally by engaging in multi-disciplinary and innovative education programs, research initiatives, and bilateral partnerships that provide opportunities for trainees, faculty, and staff to contribute to sustainable health initiatives and to address health inequities facing the world today.

All-Immu, Infect Dis, Logist-Op, MF Med, Medicine, Neonat, OB-GYN, Ortho, Ped Surg, Peds, Radiol

+1 310-312-0531

https://vfapp.org/f1a4

University of California San Francisco: Francis I. Proctor Foundation for Ophthalmology

Aims to prevent blindness worldwide through research and teaching focused on infectious and inflammatory eye disease.

Ophth-Opt, Pub Health

+1 415-476-1442

https://vfapp.org/cf47

University of California San Francisco: Institute for Global Health Sciences

Dedicates its efforts to improving health and reducing the burden of disease in the world's most vulnerable populations by integrating expertise in the health, social, and biological sciences to train global health leaders and develop solutions to the most pressing health challenges.

Infect Dis, OB-GYN, Pub Health

+1 415-476-5494

https://vfapp.org/6587

University of Colorado: Global Emergency Care Initiative

Strives to sustainably improve emergency care outcomes in low- and middle-income communities worldwide by linking cutting-edge academics with excellent on-the-ground implementation.

ER Med

https://vfapp.org/417a

University of Michigan: Department of Surgery Global Health

Improves the health of patients, populations and communities through excellence in education, patient care, community service, research and technology development, and through leadership activities.

Anesth, Ortho, Surg

+1 734-936-5732

https://vfapp.org/2fd8

University of Pennsylvania Perelman School of Medicine Center for Global Health

Aims to improve health equity worldwide – through enhanced public health awareness and access to care, discovery and outcomes based research, and comprehensive educational programs grounded in partnership.

+1 215-898-0848

https://vfapp.org/cb57

University of Utah Global Health

Supports local organizations in their quest to improve quality of life in their communities all over the world.

Anesth, CT Surg, CV Med, Crit-Care, Dent-OMFS, ENT, ER Med, Infect Dis, OB-GYN, Ophth-Opt, Ped Surg, Ped Surg, Peds, Plast, Pub Health, Surg, Urol

+1 801-585-1509

https://vfapp.org/bacd

USAID: Maternal and Child Survival Program

Works to prevent child and maternal deaths.

Infect Dis, MF Med, Neonat, OB-GYN, Peds

https://vfapp.org/6fcf

USAID: Maternal and Child Health Integrated Program

Works to improve the health of women and their families, including programs for maternal, newborn, and child health, immunization, family planning, nutrition, malaria, and HIV/AIDS.

All-Immu, General, Infect Dis, MF Med

+1 202-835-3136

https://vfapp.org/4415

Vision Care

Restores sight and helps patients get regular treatment at short-term eye camps and long-term base clinics by having doctors, missionaries, volunteers, and sponsors work together.

Ophth-Opt

+1 212-769-3056

https://vfapp.org/9d7c

Vitamin Angels

Helps at-risk populations in need—specifically pregnant women, new mothers, and children under age five—to gain access to life-changing vitamins and minerals.

General, Nutr

+1 805-564-8400

https://vfapp.org/7da1

Voluntary Service Overseas (VSO)
Works with health workers, communities, and governments to improve health services and rights for women, babies, youth, people with disabilities, and prisoners.

General, MF Med, OB-GYN

+44 20 8780 7500

https://vfapp.org/213d

Volunteers Initiative Nepal (VIN)
Empowers marginalized communities through equitable, inclusive, and holistic development programs in areas such as women's empowerment, children's development, youth empowerment, public health/healthcare, environmental conservation, and DRR.

General, Geri, Medicine, Path, Peds, Pub Health

+977 1-4362560

https://vfapp.org/92be

VOSH (Volunteer Optometric Services to Humanity) International
Facilitates the provision and the sustainability of vision care worldwide for people who can neither afford nor obtain such care.

Ophth-Opt

https://vfapp.org/a149

Washington Nepal Health Foundation (WNHF)
Provides reconstructive surgical services and medical/psychological support to underprivileged children with congenital and traumatic deformities such as burn injuries and cleft lips.

Anesth, Plast

+1 202-785-3175

https://vfapp.org/4cd3

Watsi
Uses technology to make healthcare a reality for those who might not otherwise be able to afford it.

Pub Health, Surg

+1 256-792-8747

https://vfapp.org/41a3

White Ribbon Alliance, The
Leads a movement for reproductive, maternal, and newborn health and accelerates progress by putting citizens at the center of global, national, and local health efforts.

MF Med, OB-GYN

+1 202-204-0324

https://vfapp.org/496b

Women Orthopaedist Global Outreach (WOGO)
Provides free, life-altering orthopedic surgery that eliminates debilitating arthritis and restores disabled joints so that women can reclaim their ability to care for themselves, their families, and their communities.

Anesth, Ortho, Rehab, Surg

+1 844-588-9646

https://vfapp.org/6386

Women's Foundation Nepal, The
Helps women and children in Nepal who are victims of violence, abuse, and poverty.

Dent-OMFS, Ophth-Opt

+977 1-5155160

https://vfapp.org/b251

Women's Refugee Commission
Seeks to improve lives by protecting the rights of women, children, and youth displaced by conflict and crisis through researching their needs, identifying solutions, and advocating for programs and policies to strengthen their resilience.

General, MF Med, Neonat, OB-GYN, Peds, Psych

+1 212-551-3115

https://vfapp.org/3d8f

World Health Organization, The (WHO)
The United Nations' agency for health provides leadership on global health matters, shapes the health research agenda, setting norms and standards, articulates evidence-based policy options, provides technical support and monitoring to countries, and assesses health trends.

ER Med, General, Infect Dis, Logist-Op, MF Med, OB-GYN, Peds, Psych, Pub Health

+41 22 791 21 11

https://vfapp.org/c476

World Medical Relief
Facilitates the distribution of surplus medical resources where they are needed.

Logist-Op

+1 313-866-5333

https://vfapp.org/72dc

World Vision International
Works with vulnerable communities around the world to overcome poverty and injustice with child-focused programs.

ER Med, General, Infect Dis, MF Med, Nutr, OB-GYN, Peds

+1 626-303-8811

https://vfapp.org/2642

Worldwide Healing Hands
Works to improve the quality of healthcare for women and children in the most underserved areas of the world and to stop the preventable deaths of mothers.

General, MF Med, Neonat, OB-GYN

+1 707-279-8733

https://vfapp.org/b331

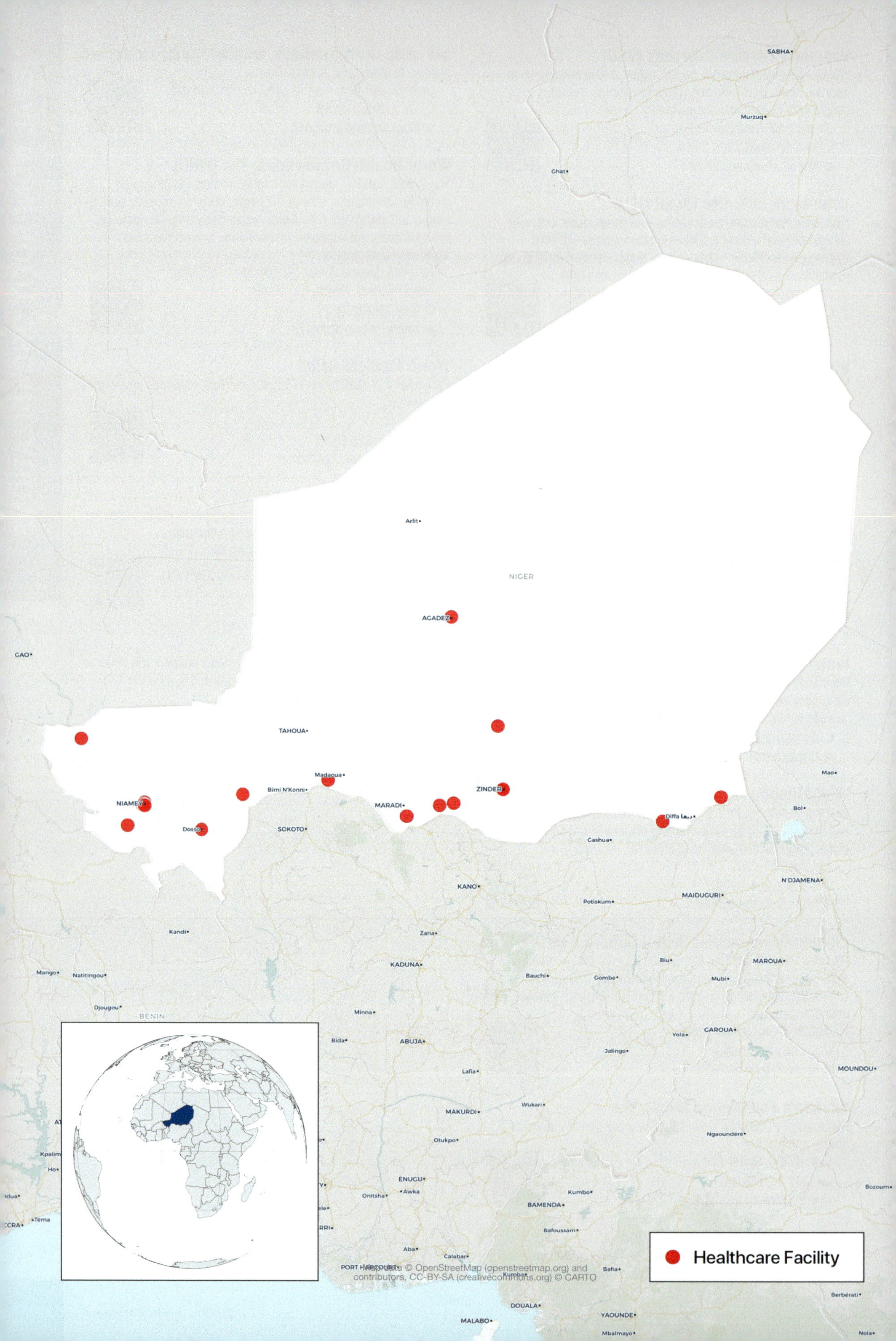
SABHA
Murzuq
Ghat
Arlit
NIGER
AGADEZ
GAO
TAHOUA
Madaoua
Birni N'Konni
NIAMEY
Dosso
SOKOTO
MARADI
ZINDER
Diffa
Mao
Bol
Gashua
N'DJAMENA
KANO
MAIDUGURI
Potiskum
Kandi
Zaria
KADUNA
Bauchi
Gombe
Biu
MAROUA
Mubi
Mango
Natitingou
Djougou
BENIN
Minna
Bida
ABUJA
Yola
GAROUA
Jalingo
Lafia
MOUNDOU
Wukari
MAKURDI
Ngaoundéré
Otukpo
ENUGU
Awka
Onitsha
Kumbo
BAMENDA
Bafoussam
Bozoum
Aba
Calabar
PORT HARCOURT
Bafia
Kumba
DOUALA
YAOUNDE
MALABO
Mbalmayo
Berbérati
Nola
Tema
© OpenStreetMap (openstreetmap.org) and contributors, CC-BY-SA (creativecommons.org) © CARTO
Healthcare Facility

Niger

The Republic of Niger is a landlocked West African country with a population of about 22.8 million mostly living in rural areas. The country's name stems from the presence of the Niger River that winds through the country. The Niger landscape is unique, composed predominantly of desert plains and sand dunes. The terrain is matched by a desert-like climate: hot, dry, and dusty, with extreme heat sometimes reaching 46 degrees Celsius. A predominantly Muslim country, Niger has a variety of linguistic groups, such as Hausa, a name which also refers to its largest ethnic group.

Following its independence from France in 1960, the country experienced several periods of violence and coups. To this day, access to basic rights remain a problem in Niger; slavery was banned only in 2003. About 41 percent of the population live in extreme poverty.

Despite extreme poverty, life expectancy and child mortality rates have been improving over the decades. The leading causes of death include diarrheal diseases, malaria, lower respiratory infections, neonatal disorders, measles, meningitis, tuberculosis, and invasive nontyphoidal salmonella (iNTS). Non-communicable diseases such as stroke, ischemic heart diseases, and congenital defects have also increased to contribute to a significant number of deaths over time. Malnutrition is the main risk factor for death and disability, as 42 percent of children under age five suffer from chronic malnutrition, and about 10 percent suffer from acute malnutrition. Pediatric ailments persist due to a young population, with death from neonatal disorders rising dramatically. Niger has the highest fertility rate in the world, with approximately seven children per woman.

22.8M
Population

$555
GDP Per Capita

62 years
Life Expectancy
↑ Improving

4.3
Doctors/100k
Physician Density

39
Beds/100k
Hospital Bed Density

509
Deaths/100k
Maternal Mortality

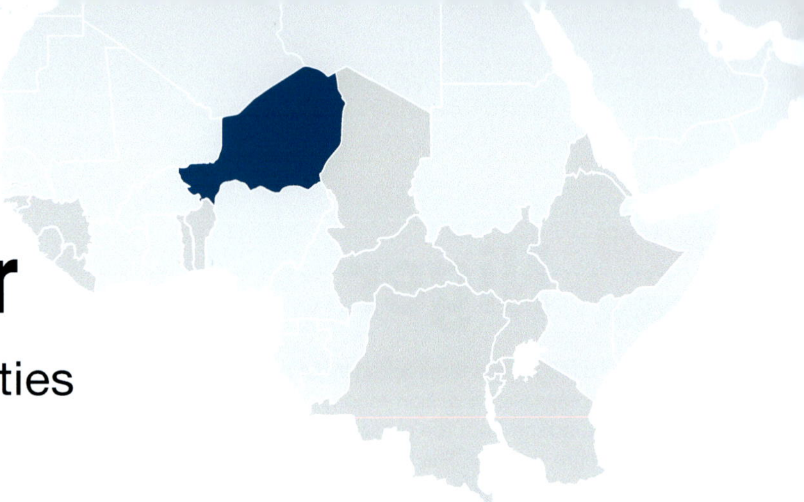

Niger

Healthcare Facilities

Aguié Public Hospital
Aguié, Niger
https://vfapp.org/8485

Centre Hospitalier Régional
Diffa, Niger
https://vfapp.org/541e

Centre Hospitalier Régional Agadez
Agadez, Niger
https://vfapp.org/6a3d

Centre Mère et Enfant
Zinder, Niger
https://vfapp.org/58aa

Centre Pilote Tessaoua pour la Chirurgie Rurale
Tessaoua, Niger
https://vfapp.org/4354

CHU de Lamordé
Niamey, Niger
https://vfapp.org/ea85

CURE Niger
Boulevard Ibraim Baré Maïnassara, Niamey, Niamey, Niger
https://vfapp.org/1224

Galmi Hospital
Madaoua RN 1, Galmi, Niger
https://vfapp.org/8a64

Hospital at Madarounfa
Madarounfa, Madarounfa, Niger
https://vfapp.org/cb93

Hospital at Say
Say, Niger
https://vfapp.org/42b3

Hôpital d'Ayorou
N 1, Ayorou, Tillabéri, Niger
https://vfapp.org/8b3c

Hôpital de District Tânout
Tânout, Niger
https://vfapp.org/2a86

Hôpital de Gawèye
Rue KI – 10, Niamey, Niger
https://vfapp.org/cfd3

Hôpital District Sanitaire de Togone
Dogondoutchi, Niger
https://vfapp.org/7eb5

Hôpital Militaire de Niamey
Corniche de Gamkale, Niamey, Niamey, Niger
https://vfapp.org/dc6c

Hôpital National de Niamey
Avenue François Mitterrand, Niamey, Niamey, Niger
https://vfapp.org/b7bc

Hôpital Regional de Dosso
Dosso, Niger
https://vfapp.org/cb4c

Hôpital Regional de Zinder
N 1, Zinder, Mirriah, Niger
https://vfapp.org/1bc9

The Kirker Hospital
Maine-Soroa, Niger
https://vfapp.org/5b18

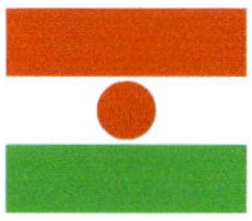

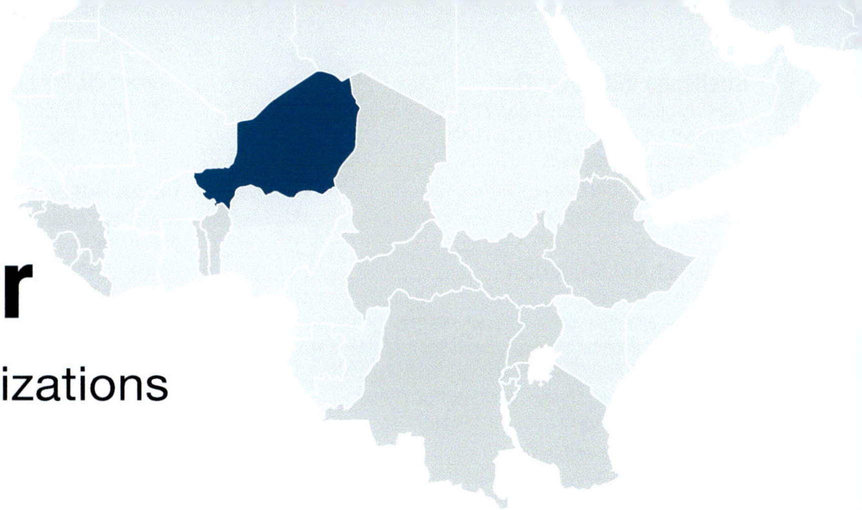

Niger

Nonprofit Organizations

Abt Associates

Seeks to improve the quality of life and economic well-being of people worldwide, while striving to meet and exceed the highest professional standards.

General, Logist-Op, MF Med, OB-GYN, Peds

+1 212-779-7700

https://vfapp.org/cec2

Action Against Hunger

Aims to end life-threatening hunger for good through treating and preventing malnutrition across more than forty-five countries.

+1 212-967-7800

https://vfapp.org/2dbc

Advance Family Planning

Aims to achieve global expansion and access to quality contraceptive information, services, and supplies through financial investment and political commitment.

General, MF Med, Pub Health

+1 410-502-8715

https://vfapp.org/7478

Africa CDC

Aims to strengthen the capacity and capability of Africa's public health institutions as well as partnerships to detect and respond quickly and effectively to disease threats and outbreaks, based on data-driven interventions and programs.

Infect Dis, Logist-Op, Pub Health

+251 11 551 7700

https://vfapp.org/339c

Alliance for International Medical Action, The (ALIMA)

Provides quality medical care to vulnerable populations, partnering with and developing national medical organizations and conducting medical research to bring innovation to twelve African countries where ALIMA works.

ER Med, General, Infect Dis, Logist-Op, MF Med, OB-GYN, Path, Peds, Psych, Pub Health

+1 646-619-9074

https://vfapp.org/1c11

Americares

Saves lives and improves health for people affected by poverty or disaster and responds with life-changing medicine, medical supplies, and health programs including domestic and global medical clinics.

All-Immu, ER Med, General, Infect Dis, MF Med, Nutr

+1 203-658-9500

https://vfapp.org/e567

AO Alliance

Builds solutions to lessen the burden of injuries in low- and middle-income countries, while enhancing the care of the injured to reduce human suffering, disability, and poverty.

Ortho, Surg

https://vfapp.org/8cd5

BroadReach

Collaborates with governments, multinational health organizations, donors, and private sector companies to affect healthcare reform and solve the world's biggest health challenges.

Logist-Op

+27 21 514 8300

https://vfapp.org/7812

CARE

Works around the globe to save lives, defeat poverty, and achieve social justice.

ER Med, General

+1 800-422-7385

https://vfapp.org/7232

Carter Center, The

Seeks to prevent and resolve conflicts, enhance freedom and democracy, and improve health, while remaining committed to human rights and the alleviation of human suffering.

Infect Dis, MF Med, Ophth-Opt

+1 800-550-3560

https://vfapp.org/6556

Center for Strategic and International Studies (CSIS) Commission on Strengthening America's Health Security

Brings together a distinguished and diverse group of high-level opinion leaders bridging security and health, with the core aim to chart a bold vision for the future of U.S. leadership in global health.

ER Med, Infect Dis, MF Med, Pub Health

+1 202-887-0200

https://vfapp.org/6d7f

Challenge Initiative, The

Seeks to rapidly and sustainably scale up proven reproductive health solutions among the urban poor.

MF Med, OB-GYN, Peds

📞 +1 410-502-8715

🌐 https://vfapp.org/2f77

Christian Aid Ministries

Strives to be a trustworthy and efficient channel for Amish, Mennonite, and other conservative Anabaptist groups and individuals to minister to physical and spiritual needs around the world.

CT Surg, ER Med, Logist-Op, Ortho, Pub Health

📞 +1 330-893-2428

🌐 https://vfapp.org/7b33

Christian Blind Mission (CBM)

Aims to improve the quality of life of persons with disabilities in the poorest countries, addressing poverty as a cause, and a consequence, of disability, and working in partnership to create a society for all.

ENT, General, Infect Dis, OB-GYN, Ophth-Opt, Ortho, Peds, Psych, Rehab, Surg

📞 +49 6251 131131

🌐 https://vfapp.org/3824

Christian Connections for International Health (CCIH)

Promotes global health and wholeness from a Christian perspective.

All-Immu, General, Infect Dis, MF Med, Neonat, OB-GYN, Psych

📞 +1 703-923-8960

🌐 https://vfapp.org/fa5d

Concern Worldwide

Seeks to permanently transform the lives of people living in extreme poverty, tackling its root causes, and building resilience.

Logist-Op, MF Med, Nutr, OB-GYN

📞 +353 1 417 7700

🌐 https://vfapp.org/77e9

Core Group

Aims to improve and expand community health practices for underserved populations, especially women and children, through collaborative action and learning.

General, Infect Dis, MF Med, Medicine, OB-GYN, Peds, Pub Health

📞 +1 202-380-3400

🌐 https://vfapp.org/9de3

CURE

Operates charitable hospitals and programs in underserved countries worldwide where patients receive surgical treatment, based in Christian ministry.

Anesth, Neurosurg, Ortho, Ped Surg, Peds, Rehab, Surg

📞 +1 616-512-3105

🌐 https://vfapp.org/aa16

Developing Country NGO Delegation: Global Fund to Fight AIDS, TB & Malaria

Works to strengthen the engagement of civil society actors and organizations in developing countries to contribute toward achieving a world in which AIDS, TB, and Malaria are no longer global, public health, and human rights threats.

Infect Dis, Pub Health

📞 +254 20 2515790

🌐 https://vfapp.org/3149

Direct Relief

Improves the health and lives of people affected by poverty or emergency situations by mobilizing and providing essential medical resources needed for their care.

ER Med, Logist-Op

📞 +1 805-964-4767

🌐 https://vfapp.org/58e5

Doctors Without Borders/Médecins Sans Frontières

Responds to emergencies and provides lifesaving medical care where needed most, including during disasters, conflicts, and epidemics.

Anesth, Crit-Care, ER Med, General, Infect Dis, Nutr, OB-GYN, Ped Surg, Peds, Psych, Pub Health, Surg

📞 +1 212-679-6800

🌐 https://vfapp.org/f363

eHealth Africa

Builds stronger health systems in Africa through the design and implementation of data-driven solutions, responding to local needs and providing underserved communities with the necessary tools to lead healthier lives.

Logist-Op, Path

🌐 https://vfapp.org/db6a

Enabel

As the development agency of the Belgian federal government, charged with implementing Belgium's international development policy, carries out public service assignments in Belgium and abroad pursuant to the 2030 Agenda for Sustainable Development.

General, Infect Dis, Logist-Op, MF Med, OB-GYN, Peds, Pub Health

📞 +32 2 505 37 00

🌐 https://vfapp.org/5af7

END Fund, The

Aims to control and eliminate the most prevalent neglected diseases among the world's poorest and most vulnerable people.

Infect Dis

📞 +1 646-690-9775

🌐 https://vfapp.org/2614

EngenderHealth

Works to implement high-quality, gender-equitable programs that advance sexual and reproductive health and rights.

General, MF Med, OB-GYN, Peds

📞 +1 202-902-2000

🌐 https://vfapp.org/1cb2

Eye Foundation of America

Works toward a world without childhood blindness.

Ophth-Opt

📞 +1 304-599-0705

🌐 https://vfapp.org/a7eb

USAID: Fistula Care Plus

A fistula repair and prevention project from USAID that builds on, enhances, and expands the work undertaken by the previous Fistula Care project (2007–2013), with attention to new areas of focus so that obstetric fistula can become a rare event for future generations.

MF Med, OB-GYN, Surg

+1 202-902-2000

https://vfapp.org/a7cd

Fistula Foundation

Aims to engage the support of people worldwide who are eager to see the day when no woman suffers from obstetric fistula. Raises and directs funds to doctors and hospitals providing life-transforming surgery to women in need.

OB-GYN

+1 408-249-9596

https://vfapp.org/e958

Global Clubfoot Initiative (GCI)

Promotes and resources the treatment of children with clubfoot in developing countries using the Ponseti technique.

Ortho, Ped Surg

https://vfapp.org/f229

Global Oncology (GO)

Brings the best in cancer care to underserved patients around the world and collaborates across geographic, professional, and academic borders to improve cancer care, research, and education.

Heme-Onc, Path, Rad-Onc

https://vfapp.org/fcb8

GOAL

Works with the most vulnerable communities to help them respond to and recover from humanitarian crises, and to assist them in building transcendent solutions to mitigate poverty and vulnerability.

ER Med, General, Pub Health

+353 1 280 9779

https://vfapp.org/bbea

Health Equity Initiative

Aims to build and sustain a global community that engages across sectors and disciplines to advance health equity.

Pub Health

https://vfapp.org/e2e2

Helen Keller International

Seeks to eliminate preventable vision loss, malnutrition, and diseases of poverty.

Infect Dis, Nutr, OB-GYN, Ophth-Opt, Peds

+1 212-532-0544

https://vfapp.org/b654

Hope Walks

Frees children, families, and communities from the burden of clubfoot, inspired by the Christian faith.

Ortho, Ped Surg, Peds, Rehab

+1 717-502-4400

https://vfapp.org/f6d4

Humanity & Inclusion

Works alongside people with disabilities and vulnerable populations, taking action and bearing witness in order to respond to their essential needs, improve their living conditions and health, and promote respect for their dignity and fundamental rights.

General, Infect Dis, MF Med, Medicine, Ortho, Peds, Psych, Pub Health, Rehab

+1 301-891-2138

https://vfapp.org/16b7

Humanity First

Provides aid and assistance to those in need, offering sustainable development solutions to society while providing and empowering local communities with the resources to help themselves.

ER Med, General, MF Med, Ophth-Opt

+44 20 8417 0082

https://vfapp.org/13cc

IMA World Health

Works to build healthier communities by collaborating with key partners to serve vulnerable people with a focus on health, healing, and well-being for all.

Infect Dis, MF Med, Nutr, OB-GYN, Pub Health

+1 202-888-6200

https://vfapp.org/8316

International Agency for the Prevention of Blindness (IAPB), The

Leads international efforts in blindness-prevention activities, works toward a world where no one is needlessly visually impaired, and ensures that everyone has access to the best possible standard of eye health.

Infect Dis, Ophth-Opt, Pub Health

https://vfapp.org/87a2

International Federation of Gynecology and Obstetrics (FIGO)

Implements global projects on specific women's health issues.

MF Med, Medicine, Neonat, OB-GYN, Surg, Urol

+44 20 7928 1166

https://vfapp.org/c4b4

International Federation of Red Cross and Red Crescent Societies (IFRC)

Coordinates and directs international assistance following natural and man-made disasters in nonconflict situations through the world's largest humanitarian and development network. Provides disaster-preparedness programs, healthcare activities, and promotes humanitarian values.

ER Med, General, Infect Dis, Nutr

+1 212-338-0161

https://vfapp.org/b4ee

International Learning Movement (ILM UK)

Supports some of the world's poorest people in developing countries with core projects in education, safe drinking water, and healthcare.

General, Ophth-Opt

+44 1254 265451

https://vfapp.org/b974

International Organization for Migration (IOM) – The UN Migration Agency

Promotes evidence-informed policies and holistic, preventive, and curative health programs that are beneficial, accessible, and equitable for vulnerable migrants.

General, Infect Dis, OB-GYN

+27 12 342 2789

https://vfapp.org/621a

International Organization for Women and Development (IOWD)

Provides underserved women and children in low-income countries with free medical and surgical services and care.

Anesth, MF Med, Neonat, OB-GYN, Ped Surg, Peds, Surg
+1 516-764-6370
https://vfapp.org/8ecb

International Relief Teams
Helps families survive and recover after a disaster by delivering timely and effective assistance through programs that improve their health and well-being while also providing a hopeful future for underserved communities.
Dent-OMFS, ER Med, General, Nutr, Ophth-Opt
+1 619-284-7979
https://vfapp.org/ffd5

International Rescue Committee (IRC)
Responds to the world's worst humanitarian crises and helps people whose lives and livelihoods are shattered by conflict and disaster to survive, recover, and gain control of their future.
ER Med, General, Infect Dis, MF Med, Peds
+1 212-551-3000
https://vfapp.org/5d24

Intersos
Provides emergency medical assistance to victims of armed conflicts, natural disasters, and extreme exclusion, with particular attention to the protection of the most vulnerable people.
ER Med, General, Nutr
+39 06 853 7431
https://vfapp.org/dbac

InterSurgeon
Fosters collaborative partnerships in the field of global surgery that will advance clinical care, teaching, training, research, and the provision and maintenance of medical equipment.
ENT, Neurosurg, Ortho, Ped Surg, Plast, Surg, Urol
https://vfapp.org/6f8a

IntraHealth International
Improves the performance of health workers and strengthens the systems in which they work.
CV Med, Endo, General, Infect Dis, MF Med, Neonat, Nutr, OB-GYN
+1 919-313-3554
https://vfapp.org/ddc8

Ipas
Focuses efforts on women and girls who want contraception or abortion, and builds programs around their needs and how best to support them.
OB-GYN
https://vfapp.org/8e39

Jhpiego
Creates and delivers transformative healthcare solutions that save lives in partnership with national governments, health experts, and local communities.
General, Infect Dis, OB-GYN, Surg
+1 410-537-1800
https://vfapp.org/45b8

John Snow, Inc. (JSI)
Aims to improve the health and well-being of underserved and vulnerable people and communities throughout the world.
General, Infect Dis, Logist-Op, MF Med, OB-GYN, Peds, Psych, Pub Health
+1 617-482-9485
https://vfapp.org/ba78

Johns Hopkins Center for Communication Programs
Believes in the power of communication to save lives, by empowering people to adopt healthy behaviors for themselves, their families, and their communities.
General, Infect Dis, Logist-Op, OB-GYN, Pub Health
+1 410-659-6300
https://vfapp.org/1bf9

Joint United Nations Programme on HIV/AIDS (UNAIDS)
Aims to place people living with HIV and people affected by the virus at the decision-making table and at the center of designing, delivering, and monitoring the AIDS response.
Infect Dis
+41 22 791 36 66
https://vfapp.org/464a

Leprosy Mission England and Wales, The
Leads the fight against leprosy by supporting people living with leprosy today and serving future generations by working to end the transmission of the disease.
Infect Dis, Pub Health
https://vfapp.org/4c67

Lions Clubs International
Empowers volunteers to serve their communities, meet humanitarian needs, encourage peace, and promote international understanding through Lions clubs.
Heme-Onc, Medicine, Nutr, Ophth-Opt
+1 630-571-5466
https://vfapp.org/7b12

London School of Hygiene & Tropical Medicine: Health in Humanitarian Crises Centre
Advances health and health equity in crisis-affected countries through research, education, and translation of knowledge into policy and practice.
ER Med, Infect Dis, Pub Health
+44 20 7636 8636
https://vfapp.org/96ad

MAP International
Provides medicines and health supplies to those in need around the world so they might experience life to the fullest.
Logist-Op
+1 800-225-8550
https://vfapp.org/deed

Marie Stopes International
Provides the contraception and safe abortion services that enable women all over the world to choose their own futures.
Infect Dis, MF Med, Neonat, OB-GYN, Pub Health
+44 20 7636 6200
https://vfapp.org/9525

Médecins du Monde/Doctors of the World
Provides care, bears witness, and supports social change worldwide with innovative medical programs and evidence-based advocacy initiatives.
ER Med, General, Infect Dis, MF Med, Neonat,

OB-GYN, Peds, Pub Health
📞 +33 1 44 92 15 15
🌐 https://vfapp.org/a43d

Medical Care Development International (MCD International)
Works to strengthen health systems through innovative, sustainable interventions.
Infect Dis, Logist-Op, OB-GYN, Pub Health
📞 +1 301-562-1920
🌐 https://vfapp.org/dc5c

Medici Per I Diritti Umani (MEDU)
Treats and brings medical aid to the most vulnerable populations, and—starting from medical practice—denounces violations of human rights and, in particular, exclusion from access to treatment.
ER Med, General, Psych, Pub Health
📞 +39 06 9784 4892
🌐 https://vfapp.org/5384

MedShare
Aims to improve the quality of life of people, communities, and the planet by sourcing and directly delivering surplus medical supplies and equipment to communities in need around the world.
Logist-Op
📞 +1 770-323-5858
🌐 https://vfapp.org/c8bc

Mérieux Foundation
Committed to fighting infectious diseases that affect developing countries by capacity building, particularly in clinical laboratories, and focusing on diagnosis.
Logist-Op, Path
📞 +33 4 72 40 79 79
🌐 https://vfapp.org/a23a

NCD Alliance
Unites and strengthens civil society to stimulate collaborative advocacy, action, and accountability for NCD (noncommunicable disease) prevention and control.
All-Immu, CV Med, General, Heme-Onc, Medicine, Peds, Psych
📞 +41 22 809 18 11
🌐 https://vfapp.org/abdd

Operation Fistula
Exists to end obstetric fistula by building models of care that serve every woman, everywhere.
MF Med, OB-GYN, Surg
📞 +1 512-687-3479
🌐 https://vfapp.org/ce8e

Pan-African Academy of Christian Surgeons (PAACS)
Exists to train and support African surgeons to provide excellent, compassionate care to those most in need, inspired by the Christian faith.
Anesth, CT Surg, Neurosurg, OB-GYN, Ortho, Ped Surg, Plast, Surg
📞 +1 847-571-9926
🌐 https://vfapp.org/85ba

Pathfinder International
Champions sexual and reproductive health and rights worldwide, mobilizing communities most in need to break through barriers and forge paths to a healthier future.
OB-GYN
📞 +1 617-924-7200
🌐 https://vfapp.org/a7b3

Pharmacists Without Borders Canada
Provides pharmaceutical and technical assistance in the implementation or improvement of community and hospital pharmacies internationally.
📞 +1 514-842-8923
🌐 https://vfapp.org/7658

PSI – Population Services International
Dedicates efforts to improving the health of people in the developing world by focusing on challenges such as a lack of family planning, HIV/AIDS, barriers to maternal health, and the greatest threats to children under the age of 5, including malaria, diarrhea, pneumonia, and malnutrition.
Infect Dis, MF Med, OB-GYN, Peds
📞 +1 202-785-0072
🌐 https://vfapp.org/ffe3

RestoringVision
Empowers lives by restoring vision for millions of people in need.
Ophth-Opt
📞 +1 209-980-7323
🌐 https://vfapp.org/e121

Rockefeller Foundation, The
Works to promote the well-being of humanity.
Logist-Op, Nutr, Pub Health
📞 +1 212-869-8500
🌐 https://vfapp.org/5424

Rotary International
Provides service to others, improves lives, and advances world understanding, goodwill, and peace through its fellowship of business, professional, and community leaders.
ER Med, General, Infect Dis, MF Med, OB-GYN
🌐 https://vfapp.org/8fb5

Samaritan's Purse International Disaster Relief
Provides spiritual and physical aid to hurting people around the world, such as victims of war, poverty, natural disasters, disease, and famine, based in Christian ministry.
Anesth, CT Surg, Crit-Care, Dent-OMFS, Derm, ENT, ER Med, Endo, GI, General, Heme-Onc, Infect Dis, MF Med, Neonat, Nephro, Neuro, Neurosurg, Nutr, OB-GYN, Ophth-Opt, Ortho, Path, Ped Surg, Peds, Plast, Psych, Pulm-Critic, Radiol, Rehab, Rheum, Surg, Urol, Vasc Surg
📞 +1 800-528-1980
🌐 https://vfapp.org/87e3

Sanofi Espoir Foundation
Contributes to reducing health inequalities among populations that need it most by applying a socially responsible approach focused on fighting childhood cancers in low-income countries, improving maternal and newborn health, and improving access to care.
ER Med, OB-GYN, Peds
📞 +33 1 53 77 91 38
🌐 https://vfapp.org/943b

SATMED
Serves non-governmental organizations, hospitals, medical

universities, and other healthcare providers active in resource-poor areas, by providing open-access e-health services for the health community.

Logist-Op

https://vfapp.org/b8d5

Save the Children

Gives children around the world a healthy start in life, the opportunity to learn, and protection from harm.

All-Immu, Crit-Care, ER Med, General, Infect Dis, MF Med, Medicine, Neonat, OB-GYN, Peds, Psych, Pub Health

+1 800-728-3843

https://vfapp.org/2e73

SIGN Fracture Care International

Builds orthopedic capacity around the world and provides the injured poor access to fracture surgery by donating orthopedic education and implant systems to surgeons in developing countries.

Ortho, Rehab, Surg

+1 509-371-1107

https://vfapp.org/123d

Smile Train

Seeks to give every child with a cleft the opportunity for a healthy, productive life by providing free cleft repair surgery and comprehensive cleft care in their own communities.

Dent-OMFS, ENT, Plast

+1 800-932-9541

https://vfapp.org/f21d

Solthis

Improves disease prevention and access to quality care by strengthening the health systems and services of the countries served.

General, Infect Dis, Logist-Op, MF Med, Neonat, Path

+33 1 81 70 17 90

https://vfapp.org/a71d

Swiss Tropical and Public Health Institute

Contributes to the improvement of the health of populations internationally, nationally, and locally through excellence in research, education, and services.

Infect Dis, Pub Health

+41 61 284 81 11

https://vfapp.org/2ee4

Task Force for Global Health, The

Consists of programs and focus areas that cover a range of global health issues including neglected tropical diseases, infectious diseases, vaccines, field epidemiology, public health informatics, health workforce development, and global health ethics.

Infect Dis, Logist-Op, Medicine, Ophth-Opt, Peds

+1 404-371-0466

https://vfapp.org/714c

Tearfund

Responds to crisis and partners with local churches to bring restoration to those living in poverty, inspired by the Christian faith.

ER Med, Logist-Op

+44 20 3906 3906

https://vfapp.org/f6cf

Turing Foundation

Aims to contribute toward a better world and a better society by focusing on efforts such as health, art, education, and nature.

Infect Dis

+31 20 520 0010

https://vfapp.org/6bcc

U.S. President's Malaria Initiative (PMI)

Supports low-income countries to help control and eliminate malaria through cost-effective, lifesaving malaria interventions.

Infect Dis, MF Med, OB-GYN

+1 202-712-0000

https://vfapp.org/dc8b

Union for International Cancer Control (UICC)

Unites and supports the cancer community to reduce the global cancer burden, promote greater equity, and ensure that cancer control continues to be a priority in the world health and development agenda.

Heme-Onc, Pub Health

+41 22 809 18 11

https://vfapp.org/88b1

United Nations Children's Fund (UNICEF)

Works in over 190 countries and territories to save children's lives, to defend their rights, and to help them fulfill their potential, from early childhood through adolescence.

All-Immu, Infect Dis, MF Med, Neonat, Nutr, OB-GYN, Ped Surg, Peds, Pub Health

https://vfapp.org/42d7

United Nations High Commissioner for Refugees (UNHCR)

Safeguards the rights and well-being of people who have been forced to flee, ensuring that everybody has the right to seek asylum and find safe refuge in another country, with the goal of seeking lasting solutions.

General, MF Med, Medicine, OB-GYN, Peds, Psych, Pub Health

https://vfapp.org/6636

United Nations Office for the Coordination of Humanitarian Affairs (OCHA)

Contributes to principled and effective humanitarian response through coordination, advocacy, policy, information management, and humanitarian financing tools and services, by leveraging functional expertise throughout the organization.

Logist-Op

https://vfapp.org/22b8

United Nations Population Fund (UNFPA)

Supports reproductive healthcare for women and youth in more than 150 countries, focusing on delivering a world where every pregnancy is wanted, every childbirth is safe, and every young person's potential is fulfilled.

Infect Dis, MF Med, Neonat, OB-GYN, Peds, Pub Health

+1 212-963-6008

https://vfapp.org/c969

United States Agency for International Development (USAID)

Promotes and demonstrates democratic values abroad and advances a free, peaceful, and prosperous world. Leads the U.S.

government's international development and disaster assistance through partnerships and investments that save lives.

ER Med, Infect Dis, MF Med, OB-GYN, Peds

+1 202-712-0000

https://vfapp.org/9a99

University of California San Francisco: Francis I. Proctor Foundation for Ophthalmology

Aims to prevent blindness worldwide through research and teaching focused on infectious and inflammatory eye disease.

Ophth-Opt, Pub Health

+1 415-476-1442

https://vfapp.org/cf47

USAID: Human Resources for Health 2030 (HRH2030)

Helps low- and middle-income countries develop the health workforce needed to prevent maternal and child deaths, support the goals of Family Planning 2020, control the HIV/AIDS epidemic, and protect communities from infectious diseases.

Logist-Op

+1 202-955-3300

https://vfapp.org/9ea8

Vision Outreach International

Advocates for helping the blind in underserved regions of the world and empowers the poor through sight restoration.

Ophth-Opt

+1 269-428-3300

https://vfapp.org/9721

West African Health Organization

Aims to attain high standards and protection of health of the people in West Africa through harmonization of policies of the member states to combat health problems.

Infect Dis, MF Med, OB-GYN

+226 20 97 01 00

https://vfapp.org/7363

World Health Organization, The (WHO)

The United Nations' agency for health provides leadership on global health matters, shapes the health research agenda, setting norms and standards, articulates evidence-based policy options, provides technical support and monitoring to countries, and assesses health trends.

ER Med, General, Infect Dis, Logist-Op, MF Med, OB-GYN, Peds, Psych, Pub Health

+41 22 791 21 11

https://vfapp.org/c476

World Medical Relief

Facilitates the distribution of surplus medical resources where they are needed.

Logist-Op

+1 313-866-5333

https://vfapp.org/72dc

World Vision International

Works with vulnerable communities around the world to overcome poverty and injustice with child-focused programs.

ER Med, General, Infect Dis, MF Med, Nutr, OB-GYN, Peds

+1 626-303-8811

https://vfapp.org/2642

Worldwide Fistula Fund

Protects and restores the health and dignity of the world's most vulnerable women by preventing and treating devastating childbirth injuries.

OB-GYN

+1 847-592-2438

https://vfapp.org/8813

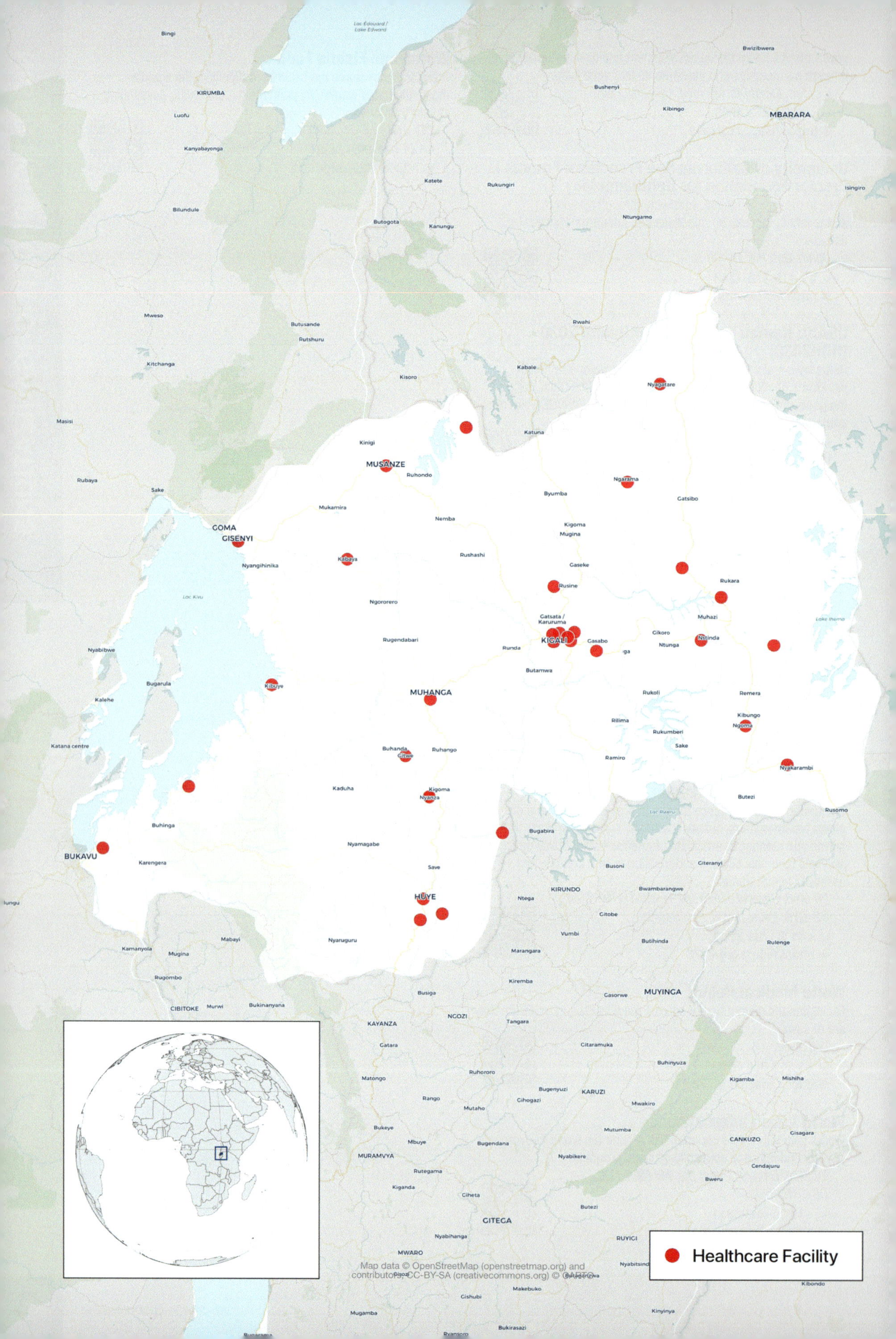

Lac Édouard / Lake Edward
Bingi
Bwizibwera
KIRUMBA
Bushenyi
Kibingo
MBARARA
Luofu
Kanyabayonga
Katete
Rukungiri
Isingiro
Bilundule
Butogota
Kanungu
Ntungamo
Mweso
Butusande
Rutshuru
Rwahi
Kitchanga
Kabale
Kisoro
Nyagatare
Masisi
Kinigi
Katuna
MUSANZE
Ruhondo
Rubaya
Ngarama
Sake
Byumba
Mukamira
Gatsibo
Nemba
GOMA
GISENYI
Kigoma
Mugina
Rushashi
Kabaya
Gaseke
Nyangihinika
Rusine
Rukara
Lac Kivu
Ngororero
Gatsata / Karuruma
Muhazi
Lake Ihema
Rugendabari
KIGALI
Gasabo
Gikoro
Ntunga
Nstinda
Nyabibwe
Runda
Butamwa
Bugarula
Kibuye
MUHANGA
Rukoli
Remera
Kalehe
Rilima
Kibungo
Ngoma
Rukumberi
Katana centre
Buhanda
Gitwe
Ruhango
Sake
Ramiro
Nyakarambi
Kaduha
Kigoma
Nyanza
Butezi
Rusomo
Lac Rweru
Buhinga
Bugabira
Nyamagabe
BUKAVU
Karengera
Busoni
Giteranyi
Save
KIRUNDO
Bwambarangwe
HUYE
Ntega
Gitobe
Vumbi
Butihinda
Rulenge
Mabayi
Nyaruguru
Kamanyola
Mugina
Marangara
Rugombo
Kiremba
Busiga
Gasorwe
MUYINGA
CIBITOKE
Murwi
Bukinanyana
KAYANZA
NGOZI
Tangara
Gatara
Citaramuka
Buhinyuza
Matongo
Ruhororo
Kigamba
Mishiha
Bugenyuzi
KARUZI
Rango
Gihogazi
Mutaho
Mwakiro
Bukeye
Mutumba
Gisagara
Mbuye
Bugendana
CANKUZO
MURAMVYA
Nyabikere
Rutegama
Cendajuru
Kiganda
Giheta
Bweru
Butezi
GITEGA
Nyabihanga
RUYIGI
MWARO
Nyabitsinda
Makebuko
Gishubi
Kibondo
Mugamba
Kinyinya
Bukirasazi
Ryansoro
Healthcare Facility
Map data © OpenStreetMap (openstreetmap.org) and contributors, CC-BY-SA (creativecommons.org)

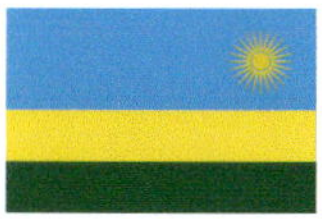

Rwanda

The Republic of Rwanda is a landlocked country just south of the equator in East-Central Africa. While small geographically, the country is home to 12.7 million people, making it one of Africa's most densely populated countries. Rwanda has been highly influenced by Christianity. Its three official languages are Kinyarwanda, English, and French. Rwanda, also called "the land of a thousand hills," is widely known for its nature and wildlife, especially the protected gorillas of Volcanoes National Park.

Rwanda's history has been marked by tension between the Hutu and Tutsi ethnic groups and the brutal genocide of the 1990s. Since the end of the genocide, Rwanda has undergone a period of reconstruction and worked to turn a new chapter, having greatly improved its political stability and economic conditions. This primarily agricultural country has significantly reduced its poverty rate from 59 percent to 39 percent between 2001 and 2014. Rwanda has also made improvements in its social policies, such as near-universal primary school enrollment. At its current rate, the country strives to reach middle-income status by 2035 and high-income status by 2050.

For both males and females, life expectancy has steadily increased. Similarly, child mortality rates have declined by over two-thirds. While some health indicators have improved, the population experiences high levels of death caused by lower respiratory infections, neonatal disorders, tuberculosis, diarrheal diseases, malaria, and HIV/AIDS. Nearly 100 percent of the country is at risk of contracting malaria. Death due to non-communicable diseases is also significant, with congenital defects, stroke, ischemic heart disease, and cirrhosis causing substantial mortality. Rates of cirrhosis, which may be caused by excessive alcohol consumption, are significantly higher than those of other countries in the region. Road injuries also cause significant numbers of deaths in Rwanda.

12.7M
Population

$802
GDP Per Capita

69 years
Life Expectancy
↑ Improving

13.4
Doctors/100k
Physician Density

160
Beds/100k
Hospital Bed Density

248
Deaths/100k
Maternal Mortality

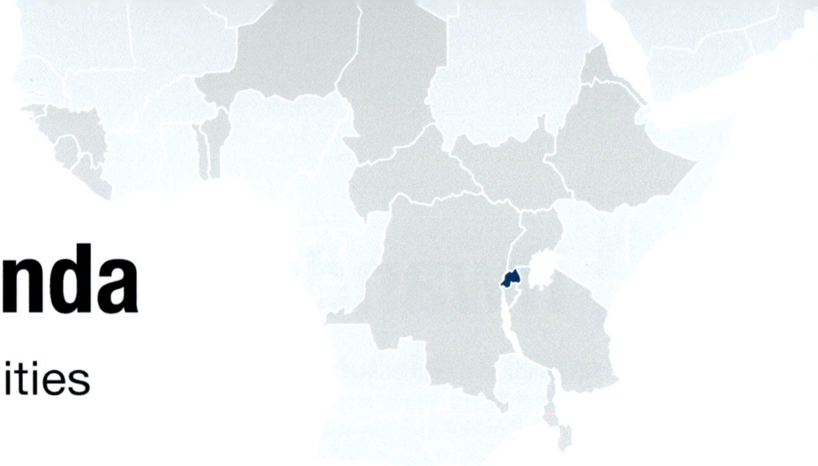

Rwanda

Healthcare Facilities

Baho International Hospital
KG 9 Ave 42, Kigali, Kigali, Rwanda
https://vfapp.org/f628

Butaro Hospital
NR21, Butaro, Majyaruguru, Rwanda
https://vfapp.org/f85b

Gahini Hospital
NR24, Urugarama, Iburasirasuba, Rwanda
https://vfapp.org/57ba

Gakoma
DR90, Mamba, Amajyepfo, Rwanda
https://vfapp.org/f2b1

Gihundwe District Hospital
Cyangugu, Rwanda
https://vfapp.org/36f2

Gisenyi District Hospital
Gisenyi, Rwanda
https://vfapp.org/e48b

Gitwe Hospital
NR6, Bwerama, Amajyepfo, Rwanda
https://vfapp.org/e2c9

HVP Gatagara
Kigali, Rwanda
https://vfapp.org/ce4b

Hôpital La Croix du Sud
KG 201 St, Kigali, Rwanda
https://vfapp.org/3b84

Kabaya Hospital
Kabaya, Rwanda
https://vfapp.org/b4bd

Kabgayi District Hospital
Kabgayi – Cyakabiri, Gitarama, Rwanda
https://vfapp.org/f3a2

Karongi Hospital
NR11, Bwishyura, Iburengerazuba, Rwanda
https://vfapp.org/f59c

Kibagabaga Hospital
KG 265 Street, Kinyinya, Umujyi wa Kigali, Rwanda
https://vfapp.org/a2d3

Kibilizi
DR107, Kibilizi, Amajyepfo, Rwanda
https://vfapp.org/acdb

Kibogora Hospital
NR11, Kanjongo, Iburengerazuba, Rwanda
https://vfapp.org/dcd8

King Faisal Hospital
KG 544 St, Kigali, Rwanda
https://vfapp.org/c1c3

Kirehe District Hospital
NR4, Mukarange, Iburasirasuba, Rwanda
https://vfapp.org/cd7c

Kiziguro Hospital
NR24, Nyakayaga, Iburasirasuba, Rwanda
https://vfapp.org/f88c

Muhima Hospital
Kigali, Rwanda
https://vfapp.org/8a12

Mukura Hospital
Mukura, Rwanda
https://vfapp.org/2462

Musanze Hospital
Ruhengeri – Gisenyi Road, Muhoza, Majyaruguru, Rwanda
https://vfapp.org/1cfa

Ngarama Hospital
Nyagahita – Ngarama Road, Ngarama, Rwanda
https://vfapp.org/6c45

Nyagatare Hospital
Nyagatare, Rwanda
https://vfapp.org/d15c

Nyanza District Hospital
Nyanza, Busasamana, Rwanda
https://vfapp.org/9d3c

Nyanza Hospital
NR6, Busasamana, Amajyepfo, Rwanda
https://vfapp.org/5452

Rwamagana Hospital
Rwamagana-Kayonza Road, Kigabiro, Iburasirasuba, Rwanda
https://vfapp.org/3399

Rwanda Military Hospital
Street KK739ST Kanombe,
Kicukiro District, Kigali,
Rwanda
⊕ https://vfapp.org/8253

Rwanda Red Cross
KG 15 Ave, Kigali, Rwanda
⊕ https://vfapp.org/ef3a

Rwinkwavu Hospital
Rwinkwavu, Rwanda
⊕ https://vfapp.org/2ad6

University Teaching Hospital of Butare
Avenue de l'Universite, Ngoma,
Amajvepfo, Rwanda
⊕ https://vfapp.org/e5b8

University Teaching Hospital of Kigali
KN 4 Ave, Kigali, Rwanda
⊕ https://vfapp.org/4a8b

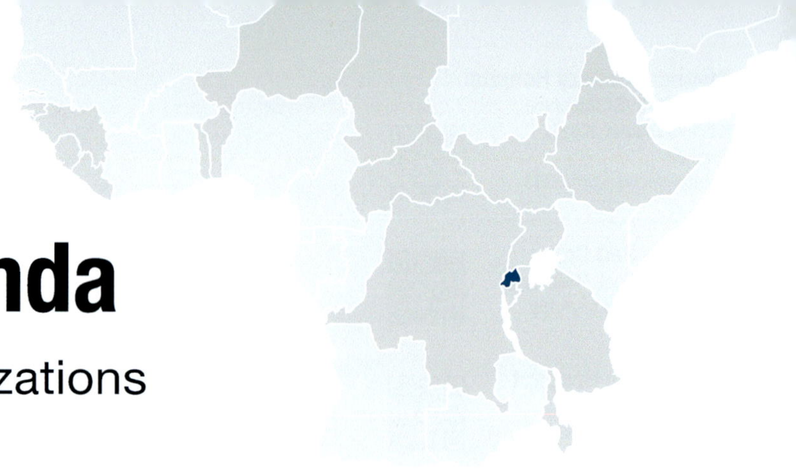

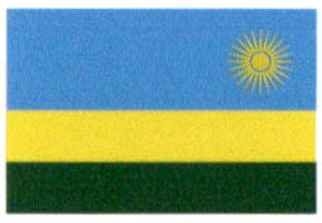

Rwanda

Nonprofit Organizations

A Broader View Volunteers
Provides developing countries around the world with significant volunteer programs that both aid the neediest communities and forge a lasting bond between those volunteering and those they have helped.

Dent-OMFS, ER Med, Infect Dis, MF Med
📞 +1 215-780-1845
🌐 https://vfapp.org/3bec

Abt Associates
Seeks to improve the quality of life and economic well-being of people worldwide, while striving to meet and exceed the highest professional standards.

General, Logist-Op, MF Med, OB-GYN, Peds
📞 +1 212-779-7700
🌐 https://vfapp.org/cec2

Aceso Global
Provides strategic healthcare advisory services in low- and middle-income countries to design and deliver highly customized, evidence-based solutions that address the complex nature of healthcare systems, with a goal to strengthen and provide affordable, high-quality care to all.

Logist-Op, Pub Health
📞 +1 202-758-2636
🌐 https://vfapp.org/b3b7

Action Kibogora
Works to redevelop and rebuild the maternity and neonatology wards at Kibogora Hospital.

Logist-Op, MF Med, Neonat, Peds
🌐 https://vfapp.org/29f9

Adventist Health International
Focuses on upgrading and managing mission hospitals by providing governance, consultation, and technical assistance to a number of affiliated Seventh-Day Adventist hospitals throughout Africa, Asia, and the Americas.

Dent-OMFS, General, Pub Health
📞 +1 909-558-5610
🌐 https://vfapp.org/16aa

Africa CDC
Aims to strengthen the capacity and capability of Africa's public health institutions as well as partnerships to detect and respond quickly and effectively to disease threats and outbreaks, based on data-driven interventions and programs.

Infect Dis, Logist-Op, Pub Health
📞 +251 11 551 7700
🌐 https://vfapp.org/339c

Africa Humanitarian Action (AHA)
Responds to crises, conflicts, and disasters in Africa, while informing and advising the international community, governments, civil society, and the private sector on humanitarian issues of concern to Africa. Supports institutional and organizational development efforts.

General, Infect Dis, MF Med, Nutr, OB-GYN
📞 +251 11 660 4800
🌐 https://vfapp.org/3ca2

Africa Indoor Residual Spraying Project (AIRS)
Aims to protect millions of people in Africa from malaria by spraying insecticide on the walls, ceilings, and other indoor resting places of mosquitoes that transmit malaria.

Infect Dis
📞 +1 301-347-5000
🌐 https://vfapp.org/9bd1

African Field Epidemiology Network (AFENET)
Strengthens field epidemiology and public health laboratory capacity to contribute effectively to addressing epidemics and other major public health problems in Africa.

All-Immu, Infect Dis, Path, Pub Health
🌐 https://vfapp.org/df2e

Africa Inland Mission International
Seeks to establish churches and community development programs including health care projects, based in Christian ministry.

Anesth, Dent-OMFS, ER Med, General, MF Med, Medicine, OB-GYN, OB-GYN, Ophth-Opt, Ped Surg, Peds, Rehab
🌐 https://vfapp.org/f2f6

Against Malaria Foundation
Helps protect people from malaria. Funds anti-malaria nets, specifically long-lasting insecticidal nets (LLINs), and works with distribution partners to ensure they are used. Tracks and reports on net use and malaria case data.

Infect Dis
📞 +44 20 7371 8735
🌐 https://vfapp.org/337d

AIDS Healthcare Foundation
Provides cutting-edge HIV/AIDS medical care and advocacy to over one million people in forty-three countries.
Infect Dis
+1 323-860-5200
https://vfapp.org/b27c

ALIGHT
Works closely with refugees, trafficked persons, economic migrants, and other displaced persons to co-design solutions that help them build full and fulfilling lives by providing healthcare, clean water, shelter protection, and economic opportunity.
ER Med, General, Infect Dis, MF Med, Neonat, Peds
+1 800-875-7060
https://vfapp.org/5993

Amref Health Africa
Serves millions of people across thirty-five countries in Sub-Saharan Africa, strengthening health systems, and training African health workers to respond to the continent's most critical health issues.
All-Immu, General, Infect Dis, Logist-Op, MF Med, OB-GYN, Path, Pub Health, Surg
+254 20 6993000
https://vfapp.org/6985

AO Alliance
Builds solutions to lessen the burden of injuries in low- and middle-income countries, while enhancing the care of the injured to reduce human suffering, disability, and poverty.
Ortho, Surg
https://vfapp.org/8cd5

Association of Medical Doctors of Asia (AMDA)
Strives to support people affected by disasters and economic distress on their road to recovery, establishing a true partnership with special emphasis on local initiative.
ER Med, Logist-Op, Pub Health
+81 86-252-6051
https://vfapp.org/e3d4

Avinta Care
Offers quality healthcare while providing a full suite of services from diagnosis to treatment, specializing in fertility and dermatology.
Derm, MF Med, OB-GYN, Path
https://vfapp.org/52a6

Benjamin H. Josephson, MD Fund
Provides healthcare professionals with the financial resources necessary to deliver medical services for those in need throughout the world.
General, OB-GYN
+1 908-522-2853
https://vfapp.org/6acc

Bill & Melinda Gates Foundation
Focuses on global issues, from poverty to health, to education, offering the opportunity to dramatically improve the quality of life for billions of people, by building partnerships that bring together resources, expertise, and vision to identify issues, find answers, and drive change.
All-Immu, General, Infect Dis, MF Med, Neonat, OB-GYN, Pub Health
https://vfapp.org/7cf2

Boston Cardiac Foundation, The
Provides advanced medical technologies and cardiac care such as pacemaker implantation to patients around the world who would otherwise not have access to these services.
Anesth, CT Surg, CV Med, Crit-Care
+1 781-662-6404
https://vfapp.org/8fd3

Boston Children's Hospital: Global Health Program
Helps solve pediatric global health care challenges by transferring expertise through long-term partnerships with scalable impact, while working in the field to strengthen healthcare systems, advocate, research and provide care delivery or education as a way of sustainably improving the health of children worldwide.
Anesth, CV Med, Crit-Care, ER Med, Heme-Onc, Infect Dis, Medicine, Nutr, Palliative, Ped Surg, Peds
+1 617-919-6438
https://vfapp.org/f9f8

Breast Cancer Initiative East Africa Inc. (BCIEA)
Seeks to ensure that through advocacy, awareness, education, empowerment, access to treatment support, and research, patients do not face breast cancer with fear or helplessly alone.
OB-GYN
+1 281-818-6241
https://vfapp.org/6c82

Bridge to Health Medical and Dental
Seeks to provide health care to those who need it most based on a philosophy of partnership, education, and community development. Strives to bring solutions to global health issues in underserved communities through clinical outreach and medical and dental training.
Dent-OMFS, General, Infect Dis, MF Med, OB-GYN, Ophth-Opt, Ortho, Pub Health, Radiol
https://vfapp.org/bb2c

Bridge2Aid Australia
Seeks to provide access to simple, safe, emergency dental treatment for all.
Anesth, Dent-OMFS
+255 754 033 003
https://vfapp.org/a899

Brigham and Women's Center for Surgery and Public Health
Advances the science of surgical care delivery by studying effectiveness, quality, equity, and value at the population level, and develops surgeon-scientists committed to excellence in these areas.
Anesth, ER Med, Infect Dis, Pub Health, Surg
+1 617-525-7300
https://vfapp.org/5d64

Brigham and Women's Hospital Global Health Hub
Cares for patients in underserved settings, provides education to staff who work in those areas to create sustainable change, and conducts research designed to improve health in such settings.
General, Infect Dis
https://vfapp.org/a8a3

Canadian Network for International Surgery, The
Aims to improve maternal health, increase safety, and build local capacity in low-income countries by creating and providing surgical and midwifery courses, training domestically, and transferring skills.
Logist-Op, Surg
+1 877-217-8856
https://vfapp.org/86ff

CARE
Works around the globe to save lives, defeat poverty, and achieve social justice.
ER Med, General
+1 800-422-7385
https://vfapp.org/7232

CareMe E-Clinic
Uses digital technology, partners with healthcare providers, raises awareness around noncommunicable diseases, and provides healthcare to patients with chronic ailments from underserved communities across Rwanda.
CV Med, Pub Health
+250 781 297 139
https://vfapp.org/85c5

Carter Center, The
Seeks to prevent and resolve conflicts, enhance freedom and democracy, and improve health, while remaining committed to human rights and the alleviation of human suffering.
Infect Dis, MF Med, Ophth-Opt
+1 800-550-3560
https://vfapp.org/6556

Centre de Chirurgie Orthopédique Pédiatrique et de Réhabilitation Sainte Marie de Rilima
Works to promote health and rehabilitative assistance of children with disabilities as well as to promote awareness about disability.
Anesth, General, Medicine, Ortho, Path, Ped Surg, Rehab
+250 783 312 831
https://vfapp.org/567b

Centre Marembo
Supports homeless girls in Kigali, providing shelter, education, counseling, and skills training.
General, Infect Dis, OB-GYN, Path, Peds
+250 788 505 355
https://vfapp.org/e8e4

Chain of Hope
Provides lifesaving heart operations for children around the world and supports the development of cardiac services in numerous developing and war-torn countries.
Anesth, CT Surg, CV Med, Crit-Care, Ped Surg, Peds, Pulm-Critic, Surg
+44 20 7351 1978
https://vfapp.org/1b1b

Christian Blind Mission (CBM)
Aims to improve the quality of life of persons with disabilities in the poorest countries, addressing poverty as a cause, and a consequence, of disability, and working in partnership to create a society for all.
ENT, General, Infect Dis, OB-GYN, Ophth-Opt, Ortho, Peds, Psych, Rehab, Surg
+49 6251 131131
https://vfapp.org/3824

Christian Connections for International Health (CCIH)
Promotes global health and wholeness from a Christian perspective.
All-Immu, General, Infect Dis, MF Med, Neonat, OB-GYN, Psych
+1 703-923-8960
https://vfapp.org/fa5d

Christian Health Service Corps
Brings Christian doctors, health professionals, and health educators who are committed to serving the poor to places that have little or no access to healthcare.
Anesth, Dent-OMFS, General, Medicine, Peds, Surg
+1 903-962-4000
https://vfapp.org/da57

Cleft Africa
Strives to provide underserved Africans with cleft lips and palates with access to the best possible treatment for their condition, so that they can live a life free of the health problems caused by cleft.
Anesth, Dent-OMFS, Ped Surg, Surg
https://vfapp.org/8298

Clinton Health Access Initiative (CHAI)
Aims to save lives and reduce the burden of disease in low- and middle-income countries. Works with partners to strengthen the capabilities of governments and the private sector to create and sustain high-quality health systems.
General, Heme-Onc, Infect Dis, Logist-Op, MF Med, Medicine, Neonat, Nutr, OB-GYN, Path, Peds, Rad-Onc
+1 617-774-0110
https://vfapp.org/9ed7

Concern Worldwide
Seeks to permanently transform the lives of people living in extreme poverty, tackling its root causes, and building resilience.
Logist-Op, MF Med, Nutr, OB-GYN
+353 1 417 7700
https://vfapp.org/77e9

Creighton University School of Medicine: Global Surgery Fellowship
Aims to significantly impact the absence of acute surgical care in developing countries by providing free surgery to underserved patients and surgical training for developing country trainees.
Anesth, Ped Surg, Surg
+1 402-250-6196
https://vfapp.org/777f

Developing Country NGO Delegation: Global Fund to Fight AIDS, TB & Malaria
Works to strengthen the engagement of civil society actors and organizations in developing countries to contribute toward achieving a world in which AIDS, TB, and Malaria are no longer global, public health, and human rights threats.
Infect Dis, Pub Health
+254 20 2515790
https://vfapp.org/3149

Direct Relief
Improves the health and lives of people affected by poverty or emergency situations by mobilizing and providing essential

medical resources needed for their care.

ER Med, Logist-Op

+1 805-964-4767

https://vfapp.org/58e5

Doctors Worldwide

Focuses on health access, health improvement, and health emergencies to serve communities in need so they can build healthier and happier futures.

Dent-OMFS, ER Med, General, MF Med, Palliative, Peds

+44 7308 139100

https://vfapp.org/99cd

Duke University: Global Health Institute

Sparks innovation in global health research and education, and brings together knowledge and resources to address the most important global health issues of our time.

All-Immu, Infect Dis, MF Med, OB-GYN, Pub Health

+1 919-681-7760

https://vfapp.org/c4cd

Edwards Lifesciences

Provides innovative solutions for people fighting cardiovascular disease, as a global leader in patient-focused medical innovations for structural heart disease, as well as critical care and surgical monitoring.

Anesth, CT Surg, CV Med, Crit-Care, Ped Surg, Peds, Pulm-Critic, Surg, Vasc Surg

+1 949-250-5176

https://vfapp.org/d671

Elizabeth Glaser Pediatric AIDS Foundation

Seeks to end global pediatric HIV/AIDS through prevention and treatment programs, research, and advocacy.

Infect Dis, Nutr, OB-GYN, Peds

+1 888-499-4673

https://vfapp.org/d6ec

Enabel

As the development agency of the Belgian federal government, charged with implementing Belgium's international development policy, carries out public service assignments in Belgium and abroad pursuant to the 2030 Agenda for Sustainable Development.

General, Infect Dis, Logist-Op, MF Med, OB-GYN, Peds, Pub Health

+32 2 505 37 00

https://vfapp.org/5af7

END Fund, The

Aims to control and eliminate the most prevalent neglected diseases among the world's poorest and most vulnerable people.

Infect Dis

+1 646-690-9775

https://vfapp.org/2614

Eugène Gasana Jr. Foundation

Provides the opportunity for compassionate and quality cancer care for children in developing nations.

Anesth, Heme-Onc, Ped Surg, Peds

+1 800-691-5412

https://vfapp.org/27cb

Eye Care Foundation

Helps prevent and cure avoidable blindness and visual impairment in low-income countries.

Ophth-Opt, Surg

+31 20 647 3879

https://vfapp.org/c8f9

Fondation d'Harcourt

Promotes national and international projects and partnerships in the fields of mental health and psychosocial support; provides grants to organizations with specific expertise in mental health or psychosocial support to implement projects, and provides direct services.

Psych, Pub Health

+41 22 716 00 23

https://vfapp.org/4a8a

Foundation for Special Surgery

Provides high-quality, complex surgical care by increasing surgical expertise in Africa through the participation of surgeons across various specialties to provide premium care and skills transfer/ education to benefit patients.

Anesth, CT Surg, ENT, Endo, Neurosurg, Plast, Surg, Urol

+1 301-787-8914

https://vfapp.org/53db

Fracarita International

Provides support and services in the fields of mental healthcare, care for people with a disability, and education.

Psych, Rehab

https://vfapp.org/8d3c

Fred Hollows Foundation, The

Works toward a world in which no person is needlessly blind or vision impaired.

Ophth-Opt, Pub Health, Surg

+1 646-374-0445

https://vfapp.org/73e5

Glo Good Foundation

Committed to building oral-health initiatives in underserved populations globally by educating families on the importance of taking care of their oral health and training local dentists to facilitate the delivery of care when needed.

Dent-OMFS, Nutr

+1 212-734-6111

https://vfapp.org/38bd

Global Alliance to Prevent Prematurity and Stillbirth (GAPPS)

Seeks to improve birth outcomes worldwide by reducing the burden of premature birth and stillbirth.

All-Immu, Infect Dis, MF Med, Neonat, Neonat, OB-GYN

+1 206-413-7954

https://vfapp.org/3f74

Global Clubfoot Initiative (GCI)

Promotes and resources the treatment of children with clubfoot in developing countries using the Ponseti technique.

Ortho, Ped Surg

https://vfapp.org/f229

Global Health Corps
Mobilizes a diverse community of leaders to build the movement for global health equity, working toward a world where every person lives a healthy life.
ER Med, General, Pub Health
https://vfapp.org/31c6

Global Ministries – The United Methodist Church
As the worldwide mission and development agency of The United Methodist Church, Global Ministries works with more than 300 hospitals and clinics around the world through its Global Health Unit.
Anesth, CT Surg, CV Med, Crit-Care, Dent-OMFS, Derm, ER Med, GI, General, Infect Dis, Logist-Op, MF Med, Medicine, Neonat, Nephro, Nutr, OB-GYN, Ophth-Opt, Ortho, Palliative, Peds, Pod, Psych, Pub Health, Rehab, Rheum, Surg, Urol
+1 800-862-4246
https://vfapp.org/1723

Global Offsite Care
Aims to be a catalyst for increasing access to specialized healthcare for all, and provides technology platforms to doctors and clinics around the world through rotary club–sponsored telemedicine projects.
Crit-Care, ER Med, General, Pulm-Critic
+1 707-827-1524
https://vfapp.org/61b5

Global Oncology (GO)
Brings the best in cancer care to underserved patients around the world and collaborates across geographic, professional, and academic borders to improve cancer care, research, and education.
Heme-Onc, Path, Rad-Onc
https://vfapp.org/fcb8

HEAL Africa
Compassionately serves vulnerable people and communities in the Democratic Republic of the Congo through a holistic approach to healthcare, education, community action, and leadership development in response to changing needs.
Medicine, OB-GYN, Ortho, Peds, Surg
+1 816-536-3751
https://vfapp.org/cf5d

Health Builders
Strengthens management, improves clinical care, and builds healthcare infrastructure in Rwanda so every person has access to high-quality healthcare, allowing them to live dignified, healthy, and prosperous lives.
General, Logist-Op, MF Med, Medicine, Neonat, Nutr, OB-GYN, Path, Peds
+1 303-598-5320
https://vfapp.org/571f

Health Equity Initiative
Aims to build and sustain a global community that engages across sectors and disciplines to advance health equity.
Pub Health
https://vfapp.org/e2e2

Health Poverty Action
Works in partnership with people around the world who are pursuing change in their own communities to demand health justice and challenge power imbalances.
ER Med, General, Infect Dis, Psych, Pub Health
+44 20 7840 3777
https://vfapp.org/ee58

Health Volunteers Overseas (HVO)
Improves the availability and quality of healthcare through the education, training, and professional development of the health workforce in resource-scarce countries.
All-Immu, Anesth, CV Med, Dent-OMFS, Derm, ENT, ER Med, Endo, GI, Heme-Onc, Infect Dis, Medicine, Medicine, Nephro, Neuro, OB-GYN, Ophth-Opt, Ortho, Peds, Plast, Psych, Pulm-Critic, Rehab, Rheum, Surg
+1 202-296-0928
https://vfapp.org/42b2

Health[e] Foundation
Supports health professionals and community workers in the world's most vulnerable societies to ensure quality health for everyone in need by providing digital education and information, using e-learning and m-health.
Logist-Op
https://vfapp.org/b73b

Heart to Heart International
Strengthens communities through improving health access, providing humanitarian development, and administering crisis relief worldwide. Engages volunteers, collaborates with partners, and deploys resources to achieve this mission.
Anesth, ER Med, General, Logist-Op, Medicine, Path, Path, Peds, Psych, Pub Health, Surg
+1 913-764-5200
https://vfapp.org/aacb

Helping Hands for Rwanda (HHFR)
Brings quality education and healthcare to the Rwandese people.
Anesth, CT Surg, CV Med, Crit-Care, General, Medicine
+250 7833663934
https://vfapp.org/b981

Himalayan Cataract Project
Works to cure needless blindness with the highest quality care at the lowest cost.
Anesth, Ophth-Opt, Surg
+1 888-287-8530
https://vfapp.org/3b3d

His Hands on Africa
Brings hope and healing to underserved communities in Africa by mobilizing Christian dentists to provide communities with dental care, based in Christian ministry.
Dent-OMFS
+1 818-350-3887
https://vfapp.org/228c

Home de la Vierge des Pauvres (HVP) Gatagara
Provides high-quality and sustainable education as well as orthopedic and rehabilitation services to persons with physical disabilities in partnership with other stakeholders.
Anesth, Ortho, Psych, Radiol, Rehab
+250 788 300 988
https://vfapp.org/9a3f

Hope Walks
Frees children, families, and communities from the burden of

clubfoot, inspired by the Christian faith.

Ortho, Ped Surg, Peds, Rehab

+1 717-502-4400

https://vfapp.org/f6d4

Hospice Without Borders

Improves access to palliative care and hospice programs that preferentially serve marginalized, traumatized, and vulnerable populations both in the U.S. and in Rwanda.

Anesth, Palliative

https://vfapp.org/bdb6

Humanity & Inclusion

Works alongside people with disabilities and vulnerable populations, taking action and bearing witness in order to respond to their essential needs, improve their living conditions and health, and promote respect for their dignity and fundamental rights.

General, Infect Dis, MF Med, Medicine, Ortho, Peds, Psych, Pub Health, Rehab

+1 301-891-2138

https://vfapp.org/16b7

ICAP at Columbia University

Serves as global leader in supporting the scale-up of multidisciplinary HIV/AIDS prevention, care, and treatment programs based on a family-focused approach.

General, Infect Dis, MF Med, Medicine, OB-GYN, Pub Health

+1 212-342-0505

https://vfapp.org/a8ef

International Agency for the Prevention of Blindness (IAPB), The

Leads international efforts in blindness-prevention activities, works toward a world where no one is needlessly visually impaired, and ensures that everyone has access to the best possible standard of eye health.

Infect Dis, Ophth-Opt, Pub Health

https://vfapp.org/87a2

International Council of Ophthalmology

Works with ophthalmologic societies and others to enhance ophthalmic education and improve access to the highest quality eye care in order to preserve and restore vision for the people of the world.

Ophth-Opt

https://vfapp.org/ffd2

International Federation of Gynecology and Obstetrics (FIGO)

Implements global projects on specific women's health issues.

MF Med, Medicine, Neonat, OB-GYN, Surg, Urol

+44 20 7928 1166

https://vfapp.org/c4b4

International Federation of Red Cross and Red Crescent Societies (IFRC)

Coordinates and directs international assistance following natural and man-made disasters in nonconflict situations through the world's largest humanitarian and development network. Provides disaster-preparedness programs, healthcare activities, and promotes humanitarian values.

ER Med, General, Infect Dis, Nutr

+1 212-338-0161

https://vfapp.org/b4ee

International Medical Relief

Provides sustainable education, training, medical and dental care, and disaster relief and response in vulnerable communities worldwide.

Dent-OMFS, General, Infect Dis, Medicine, OB-GYN

+1 970-635-0110

https://vfapp.org/b3ed

International Medical Response

Supplements, supports, and enhances healthcare systems in communities across the world that have been incapacitated by natural disaster, extreme poverty, and/or regional conflict by sending a multidisciplinary team of healthcare professionals.

Anesth, General, OB-GYN, Surg

+1 917-324-8348

https://vfapp.org/9ccd

International Organization for Migration (IOM) – The UN Migration Agency

Promotes evidence-informed policies and holistic, preventive, and curative health programs that are beneficial, accessible, and equitable for vulnerable migrants.

General, Infect Dis, OB-GYN

+27 12 342 2789

https://vfapp.org/621a

International Organization for Women and Development (IOWD)

Provides underserved women and children in low-income countries with free medical and surgical services and care.

Anesth, MF Med, Neonat, OB-GYN, Ped Surg, Peds, Surg

+1 516-764-6370

https://vfapp.org/8ecb

IntraHealth International

Improves the performance of health workers and strengthens the systems in which they work.

CV Med, Endo, General, Infect Dis, MF Med, Neonat, Nutr, OB-GYN

+1 919-313-3554

https://vfapp.org/ddc8

Iris Global

Serves the poor, the destitute, the lost, and the forgotten by providing adoration, outreach, family, education, relief, development, healing, and the arts.

General, Infect Dis, Nutr, Pub Health

+1 530-255-2077

https://vfapp.org/37f8

IVUmed

Aims to make quality urological care available worldwide by providing medical and surgical education for physicians and nurses and treatment for thousands of children and adults.

Anesth, OB-GYN, Ped Surg, Surg, Urol

+1 801-524-0201

https://vfapp.org/e619

Jhpiego

Creates and delivers transformative healthcare solutions that save lives in partnership with national governments, health experts, and local communities.

General, Infect Dis, OB-GYN, Surg

+1 410-537-1800

https://vfapp.org/45b8

John Snow, Inc. (JSI)
Aims to improve the health and well-being of underserved and vulnerable people and communities throughout the world.
General, Infect Dis, Logist-Op, MF Med, OB-GYN, Peds, Psych, Pub Health
+1 617-482-9485
https://vfapp.org/ba78

Johns Hopkins Center for Communication Programs
Believes in the power of communication to save lives, by empowering people to adopt healthy behaviors for themselves, their families, and their communities.
General, Infect Dis, Logist-Op, OB-GYN, Pub Health
+1 410-659-6300
https://vfapp.org/1bf9

Johns Hopkins Center for Global Health
Facilitates and focuses the extensive expertise and resources of the Johns Hopkins institutions together with global collaborators to effectively address and ameliorate the world's most pressing health issues.
General, Genetics, Logist-Op, MF Med, Peds, Psych, Pub Health, Pulm-Critic
+1 410-502-9872
https://vfapp.org/54ce

Joint Aid Management (JAM)
Provides food security, nutrition, water, and sanitation to vulnerable communities in Africa in dignified and sustainable ways.
ER Med, Nutr
+27 11 548 3900
https://vfapp.org/dcac

Joint United Nations Programme on HIV/AIDS (UNAIDS)
Aims to place people living with HIV and people affected by the virus at the decision-making table and at the center of designing, delivering, and monitoring the AIDS response.
Infect Dis
+41 22 791 36 66
https://vfapp.org/464a

Kageno
Works to transform communities in need into places of hope and opportunity through an integrated model that focuses on healthcare, education, income generation, and conservation.
General, Infect Dis, MF Med, Neonat, Nutr, OB-GYN
+1 212-227-0509
https://vfapp.org/f5bd

Keep a Child Alive
Committed to improving the health and well-being of vulnerable children, young people, adults, and families around the world, with a focus on combating the physical, social, and economic impacts of HIV/AIDS.
Infect Dis, MF Med, Neonat, OB-GYN
+1 646-975-5559
https://vfapp.org/7f2f

Life for a Child
Supports the provision of the best possible health care, given local circumstances, to all children and youth with diabetes in less-resourced countries, through the strengthening of existing diabetes services.
Endo, Medicine, Peds
https://vfapp.org/d712

Light for the World
Contributes to a world in which persons with disabilities fully exercise their rights and assists persons with disabilities living in poverty.
Ophth-Opt, Rehab
+43 1 8101300
https://vfapp.org/3ff6

Lions Clubs International
Empowers volunteers to serve their communities, meet humanitarian needs, encourage peace, and promote international understanding through Lions clubs.
Heme-Onc, Medicine, Nutr, Ophth-Opt
+1 630-571-5466
https://vfapp.org/7b12

London School of Hygiene & Tropical Medicine: Health in Humanitarian Crises Centre
Advances health and health equity in crisis-affected countries through research, education, and translation of knowledge into policy and practice.
ER Med, Infect Dis, Pub Health
+44 20 7636 8636
https://vfapp.org/96ad

Management Sciences for Health (MSH)
Works with countries and communities to save lives and improve the health of the world's poorest and most vulnerable people by building strong, resilient, sustainable health systems.
Infect Dis, Logist-Op, Pub Health
+1 617-250-9500
https://vfapp.org/6aa2

MAP International
Provides medicines and health supplies to those in need around the world so they might experience life to the fullest.
Logist-Op
+1 800-225-8550
https://vfapp.org/deed

Massachusetts General Hospital Global Surgery Initiative
Aims to improve surgical education and access to advanced surgical care in resource-limited settings around the world by performing surgical operations as visitors, training local surgeons, and sharing medical technology through international partnerships across disciplines.
Anesth, Crit-Care, ER Med, Heme-Onc, Peds, Surg
+1 617-724-4093
https://vfapp.org/31b1

McGill University Health Centre: Centre for Global Surgery
Works to reduce the impact of injury by advancing surgical care through research and education in resource-limited settings.
ER Med, Logist-Op, Ped Surg, Surg
+1 514-934-1934
https://vfapp.org/7246

MCW Global
Works to address communities' pressing needs by empowering current leaders and readying leaders of tomorrow.
Dent-OMFS
+1 212-453-5811
https://vfapp.org/1547

Medical Ministry International
Provides compassionate healthcare in areas of need, inspired by the Christian faith.
CT Surg, Dent-OMFS, ENT, General, OB-GYN, Ophth-Opt, Ortho, Plast, Rehab, Surg, Urol, Vasc Surg
+1 905-545-4400
https://vfapp.org/5da6

Medical Missions for Children (MMFC)
Provides quality surgical and dental services to poor and underprivileged children and young adults in various countries throughout the world, as well as facilitates the transfer of education, knowledge, and recent innovations to the local medical communities.
Dent-OMFS, ENT, Endo, Ortho, Ped Surg, Peds, Plast
+1 508-697-5821
https://vfapp.org/1631

MedShare
Aims to improve the quality of life of people, communities, and the planet by sourcing and directly delivering surplus medical supplies and equipment to communities in need around the world.
Logist-Op
+1 770-323-5858
https://vfapp.org/c8bc

MicroResearch: Africa/Asia
Seeks to improve health outcomes in Africa by training, mentoring, and supporting local multidisciplinary health professional researchers.
Infect Dis, Nutr, OB-GYN, Psych
https://vfapp.org/13e7

MSD for Mothers
Designs scalable solutions that help end preventable maternal deaths.
MF Med, OB-GYN, Pub Health
https://vfapp.org/9f99

Multi-Agency International Training and Support (MAITS)
Improves the lives of some of the world's poorest people living with disabilities through better access to quality health and education services and support.
Neuro, Psych, Rehab
+44 20 7258 8443
https://vfapp.org/9dcd

NCD Alliance
Unites and strengthens civil society to stimulate collaborative advocacy, action, and accountability for NCD (noncommunicable disease) prevention and control.
All-Immu, CV Med, General, Heme-Onc, Medicine, Peds, Psych
+41 22 809 18 11
https://vfapp.org/abdd

Ndengera Polyclinic
Provides quality care, health education to the population, and conducts research to better the quality of health services provided.
Dent-OMFS, General, Medicine, OB-GYN, Peds
+250 784 151 010
https://vfapp.org/89cd

Northwestern University Feinberg School of Medicine: Institute for Global Health
Aims to improve access to essential surgical care by addressing the barriers to care, with multidisciplinary and bidirectional partnerships, through innovation, research, education, policy, advocacy, by training the next generation of global health leaders and building sustainable capacity in regions with health inequities.
Anesth, ER Med, Heme-Onc, Logist-Op, MF Med, OB-GYN, Ped Surg, Surg
+1 312-503-9000
https://vfapp.org/24f3

Norwegian People's Aid
Aims to improve living conditions, to create a democratic, just, and safe society.
ER Med, Logist-Op
+47 22 03 77 00
https://vfapp.org/2d8e

One Family Health
Improves access to quality essential medicines and basic healthcare services in isolated communities, using a sustainable business model to help underserved communities build health as an asset in Rwanda.
General, Logist-Op, Pub Health
+250 787 058 626
https://vfapp.org/3259

OneSight
Brings eye exams and glasses to the people who lack access to vision care.
Ophth-Opt
+1 888-935-4589
https://vfapp.org/3ecc

Open Heart International
Provides surgical interventions and best practices to the most disadvantaged communities on the planet.
CT Surg, MF Med, OB-GYN, Ophth-Opt, Plast, Surg
+61 2 9487 9295
https://vfapp.org/dab2

Operation Hernia
Provides high-quality surgery at minimal costs to patients that otherwise would not receive it.
Anesth, Ortho, Surg
https://vfapp.org/6e9a

Operation Medical
Commits efforts to promoting and providing high-quality medical care and education to communities that do not have adequate access.
Anesth, ENT, Logist-Op, OB-GYN, Ped Surg, Plast, Surg, Urol
+1 717-685-9199
https://vfapp.org/7e1b

Operation Smile
Treats patients with cleft lip and cleft palate, and creates solutions that deliver safe surgery to people where it's needed most.
Anesth, Dent-OMFS, ENT, Ped Surg, Plast
+1 757-321-7645
https://vfapp.org/5c29

Options
Believes in a world where women and children can access the high-quality health services they need, without financial burden.
Logist-Op, MF Med, Neonat, OB-GYN
+44 20 7430 1900
https://vfapp.org/3a48

OPTIVEST Foundation
Funds strategic opportunities that are holistic and collaborative, inspired by the Christian faith.
General, Nutr
https://vfapp.org/f1e6

Orbis International
Works to prevent and treat blindness through hands-on training and improved access to quality eye care.
Anesth, Ophth-Opt, Surg
+1 646-674-5500
https://vfapp.org/f2b2

Pact
Works on the ground to improve the lives of those who are challenged by poverty and marginalization, striving for a world where all people are heard, capable, and vibrant.
Infect Dis, Logist-Op, MF Med, Pub Health
+1 202-466-5666
https://vfapp.org/9a6c

Pan-African Academy of Christian Surgeons (PAACS)
Exists to train and support African surgeons to provide excellent, compassionate care to those most in need, inspired by the Christian faith.
Anesth, CT Surg, Neurosurg, OB-GYN, Ortho, Ped Surg, Plast, Surg
+1 847-571-9926
https://vfapp.org/85ba

Partners for World Health
Sorts, evaluates, repackages, and prepares supplies and equipment for distribution to individuals, communities, and healthcare facilities in need, both locally and internationally.
ER Med, General, Logist-Op
+1 207-774-5555
https://vfapp.org/982e

Partners in Health
Responds to the moral imperative to provide high-quality healthcare globally to those who need it most, while striving to ease suffering by providing a comprehensive model of care that includes access to food, transportation, housing, and other key components of healing.
CT Surg, General, Heme-Onc, Infect Dis, MF Med, Neurosurg, OB-GYN, Ortho, Plast, Psych, Urol
+1 857-880-5600
https://vfapp.org/dc9c

Pfalzklinikum
Aims to establish community-psychiatry structures in Rwanda and institute the practice of exchanging knowledge in daily medical-psychological and nursing routines.
Psych
+49 6349 9001000
https://vfapp.org/2da8

Physicians Across Continents
Provides high-quality medical care to people affected by crises and disasters.
CV Med, Dent-OMFS, Heme-Onc, MF Med, Nephro, Nephro, OB-GYN, Ped Surg, Plast, Surg
+44 20 7993 6900
https://vfapp.org/fe5d

PINCC Preventing Cervical Cancer
Seeks to prevent female-specific diseases in developing countries by utilizing low-cost and low-technology methods to create sustainable programs through patient education, medical personnel training, and facility outfitting.
OB-GYN
+1 830-708-6009
https://vfapp.org/9666

Project SOAR
Conducts HIV operations research around the world to identify practical solutions to improve HIV prevention, care, and treatment services.
ER Med, General, MF Med, OB-GYN, Psych
+1 202-237-9400
https://vfapp.org/1a77

PSI – Population Services International
Dedicates efforts to improving the health of people in the developing world by focusing on challenges such as a lack of family planning, HIV/AIDS, barriers to maternal health, and the greatest threats to children under the age of 5, including malaria, diarrhea, pneumonia, and malnutrition.
Infect Dis, MF Med, OB-GYN, Peds
+1 202-785-0072
https://vfapp.org/ffe3

RAD-AID International
Improves and optimizes access to medical imaging and radiology in low-resource regions of the world.
Rad-Onc, Radiol
https://vfapp.org/537f

RD Rwanda
Promotes social welfare through research on disease control and prevention, education and health programs, and economic development initiatives.
Genetics, Infect Dis, Logist-Op, Medicine, Nutr, OB-GYN, Path, Peds, Pub Health
+250 788 634 048
https://vfapp.org/eafd

RestoringVision
Empowers lives by restoring vision for millions of people in need.
Ophth-Opt
+1 209-980-7323
https://vfapp.org/e121

Rockefeller Foundation, The
Works to promote the well-being of humanity.
Logist-Op, Nutr, Pub Health
+1 212-869-8500
https://vfapp.org/5424

Rotary International
Provides service to others, improves lives, and advances world understanding, goodwill, and peace through its

fellowship of business, professional, and community leaders.

ER Med, General, Infect Dis, MF Med, OB-GYN

https://vfapp.org/8fb5

Rutgers New Jersey Medical School

Seeks to support and promote the global health efforts of the faculty, staff, and learners in the areas of education, research, and service through The Rutgers New Jersey Medical School's Office of Global Health.

Anesth, CV Med, Crit-Care, Neurosurg, OB-GYN, Psych

+1 732-445-4636

https://vfapp.org/8e67

Rwanda Children

Seeks to provide housing, food, family, and hope to at-risk Rwandan children, inspired by the Christian faith.

General, Peds

+1 205-392-2330

https://vfapp.org/a132

Rwanda Diabetes Association

Prevents and treats diabetes and its complications, raises awareness for diabetes in Rwanda, researches and promotes the welfare of people living with diabetes, and partners with the local government and other national/international organizations to fight diabetes.

Endo, General

+250 788 839 235

https://vfapp.org/4438

Rwanda Legacy of Hope

Supports social welfare programs in Rwanda aimed at improving living conditions and providing better education, training opportunities, and health.

ENT, Ortho, Plast, Rehab, Surg

+44 1752 651817

https://vfapp.org/ea35

Salvation Army International, The

Seeks to meet human needs through services in education, healthcare, community support, emergency response, and ministry development, inspired by the Christian faith.

Dent-OMFS, Derm, ER Med, Infect Dis, MF Med, Medicine, Nutr, OB-GYN, Ophth-Opt, Palliative, Psych, Rehab, Surg

+44 20 7332 0101

https://vfapp.org/8eb3

Samaritan's Purse International Disaster Relief

Provides spiritual and physical aid to hurting people around the world, such as victims of war, poverty, natural disasters, disease, and famine, based in Christian ministry.

Anesth, CT Surg, Crit-Care, Dent-OMFS, Derm, ENT, ER Med, Endo, GI, General, Heme-Onc, Infect Dis, MF Med, Neonat, Nephro, Neuro, Neurosurg, Nutr, OB-GYN, Ophth-Opt, Ortho, Path, Ped Surg, Peds, Plast, Psych, Pulm-Critic, Radiol, Rehab, Rheum, Surg, Urol, Vasc Surg

+1 800-528-1980

https://vfapp.org/87e3

Sanofi Espoir Foundation

Contributes to reducing health inequalities among populations that need it most by applying a socially responsible approach focused on fighting childhood cancers in low-income countries, improving maternal and newborn health, and improving access to care.

ER Med, OB-GYN, Peds

+33 1 53 77 91 38

https://vfapp.org/943b

Save A Child's Heart

Provides lifesaving cardiac treatment to children in developing countries, and trains healthcare professionals from these countries to deliver quality care in their communities.

CT Surg, CV Med, Crit-Care, Ped Surg, Peds

+1 240-223-3940

https://vfapp.org/1bef

Save the Children

Gives children around the world a healthy start in life, the opportunity to learn, and protection from harm.

All-Immu, Crit-Care, ER Med, General, Infect Dis, MF Med, Medicine, Neonat, OB-GYN, Peds, Psych, Pub Health

+1 800-728-3843

https://vfapp.org/2e73

SIGN Fracture Care International

Builds orthopedic capacity around the world and provides the injured poor access to fracture surgery by donating orthopedic education and implant systems to surgeons in developing countries.

Ortho, Rehab, Surg

+1 509-371-1107

https://vfapp.org/123d

Smile Train

Seeks to give every child with a cleft the opportunity for a healthy, productive life by providing free cleft repair surgery and comprehensive cleft care in their own communities.

Dent-OMFS, ENT, Plast

+1 800-932-9541

https://vfapp.org/f21d

Society for Family Health Rwanda

Provides health promotion interventions using evidence-based social and behavior change communication and social marketing to empower Rwandans to choose healthier lives.

Infect Dis, Logist-Op, MF Med, Nutr

+250 788 305 684

https://vfapp.org/455e

Solace Ministries

Meets the needs of widows and orphans by supporting them with health, educational, and psychological services, helping to improve their livelihoods.

General, OB-GYN, Psych

https://vfapp.org/d691

SOS Children's Villages International

Supports children through alternative care and family strengthening.

ER Med, Peds

+43 1 36824570

https://vfapp.org/aca1

Surgeons OverSeas (SOS)

Works to reduce death and disability from surgically treatable conditions in developing countries.

Anesth, Heme-Onc, Surg

https://vfapp.org/5d16

Sustainable Medical Missions
Trains and supports Indigenous healthcare and faith leaders in underdeveloped communities to treat neglected tropical diseases (NTDs) and other endemic conditions affecting the poorest community members by pairing faith-based solutions with best practices.
Infect Dis, Pub Health
+1 513-543-2896
https://vfapp.org/9165

Swiss Tropical and Public Health Institute
Contributes to the improvement of the health of populations internationally, nationally, and locally through excellence in research, education, and services.
Infect Dis, Pub Health
+41 61 284 81 11
https://vfapp.org/2ee4

Task Force for Global Health, The
Consists of programs and focus areas that cover a range of global health issues including neglected tropical diseases, infectious diseases, vaccines, field epidemiology, public health informatics, health workforce development, and global health ethics.
Infect Dis, Logist-Op, Medicine, Ophth-Opt, Peds
+1 404-371-0466
https://vfapp.org/714c

Team Heart
Addresses the burden of cardiovascular disease in Rwanda by increasing access to specialized, lifesaving cardiac care.
Anesth, CT Surg, CV Med, Crit-Care, Ped Surg, Peds, Surg
+1 617-454-4355
https://vfapp.org/798e

Tearfund
Responds to crisis and partners with local churches to bring restoration to those living in poverty, inspired by the Christian faith.
ER Med, Logist-Op
+44 20 3906 3906
https://vfapp.org/f6cf

TIP Global Health
Empowers Rwandan communities to develop integrated approaches to complex health challenges by increasing access to overall healthcare, improving healthcare quality, and fostering long-term success through economic development.
Crit-Care, General, Infect Dis, MF Med, Neonat, OB-GYN
+1 831-661-5237
https://vfapp.org/e7bc

U.S. President's Malaria Initiative (PMI)
Supports low-income countries to help control and eliminate malaria through cost-effective, lifesaving malaria interventions.
Infect Dis, MF Med, OB-GYN
+1 202-712-0000
https://vfapp.org/dc8b

Union for International Cancer Control (UICC)
Unites and supports the cancer community to reduce the global cancer burden, promote greater equity, and ensure that cancer control continues to be a priority in the world health and development agenda.
Heme-Onc, Pub Health
+41 22 809 18 11
https://vfapp.org/88b1

United Nations Children's Fund (UNICEF)
Works in over 190 countries and territories to save children's lives, to defend their rights, and to help them fulfill their potential, from early childhood through adolescence.
All-Immu, Infect Dis, MF Med, Neonat, Nutr, OB-GYN, Ped Surg, Peds, Pub Health
https://vfapp.org/42d7

United Nations Development Programme (UNDP)
Helps countries achieve the simultaneous eradication of extreme poverty and significant reduction of inequalities and exclusion using a sustainable human development approach.
Infect Dis, Logist-Op, Pub Health
https://vfapp.org/935c

United Nations High Commissioner for Refugees (UNHCR)
Safeguards the rights and well-being of people who have been forced to flee, ensuring that everybody has the right to seek asylum and find safe refuge in another country, with the goal of seeking lasting solutions.
General, MF Med, Medicine, OB-GYN, Peds, Psych, Pub Health
https://vfapp.org/6636

United Nations Population Fund (UNFPA)
Supports reproductive healthcare for women and youth in more than 150 countries, focusing on delivering a world where every pregnancy is wanted, every childbirth is safe, and every young person's potential is fulfilled.
Infect Dis, MF Med, Neonat, OB-GYN, Peds, Pub Health
+1 212-963-6008
https://vfapp.org/c969

United States Agency for International Development (USAID)
Promotes and demonstrates democratic values abroad and advances a free, peaceful, and prosperous world. Leads the U.S. government's international development and disaster assistance through partnerships and investments that save lives.
ER Med, Infect Dis, MF Med, OB-GYN, Peds
+1 202-712-0000
https://vfapp.org/9a99

United States President's Emergency Plan for AIDS Relief (PEPFAR)
The U.S. global HIV/AIDS response works to prevent new HIV infections and accelerate progress to control the global epidemic in more than 50 countries, by partnering with governments to support sustainable, integrated, and country-led responses to HIV/AIDS.
Infect Dis, Pub Health
https://vfapp.org/a57c

University of California, Berkeley: Bixby Center for Population, Health & Sustainability
Aims to help manage population growth, improve maternal health, and address the unmet need for family planning within a human rights framework.

OB-GYN
📞 +1 510-642-6915
🌐 https://vfapp.org/ff2b

University of California: Global Health Institute
Mobilizes people and resources across the University of California to advance global health research, education, and collaboration.
General, OB-GYN, Pub Health
🌐 https://vfapp.org/ee7f

University of Minnesota: Global Surgery & Disparities Program
Works to understand and improve surgical, anesthesia, and OBGYN care in underserved areas through partnerships with local providers, while training the next generation of academic global surgery leaders.
All-Immu, Dent-OMFS, ER Med, Heme-Onc, MF Med, Neurosurg, OB-GYN, Ophth-Opt, Path, Ped Surg, Plast, Surg, Urol
📞 +1 612-626-1999
🌐 https://vfapp.org/e59a

University of Utah Global Health
Supports local organizations in their quest to improve quality of life in their communities all over the world.
Anesth, CT Surg, CV Med, Crit-Care, Dent-OMFS, ENT, ER Med, Infect Dis, OB-GYN, Ophth-Opt, Ped Surg, Ped Surg, Peds, Plast, Pub Health, Surg, Urol
📞 +1 801-585-1509
🌐 https://vfapp.org/bacd

University of Virginia: Anesthesiology Department Global Health Initiatives
Educates and trains physicians, to help people achieve healthy productive lives, and advances knowledge in the medical sciences.
Anesth, Pub Health
📞 +1 434-924-2283
🌐 https://vfapp.org/1b8b

USAID: Maternal and Child Survival Program
Works to prevent child and maternal deaths.
Infect Dis, MF Med, Neonat, OB-GYN, Peds
🌐 https://vfapp.org/6fcf

USAID: Deliver Project
Builds a global supply chain to deliver lifesaving health products to people in order to enable countries to provide family planning, protect against malaria, and limit the spread of pandemic threats.
Infect Dis, Logist-Op, MF Med
📞 +1 202-712-0000
🌐 https://vfapp.org/374e

USAID: Health Policy Initiative
Provides field-level programming in health policy development and implementation.
General, Infect Dis, MF Med, OB-GYN, Peds
🌐 https://vfapp.org/8f84

USAID: Leadership, Management and Governance Project
Improves leadership, management, and governance practices to strengthen health systems and improve health for all, including vulnerable populations worldwide.
Logist-Op
🌐 https://vfapp.org/d35e

Vision for a Nation
Makes eye care accessible and aims to unlock economic growth and human potential in the world's poorest communities.
Ophth-Opt
🌐 https://vfapp.org/9c2c

Vision for the Poor
Reduces human suffering and improves quality of life through the recovery of sight by building sustainable eye hospitals in developing countries, empowering local eye specialists, funding essential ophthalmic infrastructure, and partnering with like-minded agencies.
Ophth-Opt
📞 +1 814-823-4486
🌐 https://vfapp.org/528e

Voluntary Service Overseas (VSO)
Works with health workers, communities, and governments to improve health services and rights for women, babies, youth, people with disabilities, and prisoners.
General, MF Med, OB-GYN
📞 +44 20 8780 7500
🌐 https://vfapp.org/213d

Wings of Hope for Africa Foundation
Aims to support family welfare, empowers communities, and develops self-sufficiency programs to end poverty in Burundi and Rwanda, East Africa, and in Calgary, Canada.
Infect Dis, Medicine, Peds
📞 +1 403-815-0037
🌐 https://vfapp.org/8d4e

Women's Equity in Access to Care & Treatment (WE-ACT)
Increases women's and children's access to primary healthcare and treatment in resource-limited settings at the grassroots level, while remaining committed to a locally driven, collaborative model of primary healthcare and treatment provision.
General, Infect Dis, Psych, Pub Health
📞 +1 415-655-3894
🌐 https://vfapp.org/2654

Women for Women International
Supports the most marginalized women to earn and save money, improve health and well-being, influence decisions in their home and community, and connect to networks for support.
MF Med, OB-GYN
📞 +1 202-737-7705
🌐 https://vfapp.org/768c

Women's Refugee Commission
Seeks to improve lives by protecting the rights of women, children, and youth displaced by conflict and crisis through researching their needs, identifying solutions, and advocating for programs and policies to strengthen their resilience.
General, MF Med, Neonat, OB-GYN, Peds, Psych
📞 +1 212-551-3115
🌐 https://vfapp.org/3d8f

World Blind Union (WBU)
Represents those experiencing blindness, speaking to

governments and international bodies on issues concerning visual impairments.

Ophth-Opt

🌐 https://vfapp.org/2bd3

World Compassion Fellowship (WCF)

Serves the global poor and persecuted through relief, medical care, development, and training.

CV Med, ER Med, Endo, GI, General, Infect Dis, Medicine, Nutr, OB-GYN, Ortho, Peds, Psych, Pub Health, Rehab

📞 +1 646-535-2344

🌐 https://vfapp.org/7b97

World Health Organization, The (WHO)

The United Nations' agency for health provides leadership on global health matters, shapes the health research agenda, setting norms and standards, articulates evidence-based policy options, provides technical support and monitoring to countries, and assesses health trends.

ER Med, General, Infect Dis, Logist-Op, MF Med, OB-GYN, Peds, Psych, Pub Health

📞 +41 22 791 21 11

🌐 https://vfapp.org/c476

World Relief

Brings sustainable solutions to the world's greatest problems: disasters, extreme poverty, violence, oppression, and mass displacement.

ER Med, Nutr, Psych, Pub Health

📞 +1 800-535-5433

🌐 https://vfapp.org/fbcd

World Vision International

Works with vulnerable communities around the world to overcome poverty and injustice with child-focused programs.

ER Med, General, Infect Dis, MF Med, Nutr, OB-GYN, Peds

📞 +1 626-303-8811

🌐 https://vfapp.org/2642

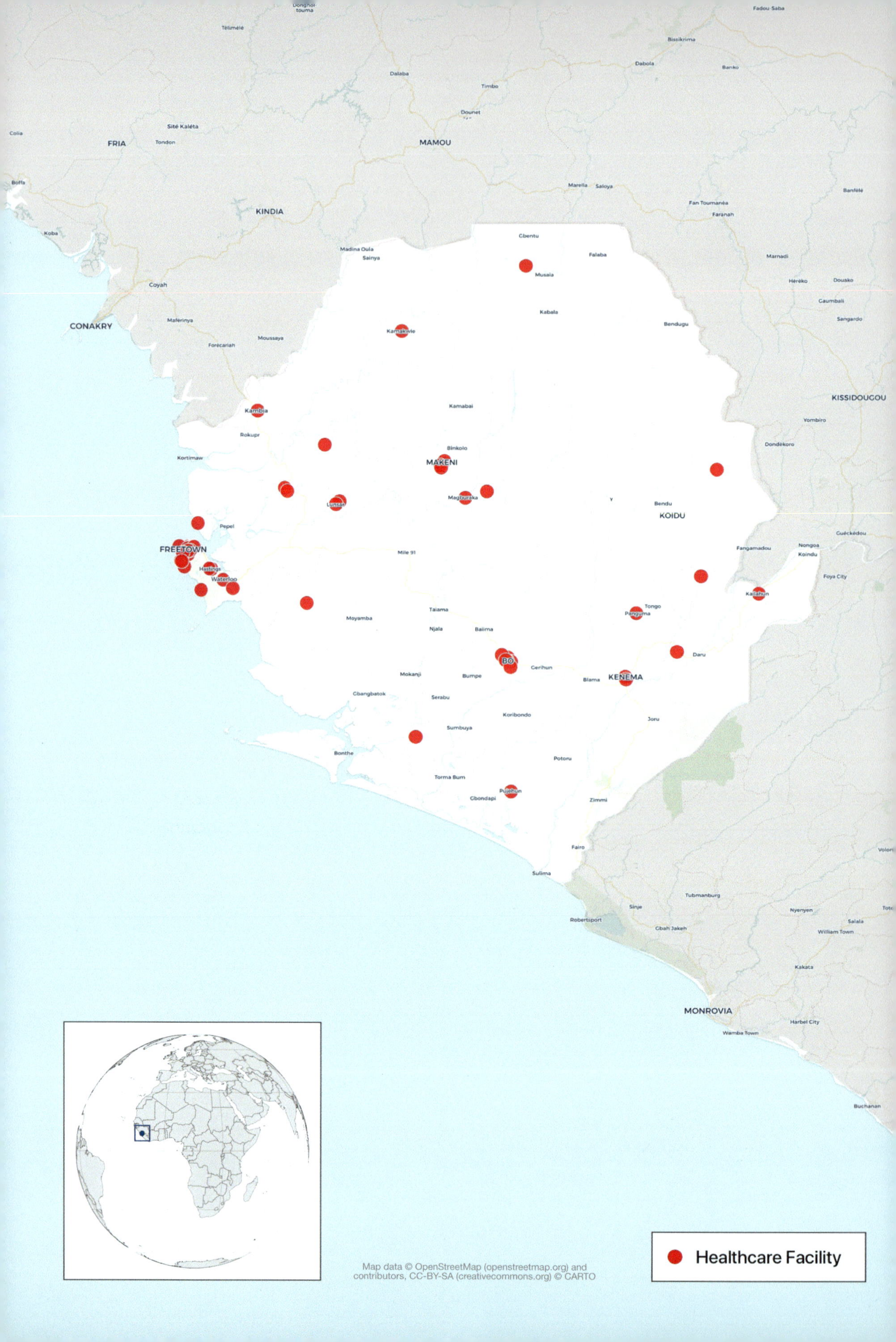

Telimele
Fadou Saba
Bissikrima
Dabola
Banko
Dalaba
Timbo
Dounet
Sité Kaléta
Colia
FRIA
Tondon
MAMOU
Boffa
Marella
Saloya
Banfèlè
KINDIA
Fan Toumanéa
Faranah
Koba
Gbentu
Madina Oula
Sainya
Falaba
Musaia
Marnadi
Coyah
Hérèko
Douako
Kabala
Gaumbali
CONAKRY
Maférinya
Bendugu
Sangardo
Kamakwie
Moussaya
Forécariah
KISSIDOUGOU
Kambia
Kamabai
Yombiro
Rokupr
Binkolo
Dondékoro
Kortimaw
MAKENI
Magburaka
Lunsar
Bendu
KOIDU
Pepel
Guéckédou
FREETOWN
Fangamadou
Nongoa
Koindu
Mile 91
Hastings
Waterloo
Foya City
Kailahun
Tongo
Panguma
Taiama
Moyamba
Njala
Baiima
Daru
BO
Gerihun
Mokanji
Bumpe
Blama
KENEMA
Gbangbatok
Serabu
Koribondo
Joru
Sumbuya
Bonthe
Potoru
Torma Bum
Pujehun
Gbondapi
Zimmi
Fairo
Voiom
Sulima
Tubmanburg
Sinje
Nyenyen
Robertsport
Salala
Gbah Jakeh
William Town
Kakata
MONROVIA
Harbel City
Wamba Town
Buchanan
Map data © OpenStreetMap (openstreetmap.org) and contributors, CC-BY-SA (creativecommons.org) © CARTO
Healthcare Facility

Sierra Leone

Located on West Africa's coast, the Republic of Sierra Leone has a population of about 6.6 million people. The Portuguese origins of the country's name translates to "Lion Mountains," referencing the hills that surround the capital of Freetown, one the largest natural harbors in the world. The primarily agricultural country has deposits of gold, diamonds, bauxite, and rutile. Large ethnic groups include the Mende and the Temne; English and Krio are the nation's official languages.

The country continues to recover from a devastating civil war that ended in 2002. Since then, Sierra Leone has had significant and impressive economic growth and was on track to reach middle-income status by 2035. However, progress was hindered by an Ebola outbreak in 2014 that infected more than 14,000 and killed nearly 4,000 people. The country is still recovering from this crisis.

While life expectancy continues to increase in Sierra Leone, it is still one of the lowest in the world at around 54 years. Likewise, although child mortality continues to decrease, the maternal mortality rate remains one of the highest in the world. The country has significantly higher rates of malaria than other countries in the same region. While some progress has been made to address illness and disease, the impact of the civil war left the country with a debilitated health system, tens of thousands of war amputees, and shortages of equipment, supplies, and doctors. Both communicable and non-communicable diseases such as malaria, lower-respiratory infections, neonatal disorders, ischemic heart disease, diarrheal diseases, stroke, HIV/AIDS, congenital defects, tuberculosis, and meningitis cause the most deaths in Sierra Leone.

6.6M
Population

$505
GDP Per Capita

54 years
Life Expectancy
↑ Improving

2.5
Doctors/100k
Physician Density

40
Beds/100k
Hospital Bed Density

1,120
Deaths/100k
Maternal Mortality

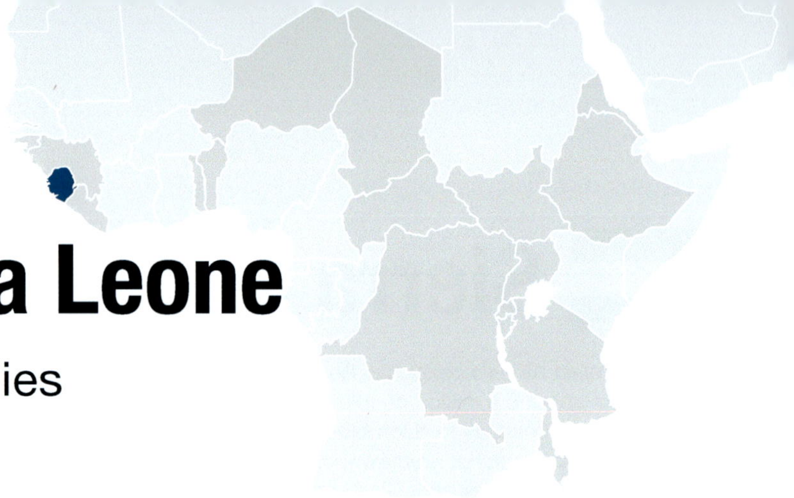

Sierra Leone

Healthcare Facilities

34 Military Hospital
Regent Road, Freetown, Western Area, Sierra Leone
https://vfapp.org/2737

Ahmadiyya Hospital
Hanga Road, Kenema, Sierra Leone
https://vfapp.org/de2d

AHS – Waterloo Hospital
New Main Motor Road, Rokel, Western Area, Sierra Leone
https://vfapp.org/77fa

ARAB Hospital
Magburaka Highway, Makeni, Bombali District, Sierra Leone
https://vfapp.org/44a5

Aspen Medical Sierra Leone Private Hospital
Bass Street, Freetown, Western Area, Sierra Leone
https://vfapp.org/9bca

Blue Shield Hospital
Ascension Town Road, Freetown, Western Area, Sierra Leone
https://vfapp.org/1c57

Bo Children's Hospital
Bo-Tiama Highway, Bo, Southern Province, Sierra Leone
https://vfapp.org/5984

Brookfields
Maboikandoh Road, Waterloo, Western Area, Sierra Leone
https://vfapp.org/f26d

China-SL Friendship Hospital, Jui
New Main Motor Road, Jui, Western Area, Sierra Leone
https://vfapp.org/b15c

Choithram Memorial Hospital
Damaya Drive, Freetown, Western Area, Sierra Leone
https://vfapp.org/b258

Connaught Hospital
Bathurst Street, Freetown, Western Area, Sierra Leone
https://vfapp.org/bb17

Curney Barnes Hospital
Cannon Street, Freetown, Western Area, Sierra Leone
https://vfapp.org/d284

EDC Unit
Moriaw Lane, Bo, Southern Province, Sierra Leone
https://vfapp.org/7c13

Emergency Hospital
Sugarland Drive, Adonkia Village, Western Area, Sierra Leone
https://vfapp.org/afaf

Gandorhun CHC
Koidu, Eastern Province, Sierra Leone
https://vfapp.org/f7f4

Goderich ETC
MMCET Road, Freetown, Western Area, Sierra Leone
https://vfapp.org/17de

Holy Mary Hospital
Holy Mary Drive, Bo, Southern Province, Sierra Leone
https://vfapp.org/28bf

Holy Spirit Hospital
Wallace Johnson Street, Makeni, Bombali District, Sierra Leone
https://vfapp.org/379a

Kailahun Government Hospital
Kailahun, Eastern Province, Sierra Leone
https://vfapp.org/bc46

Kamakwie Wesleyan Hospital
Kamakwie Makeni Rd, Bombali, Sierra Leone
https://vfapp.org/1b62

Kambia General Hospital
TAH 7, Kambia, North Western Province, Sierra Leone
https://vfapp.org/a952

Kenema Government Hospital
Combema Road, Kenema, Eastern Province, Sierra Leone
https://vfapp.org/dd2c

Kindoya Hospital
Prince Williams St., Bo, Sierra Leone
https://vfapp.org/dd99

Kingharman Maternal and Child Health Hospital
King Harman Rd, Freetown,

Sierra Leone
⊕ https://vfapp.org/91e7

Lakka Hospital ETU
St. Micheal Drive, Angola Town, Western Area, Sierra Leone
⊕ https://vfapp.org/6c83

Maforki ETU
TAH 7, Port Loko, Port Loko District, Sierra Leone
⊕ https://vfapp.org/174e

Magburaka Hospital
Police Roundabout, Magburaka, Northern Province, Sierra Leone
⊕ https://vfapp.org/2b6c

Mahera Hospital
Mahera Hospital Road, Mahera, Port Loko District, Sierra Leone
⊕ https://vfapp.org/f3ea

Makeni Regional Hospital
Aggienold Road, Makeni, Bombali District, Sierra Leone
⊕ https://vfapp.org/5bb6

Malema
Malema, Eastern Province, Sierra Leone
⊕ https://vfapp.org/f521

Mamudia MCHP
Mamudia, Koinadugu District, Sierra Leone
⊕ https://vfapp.org/685f

Masanga Hospital
Ms Road, Masanga, Northern Province, Sierra Leone
⊕ https://vfapp.org/77b4

Mattru General Hospital
Momaligie Road, Mattru Jong, Southern Province, Sierra Leone
⊕ https://vfapp.org/39ee

Mercy Hospital
Mahei Boima Road, Bo, Southern Province, Sierra Leone
⊕ https://vfapp.org/a84c

Morning Star
73 Old Railway Line, Bo, Southern Province, Sierra Leone
⊕ https://vfapp.org/7c9d

National Emergency Medical Service (NEMS)
Freetown, Sierra Leone
⊕ https://vfapp.org/b43e

Ola During Children's Hospital
Fourah Bay Road, Freetown, Western Area, Sierra Leone
⊕ https://vfapp.org/c1bf

Panguma Hospital
Minor Road, Panguma, Eastern Province, Sierra Leone
⊕ https://vfapp.org/9c77

Police Training Sch-Hastings 1 ETC
Leigh Road, Hastings, Western Area, Sierra Leone
⊕ https://vfapp.org/2c2c

Port Loko Hospital
Kandebaleh Street, Port Loko, Port Loko District, Sierra Leone
⊕ https://vfapp.org/f1f8

Pujehun Government Hospital
Gobaru, Southern Province, Sierra Leone
⊕ https://vfapp.org/bf6e

Segbwema Nixon Memorial Hospital
Male Bridge, Masahun, Eastern Province, Sierra Leone
⊕ https://vfapp.org/1969

Shuman Hospital
Tower Hill, Freetown, Sierra Leone
⊕ https://vfapp.org/1d48

Sierra Leone Police Hospital
Battery St, Freetown, Sierra Leone
⊕ https://vfapp.org/867a

St. John of God Hospital Sierra Leone
Gbinti, Sierra Leone
⊕ https://vfapp.org/d787

St. John-of-God Catholic Hospital
Lunsar-Makeni Highway, Lunsar, Port Loko District, Sierra Leone
⊕ https://vfapp.org/c2cf

St. Mary Hospital
Lunsar Makeni Hwy, Port Loko, Sierra Leone
⊕ https://vfapp.org/b3dd

Towama Old Town Hospital
Torwama Village, Kailey St., Bo, Sierra Leone
⊕ https://vfapp.org/c1fe

United Methodist Hatfield Archer Memorial Hospital
Rotifunk, Southern Province, Sierra Leone
⊕ https://vfapp.org/6b6f

York Hospital
Black Street, York, Western Area, Sierra Leone
⊕ https://vfapp.org/5fe8

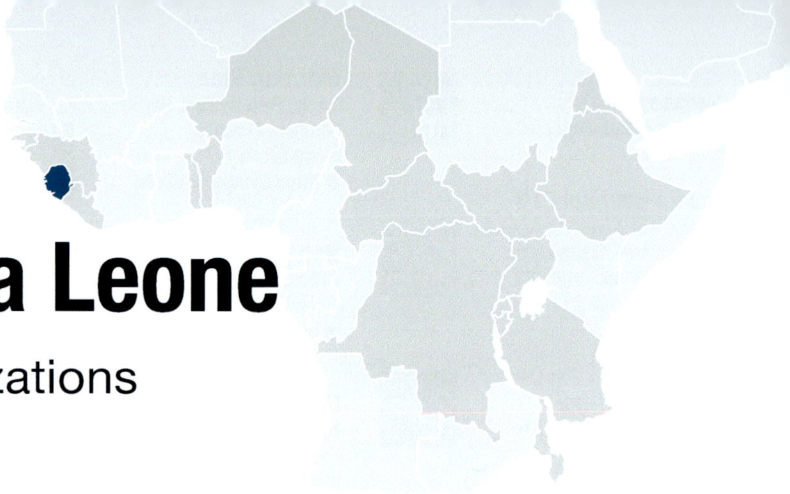

Sierra Leone

Nonprofit Organizations

Abt Associates
Seeks to improve the quality of life and economic well-being of people worldwide, while striving to meet and exceed the highest professional standards.

General, Logist-Op, MF Med, OB-GYN, Peds
+1 212-779-7700
https://vfapp.org/cec2

Action Against Hunger
Aims to end life-threatening hunger for good through treating and preventing malnutrition across more than forty-five countries.

+1 212-967-7800
https://vfapp.org/2dbc

Advance Family Planning
Aims to achieve global expansion and access to quality contraceptive information, services, and supplies through financial investment and political commitment.

General, MF Med, Pub Health
+1 410-502-8715
https://vfapp.org/7478

Adventist Health International
Focuses on upgrading and managing mission hospitals by providing governance, consultation, and technical assistance to a number of affiliated Seventh-Day Adventist hospitals throughout Africa, Asia, and the Americas.

Dent-OMFS, General, Pub Health
+1 909-558-5610
https://vfapp.org/16aa

Africa CDC
Aims to strengthen the capacity and capability of Africa's public health institutions as well as partnerships to detect and respond quickly and effectively to disease threats and outbreaks, based on data-driven interventions and programs.

Infect Dis, Logist-Op, Pub Health
+251 11 551 7700
https://vfapp.org/339c

Africa Humanitarian Action (AHA)
Responds to crises, conflicts, and disasters in Africa, while informing and advising the international community, governments, civil society, and the private sector on humanitarian issues of concern to Africa. Supports institutional and organizational development efforts.

General, Infect Dis, MF Med, Nutr, OB-GYN
+251 11 660 4800
https://vfapp.org/3ca2

Africa Uplifted
Seeks to enrich the lives of the people of Sierra Leone by promoting basic wellness, removing barriers to education, satisfying essential physical needs, and nurturing spiritual development.

General
+1 952-797-3895
https://vfapp.org/ba33

African Cultural Exchange, Inc., The
Enriches lives through humanitarian programs in culture, development, education, and healthcare.

General
+1 888-748-0843
https://vfapp.org/f238

Against Malaria Foundation
Helps protect people from malaria. Funds anti-malaria nets, specifically long-lasting insecticidal nets (LLINs), and works with distribution partners to ensure they are used. Tracks and reports on net use and malaria case data.

Infect Dis
+44 20 7371 8735
https://vfapp.org/337d

AIDS Healthcare Foundation
Provides cutting-edge HIV/AIDS medical care and advocacy to over one million people in forty-three countries.

Infect Dis
+1 323-860-5200
https://vfapp.org/b27c

AISPO
Implements international initiatives in the healthcare sector and remains involved in a variety of projects to combat poverty, social injustice, and disease in the world.

All-Immu, ER Med, GI, General, Infect Dis, Logist-Op, MF Med, Neonat, OB-GYN, Peds, Psych, Pub Health, Radiol
+39 02 2643 4481
https://vfapp.org/c9e6

Americares
Saves lives and improves health for people affected by poverty or disaster and responds with life-changing medicine, medical supplies, and health programs including domestic and global medical clinics.
All-Immu, ER Med, General, Infect Dis, MF Med, Nutr
+1 203-658-9500
https://vfapp.org/e567

Aminata Maternal Foundation
Aims to improve maternal mortality outcomes for women and girls in Sierra Leone.
MF Med, Neonat, OB-GYN
+61 413 078 495
https://vfapp.org/a9f2

Amref Health Africa
Serves millions of people across thirty-five countries in Sub-Saharan Africa, strengthening health systems, and training African health workers to respond to the continent's most critical health issues.
All-Immu, General, Infect Dis, Logist-Op, MF Med, OB-GYN, Path, Pub Health, Surg
+254 20 6993000
https://vfapp.org/6985

Aspen Management Partnership for Health (AMP Health)
Works to improve health systems and outcomes by collaborating with governments to strengthen leadership and management capabilities through public-private partnership.
Logist-Op
+1 202-736-5800
https://vfapp.org/ea78

Association of Sierra Leonean Health Professionals in the US, The (TASHPUS)
Works to improve the standard of health for the people of Sierra Leone through education, volunteerism, partnering with and empowering communities, and strengthening health systems.
General, Infect Dis, Logist-Op, Peds, Surg
+1 302-220-4410
https://vfapp.org/fcba

Austrian Doctors
Stands for a life in dignity and takes care of the health of disadvantaged people. Helps all people regardless of gender, skin color, religion or sexual orientation.
General, Infect Dis, Medicine
+1 215-780-1845
https://vfapp.org/e929

BethanyKids
Transforms the lives of African children with surgical conditions and disabilities through pediatric surgery, rehabilitation, public education, spiritual ministry, and training health professionals.
Neurosurg, Nutr, Ortho, Ped Surg, Peds, Rehab, Surg
https://vfapp.org/db4e

Bo Children's Hospital
Cares for sick children and provides health education for families in Sierra Leone.
All-Immu, Anesth, Infect Dis, MF Med, Neonat, Nutr, Peds
https://vfapp.org/6f11

BRAC USA
Seeks to empower people and communities in situations of poverty, illiteracy, disease, and social injustice. Interventions aim to achieve large-scale, positive changes through economic and social programs that enable everyone to realize their potential.
ER Med, General, Infect Dis, Logist-Op, MF Med, OB-GYN
+1 212-808-5615
https://vfapp.org/9d9e

BroadReach
Collaborates with governments, multinational health organizations, donors, and private sector companies to affect healthcare reform and solve the world's biggest health challenges.
Logist-Op
+27 21 514 8300
https://vfapp.org/7812

Carter Center, The
Seeks to prevent and resolve conflicts, enhance freedom and democracy, and improve health, while remaining committed to human rights and the alleviation of human suffering.
Infect Dis, MF Med, Ophth-Opt
+1 800-550-3560
https://vfapp.org/6556

Catholic Organization for Relief & Development Aid (CORDAID)
Provides humanitarian assistance and creates opportunities to improve security, healthcare, education, and inclusive economic growth in fragile and conflict-affected areas.
ER Med, Infect Dis, MF Med, OB-GYN, Peds, Psych
+31 70 313 6300
https://vfapp.org/8ae5

CAUSE Canada
Strives to be a catalyst for global justice as a faith-based organization that aims to provide sustainable, integrated community development in rural West Africa and Central America through authentic, collaborative long-term relationships.
General, MF Med, Neonat, OB-GYN, Peds
+1 403-678-3332
https://vfapp.org/6fc1

Centre for Global Mental Health
Closes the care gap and reduces human rights abuses experienced by people living with mental, neurological, and substance use conditions, particularly in low-resource settings.
Neuro, OB-GYN, Palliative, Peds, Psych
https://vfapp.org/a96d

Chain of Hope
Provides lifesaving heart operations for children around the world and supports the development of cardiac services in numerous developing and war-torn countries.
Anesth, CT Surg, CV Med, Crit-Care, Ped Surg, Peds, Pulm-Critic, Surg
+44 20 7351 1978
https://vfapp.org/1b1b

ChildFund Australia
Works to reduce poverty for children in many of the world's most disadvantaged communities.
ER Med, General, Peds
+1 800023600
https://vfapp.org/13df

Children & Charity International

Puts people first by providing education, leadership, and nutrition programs along with mentoring and healthcare support services to children, youth, and families.

Nutr, Peds

+1 202-234-0488

https://vfapp.org/6538

Children of the Nations

Provides holistic, Christ-centered care for orphaned children, enabling them to create positive and lasting change in their nations.

Anesth, Dent-OMFS, General, Surg

+1 360-698-7227

https://vfapp.org/cc52

Children Without Worms

Enhances the health and development of children by reducing intestinal worm infections.

Infect Dis, Pub Health

+1 404-371-0466

https://vfapp.org/6bee

Christian Aid Ministries

Strives to be a trustworthy and efficient channel for Amish, Mennonite, and other conservative Anabaptist groups and individuals to minister to physical and spiritual needs around the world.

CT Surg, ER Med, Logist-Op, Ortho, Pub Health

+1 330-893-2428

https://vfapp.org/7b33

Christian Blind Mission (CBM)

Aims to improve the quality of life of persons with disabilities in the poorest countries, addressing poverty as a cause, and a consequence, of disability, and working in partnership to create a society for all.

ENT, General, Infect Dis, OB-GYN, Ophth-Opt, Ortho, Peds, Psych, Rehab, Surg

+49 6251 131131

https://vfapp.org/3824

Christian Connections for International Health (CCIH)

Promotes global health and wholeness from a Christian perspective.

All-Immu, General, Infect Dis, MF Med, Neonat, OB-GYN, Psych

+1 703-923-8960

https://vfapp.org/fa5d

Circle of Health International (COHI)

Aligns with local, community-based organizations led and powered by women to help respond to the needs of the women and children that they serve. Helps with the provision of professional volunteers, capacity training, and procurement of requested and appropriate supplies and equipment. Raises funds for the organizations to provide the services required.

ER Med, Logist-Op, MF Med, Neonat, OB-GYN, Psych

+1 512-210-7710

https://vfapp.org/8b63

City Garden Clinic

Works to provide quality patient care with attention to clinical excellence and patient safety.

Crit-Care, General, Infect Dis, OB-GYN, Ortho, Surg, Urol

+1 405-473-3214

https://vfapp.org/dbeb

Clinton Health Access Initiative (CHAI)

Aims to save lives and reduce the burden of disease in low- and middle-income countries. Works with partners to strengthen the capabilities of governments and the private sector to create and sustain high-quality health systems.

General, Heme-Onc, Infect Dis, Logist-Op, MF Med, Medicine, Neonat, Nutr, OB-GYN, Path, Peds, Rad-Onc

+1 617-774-0110

https://vfapp.org/9ed7

Concern Worldwide

Seeks to permanently transform the lives of people living in extreme poverty, tackling its root causes, and building resilience.

Logist-Op, MF Med, Nutr, OB-GYN

+353 1 417 7700

https://vfapp.org/77e9

Curamericas Global

Partners with communities abroad to save the lives of mothers and children by providing health services and education.

General, Infect Dis, MF Med, OB-GYN, Peds, Pub Health

+1 919-510-8787

https://vfapp.org/286b

Dentaid

Seeks to treat, equip, train, and educate people in need of dental care.

Dent-OMFS

+44 1794 324249

https://vfapp.org/a183

Direct Relief

Improves the health and lives of people affected by poverty or emergency situations by mobilizing and providing essential medical resources needed for their care.

ER Med, Logist-Op

+1 805-964-4767

https://vfapp.org/58e5

Doctors with Africa (CUAMM)

Advocates for the universal right to health and promotes the values of international solidarity, justice, and peace. Works to protect and improve the well-being and health of vulnerable communities in Africa with a long-term development perspective.

ER Med, Infect Dis, MF Med, Neonat, OB-GYN, Peds

https://vfapp.org/d2fb

Doctors Without Borders/Médecins Sans Frontières (MSF)

Responds to emergencies and provides lifesaving medical care where needed most, including during disasters, conflicts, and epidemics.

Anesth, Crit-Care, ER Med, General, Infect Dis, Nutr, OB-GYN, Ped Surg, Peds, Psych, Pub Health, Surg

+1 212-679-6800

https://vfapp.org/f363

eHealth Africa
Builds stronger health systems in Africa through the design and implementation of data-driven solutions, responding to local needs and providing underserved communities with the necessary tools to lead healthier lives.

Logist-Op, Path

https://vfapp.org/db6a

EMERGENCY
Provides free, high-quality healthcare to victims of war, poverty, and landmines. Also builds hospitals and trains local staff, while pursuing human-rights-based medicine.

ER Med, Neonat, OB-GYN, Ophth-Opt, Ped Surg

+39 02 881881

https://vfapp.org/c361

Episcopal Relief & Development
Provides relief in times of disaster and promotes sustainable development by identifying and addressing the root causes of suffering.

Infect Dis, MF Med, Neonat, Nutr, Peds

+1 855-312-4325

https://vfapp.org/7cfa

eRanger
Provides sustainable solutions to transportation and medical provision such as ambulances and mobile clinics in developing countries.

ER Med, General, Logist-Op

+27 40 654 3207

https://vfapp.org/4c18

Freedom From Fistula
Helps women and girls who are injured and left incontinent following prolonged, obstructed childbirth by providing free surgical repairs for patients already suffering with fistula, as well as maternity care to prevent fistulas from happening at all.

MF Med, OB-GYN, Peds

+1 646-867-0994

https://vfapp.org/6e11

Friends of Nixon Memorial Hospital
Supports the Nixon Memorial Hospital in providing inpatient and outpatient care to the town of Segbwema and the surrounding rural villages in Sierra Leone.

General, Logist-Op, OB-GYN, Path, Peds

https://vfapp.org/545b

German Doctors
Conducts voluntary medical work in developing countries and brings help where misery is part of everyday life.

General, Infect Dis, Medicine

https://vfapp.org/21ad

Global Alliance to Prevent Prematurity and Stillbirth (GAPPS)
Seeks to improve birth outcomes worldwide by reducing the burden of premature birth and stillbirth.

All-Immu, Infect Dis, MF Med, Neonat, Neonat, OB-GYN

+1 206-413-7954

https://vfapp.org/3f74

Global Ministries – The United Methodist Church
As the worldwide mission and development agency of The United Methodist Church, Global Ministries works with more than 300 hospitals and clinics around the world through its Global Health Unit.

Anesth, CT Surg, CV Med, Crit-Care, Dent-OMFS, Derm, ER Med, GI, General, Infect Dis, Logist-Op, MF Med, Medicine, Neonat, Nephro, Nutr, OB-GYN, Ophth-Opt, Ortho, Palliative, Peds, Pod, Psych, Pub Health, Rehab, Rheum, Surg, Urol

+1 800-862-4246

https://vfapp.org/1723

Global Oncology (GO)
Brings the best in cancer care to underserved patients around the world and collaborates across geographic, professional, and academic borders to improve cancer care, research, and education.

Heme-Onc, Path, Rad-Onc

https://vfapp.org/fcb8

Global Polio Eradication Initiative
Aims to eradicate polio worldwide.

All-Immu, Logist-Op

+1 847-866-3000

https://vfapp.org/7e2c

GOAL
Works with the most vulnerable communities to help them respond to and recover from humanitarian crises, and to assist them in building transcendent solutions to mitigate poverty and vulnerability.

ER Med, General, Pub Health

+353 1 280 9779

https://vfapp.org/bbea

Hands for Africa
Provides innocent civil war victims in Africa with tools that enable them to become self-reliant, such as immediate needs like food, water, clothing, and shelter, while developing and implementing successful programs that foster self-reliance.

Ortho, Rehab

+1 714-426-2229

https://vfapp.org/19a3

Healing Hands Foundation, The
Provides high-quality surgical procedures, medical treatment, dental care, and educational support in under-resourced areas worldwide.

Anesth, Dent-OMFS, General, Ped Surg, Peds, Surg

+1 410-440-0473

https://vfapp.org/4bfc

Health Equity Initiative
Aims to build and sustain a global community that engages across sectors and disciplines to advance health equity.

Pub Health

https://vfapp.org/e2e2

Health Poverty Action
Works in partnership with people around the world who are pursuing change in their own communities to demand health justice and challenge power imbalances.

ER Med, General, Infect Dis, Psych, Pub Health

+44 20 7840 3777

https://vfapp.org/ee58

Heart to Heart International
Strengthens communities through improving health access, providing humanitarian development, and administering crisis relief worldwide. Engages volunteers, collaborates with partners, and deploys resources to achieve this mission.

Anesth, ER Med, General, Logist-Op, Medicine, Path, Path, Peds, Psych, Pub Health, Surg

+1 913-764-5200

https://vfapp.org/aacb

Heineman Medical Outreach
Provides medical and educational assistance globally to promote sustainable healthcare and enhanced living standards in underserved communities through the International Medical Outreach (IMO) program, a collaborative partnership between Heineman Medical Outreach and Atrium Health.

Anesth, CT Surg, CV Med, ER Med, General, Heme-Onc, Logist-Op, Medicine, Neonat, OB-GYN, Ped Surg, Peds, Surg, Vasc Surg

+1 704-374-0505

https://vfapp.org/389b

Helen Keller International
Seeks to eliminate preventable vision loss, malnutrition, and diseases of poverty.

Infect Dis, Nutr, OB-GYN, Ophth-Opt, Peds

+1 212-532-0544

https://vfapp.org/b654

Help Madina
Envisions a world where every citizen of Sierra Leone is healthy and has the opportunity to contribute meaningfully to society. Works hand-in-hand with the people living in the Madina district and other locations in Sierra Leone to improve people's health and well-being.

Endo, General, Geri, Infect Dis, Nutr, Ophth-Opt, Peds, Pub Health

+44 1285 711180

https://vfapp.org/86c8

Helping Children Worldwide
Supports programs that provide vulnerable children and their families with education, healthcare, and spiritual mentoring, in order to help transform communities and create sustainable futures, inspired by the Christian faith.

Heme-Onc, Infect Dis, Nutr, OB-GYN, Ped Surg, Peds

+1 703-793-9521

https://vfapp.org/c3c1

HelpMeSee
Trains local cataract specialists in Manual Small Incision Cataract Surgery (MSICS) in significant numbers, to meet the increasing demand for surgical services in the communities most impacted by cataract blindness.

Anesth, Ophth-Opt, Surg

+1 844-435-7638

https://vfapp.org/973c

Humanity & Inclusion
Works alongside people with disabilities and vulnerable populations, taking action and bearing witness in order to respond to their essential needs, improve their living conditions and health, and promote respect for their dignity and fundamental rights.

General, Infect Dis, MF Med, Medicine, Ortho, Peds, Psych, Pub Health, Rehab

+1 301-891-2138

https://vfapp.org/16b7

Humanity First
Provides aid and assistance to those in need, offering sustainable development solutions to society while providing and empowering local communities with the resources to help themselves.

ER Med, General, MF Med, Ophth-Opt

+44 20 8417 0082

https://vfapp.org/13cc

ICAP at Columbia University
Serves as global leader in supporting the scale-up of multidisciplinary HIV/AIDS prevention, care, and treatment programs based on a family-focused approach.

General, Infect Dis, MF Med, Medicine, OB-GYN, Pub Health

+1 212-342-0505

https://vfapp.org/a8ef

International Agency for the Prevention of Blindness (IAPB), The
Leads international efforts in blindness-prevention activities, works toward a world where no one is needlessly visually impaired, and ensures that everyone has access to the best possible standard of eye health.

Infect Dis, Ophth-Opt, Pub Health

https://vfapp.org/87a2

International Federation of Gynecology and Obstetrics (FIGO)
Implements global projects on specific women's health issues.

MF Med, Medicine, Neonat, OB-GYN, Surg, Urol

+44 20 7928 1166

https://vfapp.org/c4b4

International Federation of Red Cross and Red Crescent Societies (IFRC)
Coordinates and directs international assistance following natural and man-made disasters in nonconflict situations through the world's largest humanitarian and development network. Provides disaster-preparedness programs, healthcare activities, and promotes humanitarian values.

ER Med, General, Infect Dis, Nutr

+1 212-338-0161

https://vfapp.org/b4ee

International Learning Movement (ILM UK)
Supports some of the world's poorest people in developing countries with core projects in education, safe drinking water, and healthcare.

General, Ophth-Opt

+44 1254 265451

https://vfapp.org/b974

International Organization for Migration (IOM) – The UN Migration Agency
Promotes evidence-informed policies and holistic, preventive, and curative health programs that are beneficial, accessible, and equitable for vulnerable migrants.

General, Infect Dis, OB-GYN

+27 12 342 2789

https://vfapp.org/621a

International Planned Parenthood Federation (IPPF)
Leads a locally owned, globally connected civil society movement that provides and enables services and champions sexual and reproductive health and rights for all, especially

the underserved.
Infect Dis, MF Med, OB-GYN
+44 20 7939 8200
https://vfapp.org/dc97

International Rescue Committee (IRC)
Responds to the world's worst humanitarian crises and helps people whose lives and livelihoods are shattered by conflict and disaster to survive, recover, and gain control of their future.
ER Med, General, Infect Dis, MF Med, Peds
+1 212-551-3000
https://vfapp.org/5d24

International Surgical Health Initiative (ISHI)
Provides free surgical care to underserved communities worldwide, regardless of race, religion, politics, geography, or financial considerations.
Anesth, ER Med, Logist-Op, Ped Surg, Surg, Urol
+1 551-689-3632
https://vfapp.org/2374

InterSurgeon
Fosters collaborative partnerships in the field of global surgery that will advance clinical care, teaching, training, research, and the provision and maintenance of medical equipment.
ENT, Neurosurg, Ortho, Ped Surg, Plast, Surg, Urol
https://vfapp.org/6f8a

IntraHealth International
Improves the performance of health workers and strengthens the systems in which they work.
CV Med, Endo, General, Infect Dis, MF Med, Neonat, Nutr, OB-GYN
+1 919-313-3554
https://vfapp.org/ddc8

Iris Global
Serves the poor, the destitute, the lost, and the forgotten by providing adoration, outreach, family, education, relief, development, healing, and the arts.
General, Infect Dis, Nutr, Pub Health
+1 530-255-2077
https://vfapp.org/37f8

IsraAID
Supports people affected by humanitarian crisis and partners with local communities around the world to provide urgent aid, assist recovery, and reduce the risk of future disasters.
ER Med, Infect Dis, Psych, Rehab
+972 3-947-7766
https://vfapp.org/de96

IVUmed
Aims to make quality urological care available worldwide by providing medical and surgical education for physicians and nurses and treatment for thousands of children and adults.
Anesth, OB-GYN, Ped Surg, Surg, Urol
+1 801-524-0201
https://vfapp.org/e619

John Snow, Inc. (JSI)
Aims to improve the health and well-being of underserved and vulnerable people and communities throughout the world.
General, Infect Dis, Logist-Op, MF Med, OB-GYN, Peds, Psych, Pub Health
+1 617-482-9485
https://vfapp.org/ba78

Johns Hopkins Center for Communication Programs
Believes in the power of communication to save lives, by empowering people to adopt healthy behaviors for themselves, their families, and their communities.
General, Infect Dis, Logist-Op, OB-GYN, Pub Health
+1 410-659-6300
https://vfapp.org/1bf9

Joint Aid Management (JAM)
Provides food security, nutrition, water, and sanitation to vulnerable communities in Africa in dignified and sustainable ways.
ER Med, Nutr
+27 11 548 3900
https://vfapp.org/dcac

Joint United Nations Programme on HIV/AIDS (UNAIDS)
Aims to place people living with HIV and people affected by the virus at the decision-making table and at the center of designing, delivering, and monitoring the AIDS response.
Infect Dis
+41 22 791 36 66
https://vfapp.org/464a

Kambia Appeal, The
Works in collaboration with the key groups in the Kambia District to support and strengthen the existing health facilities owned and managed by the government of Sierra Leone to improve maternal and child health.
General, MF Med, Neonat, OB-GYN
https://vfapp.org/b128

King's Sierra Leone Partnership
Aims to build a strong and resilient health system in Sierra Leone.
Crit-Care, Dent-OMFS, ER Med, Infect Dis, Medicine, Path, Psych, Rehab, Surg
+44 20 7848 0981
https://vfapp.org/e4f1

Korle-Bu Neuroscience Foundation
Committed to providing medical support for brain and spinal injuries and disease to the people of Ghana and West Africa.
Anesth, Logist-Op, Neuro, Neurosurg, Rehab
+1 604-513-0029
https://vfapp.org/6695

Life for African Mothers
Aims to save the lives of pregnant women in Sub-Saharan Africa.
MF Med, Neonat, OB-GYN
+44 29 2034 3774
https://vfapp.org/fce2

Lions Clubs International
Empowers volunteers to serve their communities, meet humanitarian needs, encourage peace, and promote international understanding through Lions clubs.

Heme-Onc, Medicine, Nutr, Ophth-Opt
+1 630-571-5466
https://vfapp.org/7b12

London School of Hygiene & Tropical Medicine: Health in Humanitarian Crises Centre
Advances health and health equity in crisis-affected countries through research, education, and translation of knowledge into policy and practice.
ER Med, Infect Dis, Pub Health
+44 20 7636 8636
https://vfapp.org/96ad

London School of Hygiene & Tropical Medicine: International Centre for Eye Health
Works to improve eye health and eliminate avoidable visual impairment and blindness with a focus on low-income populations.
Logist-Op, Ophth-Opt, Pub Health
+44 20 7958 8316
https://vfapp.org/6f5f

Mama-Pikin Foundation
Helps enhance, improve, and otherwise positively contribute to the health and well-being of mothers, children, and families in Sierra Leone, West Africa.
General, MF Med, Neonat, Nutr, OB-GYN
+1 404-326-5560
https://vfapp.org/4aa6

Management Sciences for Health (MSH)
Works with countries and communities to save lives and improve the health of the world's poorest and most vulnerable people by building strong, resilient, sustainable health systems.
Infect Dis, Logist-Op, Pub Health
+1 617-250-9500
https://vfapp.org/6aa2

MAP International
Provides medicines and health supplies to those in need around the world so they might experience life to the fullest.
Logist-Op
+1 800-225-8550
https://vfapp.org/deed

Marie Stopes International
Provides the contraception and safe abortion services that enable women all over the world to choose their own futures.
Infect Dis, MF Med, Neonat, OB-GYN, Pub Health
+44 20 7636 6200
https://vfapp.org/9525

Massachusetts General Hospital Global Surgery Initiative
Aims to improve surgical education and access to advanced surgical care in resource-limited settings around the world by performing surgical operations as visitors, training local surgeons, and sharing medical technology through international partnerships across disciplines.
Anesth, Crit-Care, ER Med, Heme-Onc, Peds, Surg
+1 617-724-4093
https://vfapp.org/31b1

Maternity Foundation
Works to ensure safer childbirth for women and newborns everywhere through innovative mobile health solutions such as the Safe Delivery App, a mobile training tool for skilled birth attendants.
MF Med, OB-GYN, Pub Health
https://vfapp.org/ff4f

Maternity Worldwide
Works with communities and partners to identify and develop appropriate and effective ways to reduce maternal and newborn mortality and morbidity, facilitate communities to access quality skilled maternity care, and support the provision of quality skilled care.
MF Med, OB-GYN
+44 1273 234033
https://vfapp.org/822b

Médecins du Monde/Doctors of the World
Provides care, bears witness, and supports social change worldwide with innovative medical programs and evidence-based advocacy initiatives.
ER Med, General, Infect Dis, MF Med, Neonat, OB-GYN, Peds, Pub Health
+33 1 44 92 15 15
https://vfapp.org/a43d

Medical Assistance Sierra Leone
Supports access to healthcare and urgent medical treatment for communities and individuals in Sierra Leone.
General, Neuro
+44 118 375 1432
https://vfapp.org/3925

Medical Care Development International (MCD International)
Works to strengthen health systems through innovative, sustainable interventions.
Infect Dis, Logist-Op, OB-GYN, Pub Health
+1 301-562-1920
https://vfapp.org/dc5c

MedShare
Aims to improve the quality of life of people, communities, and the planet by sourcing and directly delivering surplus medical supplies and equipment to communities in need around the world.
Logist-Op
+1 770-323-5858
https://vfapp.org/c8bc

MENTOR Initiative
Saves lives in emergencies through tropical disease control, and helps people recover from crisis with dignity, working side by side with communities, health workers, and health authorities to leave a lasting impact.
ER Med, Infect Dis
+44 1444 412171
https://vfapp.org/3bd5

Mercy Ships
Operates hospital ships staffed by volunteers to bring hope, healing, and healthcare to underserved communities worldwide.
Anesth, Dent-OMFS, Logist-Op, Neonat, OB-GYN, Ophth-Opt, Ortho, Palliative, Plast, Psych, Surg
+1 903-939-7000
https://vfapp.org/2e99

Mercy Without Limits
Educates and empowers women and children by enabling them to have an effective and positive role in constructing a better society.

ER Med

☎ +1 855-633-3695

⊕ https://vfapp.org/c3b6

MiracleFeet
Brings low-cost treatment to every child on the planet born with clubfoot, a leading cause of physical disability.

Ortho, Peds, Rehab

☎ +1 919-240-5572

⊕ https://vfapp.org/bda8

Mission of Hope: Rotifunk Sierra Leone
Brings better healthcare, education, economic opportunities, and sustainability to mothers and children in this impoverished region.

General, OB-GYN, Peds

☎ +1 910-239-7892

⊕ https://vfapp.org/e74e

Mobility Outreach International
Enables mobility for children and adults in under-resourced areas of the world, and creates a sustainable orthopedic surgery model using local resources.

Ortho, Rehab

☎ +1 206-726-1636

⊕ https://vfapp.org/9376

Nazarene Compassionate Ministries
Partners with local churches around the world to clothe, shelter, feed, heal, educate, and live in solidarity with those in need.

General, Infect Dis, OB-GYN

☎ +1 800-310-6362

⊕ https://vfapp.org/6b4d

Operation Fistula
Exists to end obstetric fistula by building models of care that serve every woman, everywhere.

MF Med, OB-GYN, Surg

☎ +1 512-687-3479

⊕ https://vfapp.org/ce8e

Options
Believes in a world where women and children can access the high-quality health services they need, without financial burden.

Logist-Op, MF Med, Neonat, OB-GYN

☎ +44 20 7430 1900

⊕ https://vfapp.org/3a48

Pact
Works on the ground to improve the lives of those who are challenged by poverty and marginalization, striving for a world where all people are heard, capable, and vibrant.

Infect Dis, Logist-Op, MF Med, Pub Health

☎ +1 202-466-5666

⊕ https://vfapp.org/9a6c

Partners for World Health
Sorts, evaluates, repackages, and prepares supplies and equipment for distribution to individuals, communities, and healthcare facilities in need, both locally and internationally.

ER Med, General, Logist-Op

☎ +1 207-774-5555

⊕ https://vfapp.org/982e

Partners in Health
Responds to the moral imperative to provide high-quality healthcare globally to those who need it most, while striving to ease suffering by providing a comprehensive model of care that includes access to food, transportation, housing, and other key components of healing.

CT Surg, General, Heme-Onc, Infect Dis, MF Med, Neurosurg, OB-GYN, Ortho, Plast, Psych, Urol

☎ +1 857-880-5600

⊕ https://vfapp.org/dc9c

Patcha Foundation
Dedicates efforts to healthcare, securing and providing the latest and most innovative approaches to diagnosis and treatment.

ER Med, General, Logist-Op, Nutr, Palliative, Peds, Surg

☎ +1 301-850-2991

⊕ https://vfapp.org/ea4a

Practical Tools Initiative
Provides or assists in the provision of education, training, healthcare projects and all the necessary support designed to enable individuals to generate a sustainable income.

General, Logist-Op, MF Med

☎ +44 1329 829121

⊕ https://vfapp.org/16b6

Project HOPE
Works on the front lines of the world's health challenges, partnering hand-in-hand with communities, healthcare workers, and public health systems to ensure sustainable change.

CV Med, ER Med, Endo, General, Infect Dis, MF Med, Peds

☎ +1 844-349-0188

⊕ https://vfapp.org/2bd7

PSI – Population Services International
Dedicates efforts to improving the health of people in the developing world by focusing on challenges such as a lack of family planning, HIV/AIDS, barriers to maternal health, and the greatest threats to children under the age of 5, including malaria, diarrhea, pneumonia, and malnutrition.

Infect Dis, MF Med, OB-GYN, Peds

☎ +1 202-785-0072

⊕ https://vfapp.org/ffe3

RAD-AID International
Improves and optimizes access to medical imaging and radiology in low-resource regions of the world.

Rad-Onc, Radiol

⊕ https://vfapp.org/537f

RestoringVision
Empowers lives by restoring vision for millions of people in need.

Ophth-Opt

☎ +1 209-980-7323

⊕ https://vfapp.org/e121

Rockefeller Foundation, The
Works to promote the well-being of humanity.
Logist-Op, Nutr, Pub Health
+1 212-869-8500
https://vfapp.org/5424

Rotary International
Provides service to others, improves lives, and advances world understanding, goodwill, and peace through its fellowship of business, professional, and community leaders.
ER Med, General, Infect Dis, MF Med, OB-GYN
https://vfapp.org/8fb5

ROW Foundation
Works to improve the quality of training for healthcare providers, and the diagnosis and treatment available to people with epilepsy and associated psychiatric disorders in under-resourced areas of the world.
Neuro, Psych
+1 630-791-0247
https://vfapp.org/25eb

Rutgers New Jersey Medical School
Seeks to support and promote the global health efforts of the faculty, staff, and learners in the areas of education, research, and service through The Rutgers New Jersey Medical School's Office of Global Health.
Anesth, CV Med, Crit-Care, Neurosurg, OB-GYN, Psych
+1 732-445-4636
https://vfapp.org/8e67

Salvation Army International, The
Seeks to meet human needs through services in education, healthcare, community support, emergency response, and ministry development, inspired by the Christian faith.
Dent-OMFS, Derm, ER Med, Infect Dis, MF Med, Medicine, Nutr, OB-GYN, Ophth-Opt, Palliative, Psych, Rehab, Surg
+44 20 7332 0101
https://vfapp.org/8eb3

Sanofi Espoir Foundation
Contributes to reducing health inequalities among populations that need it most by applying a socially responsible approach focused on fighting childhood cancers in low-income countries, improving maternal and newborn health, and improving access to care.
ER Med, OB-GYN, Peds
+33 1 53 77 91 38
https://vfapp.org/943b

SATMED
Serves non-governmental organizations, hospitals, medical universities, and other healthcare providers active in resource-poor areas, by providing open-access e-health services for the health community.
Logist-Op
https://vfapp.org/b8d5

Save the Children
Gives children around the world a healthy start in life, the opportunity to learn, and protection from harm.
All-Immu, Crit-Care, ER Med, General, Infect Dis, MF Med, Medicine, Neonat, OB-GYN, Peds, Psych, Pub Health
+1 800-728-3843
https://vfapp.org/2e73

SEE International
Provides sustainable medical, surgical, and educational services through volunteer ophthalmic surgeons, with the objectives of restoring sight and preventing blindness to disadvantaged individuals worldwide.
Ophth-Opt, Surg
+1 805-963-3303
https://vfapp.org/6e1b

Set Free Alliance
Works with in-country partners to rescue children, provide clean water, host medical clinics, and plant churches, based in Christian ministry.
General, Peds
+1 864-469-9500
https://vfapp.org/bdb8

Shepherd's Hospice Sierra Leone, The
Promotes competent, compassionate care of patients and families of patients with life-limiting illnesses.
Palliative
+232 76 620441
https://vfapp.org/5831

Sierra Leone Missions and Development
Brings hope, help, and healing to Sierra Leone though agriculture, education, leadership training, healthcare missions, and disaster relief programs.
ER Med, General, Peds
+232 79 333364
https://vfapp.org/e6f5

Sightsavers
Prevents avoidable blindness in some of the poorest parts of the world by treating debilitating eye diseases.
Infect Dis, Ophth-Opt, Surg
+1 800-707-9746
https://vfapp.org/aa52

SIGN Fracture Care International
Builds orthopedic capacity around the world and provides the injured poor access to fracture surgery by donating orthopedic education and implant systems to surgeons in developing countries.
Ortho, Rehab, Surg
+1 509-371-1107
https://vfapp.org/123d

Smile Train
Seeks to give every child with a cleft the opportunity for a healthy, productive life by providing free cleft repair surgery and comprehensive cleft care in their own communities.
Dent-OMFS, ENT, Plast
+1 800-932-9541
https://vfapp.org/f21d

Solthis
Improves disease prevention and access to quality care by strengthening the health systems and services of the countries served.
General, Infect Dis, Logist-Op, MF Med, Neonat, Path
+33 1 81 70 17 90
https://vfapp.org/a71d

Sound Seekers
Supports people with hearing loss by enabling access to healthcare and education.

ENT
+44 7305 433250
https://vfapp.org/ef1c

Stepping Forward
Aims to be a practical and creative hub of information, support, and strategies for people affected by disability.
Rehab
https://vfapp.org/97de

Surg+ Restore
Creates pathways to sustainable health infrastructure to those living in nations where opportunities are lacking, through professional education, training of medical professionals, and purchasing of medical equipment.
Anesth, Dent-OMFS, ENT, Infect Dis, Logist-Op, Plast, Surg
+1 503-309-7572
https://vfapp.org/39cc

Surgeons OverSeas (SOS)
Works to reduce death and disability from surgically treatable conditions in developing countries.
Anesth, Heme-Onc, Surg
https://vfapp.org/5d16

Sustainable Cardiovascular Health Equity Development Alliance
Fights cardiovascular disease in underserved populations globally via education, training, and increasing interventional capacity.
CV Med, Pub Health, Radiol
+1 608-338-3357
https://vfapp.org/799c

Swiss Doctors
Aims to improve the health of populations in developing countries through medical-aid projects and training.
General, Infect Dis, Medicine
https://vfapp.org/311a

Swiss Sierra Leone Development Foundation
Provides long- and short-term support to communities in Northern Sierra Leone, such as health, education, and community development, with the continuing aim of self-sustainability.
Infect Dis, MF Med, Neonat
+41 22 364 27 93
https://vfapp.org/fea7

Swiss Tropical and Public Health Institute
Contributes to the improvement of the health of populations internationally, nationally, and locally through excellence in research, education, and services.
Infect Dis, Pub Health
+41 61 284 81 11
https://vfapp.org/2ee4

Task Force for Global Health, The
Consists of programs and focus areas that cover a range of global health issues including neglected tropical diseases, infectious diseases, vaccines, field epidemiology, public health informatics, health workforce development, and global health ethics.
Infect Dis, Logist-Op, Medicine, Ophth-Opt, Peds
+1 404-371-0466
https://vfapp.org/714c

Tearfund
Responds to crisis and partners with local churches to bring restoration to those living in poverty, inspired by the Christian faith.
ER Med, Logist-Op
+44 20 3906 3906
https://vfapp.org/f6cf

Touch of Grace
Provides world-class healthcare services, education, and research with compassion and grace to underserved communities and regions.
General
+1 240-505-0492
https://vfapp.org/dad7

Turing Foundation
Aims to contribute toward a better world and a better society by focusing on efforts such as health, art, education, and nature.
Infect Dis
+31 20 520 0010
https://vfapp.org/6bcc

U.S. President's Malaria Initiative (PMI)
Supports low-income countries to help control and eliminate malaria through cost-effective, lifesaving malaria interventions.
Infect Dis, MF Med, OB-GYN
+1 202-712-0000
https://vfapp.org/dc8b

Unforgotten Fund, The (UNFF)
Provides lifesaving humanitarian relief to UN Field Operations and projects such as water supply, sanitation and hygiene (WASH), food security, health, and shelter.
ER Med, MF Med, Nutr, OB-GYN, Peds
+1 443-668-2648
https://vfapp.org/928f

Union for International Cancer Control (UICC)
Unites and supports the cancer community to reduce the global cancer burden, promote greater equity, and ensure that cancer control continues to be a priority in the world health and development agenda.
Heme-Onc, Pub Health
+41 22 809 18 11
https://vfapp.org/88b1

United Methodist Volunteers in Mission (UMVIM)
Engages in short-term missions each year in ministries as varied as disaster response, community development, pastor training, microenterprise, agriculture, Vacation Bible School, building repair and construction, and medical/dental services.
Dent-OMFS, ER Med, General
https://vfapp.org/1ee6

United Nations Children's Fund (UNICEF)
Works in over 190 countries and territories to save children's lives, to defend their rights, and to help them fulfill their potential, from early childhood through adolescence.
All-Immu, Infect Dis, MF Med, Neonat, Nutr, OB-GYN, Ped Surg, Peds, Pub Health
https://vfapp.org/42d7

United Nations Development Programme (UNDP)
Helps countries achieve the simultaneous eradication of extreme poverty and significant reduction of inequalities and exclusion using a sustainable human development approach.
Infect Dis, Logist-Op, Pub Health
https://vfapp.org/935c

United Nations High Commissioner for Refugees (UNHCR)
Safeguards the rights and well-being of people who have been forced to flee, ensuring that everybody has the right to seek asylum and find safe refuge in another country, with the goal of seeking lasting solutions.
General, MF Med, Medicine, OB-GYN, Peds, Psych, Pub Health
https://vfapp.org/6636

United Nations Population Fund (UNFPA)
Supports reproductive healthcare for women and youth in more than 150 countries, focusing on delivering a world where every pregnancy is wanted, every childbirth is safe, and every young person's potential is fulfilled.
Infect Dis, MF Med, Neonat, OB-GYN, Peds, Pub Health
+1 212-963-6008
https://vfapp.org/c969

USAID: A2Z The Micronutrient and Child Blindness Project
Aims to increase the use of key micronutrient and blindness interventions to improve child and maternal health.
MF Med, Neonat, Nutr, Ophth-Opt, Surg
+1 202-884-8785
https://vfapp.org/c5f1

USAID: Human Resources for Health 2030 (HRH2030)
Helps low- and middle-income countries develop the health workforce needed to prevent maternal and child deaths, support the goals of Family Planning 2020, control the HIV/AIDS epidemic, and protect communities from infectious diseases.
Logist-Op
+1 202-955-3300
https://vfapp.org/9ea8

USAID: Leadership, Management and Governance Project
Improves leadership, management, and governance practices to strengthen health systems and improve health for all, including vulnerable populations worldwide.
Logist-Op
https://vfapp.org/d35e

Village Medical Project for Sierra Leone
Provides free medical treatment to local community members in Sierra Leone.
General, OB-GYN, Peds
+1 250-616-8594
https://vfapp.org/61f8

Vision Aid Overseas
Enables people living in poverty to access affordable glasses and eye care.
Ophth-Opt
+44 1293 535016
https://vfapp.org/c695

Vision Outreach International
Advocates for helping the blind in underserved regions of the world and empowers the poor through sight restoration.
Ophth-Opt
+1 269-428-3300
https://vfapp.org/9721

Vitamin Angels
Helps at-risk populations in need—specifically pregnant women, new mothers, and children under age five—to gain access to life-changing vitamins and minerals.
General, Nutr
+1 805-564-8400
https://vfapp.org/7da1

Voluntary Service Overseas (VSO)
Works with health workers, communities, and governments to improve health services and rights for women, babies, youth, people with disabilities, and prisoners.
General, MF Med, OB-GYN
+44 20 8780 7500
https://vfapp.org/213d

Watsi
Uses technology to make healthcare a reality for those who might not otherwise be able to afford it.
Pub Health, Surg
+1 256-792-8747
https://vfapp.org/41a3

West Africa Fistula Foundation (WAFF)
Works to bring value back to the lives of the women of Sierra Leone by providing them with access to education and resources to help reduce the number of new fistulas and to surgically remedy those that already exist.
Anesth, MF Med, OB-GYN
+1 903-463-9400
https://vfapp.org/a2ed

West African Education and Medical Mission (WAEMM)
Works to help people access healthcare in Sierra Leone and oversees 14 hospitals and 40 clinics across the country, helping to support the ongoing problem of medical supply shortages.
General, MF Med, Nutr, Ophth-Opt
+232 88 280093
https://vfapp.org/13f3

Willing and Abel
Seeks to provide connections between children in developing nations and specialist centers, helping with visas, passports, transportation, and finances.
Anesth, Dent-OMFS, Ped Surg
https://vfapp.org/9dc7

Women and Children First
Pioneers approaches that support communities to solve problems themselves.
MF Med, Neonat, OB-GYN, Peds
+44 20 7700 6309
https://vfapp.org/cdc9

Women's Refugee Commission
Seeks to improve lives by protecting the rights of women, children, and youth displaced by conflict and crisis through researching their needs, identifying solutions, and advocating for programs and

policies to strengthen their resilience.

General, MF Med, Neonat, OB-GYN, Peds, Psych

📞 +1 212-551-3115

🌐 https://vfapp.org/3d8f

World Changing Centre

Aims to provide children and young people in Sierra Leone with a better quality of life and improve standards of living in the community through education, healthcare, and sanitation activities.

General, Peds

📞 +256 3017339929

🌐 https://vfapp.org/28bb

World Health Organization, The (WHO)

The United Nations' agency for health provides leadership on global health matters, shapes the health research agenda, setting norms and standards, articulates evidence-based policy options, provides technical support and monitoring to countries, and assesses health trends.

ER Med, General, Infect Dis, Logist-Op, MF Med, OB-GYN, Peds, Psych, Pub Health

📞 +41 22 791 21 11

🌐 https://vfapp.org/c476

World Hope International

Empowers the poorest individuals around the world so they can become agents of change within their communities, by offering resources and knowledge.

Infect Dis, Logist-Op, MF Med, OB-GYN, Peds

📞 +1 703-923-9414

🌐 https://vfapp.org/a4b8

World Medical Relief

Facilitates the distribution of surplus medical resources where they are needed.

Logist-Op

📞 +1 313-866-5333

🌐 https://vfapp.org/72dc

World Vision International

Works with vulnerable communities around the world to overcome poverty and injustice with child-focused programs.

ER Med, General, Infect Dis, MF Med, Nutr, OB-GYN, Peds

📞 +1 626-303-8811

🌐 https://vfapp.org/2642

Worldwide Healing Hands

Works to improve the quality of healthcare for women and children in the most underserved areas of the world and to stop the preventable deaths of mothers.

General, MF Med, Neonat, OB-GYN

📞 +1 707-279-8733

🌐 https://vfapp.org/b331

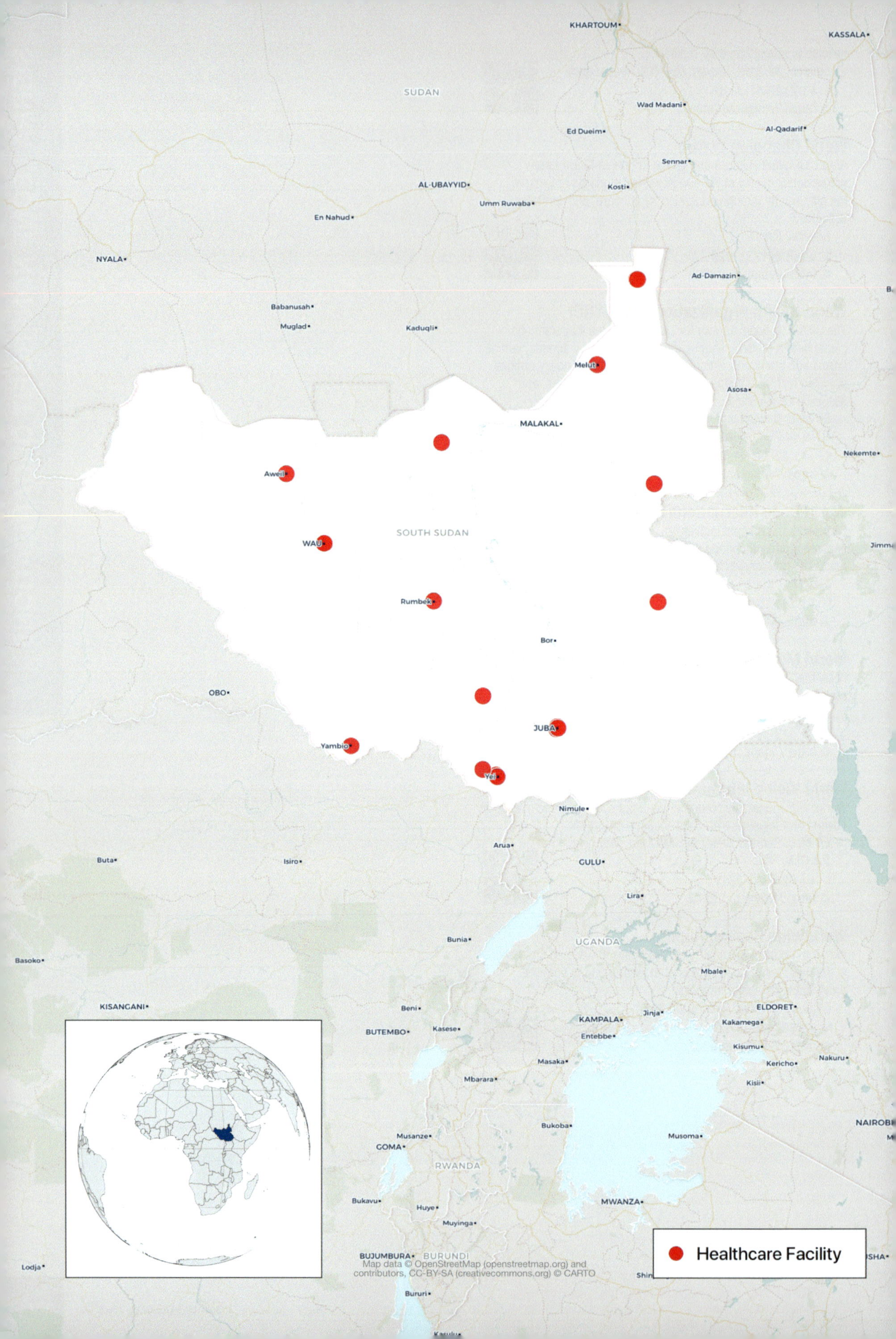

KHARTOUM
KASSALA
SUDAN
Wad Madani
Ed Dueim
Al-Qadarif
Sennar
AL-UBAYYID
Kosti
Umm Ruwaba
En Nahud
NYALA
Ad-Damazin
Babanusah
Muglad
Kaduqli
Melut
Asosa
MALAKAL
Nekemte
Aweil
SOUTH SUDAN
WAU
Rumbek
Bor
OBO
JUBA
Yambio
Yei
Nimule
Arua
Buta
Isiro
GULU
Lira
Bunia
UGANDA
Basoko
Mbale
KISANGANI
Beni
ELDORET
KAMPALA
Jinja
BUTEMBO
Kasese
Kakamega
Entebbe
Kisumu
Masaka
Nakuru
Kericho
Mbarara
Kisii
Bukoba
NAIROBI
Musanze
Musoma
GOMA
RWANDA
Bukavu
MWANZA
Huye
Muyinga
BUJUMBURA
BURUNDI
Lodja
Bururi
Healthcare Facility
Map data © OpenStreetMap (openstreetmap.org) and contributors, CC-BY-SA (creativecommons.org) © CARTO

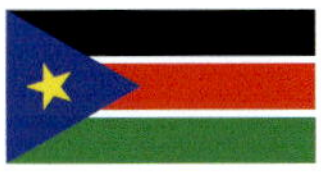

South Sudan

The Republic of South Sudan is a landlocked nation in East-Central Africa whose bordering neighbors are Sudan, Ethiopia, Kenya, the Democratic Republic of the Congo, Uganda, and the Central African Republic. South Sudan is one of the most culturally diverse countries in sub-Saharan Africa, with a population of about 10.6 million people and more than 60 different major ethnic groups. About 20 percent of the population lives in urban areas, including Juba, the capital. South Sudan is also home to the second largest animal migration in the world: a significant movement of antelopes, specifically the tiang and white-eared kob.

South Sudan is also Africa's newest country, a distinction achieved after it won independence from Sudan in July 2011. The country's newfound nationhood followed an agreement that ended Africa's longest-running civil war. Yet the violent conflict did not stop: In 2013, another civil war broke out, leading to large-scale conflict that devastated the economy. During the war, more than a third of the population was forced to leave their homes, resulting in a poverty rate that rose from 51 percent to 82 percent between 2009 and 2016.

The ongoing instability has affected health in South Sudan. Severe acute food insecurity is pervasive, and more than half the population requires some form of humanitarian assistance. The average life expectancy is only 58 years, and the under-five mortality rate is about 97 deaths per 1,000 live births. Diseases contributing to the most deaths in South Sudan include neonatal disorders, lower respiratory infections, diarrheal diseases, malaria, HIV/AIDS, tuberculosis, protein-energy malnutrition, and meningitis. Non-communicable diseases such as congenital defects, stroke, and ischemic heart disease have also increased, causing significant deaths in the country. Overall, the healthcare system suffers from an extreme shortage of professionals, forcing the country at times to rely on inadequately trained or low-skilled health workers. The country's hospital infrastructure remains insufficiently developed.

10.6M
Population

$1,120
GDP Per Capita

58 years
Life Expectancy
↑ Improving

1.5
Doctors/100k
Physician Density

1,150
Deaths/100k
Maternal Mortality

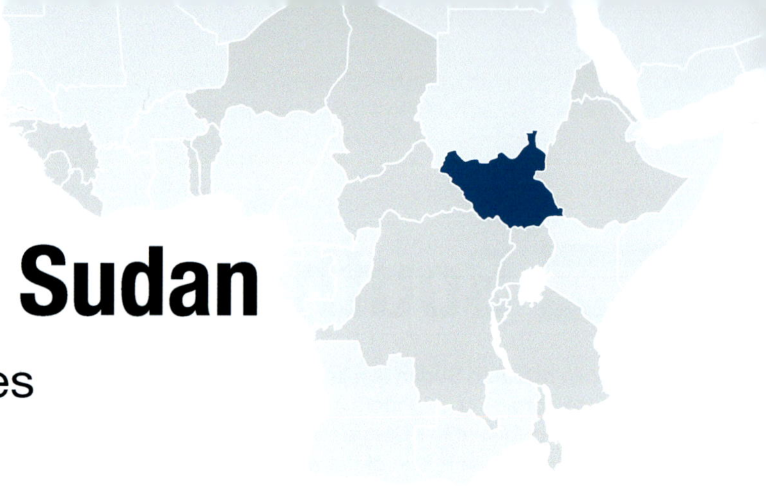

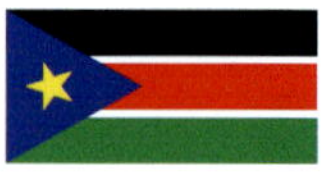

South Sudan

Healthcare Facilities

Al Amin Hospital
Juba, South Sudan
https://vfapp.org/4fb2

Al Sabbah Children's Hospital
Gombura Street, Juba, Central Equatoria, South Sudan
https://vfapp.org/9adb

Aweil Civil Hospital
Wau-Aweil, Aweil, Northern Bahr el Ghazal, South Sudan
https://vfapp.org/bc8e

Bentiu Hospital
Bentiu-Leer, Mir Mir, Unity, South Sudan
https://vfapp.org/229e

Comboni Hospital
Wau-Raja, Wau, Western Bahr el Ghazal, South Sudan
https://vfapp.org/a2a6

Goli Hospital
Yei Maridi, Goli, Central Equatoria, South Sudan
https://vfapp.org/b1fc

Government Hospital at Naseer
Nasser-Ethiopia, Jikmir, Upper Nile, South Sudan
https://vfapp.org/ef7a

His House of Hope Hospital
Yei Maridi, Yei, Central Equatoria, South Sudan
https://vfapp.org/dcdb

Hospital Yambio
Yambio, South Sudan
https://vfapp.org/6953

Juba Teaching Hospital
Unity Avenue, Juba, Central Equatoria, South Sudan
https://vfapp.org/6856

Juba Military Hospital
Hamia Road, Juba, Central Equatoria, South Sudan
https://vfapp.org/a6b4

Lakes State Hospital
Rumbek, South Sudan
https://vfapp.org/4b47

Lui Hospital
Juba-Mundri, Lui, Western Equatoria, South Sudan
https://vfapp.org/6fe7

Melut Hospital
Melut – Mabek Track, Melut, Upper Nile, South Sudan
https://vfapp.org/8693

MSF Hospital
Boma-Pibor, Pibor, Jonglei, South Sudan
https://vfapp.org/65a5

Police Hospital
Juba University Road, Juba, Central Equatoria, South Sudan
https://vfapp.org/e6df

Renk Civil Hospital
Renk-Kosti, Renk, Upper Nile, South Sudan
https://vfapp.org/8218

Renk Military Hospital
Renk-Kosti, Renk, Upper Nile, South Sudan
https://vfapp.org/cd86

UNMISS Hospital
Juba, Central Equatoria, South Sudan
https://vfapp.org/eac7

Usratuna PHCC
Usratuna Road, Juba, Central Equatoria, South Sudan
https://vfapp.org/f89c

Wau Teaching Hospital
Wau, South Sudan
https://vfapp.org/1f35

Yei Civil Hospital
Congo Road, Yei, Central Equatoria, South Sudan
https://vfapp.org/77b1

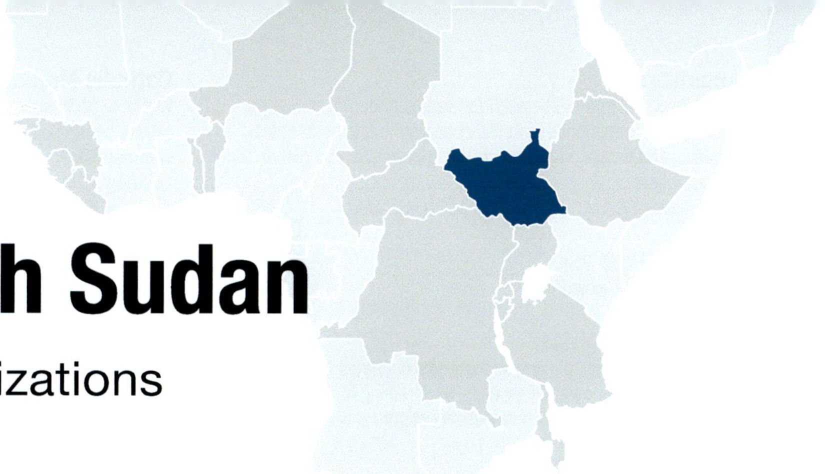

South Sudan

Nonprofit Organizations

Abt Associates
Seeks to improve the quality of life and economic well-being of people worldwide, while striving to meet and exceed the highest professional standards.

General, Logist-Op, MF Med, OB-GYN, Peds

+1 212-779-7700

https://vfapp.org/cec2

Action Against Hunger
Aims to end life-threatening hunger for good through treating and preventing malnutrition across more than forty-five countries.

+1 212-967-7800

https://vfapp.org/2dbc

Advance Family Planning
Aims to achieve global expansion and access to quality contraceptive information, services, and supplies through financial investment and political commitment.

General, MF Med, Pub Health

+1 410-502-8715

https://vfapp.org/7478

Africa CDC
Aims to strengthen the capacity and capability of Africa's public health institutions as well as partnerships to detect and respond quickly and effectively to disease threats and outbreaks, based on data-driven interventions and programs.

Infect Dis, Logist-Op, Pub Health

+251 11 551 7700

https://vfapp.org/339c

Africa Humanitarian Action (AHA)
Responds to crises, conflicts, and disasters in Africa, while informing and advising the international community, governments, civil society, and the private sector on humanitarian issues of concern to Africa. Supports institutional and organizational development efforts.

General, Infect Dis, MF Med, Nutr, OB-GYN

+251 11 660 4800

https://vfapp.org/3ca2

African Field Epidemiology Network (AFENET)
Strengthens field epidemiology and public health laboratory capacity to contribute effectively to addressing epidemics and other major public health problems in Africa.

All-Immu, Infect Dis, Path, Pub Health

https://vfapp.org/df2e

Africa Inland Mission International
Seeks to establish churches and community development programs including health care projects, based in Christian ministry.

Anesth, Dent-OMFS, ER Med, General, MF Med, Medicine, OB-GYN, OB-GYN, Ophth-Opt, Ped Surg, Peds, Rehab

https://vfapp.org/f2f6

AISPO
Implements international initiatives in the healthcare sector and remains involved in a variety of projects to combat poverty, social injustice, and disease in the world.

All-Immu, ER Med, GI, General, Infect Dis, Logist-Op, MF Med, Neonat, OB-GYN, Peds, Psych, Pub Health, Radiol

+39 02 2643 4481

https://vfapp.org/c9e6

Alaska Sudan Medical Project
Works to provide vital humanitarian aid to a remote, isolated region in South Sudan with the mission of saving lives through health, water, and agriculture.

Crit-Care, ER Med, General, Infect Dis, Medicine, Nutr, Surg

+1 907-250-5022

https://vfapp.org/7c19

ALIGHT
Works closely with refugees, trafficked persons, economic migrants, and other displaced persons to co-design solutions that help them build full and fulfilling lives by providing healthcare, clean water, shelter protection, and economic opportunity.

ER Med, General, Infect Dis, MF Med, Neonat, Peds

+1 800-875-7060

https://vfapp.org/5993

Alliance for International Medical Action, The (ALIMA)
Provides quality medical care to vulnerable populations, partnering with and developing national medical organizations and conducting medical research to bring innovation to twelve African countries where ALIMA works.

ER Med, General, Infect Dis, Logist-Op, MF Med, OB-GYN, Path, Peds, Psych, Pub Health

+1 646-619-9074

https://vfapp.org/1c11

Americares
Saves lives and improves health for people affected by poverty or disaster and responds with life-changing medicine, medical supplies, and health programs including domestic and global medical clinics.
All-Immu, ER Med, General, Infect Dis, MF Med, Nutr
+1 203-658-9500
https://vfapp.org/e567

Amref Health Africa
Serves millions of people across thirty-five countries in Sub-Saharan Africa, strengthening health systems, and training African health workers to respond to the continent's most critical health issues.
All-Immu, General, Infect Dis, Logist-Op, MF Med, OB-GYN, Path, Pub Health, Surg
+254 20 6993000
https://vfapp.org/6985

BRAC USA
Seeks to empower people and communities in situations of poverty, illiteracy, disease, and social injustice. Interventions aim to achieve large-scale, positive changes through economic and social programs that enable everyone to realize their potential.
ER Med, General, Infect Dis, Logist-Op, MF Med, OB-GYN
+1 212-808-5615
https://vfapp.org/9d9e

BroadReach
Collaborates with governments, multinational health organizations, donors, and private sector companies to affect healthcare reform and solve the world's biggest health challenges.
Logist-Op
+27 21 514 8300
https://vfapp.org/7812

Buckeye Clinic in South Sudan
Improves the health of persons living in Piol, Twic East County, South Sudan, and surrounding villages, with a primary focus on maternal and child health.
General, MF Med, OB-GYN, Peds
https://vfapp.org/6ef2

Canadian Network for International Surgery, The
Aims to improve maternal health, increase safety, and build local capacity in low-income countries by creating and providing surgical and midwifery courses, training domestically, and transferring skills.
Logist-Op, Surg
+1 877-217-8856
https://vfapp.org/86ff

CARE
Works around the globe to save lives, defeat poverty, and achieve social justice.
ER Med, General
+1 800-422-7385
https://vfapp.org/7232

Carter Center, The
Seeks to prevent and resolve conflicts, enhance freedom and democracy, and improve health, while remaining committed to human rights and the alleviation of human suffering.
Infect Dis, MF Med, Ophth-Opt
+1 800-550-3560
https://vfapp.org/6556

Catholic Medical Mission Board (CMMB)
Works in partnership globally to deliver locally sustainable, quality health solutions to women, children, and their communities.
General, MF Med, Peds
+1 800-678-5659
https://vfapp.org/9498

Catholic Organization for Relief & Development Aid (CORDAID)
Provides humanitarian assistance and creates opportunities to improve security, healthcare, education, and inclusive economic growth in fragile and conflict-affected areas.
ER Med, Infect Dis, MF Med, OB-GYN, Peds, Psych
+31 70 313 6300
https://vfapp.org/8ae5

Christian Aid Ministries
Strives to be a trustworthy and efficient channel for Amish, Mennonite, and other conservative Anabaptist groups and individuals to minister to physical and spiritual needs around the world.
CT Surg, ER Med, Logist-Op, Ortho, Pub Health
+1 330-893-2428
https://vfapp.org/7b33

Christian Blind Mission (CBM)
Aims to improve the quality of life of persons with disabilities in the poorest countries, addressing poverty as a cause, and a consequence, of disability, and working in partnership to create a society for all.
ENT, General, Infect Dis, OB-GYN, Ophth-Opt, Ortho, Peds, Psych, Rehab, Surg
+49 6251 131131
https://vfapp.org/3824

Comitato Collaborazione Medica (CCM)
Supports development processes that safeguard and promote the right to health with a global approach, working on health needs and influencing socio-economic factors, identifying poverty as the main cause for the lack of health.
All-Immu, General, Infect Dis, MF Med, OB-GYN
+39 011 660 2793
https://vfapp.org/4272

Concern Worldwide
Seeks to permanently transform the lives of people living in extreme poverty, tackling its root causes, and building resilience.
Logist-Op, MF Med, Nutr, OB-GYN
+353 1 417 7700
https://vfapp.org/77e9

Confident Children Out of Conflict
Provides vulnerable children with a safe space to sleep, eat, learn, and play to help them develop into young adults, fulfilling their potential, and supports households to develop a protective environment for safe reintegration of these children into communities.
All-Immu, General, Peds, Psych
+211 955 065 445
https://vfapp.org/daf7

Core Group
Aims to improve and expand community health practices for underserved populations, especially women and children, through collaborative action and learning.

General, Infect Dis, MF Med, Medicine, OB-GYN, Peds, Pub Health

+1 202-380-3400

https://vfapp.org/9de3

Deng Foundation

Strives to provide the children of Aweil East, South Sudan, with access to clean water, basic healthcare, and the proper educational infrastructure to have a better childhood. Also works to fight malaria in the South Sudan.

General, Peds, Pub Health

+1 605-216-1327

https://vfapp.org/d89c

Direct Relief

Improves the health and lives of people affected by poverty or emergency situations by mobilizing and providing essential medical resources needed for their care.

ER Med, Logist-Op

+1 805-964-4767

https://vfapp.org/58e5

Doctors with Africa (CUAMM)

Advocates for the universal right to health and promotes the values of international solidarity, justice, and peace. Works to protect and improve the well-being and health of vulnerable communities in Africa with a long-term development perspective.

ER Med, Infect Dis, MF Med, Neonat, OB-GYN, Peds

https://vfapp.org/d2fb

Doctors Without Borders/Médecins Sans Frontières (MSF)

Responds to emergencies and provides lifesaving medical care where needed most, including during disasters, conflicts, and epidemics.

Anesth, Crit-Care, ER Med, General, Infect Dis, Nutr, OB-GYN, Ped Surg, Peds, Psych, Pub Health, Surg

+1 212-679-6800

https://vfapp.org/f363

END Fund, The

Aims to control and eliminate the most prevalent neglected diseases among the world's poorest and most vulnerable people.

Infect Dis

+1 646-690-9775

https://vfapp.org/2614

Episcopal Relief & Development

Provides relief in times of disaster and promotes sustainable development by identifying and addressing the root causes of suffering.

Infect Dis, MF Med, Neonat, Nutr, Peds

+1 855-312-4325

https://vfapp.org/7cfa

Finn Church Aid

Supports people in the most vulnerable situations within fragile and disaster-affected regions in three thematic priority areas: right to peace, livelihood, and education.

ER Med, Psych, Pub Health

+358 20 7871201

https://vfapp.org/9623

Fistula Foundation

Aims to engage the support of people worldwide who are eager to see the day when no woman suffers from obstetric fistula. Raises and directs funds to doctors and hospitals providing life-transforming surgery to women in need.

OB-GYN

+1 408-249-9596

https://vfapp.org/e958

Friends of UNFPA

Promotes the health, dignity, and rights of women and girls around the world by supporting the lifesaving work of UNFPA, the United Nations reproductive health and rights agency, through education, advocacy, and fundraising.

MF Med, OB-GYN

+1 646-649-9100

https://vfapp.org/2a3a

Global Alliance to Prevent Prematurity and Stillbirth (GAPPS)

Seeks to improve birth outcomes worldwide by reducing the burden of premature birth and stillbirth.

All-Immu, Infect Dis, MF Med, Neonat, Neonat, OB-GYN

+1 206-413-7954

https://vfapp.org/3f74

Global Ministries – The United Methodist Church

As the worldwide mission and development agency of The United Methodist Church, Global Ministries works with more than 300 hospitals and clinics around the world through its Global Health Unit.

Anesth, CT Surg, CV Med, Crit-Care, Dent-OMFS, Derm, ER Med, GI, General, Infect Dis, Logist-Op, MF Med, Medicine, Neonat, Nephro, Nutr, OB-GYN, Ophth-Opt, Ortho, Palliative, Peds, Pod, Psych, Pub Health, Rehab, Rheum, Surg, Urol

+1 800-862-4246

https://vfapp.org/1723

Global Oncology (GO)

Brings the best in cancer care to underserved patients around the world and collaborates across geographic, professional, and academic borders to improve cancer care, research, and education.

Heme-Onc, Path, Rad-Onc

https://vfapp.org/fcb8

Global Polio Eradication Initiative

Aims to eradicate polio worldwide.

All-Immu, Logist-Op

+1 847-866-3000

https://vfapp.org/7e2c

GOAL

Works with the most vulnerable communities to help them respond to and recover from humanitarian crises, and to assist them in building transcendent solutions to mitigate poverty and vulnerability.

ER Med, General, Pub Health

+353 1 280 9779

https://vfapp.org/bbea

Grassroot Soccer

Leverages the power of soccer to educate, inspire, and mobilize at risk youth in developing countries to overcome their greatest health challenges, live healthier more productive lives, and be

agents for change in their communities.
Infect Dis
☏ +1 603-277-9685
⊕ https://vfapp.org/3521

Healing Kadi Foundation
Works with the people of South Sudan and Uganda to provide sustainable high-quality healthcare, education for local healthcare providers, and psychological and spiritual counseling.
All-Immu, Dent-OMFS, General, Infect Dis, MF Med, Neonat, OB-GYN, Peds, Psych
☏ +1 951-315-7070
⊕ https://vfapp.org/a7f1

Health Link South Sudan
Contributes toward the reduction and elimination of absolute poverty and social inequalities by promoting social justice, equity, and the dignity of the human person.
General, Infect Dis, Medicine, OB-GYN, Peds, Psych
☏ +211 922 000 991
⊕ https://vfapp.org/38fd

Health Outreach to the Middle East (H.O.M.E.)
Offers physical and Christian-inspired spiritual healing to people in need in the Middle East, providing medical care and education.
Anesth, Dent-OMFS, ER Med, General, Geri, Infect Dis, MF Med, Medicine, OB-GYN, Path, Peds, Psych, Surg
☏ +1 609-579-8681
⊕ https://vfapp.org/134e

HealthNet TPO
Aims to facilitate and strengthen communities and help them to regain control and maintain their health and well-being, believing that even the most vulnerable people have the inner strength to rebuild a better future for themselves.
Crit-Care, General, Infect Dis, Logist-Op, Medicine, OB-GYN, Ophth-Opt, Peds, Psych, Pub Health, Surg
☏ +31 20 620 0005
⊕ https://vfapp.org/67d6

HEART (High-Quality Technical Assistance for Results)
Works to support the use of evidence and expert advice in policymaking in the areas of international development, health, nutrition, education, social protection, and water and sanitation (WASH).
General, Infect Dis, Infect Dis, Logist-Op, MF Med, Medicine, Nutr, OB-GYN, Peds, Psych
☏ +44 1865 207333
⊕ https://vfapp.org/c491

HelpAge International
Works to ensure that people everywhere understand how much older people contribute to society and that they must enjoy their right to healthcare, social services, economic, and physical security.
General, Geri, Infect Dis, Medicine, Pub Health
☏ +44 20 7148 7623
⊕ https://vfapp.org/5d91

Hope and Healing International
Gives hope and healing to children and families trapped by poverty and disability.
General, Nutr, Ophth-Opt, Peds, Rehab
☏ +1 905-640-6464
⊕ https://vfapp.org/c638

Hope Health Action
Facilitates sustainable, lifesaving health, and disability care for the world's most vulnerable, without any discrimination.
ER Med, MF Med, Neonat, Nutr, OB-GYN, Peds, Rehab
☏ +44 20 8462 5256
⊕ https://vfapp.org/86f7

ICAP at Columbia University
Serves as global leader in supporting the scale-up of multidisciplinary HIV/AIDS prevention, care, and treatment programs based on a family-focused approach.
General, Infect Dis, MF Med, Medicine, OB-GYN, Pub Health
☏ +1 212-342-0505
⊕ https://vfapp.org/a8ef

IMA World Health
Works to build healthier communities by collaborating with key partners to serve vulnerable people with a focus on health, healing, and well-being for all.
Infect Dis, MF Med, Nutr, OB-GYN, Pub Health
☏ +1 202-888-6200
⊕ https://vfapp.org/8316

In Deed and Truth Ministries
Serves the community of Tonj, South Sudan, through medical care, pastoral training, and discipleship.
All-Immu, ER Med, General, OB-GYN
☏ +1 760-707-7367
⊕ https://vfapp.org/f9ce

International Council of Ophthalmology
Works with ophthalmologic societies and others to enhance ophthalmic education and improve access to the highest quality eye care in order to preserve and restore vision for the people of the world.
Ophth-Opt
⊕ https://vfapp.org/ffd2

International Federation of Red Cross and Red Crescent Societies (IFRC)
Coordinates and directs international assistance following natural and man-made disasters in nonconflict situations through the world's largest humanitarian and development network. Provides disaster-preparedness programs, healthcare activities, and promotes humanitarian values.
ER Med, General, Infect Dis, Nutr
☏ +1 212-338-0161
⊕ https://vfapp.org/b4ee

International Medical Corps
Seeks to improve quality of life through health interventions and related activities that strengthen underserved communities worldwide, with the flexibility to respond rapidly to emergencies and offer medical services and training to people at the highest risk.
ER Med, General, Infect Dis, Nutr, OB-GYN, Peds, Pub Health, Surg
☏ +1 310-826-7800
⊕ https://vfapp.org/a8a5

International Organization for Migration (IOM) – The UN Migration Agency
Promotes evidence-informed policies and holistic, preventive, and curative health programs that are beneficial, accessible, and equitable for vulnerable migrants.

General, Infect Dis, OB-GYN
+27 12 342 2789
https://vfapp.org/621a

International Rescue Committee (IRC)
Responds to the world's worst humanitarian crises and helps people whose lives and livelihoods are shattered by conflict and disaster to survive, recover, and gain control of their future.
ER Med, General, Infect Dis, MF Med, Peds
+1 212-551-3000
https://vfapp.org/5d24

International Trachoma Initiative (iTi)
Works toward a world free from trachoma, a preventable cause of blindness, and provides comprehensive support to national ministries of health and governmental and nongovernmental organizations to implement a comprehensive approach to fight trachoma.
Infect Dis, Ophth-Opt
+1 404-371-0466
https://vfapp.org/3278

Intersos
Provides emergency medical assistance to victims of armed conflicts, natural disasters, and extreme exclusion, with particular attention to the protection of the most vulnerable people.
ER Med, General, Nutr
+39 06 853 7431
https://vfapp.org/dbac

InterSurgeon
Fosters collaborative partnerships in the field of global surgery that will advance clinical care, teaching, training, research, and the provision and maintenance of medical equipment.
ENT, Neurosurg, Ortho, Ped Surg, Plast, Surg, Urol
https://vfapp.org/6f8a

IntraHealth International
Improves the performance of health workers and strengthens the systems in which they work.
CV Med, Endo, General, Infect Dis, MF Med, Neonat, Nutr, OB-GYN
+1 919-313-3554
https://vfapp.org/ddc8

IsraAID
Supports people affected by humanitarian crisis and partners with local communities around the world to provide urgent aid, assist recovery, and reduce the risk of future disasters.
ER Med, Infect Dis, Psych, Rehab
+972 3-947-7766
https://vfapp.org/de96

Jesus Harvesters Ministries
Reaches communities through medical clinics, dental care, veterinarian outreach, pastor training, and community service, based in Christian ministry.
Dent-OMFS, General, Infect Dis
https://vfapp.org/8a23

Jewish World Watch
Brings help and healing to survivors of mass atrocities around the globe and seeks to inspire people of all faiths and cultures to join the ongoing fight against genocide.
ER Med, Logist-Op, OB-GYN, Peds
+1 818-501-1836
https://vfapp.org/8c92

Jhpiego
Creates and delivers transformative healthcare solutions that save lives in partnership with national governments, health experts, and local communities.
General, Infect Dis, OB-GYN, Surg
+1 410-537-1800
https://vfapp.org/45b8

John Snow, Inc. (JSI)
Aims to improve the health and well-being of underserved and vulnerable people and communities throughout the world.
General, Infect Dis, Logist-Op, MF Med, OB-GYN, Peds, Psych, Pub Health
+1 617-482-9485
https://vfapp.org/ba78

Joint Aid Management (JAM)
Provides food security, nutrition, water, and sanitation to vulnerable communities in Africa in dignified and sustainable ways.
ER Med, Nutr
+27 11 548 3900
https://vfapp.org/dcac

Joint United Nations Programme on HIV/AIDS (UNAIDS)
Aims to place people living with HIV and people affected by the virus at the decision-making table and at the center of designing, delivering, and monitoring the AIDS response.
Infect Dis
+41 22 791 36 66
https://vfapp.org/464a

Kajo Keji Health Training Institute (KKHTI)
Addresses the severe shortage of medical personnel in South Sudan by training quality healthcare workers.
General, Infect Dis, MF Med
+211 954 338 623
https://vfapp.org/ff59

Light for the World
Contributes to a world in which persons with disabilities fully exercise their rights and assists persons with disabilities living in poverty.
Ophth-Opt, Rehab
+43 1 8101300
https://vfapp.org/3ff6

Lions Clubs International
Empowers volunteers to serve their communities, meet humanitarian needs, encourage peace, and promote international understanding through Lions clubs.
Heme-Onc, Medicine, Nutr, Ophth-Opt
+1 630-571-5466
https://vfapp.org/7b12

London School of Hygiene & Tropical Medicine: Health in Humanitarian Crises Centre
Advances health and health equity in crisis-affected countries through research, education, and translation of knowledge into policy and practice.
ER Med, Infect Dis, Pub Health
+44 20 7636 8636
https://vfapp.org/96ad

MAGNA International
Helps those who are suffering or recovering from conflicts and disasters by reducing the risks of diseases and treating them immediately.
ER Med, General, Infect Dis, Peds, Surg
+421 2/381 046 69
https://vfapp.org/58f4

Management Sciences for Health (MSH)
Works with countries and communities to save lives and improve the health of the world's poorest and most vulnerable people by building strong, resilient, sustainable health systems.
Infect Dis, Logist-Op, Pub Health
+1 617-250-9500
https://vfapp.org/6aa2

MAP International
Provides medicines and health supplies to those in need around the world so they might experience life to the fullest.
Logist-Op
+1 800-225-8550
https://vfapp.org/deed

Medair
Works to relieve human suffering in some of the world's most remote and devasted places, saving lives in emergencies and helping people in crises survive and recover, inspired by the Christian faith.
ER Med, General, Logist-Op, MF Med, Pub Health
+41 21 694 35 35
https://vfapp.org/5b33

Médecins du Monde/Doctors of the World
Provides care, bears witness, and supports social change worldwide with innovative medical programs and evidence-based advocacy initiatives.
ER Med, General, Infect Dis, MF Med, Neonat, OB-GYN, Peds, Pub Health
+33 1 44 92 15 15
https://vfapp.org/a43d

MedShare
Aims to improve the quality of life of people, communities, and the planet by sourcing and directly delivering surplus medical supplies and equipment to communities in need around the world.
Logist-Op
+1 770-323-5858
https://vfapp.org/c8bc

MENTOR Initiative
Saves lives in emergencies through tropical disease control, and helps people recover from crisis with dignity, working side by side with communities, health workers, and health authorities to leave a lasting impact.
ER Med, Infect Dis
+44 1444 412171
https://vfapp.org/3bd5

Mercy Ships
Operates hospital ships staffed by volunteers to bring hope, healing, and healthcare to underserved communities worldwide.
Anesth, Dent-OMFS, Logist-Op, Neonat, OB-GYN, Ophth-Opt, Ortho, Palliative, Plast, Psych, Surg
+1 903-939-7000
https://vfapp.org/2e99

MiracleFeet
Brings low-cost treatment to every child on the planet born with clubfoot, a leading cause of physical disability.
Ortho, Peds, Rehab
+1 919-240-5572
https://vfapp.org/bda8

Norwegian People's Aid
Aims to improve living conditions, to create a democratic, just, and safe society.
ER Med, Logist-Op
+47 22 03 77 00
https://vfapp.org/2d8e

Options
Believes in a world where women and children can access the high-quality health services they need, without financial burden.
Logist-Op, MF Med, Neonat, OB-GYN
+44 20 7430 1900
https://vfapp.org/3a48

Pact
Works on the ground to improve the lives of those who are challenged by poverty and marginalization, striving for a world where all people are heard, capable, and vibrant.
Infect Dis, Logist-Op, MF Med, Pub Health
+1 202-466-5666
https://vfapp.org/9a6c

Partners in Compassionate Care
Works to provide hope, medical care, and healing to the people of South Sudan, based in Christian ministry.
General, Ophth-Opt
+1 616-356-2464
https://vfapp.org/74e2

Pharmacists Without Borders Canada
Provides pharmaceutical and technical assistance in the implementation or improvement of community and hospital pharmacies internationally.
+1 514-842-8923
https://vfapp.org/7658

Poole Africa Link
Provides a link of training for doctors, nurses, midwives, and student nurses between Poole Hospital NHS Foundation Trust and Wau Hospital in South Sudan.
Logist-Op, OB-GYN
+44 1202 448182
https://vfapp.org/1f6f

Première Urgence International
Helps civilians who are marginalized or excluded as a result of natural disasters, war, or economic collapse.
ER Med, General, MF Med, Peds, Psych
+53 119997400027
https://vfapp.org/62ba

Real Medicine Foundation (RMF)
Provides humanitarian support to people living in disaster and poverty-stricken areas, focusing on the person as a whole by providing medical/physical, emotional, economic, and social support.
ER Med, General, Infect Dis, Nutr, Peds, Psych
+44 20 8638 0637
https://vfapp.org/d45a

Relief International
Helps people in fragile settings achieve good health and nutrition by delivering primary healthcare and emergency treatment, and builds local capacity to ensure that communities in vulnerable situations have the access to the quality care they need to live healthy lives.

ER Med, General, MF Med, Neonat, OB-GYN, Peds, Psych

☏ +1 202-639-8660

🌐 https://vfapp.org/1522

RestoringVision
Empowers lives by restoring vision for millions of people in need.

Ophth-Opt

☏ +1 209-980-7323

🌐 https://vfapp.org/e121

Rotary International
Provides service to others, improves lives, and advances world understanding, goodwill, and peace through its fellowship of business, professional, and community leaders.

ER Med, General, Infect Dis, MF Med, OB-GYN

🌐 https://vfapp.org/8fb5

Sanofi Espoir Foundation
Contributes to reducing health inequalities among populations that need it most by applying a socially responsible approach focused on fighting childhood cancers in low-income countries, improving maternal and newborn health, and improving access to care.

ER Med, OB-GYN, Peds

☏ +33 1 53 77 91 38

🌐 https://vfapp.org/943b

Save Lives Initiative
Moves to save and improve the lives of people less privileged in the Republic of South Sudan, through participation and empowerment.

General, OB-GYN

☏ +211 928 000 802

🌐 https://vfapp.org/23c4

Save the Children
Gives children around the world a healthy start in life, the opportunity to learn, and protection from harm.

All-Immu, Crit-Care, ER Med, General, Infect Dis, MF Med, Medicine, Neonat, OB-GYN, Peds, Psych, Pub Health

☏ +1 800-728-3843

🌐 https://vfapp.org/2e73

Sightsavers
Prevents avoidable blindness in some of the poorest parts of the world by treating debilitating eye diseases.

Infect Dis, Ophth-Opt, Surg

☏ +1 800-707-9746

🌐 https://vfapp.org/aa52

SIGN Fracture Care International
Builds orthopedic capacity around the world and provides the injured poor access to fracture surgery by donating orthopedic education and implant systems to surgeons in developing countries.

Ortho, Rehab, Surg

☏ +1 509-371-1107

🌐 https://vfapp.org/123d

South Sudan Medical Relief
Provides the best possible health care in a remote area in South Sudan, primarily offering clinical services and ongoing training, and striving for increased equity in healthcare access across many areas of primary and consultant healthcare.

General, Infect Dis, OB-GYN, Peds

☏ +61 3 6352 3560

🌐 https://vfapp.org/c475

South Sudan Villages Clinic, Inc.
Aims to provide curative and preventive care to people in the county of Korok East and surrounding villages in South Sudan.

Dent-OMFS, General, Infect Dis, OB-GYN, Ophth-Opt, Peds, Pub Health

☏ +1 716-715-5840

🌐 https://vfapp.org/4554

Southern Sudan Healthcare Organization
Provides healthcare services, medical supplies, and education to uplift the people of South Sudan and brings hope to where it is lost.

General, MF Med, Neonat, OB-GYN, Peds

☏ +1 517-243-3118

🌐 https://vfapp.org/cd91

Sudan Relief Fund
Brings aid in the form of food, clothing, shelter, and medical attention to the people of South Sudan.

ER Med, General, Nutr

☏ +1 888-488-0348

🌐 https://vfapp.org/542a

Task Force for Global Health, The
Consists of programs and focus areas that cover a range of global health issues including neglected tropical diseases, infectious diseases, vaccines, field epidemiology, public health informatics, health workforce development, and global health ethics.

Infect Dis, Logist-Op, Medicine, Ophth-Opt, Peds

☏ +1 404-371-0466

🌐 https://vfapp.org/714c

Tearfund
Responds to crisis and partners with local churches to bring restoration to those living in poverty, inspired by the Christian faith.

ER Med, Logist-Op

☏ +44 20 3906 3906

🌐 https://vfapp.org/f6cf

Terre Des Hommes
Works to improve the conditions of the most vulnerable children worldwide by improving the health of children under the age of 3, protecting migrant children, providing humanitarian aid to children and their families in times of crisis, and preventing child exploitation.

ER Med, MF Med, Neonat, OB-GYN, Ped Surg, Peds

☏ +41 58 611 06 66

🌐 https://vfapp.org/2689

Unforgotten Fund, The (UNFF)
Provides lifesaving humanitarian relief to UN Field Operations and projects such as water supply, sanitation and hygiene (WASH), food security, health, and shelter.

ER Med, MF Med, Nutr, OB-GYN, Peds

☏ +1 443-668-2648

🌐 https://vfapp.org/928f

United Nations Children's Fund (UNICEF)
Works in over 190 countries and territories to save children's lives, to defend their rights, and to help them fulfill their potential, from early childhood through adolescence.
All-Immu, Infect Dis, MF Med, Neonat, Nutr, OB-GYN, Ped Surg, Peds, Pub Health
https://vfapp.org/42d7

United Nations Development Programme (UNDP)
Helps countries achieve the simultaneous eradication of extreme poverty and significant reduction of inequalities and exclusion using a sustainable human development approach.
Infect Dis, Logist-Op, Pub Health
https://vfapp.org/935c

United Nations High Commissioner for Refugees (UNHCR)
Safeguards the rights and well-being of people who have been forced to flee, ensuring that everybody has the right to seek asylum and find safe refuge in another country, with the goal of seeking lasting solutions.
General, MF Med, Medicine, OB-GYN, Peds, Psych, Pub Health
https://vfapp.org/6636

United Nations Office for the Coordination of Humanitarian Affairs (OCHA)
Contributes to principled and effective humanitarian response through coordination, advocacy, policy, information management, and humanitarian financing tools and services, by leveraging functional expertise throughout the organization.
Logist-Op
https://vfapp.org/22b8

United Nations Population Fund (UNFPA)
Supports reproductive healthcare for women and youth in more than 150 countries, focusing on delivering a world where every pregnancy is wanted, every childbirth is safe, and every young person's potential is fulfilled.
Infect Dis, MF Med, Neonat, OB-GYN, Peds, Pub Health
+1 212-963-6008
https://vfapp.org/c969

United States Agency for International Development (USAID)
Promotes and demonstrates democratic values abroad and advances a free, peaceful, and prosperous world. Leads the U.S. government's international development and disaster assistance through partnerships and investments that save lives.
ER Med, Infect Dis, MF Med, OB-GYN, Peds
+1 202-712-0000
https://vfapp.org/9a99

United States President's Emergency Plan for AIDS Relief (PEPFAR)
The U.S. global HIV/AIDS response works to prevent new HIV infections and accelerate progress to control the global epidemic in more than 50 countries, by partnering with governments to support sustainable, integrated, and country-led responses to HIV/AIDS.
Infect Dis, Pub Health
https://vfapp.org/a57c

University of British Columbia - Faculty of Medicine: Branch for International Surgical Care
Aims to advance sustainable improvements in the delivery of surgical care in the world's most underserved countries by building capacity within the field of surgery through the provision of care in low-resource settings.
Anesth, ER Med, Neurosurg, Surg, Urol
+1 604-875-4111
https://vfapp.org/4164

USAID: A2Z The Micronutrient and Child Blindness Project
Aims to increase the use of key micronutrient and blindness interventions to improve child and maternal health.
MF Med, Neonat, Nutr, Ophth-Opt, Surg
+1 202-884-8785
https://vfapp.org/c5f1

USAID: Deliver Project
Builds a global supply chain to deliver lifesaving health products to people in order to enable countries to provide family planning, protect against malaria, and limit the spread of pandemic threats.
Infect Dis, Logist-Op, MF Med
+1 202-712-0000
https://vfapp.org/374e

USAID: Maternal and Child Health Integrated Program
Works to improve the health of women and their families, including programs for maternal, newborn, and child health, immunization, family planning, nutrition, malaria, and HIV/AIDS.
All-Immu, General, Infect Dis, MF Med
+1 202-835-3136
https://vfapp.org/4415

Village Help for South Sudan
Delivers education, opportunity, healthcare, and sanitation to remote areas of South Sudan.
General, Neonat, OB-GYN
+1 781-929-3925
https://vfapp.org/41c2

Vitamin Angels
Helps at-risk populations in need—specifically pregnant women, new mothers, and children under age five—to gain access to life-changing vitamins and minerals.
General, Nutr
+1 805-564-8400
https://vfapp.org/7da1

Watsi
Uses technology to make healthcare a reality for those who might not otherwise be able to afford it.
Pub Health, Surg
+1 256-792-8747
https://vfapp.org/41a3

Women for Women International
Supports the most marginalized women to earn and save money, improve health and well-being, influence decisions in their home and community, and connect to networks for support.
MF Med, OB-GYN
+1 202-737-7705
https://vfapp.org/768c

Women's Refugee Commission
Seeks to improve lives by protecting the rights of women, children, and youth displaced by conflict and crisis through researching their needs, identifying solutions, and advocating for programs and policies to strengthen their resilience.

General, MF Med, Neonat, OB-GYN, Peds, Psych

+1 212-551-3115

https://vfapp.org/3d8f

World Gospel Mission
Mobilizes volunteers to help transform communities through healthcare and education, based in Christian ministry.

ER Med, General

+1 765-664-7331

https://vfapp.org/efa4

World Health Organization, The (WHO)
The United Nations' agency for health provides leadership on global health matters, shapes the health research agenda, setting norms and standards, articulates evidence-based policy options, provides technical support and monitoring to countries, and assesses health trends.

ER Med, General, Infect Dis, Logist-Op, MF Med, OB-GYN, Peds, Psych, Pub Health

+41 22 791 21 11

https://vfapp.org/c476

World Relief
Brings sustainable solutions to the world's greatest problems: disasters, extreme poverty, violence, oppression, and mass displacement.

ER Med, Nutr, Psych, Pub Health

+1 800-535-5433

https://vfapp.org/fbcd

World Vision International
Works with vulnerable communities around the world to overcome poverty and injustice with child-focused programs.

ER Med, General, Infect Dis, MF Med, Nutr, OB-GYN, Peds

+1 626-303-8811

https://vfapp.org/2642

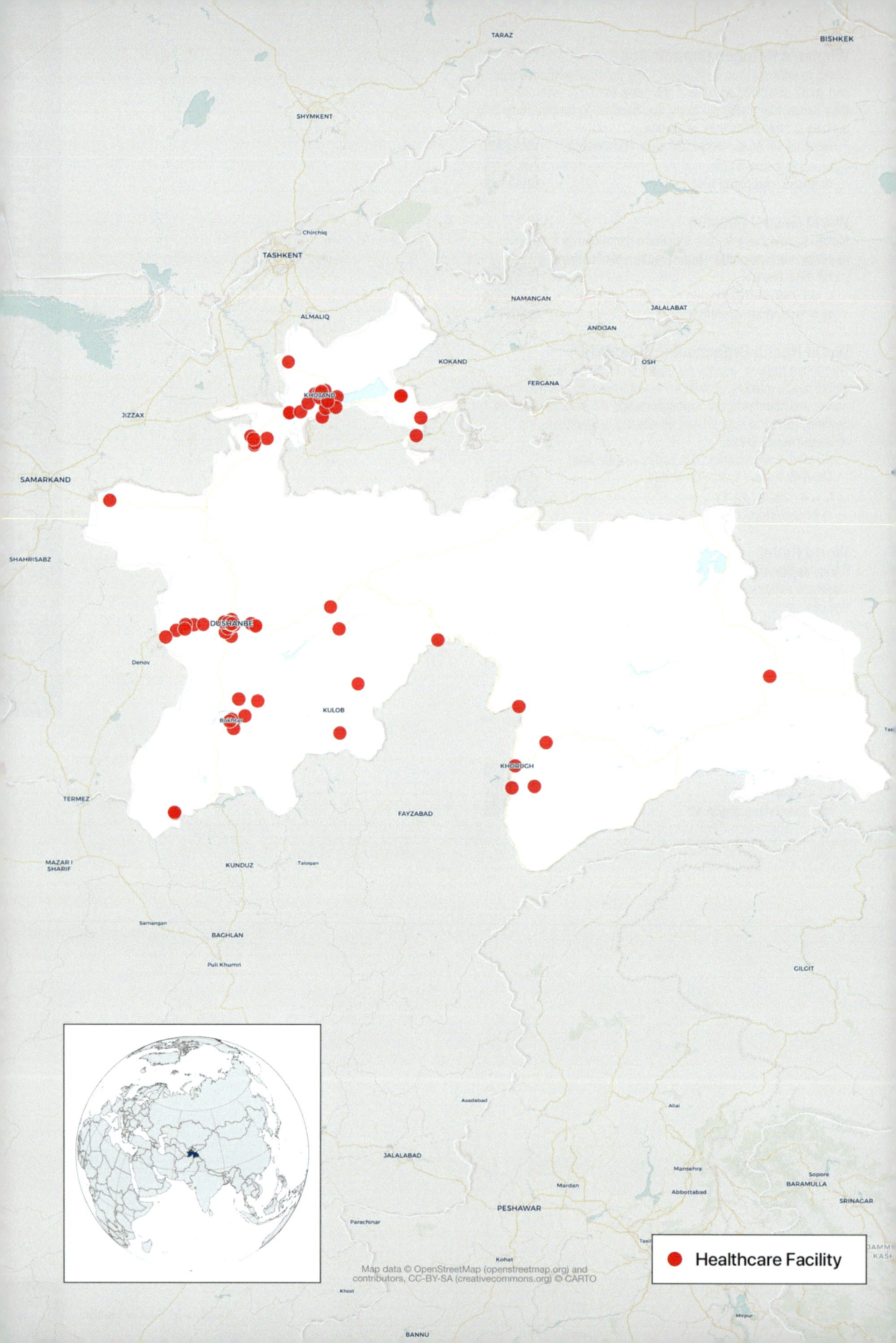
TARAZ
BISHKEK
SHYMKENT
Chirchiq
TASHKENT
NAMANGAN
JALALABAT
ALMALIQ
ANDIJAN
KOKAND
OSH
KHUJAND
FERGANA
JIZZAX
SAMARKAND
SHAHRISABZ
DUSHANBE
Denov
KULOB
Bokhtar
KHORUGH
TERMEZ
FAYZABAD
MAZAR I SHARIF
KUNDUZ
Taloqan
Samangan
BAGHLAN
Puli Khumri
GILGIT
Asadabad
Allai
JALALABAD
Mansehra
Sopore
BARAMULLA
Mardan
Abbottabad
SRINAGAR
PESHAWAR
Parachinar
Kohat
Khost
BANNU
Mirpur
Map data © OpenStreetMap (openstreetmap.org) and contributors, CC-BY-SA (creativecommons.org) © CARTO
Healthcare Facility

Tajikistan

The Republic of Tajikistan is a mountainous, landlocked country in Central Asia. The country's history is ancient: The Silk Road once passed through Tajikistan. In a population of 8.9 million people, 90 percent live in lower elevations, predominantly in settlements called qishlaqs, with population density increasing from east to west. The population is overwhelmingly of the Tajik ethnicity, and the majority of Tajikistanis are Muslim. The nation is rich in mineral resources such as iron, lead, zinc, salt, fluorite, and precious stones.

The country is relatively young, having broken off from the Soviet Union in 1991. Shortly after independence, anti-government demonstrations sparked a five-year civil war ending in 1997. Despite the turmoil, Tajikistan has since increased its political stability and made significant economic progress. Over two decades, from 2000 to 2018, the country dramatically decreased poverty rates from 83 percent to 27 percent.

Tajikistan must still work to repair its healthcare system after infrastructure damage from the civil war and decades of underinvestment. The country continues to have the lowest health expenditure in the WHO European Region. Since its civil war, Tajikistan has made gains in life expectancy, hitting a plateau of around 71 years. Likewise, the under-five mortality rate has improved, dropping from over 90 deaths per 1,000 live births in the early 1990s to under 50 deaths per 1,000 live births in 2019. Lower respiratory infections, neonatal disorders, and diarrheal diseases continue to cause a significant number of deaths, but have improved over time. Significantly, non-communicable diseases contribute most to death in Tajikistan, with ischemic heart disease, stroke, cirrhosis, congenital defects, diabetes, hypertensive heart disease, stomach cancer, and COPD causing the most deaths.

8.9M
Population

$871
GDP Per Capita

71 years
Life Expectancy
↑ Improving

210.3
Doctors/100k
Physician Density

467
Beds/100k
Hospital Bed Density

17
Deaths/100k
Maternal Mortality

Tajikistan

Healthcare Facilities

Abu Ibn Sino Hospital
Street Foteh Niyozi 34,
Dushanbe, Tajikistan
⊕ https://vfapp.org/ccc3

Avis Hospital
Budyonniy Street, Istaravshan,
Sughd Region, Tajikistan
⊕ https://vfapp.org/d8fe

Avis Siti
M34, Rugund, Sughd Province,
Tajikistan
⊕ https://vfapp.org/3759

Bactria Hospital
Sina Street, Ismoili Somoni,
Khatlon Province, Tajikistan
⊕ https://vfapp.org/15b5

Bemorkhonai Kariyai Bolo Maternity Hospital
Borbad Street, Tursunzoda,
Districts of Republican
Subordination, Tajikistan
⊕ https://vfapp.org/fa8d

Cardiac Hospital Khujand
Avenue Rahmon Nabieva,
Khujand, Sughd Province,
Tajikistan
⊕ https://vfapp.org/b517

Central District Hospital Munimabad
RJ033, Muminabad, Khatlon
Province, Tajikistan
⊕ https://vfapp.org/1af8

Central Hospital
20th Anniversary of
Independence Street, Vahdat,
Districts of Republican
Subordination, Tajikistan
⊕ https://vfapp.org/5391

Central Hospital at Vahdat
20-Solagii Istiglaliyyat Str 39,
Vahdat 735400, Tajikistan
⊕ https://vfapp.org/7efb

Central Hospital of Gonchi District
Ghonchi, Sughd Province,
Tajikistan
⊕ https://vfapp.org/fecb

Central Hospital of Rogun
Gidrostroiteley Avenue,
Rogun, Districts of Republican
Subordination,
Tajikistan
⊕ https://vfapp.org/d64f

Central Hospital of Sharinav
Otdel Street, Shahrinav,
Districts of Republican
Subordination, Tajikistan
⊕ https://vfapp.org/82b9

CGB
Istiqlol Street, Guliston, Sughd,
Tajikistan
⊕ https://vfapp.org/3121

Children's Clinical Hospital of Khujand
S. Khofiz Street,
Khujand, Sughd Region,
Tajikistan
⊕ https://vfapp.org/dc4e

Children's Hospital of Bokhtar
86 Ayni Street, Bokhtar, Khatlon
Province, Tajikistan
⊕ https://vfapp.org/ab3b

Children's Hospital of Panjakent
Tereshkova Street,
Panjakent, Sughd Region,
Tajikistan
⊕ https://vfapp.org/a998

Children's Infectious Disease Clinical Hospital
Sheroz Street,
Dushanbe, Dushanbe,
Tajikistan
⊕ https://vfapp.org/4d89

Children's Surgery Hospital
Jalal Ikromi Street,
Dushanbe, Dushanbe,
Tajikistan
⊕ https://vfapp.org/5c2c

Chinor Hospital
Frunze Street,
Khistevarz, Sughd Region,
Tajikistan
⊕ https://vfapp.org/99db

Chorku Hospital
Chorku, Sughd Province,
Tajikistan
⊕ https://vfapp.org/3c53

City Center for Skin and Venereal Diseases
Rahmon Nabiev Street,
Dushanbe, Dushanbe,
Tajikistan
⊕ https://vfapp.org/11c4

City Clinical Hospital #5
Samadi Ghani Street, Dushanbe, Dushanbe, Tajikistan
https://vfapp.org/8fb1

City Hospital
Academics Rajabov Street, Dushanbe, Tajikistan
https://vfapp.org/82e9

City Hospital
Mir Street, D.C. Olimov, Sughd Province, Tajikistan
https://vfapp.org/6ac5

City Hospital #1
Gagarin Street, Khujand, Tajikistan
https://vfapp.org/ce81

City Hospital #2 of Khujand
Rahbara Kasymova Street, Khujand, Sughd Region, Tajikistan
https://vfapp.org/9c1e

City Hospital #7
Abay Street, Dushanbe, Dushanbe, Tajikistan
https://vfapp.org/3775

City Maternity Hospital
1 Kucha, Khujand, Sughd, Tajikistan
https://vfapp.org/28f5

CRCB
M34, Istaravshan, Sughd, Tajikistan
https://vfapp.org/9222

Davo Hospital
Ayni Street, Bokhtar, Khatlon Province, Tajikistan
https://vfapp.org/75f5

District Central Hospital of Bustan
RB14, Bustan, Sughd Province, Tajikistan
https://vfapp.org/ea96

Gafurov District Hospital
Gafurov Avenue, Khujand, Sughd Province, Tajikistan
https://vfapp.org/97fc

Murghab District Hospital
RB 05, Murgab, Gorno-Badakhshan Autonomous Oblast, Tajikistan
https://vfapp.org/3a22

Dushanbe Municipal Emergency Clinic Hospital
Sadriddin Aini Street, Dushanbe, Dushanbe, Tajikistan
https://vfapp.org/e7a2

Emergency Station
M. Tanburi Street, Khujand, Viloyati Sughd, Tajikistan
https://vfapp.org/5fdb

Eshdavlat Doctor
Teshiktosh, Viloyati Khatlon, Tajikistan
https://vfapp.org/671c

Eye Hospital of Bokhtar
N. Huvaydulloev Street, Bokhtar, Khatlon Province, Tajikistan
https://vfapp.org/fd37

Gastroenterology Center
Ismoili Somoni Street, Dushanbe, Dushanbe, Tajikistan
https://vfapp.org/3975

Gorodskaya Bolnitsa Chkalovska Hospital
Hospital Patrice Lumumby Street, Bostan, Sughd Province, Tajikistan
https://vfapp.org/d6c6

GU Republican Scientific and Clinical Center of Urology
Dushanbe, Tajikistan
https://vfapp.org/dd9a

Gulakandoz Hospital
Davron Samadov, Gulakandoz, Sughd Province, Tajikistan
https://vfapp.org/961f

Hospital at Ispechak
Alisher Navoi Street, Dushanbe, Dushanbe, Tajikistan
https://vfapp.org/f724

Hospital at Istaravshan
Budyonniy Street, Istaravshan, Sughd Region, Tajikistan
https://vfapp.org/b9b8

Hospital at Kazanguzar
Zagertut-Zagerti, Khatlon Province, Tajikistan
https://vfapp.org/4e9e

Hospital at Kuliev
RJ04, Navabad, Gorno-Badakhshan Autonomous Oblast, Tajikistan
https://vfapp.org/83c1

Hospital at Machiton
RB01, Rugund, Sughd Province, Tajikistan
https://vfapp.org/4f88

Hospital at Ozodii-Shark
Ozodii-Shark, Khatlon Province, Tajikistan
https://vfapp.org/2feb

Hospital at Qurgonteppa
2 Sino Street, Bokhtar, Khatlon Province, Tajikistan
https://vfapp.org/84e7

Hospital at Rasulov
Zhdanov Street, Ghafurov, Sughd Region, Tajikistan
https://vfapp.org/5473

Hospital at Rŭshan
Rŭshan, Tajikistan
https://vfapp.org/1798

Hospital at Shakhrinaw
Otdel Street, Shahrinav, Districts of Republican Subordination, Tajikistan
https://vfapp.org/486b

Hospital at Shichozg
Karamshoev Street, Pish, Gorno-Badakhshan Autonomous Oblast, Tajikistan
https://vfapp.org/49ef

Hospital at Stakhanov
PJ042, Dushanbe, Dushanbe, Tajikistan
https://vfapp.org/5cbb

Hospital at Teshiktosh
Teshiktosh, Khatlon Province, Tajikistan
https://vfapp.org/2213

Hospital at Yogodka
32 MKR, Khujand, Sughd Province, Tajikistan
⊕ https://vfapp.org/cc2d

Hospital for Infectious Disease
2th Makhalla, Khujand, Sughd Province, Tajikistan
⊕ https://vfapp.org/cb54

Hospital of Infectious Diseases
M34, Rugund, Sughd Province, Tajikistan
⊕ https://vfapp.org/fd4e

Hospital of Mirza-ali
RJ036, Sari Chashma Jamoat, Khatlon Province, Tajikistan
⊕ https://vfapp.org/f2cd

Hospital of Sarband
RJ057, Levakant, Khatlon Province, Tajikistan
⊕ https://vfapp.org/c1a2

Hospital Sugh Region
84 Sharq Street, Khujand, Sughd Region, Tajikistan
⊕ https://vfapp.org/7f77

Infectious Disease Clinical Hospital of Dushanbe
Ismoili Somoni Avenue, Dushanbe, Dushanbe, Tajikistan
⊕ https://vfapp.org/13c5

Infectious Diseases Children's Hospital
20 Sheroz Street, 734025, Dushanbe, Tajikistan
⊕ https://vfapp.org/619e

Isfara Hospital
RB16, Isfara, Sughd Province, Tajikistan
⊕ https://vfapp.org/9943

Isham Hospital
PB02, Otkanoq, Districts of Republican Subordination, Tajikistan
⊕ https://vfapp.org/78c6

Istiklol Hospital
6A Nemat Karaboev Avenue, Dushanbe, Dushanbe, Tajikistan
⊕ https://vfapp.org/ede8

Khatlon Medical Center
Ayni Street, Bokhtar, Khatlon Province, Tajikistan
⊕ https://vfapp.org/9c93

Kulundinskaya Gorodskaya Bol'nitsa
Интернационал, Кыргызстан, Tajikistan
⊕ https://vfapp.org/86e3

Maternity Hospital #2
Husseinzoda Street 5, Dushanbe, Tajikistan
⊕ https://vfapp.org/1d27

Military Hospital
Rudaki Avenue, Dushanbe, Dushanbe, Tajikistan
⊕ https://vfapp.org/8fbf

Military Medical
Dushanbe, Tajikistan
⊕ https://vfapp.org/15a7

National Medical Center
Sharaf Street, Dushanbe, Dushanbe, Tajikistan
⊕ https://vfapp.org/ae8f

Nov Maternity Hospital
Lenin Street, Nov, Sughd, Tajikistan
⊕ https://vfapp.org/ac7b

Oncology Hospital
Narrow Street N. Huvaydulloev, Bokhtar, Khatlon Region, Tajikistan
⊕ https://vfapp.org/dab7

Pakhtaobod Hospital
RJ02, Zarbdor, Districts of Republican Subordination, Tajikistan
⊕ https://vfapp.org/88f4

Paradise Hospital
Lenin Street, Nov, Sughd Region, Tajikistan
⊕ https://vfapp.org/2222

Physiotherapeutic Hospital of Khujand
Avenue Rahmon Nabieva, Khujand, Sughd Province, Tajikistan
⊕ https://vfapp.org/8ee6

Psychiatric Hospital of Khujand
Lunacharsky Street, Khujand, Sughd Region, Tajikistan
⊕ https://vfapp.org/b5af

Qal'ai Khumb Hospital
Shohmansur Street, Kalai Khumb, Gorno-Badakhshan Autonomous Oblast, Tajikistan
⊕ https://vfapp.org/afd5

Regional Hospital Karabollo
Vahdat Street 1, Bokhtar, Khatlon Province, Tajikistan
⊕ https://vfapp.org/bc3f

Regional Maternity Hospital
Nabiev Street, Khujand, Sughd, Tajikistan
⊕ https://vfapp.org/da3e

Regional Psychiatric Hospital
Roshtqala Road, Barjangal, Gorno-Badakhshan Autonomous Oblast, Tajikistan
⊕ https://vfapp.org/9129

Roddom Hospital
Istaravshan, Tajikistan
⊕ https://vfapp.org/96c9

Roddom Regional Hospital
Lenin Street, Khorog, Gorno-Badakhshan Autonomous Oblast, Tajikistan
⊕ https://vfapp.org/1fa4

Russian Military Hospital
126 Khanzhin Street, Dushanbe, Dushanbe, Tajikistan
⊕ https://vfapp.org/5777

Shaydon Hospital
Sari Khosor, Sari Khosor – Shahidon, Вилояти Хатлон, Tajikistan
⊕ https://vfapp.org/e31d

SHIFO Medical Center
Druzhba Narodov Street, Dushanbe, Dushanbe, Tajikistan
⊕ https://vfapp.org/a2b4

Skin Hospital
Saida Valiyeva Street, Khujand, Sughd Region, Tajikistan
⊕ https://vfapp.org/a5a4

Solim Med
Omar Khayam Street, Dushanbe, Tajikistan
https://vfapp.org/ab43

State Epidemiological Service of the Republic of Tajikistan
Saida Valiyeva Street, Khujand, Sughd, Tajikistan
https://vfapp.org/8bf7

State Unitary Enterprise Tajik Railway Hospital
Moensho Nazarshoev Street, Dushanbe, Dushanbe, Tajikistan
https://vfapp.org/bf99

Sughd Regional Hospital Khujand
Severnaya Street, Khujand, Sughd Region, Tajikistan
https://vfapp.org/4373

Tadzhikskiy Gosudarstvennyy Meditsinskiy Universitet
Shamsi Street, Dushanbe, Dushanbe, Tajikistan
https://vfapp.org/4414

Tuberculosis Hospital
RB 13, Khujand, Sughd, Tajikistan
https://vfapp.org/5bb7

Vodnik Hospital
Bahor Street, Khujand, Sughd Region, Tajikistan
https://vfapp.org/d679

Tajikistan

Nonprofit Organizations

Abt Associates
Seeks to improve the quality of life and economic well-being of people worldwide, while striving to meet and exceed the highest professional standards.

General, Logist-Op, MF Med, OB-GYN, Peds

+1 212-779-7700

https://vfapp.org/cec2

AFEW International
Aims to improve the health of populations in Eastern Europe and Central Asia, and strives to promote health and increase access to prevention, treatment, and care for HIV, TB, viral hepatitis, and SRHR.

Infect Dis, Pub Health

+31 20 638 1718

https://vfapp.org/19c6

American International Health Alliance (AIHA)
Strengthens health systems and workforce capacity worldwide through locally-driven, peer-to-peer institutional partnerships.

CV Med, ER Med, Infect Dis, Medicine, OB-GYN

+1 202-789-1136

https://vfapp.org/69fd

Center for Strategic and International Studies (CSIS) Commission on Strengthening America's Health Security
Brings together a distinguished and diverse group of high-level opinion leaders bridging security and health, with the core aim to chart a bold vision for the future of U.S. leadership in global health.

ER Med, Infect Dis, MF Med, Pub Health

+1 202-887-0200

https://vfapp.org/6d7f

Christian Aid Ministries
Strives to be a trustworthy and efficient channel for Amish, Mennonite, and other conservative Anabaptist groups and individuals to minister to physical and spiritual needs around the world.

CT Surg, ER Med, Logist-Op, Ortho, Pub Health

+1 330-893-2428

https://vfapp.org/7b33

Developing Country NGO Delegation: Global Fund to Fight AIDS, TB & Malaria
Works to strengthen the engagement of civil society actors and organizations in developing countries to contribute toward achieving a world in which AIDS, TB, and Malaria are no longer global, public health, and human rights threats.

Infect Dis, Pub Health

+254 20 2515790

https://vfapp.org/3149

Direct Relief
Improves the health and lives of people affected by poverty or emergency situations by mobilizing and providing essential medical resources needed for their care.

ER Med, Logist-Op

+1 805-964-4767

https://vfapp.org/58e5

Doctors Without Borders/Médecins Sans Frontières (MSF)
Responds to emergencies and provides lifesaving medical care where needed most, including during disasters, conflicts, and epidemics.

Anesth, Crit-Care, ER Med, General, Infect Dis, Nutr, OB-GYN, Ped Surg, Peds, Psych, Pub Health, Surg

+1 212-679-6800

https://vfapp.org/f363

Elton John Aids Foundation
Seeks to address and overcome the stigma, discrimination, and neglect that prevents ending AIDS by funding local experts to challenge discrimination, prevent infections, and provide treatment.

Infect Dis, Pub Health

+1 212-219-0670

https://vfapp.org/9d31

Gift of Life International
Provides lifesaving cardiac treatment to children in developing countries while developing sustainable pediatric cardiac programs by implementing screening, surgical, and training missions.

Anesth, CT Surg, CV Med, Crit-Care, Ped Surg, Peds, Pulm-Critic

+1 855-734-3278

https://vfapp.org/f2f9

Global Oncology (GO)
Brings the best in cancer care to underserved patients around the world and collaborates across geographic, professional, and

academic borders to improve cancer care, research, and education.

Heme-Onc, Path, Rad-Onc

https://vfapp.org/fcb8

Health Equity Initiative

Aims to build and sustain a global community that engages across sectors and disciplines to advance health equity.

Pub Health

https://vfapp.org/e2e2

HealthProm

Works with local partners to promote health and social care for vulnerable children and their families.

General, MF Med, Peds, Pub Health

+44 20 7832 5832

https://vfapp.org/153d

Healthy Developments

Provides Germany-supported health and social protection programs around the globe in a collaborative knowledge management process.

All-Immu, General, Infect Dis, Logist-Op, MF Med

https://vfapp.org/dc31

ICAP at Columbia University

Serves as global leader in supporting the scale-up of multidisciplinary HIV/AIDS prevention, care, and treatment programs based on a family-focused approach.

General, Infect Dis, MF Med, Medicine, OB-GYN, Pub Health

+1 212-342-0505

https://vfapp.org/a8ef

International Federation of Red Cross and Red Crescent Societies (IFRC)

Coordinates and directs international assistance following natural and man-made disasters in nonconflict situations through the world's largest humanitarian and development network. Provides disaster-preparedness programs, healthcare activities, and promotes humanitarian values.

ER Med, General, Infect Dis, Nutr

+1 212-338-0161

https://vfapp.org/b4ee

International Organization for Migration (IOM) – The UN Migration Agency

Promotes evidence-informed policies and holistic, preventive, and curative health programs that are beneficial, accessible, and equitable for vulnerable migrants.

General, Infect Dis, OB-GYN

+27 12 342 2789

https://vfapp.org/621a

International Planned Parenthood Federation (IPPF)

Leads a locally owned, globally connected civil society movement that provides and enables services and champions sexual and reproductive health and rights for all, especially the underserved.

Infect Dis, MF Med, OB-GYN

+44 20 7939 8200

https://vfapp.org/dc97

IntraHealth International

Improves the performance of health workers and strengthens the systems in which they work.

CV Med, Endo, General, Infect Dis, MF Med, Neonat, Nutr, OB-GYN

+1 919-313-3554

https://vfapp.org/ddc8

John Snow, Inc. (JSI)

Aims to improve the health and well-being of underserved and vulnerable people and communities throughout the world.

General, Infect Dis, Logist-Op, MF Med, OB-GYN, Peds, Psych, Pub Health

+1 617-482-9485

https://vfapp.org/ba78

Joint United Nations Programme on HIV/AIDS (UNAIDS)

Aims to place people living with HIV and people affected by the virus at the decision-making table and at the center of designing, delivering, and monitoring the AIDS response.

Infect Dis

+41 22 791 36 66

https://vfapp.org/464a

Life for a Child

Supports the provision of the best possible health care, given local circumstances, to all children and youth with diabetes in less-resourced countries, through the strengthening of existing diabetes services.

Endo, Medicine, Peds

https://vfapp.org/d712

Lions Clubs International

Empowers volunteers to serve their communities, meet humanitarian needs, encourage peace, and promote international understanding through Lions clubs.

Heme-Onc, Medicine, Nutr, Ophth-Opt

+1 630-571-5466

https://vfapp.org/7b12

Management Sciences for Health (MSH)

Works with countries and communities to save lives and improve the health of the world's poorest and most vulnerable people by building strong, resilient, sustainable health systems.

Infect Dis, Logist-Op, Pub Health

+1 617-250-9500

https://vfapp.org/6aa2

MedShare

Aims to improve the quality of life of people, communities, and the planet by sourcing and directly delivering surplus medical supplies and equipment to communities in need around the world.

Logist-Op

+1 770-323-5858

https://vfapp.org/c8bc

Norwegian People's Aid

Aims to improve living conditions, to create a democratic, just, and safe society.

ER Med, Logist-Op

+47 22 03 77 00

https://vfapp.org/2d8e

Operation Fistula
Exists to end obstetric fistula by building models of care that serve every woman, everywhere.
MF Med, OB-GYN, Surg
+1 512-687-3479
https://vfapp.org/ce8e

Operation Mercy
Serves the poor and marginalized through community development and humanitarian aid projects.
General, MF Med, OB-GYN, Peds, Psych, Pub Health, Rehab
+46 19 22 41 61
https://vfapp.org/81c5

PASHA
Creates opportunities to improve health among vulnerable populations around the world, by bringing together diverse individuals with various areas of expertise and engaging them in solving local and global health challenges.
Derm, Logist-Op, Ophth-Opt, Ortho
+1 310-400-0205
https://vfapp.org/efbc

Pharmacists Without Borders Canada
Provides pharmaceutical and technical assistance in the implementation or improvement of community and hospital pharmacies internationally.
+1 514-842-8923
https://vfapp.org/7658

RestoringVision
Empowers lives by restoring vision for millions of people in need.
Ophth-Opt
+1 209-980-7323
https://vfapp.org/e121

Rockefeller Foundation, The
Works to promote the well-being of humanity.
Logist-Op, Nutr, Pub Health
+1 212-869-8500
https://vfapp.org/5424

Rotary International
Provides service to others, improves lives, and advances world understanding, goodwill, and peace through its fellowship of business, professional, and community leaders.
ER Med, General, Infect Dis, MF Med, OB-GYN
https://vfapp.org/8fb5

Save A Child's Heart
Provides lifesaving cardiac treatment to children in developing countries, and trains healthcare professionals from these countries to deliver quality care in their communities.
CT Surg, CV Med, Crit-Care, Ped Surg, Peds
+1 240-223-3940
https://vfapp.org/1bef

Save the Children
Gives children around the world a healthy start in life, the opportunity to learn, and protection from harm.
All-Immu, Crit-Care, ER Med, General, Infect Dis, MF Med, Medicine, Neonat, OB-GYN, Peds, Psych, Pub Health
+1 800-728-3843
https://vfapp.org/2e73

Task Force for Global Health, The
Consists of programs and focus areas that cover a range of global health issues including neglected tropical diseases, infectious diseases, vaccines, field epidemiology, public health informatics, health workforce development, and global health ethics.
Infect Dis, Logist-Op, Medicine, Ophth-Opt, Peds
+1 404-371-0466
https://vfapp.org/714c

Union for International Cancer Control (UICC)
Unites and supports the cancer community to reduce the global cancer burden, promote greater equity, and ensure that cancer control continues to be a priority in the world health and development agenda.
Heme-Onc, Pub Health
+41 22 809 18 11
https://vfapp.org/88b1

United Nations Children's Fund (UNICEF)
Works in over 190 countries and territories to save children's lives, to defend their rights, and to help them fulfill their potential, from early childhood through adolescence.
All-Immu, Infect Dis, MF Med, Neonat, Nutr, OB-GYN, Ped Surg, Peds, Pub Health
https://vfapp.org/42d7

United Nations Development Programme (UNDP)
Helps countries achieve the simultaneous eradication of extreme poverty and significant reduction of inequalities and exclusion using a sustainable human development approach.
Infect Dis, Logist-Op, Pub Health
https://vfapp.org/935c

United Nations High Commissioner for Refugees (UNHCR)
Safeguards the rights and well-being of people who have been forced to flee, ensuring that everybody has the right to seek asylum and find safe refuge in another country, with the goal of seeking lasting solutions.
General, MF Med, Medicine, OB-GYN, Peds, Psych, Pub Health
https://vfapp.org/6636

United Nations Population Fund (UNFPA)
Supports reproductive healthcare for women and youth in more than 150 countries, focusing on delivering a world where every pregnancy is wanted, every childbirth is safe, and every young person's potential is fulfilled.
Infect Dis, MF Med, Neonat, OB-GYN, Peds, Pub Health
+1 212-963-6008
https://vfapp.org/c969

University of Illinois at Chicago: Center for Global Health
Aims to improve the health of populations around the world and reduce health disparities by collaboratively conducting trans-disciplinary research, training the next generations of global health leaders, and building the capacities of global and local partners.
Pub Health
+1 312-355-4116
https://vfapp.org/b749

USAID: Leadership, Management and Governance Project

Improves leadership, management, and governance practices to strengthen health systems and improve health for all, including vulnerable populations worldwide.

Logist-Op

🌐 https://vfapp.org/d35e

USAID: Maternal and Child Health Integrated Program

Works to improve the health of women and their families, including programs for maternal, newborn, and child health, immunization, family planning, nutrition, malaria, and HIV/AIDS.

All-Immu, General, Infect Dis, MF Med

📞 +1 202-835-3136

🌐 https://vfapp.org/4415

USAID: TB Care II

Focuses on tuberculosis care and treatment.

Infect Dis

📞 +1 301-654-8338

🌐 https://vfapp.org/57d4

Vision Care

Restores sight and helps patients get regular treatment at short-term eye camps and long-term base clinics by having doctors, missionaries, volunteers, and sponsors work together.

Ophth-Opt

📞 +1 212-769-3056

🌐 https://vfapp.org/9d7c

World Health Organization, The (WHO)

The United Nations' agency for health provides leadership on global health matters, shapes the health research agenda, setting norms and standards, articulates evidence-based policy options, provides technical support and monitoring to countries, and assesses health trends.

ER Med, General, Infect Dis, Logist-Op, MF Med, OB-GYN, Peds, Psych, Pub Health

📞 +41 22 791 21 11

🌐 https://vfapp.org/c476

World Medical Relief

Facilitates the distribution of surplus medical resources where they are needed.

Logist-Op

📞 +1 313-866-5333

🌐 https://vfapp.org/72dc

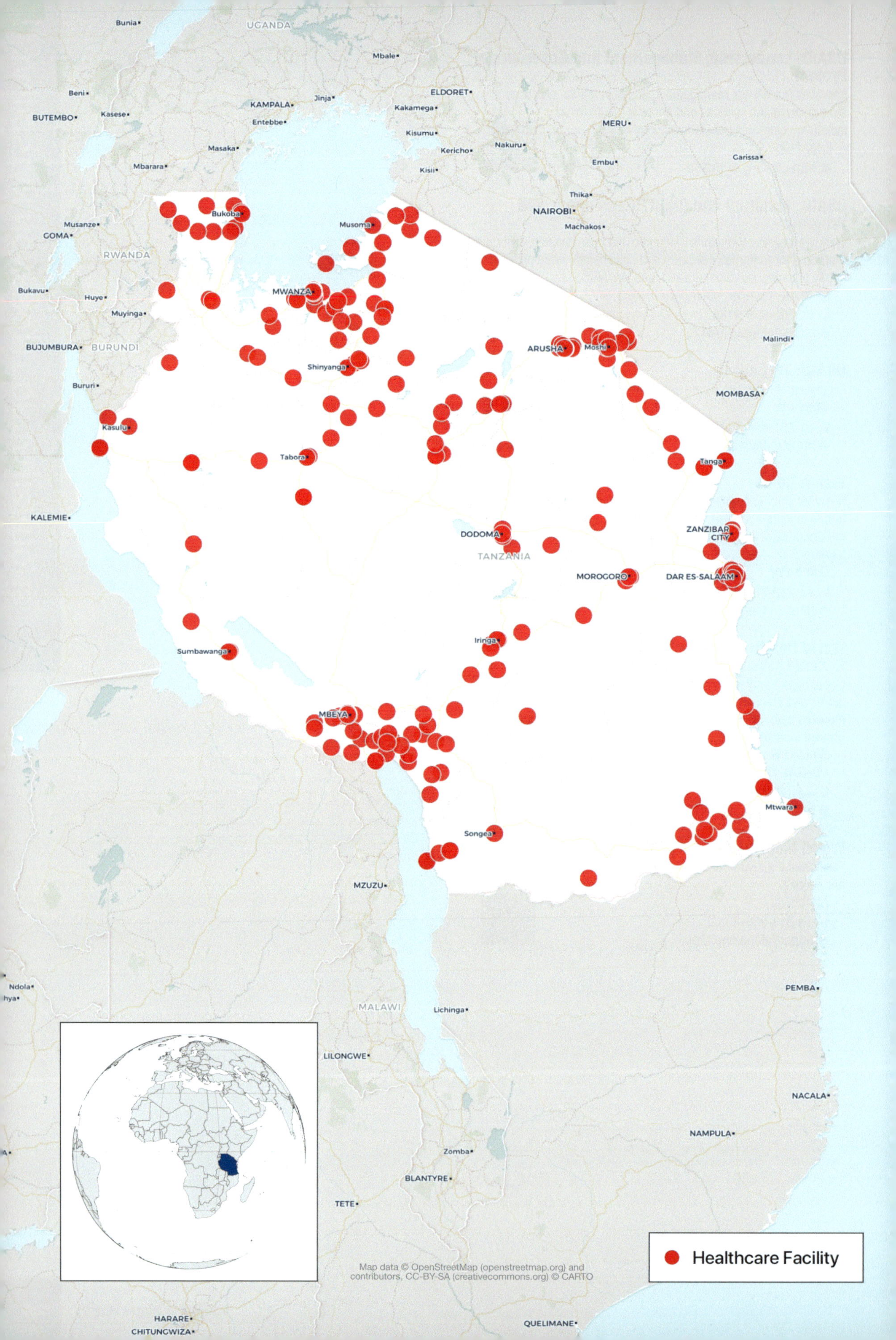

UGANDA
RWANDA
BURUNDI
TANZANIA
MALAWI
KAMPALA
NAIROBI
MWANZA
ARUSHA
Moshi
DODOMA
MOROGORO
DAR ES-SALAAM
ZANZIBAR CITY
Tanga
MOMBASA
MBEYA
Iringa
Songea
Mtwara
Tabora
Shinyanga
Musoma
Bukoba
Kasulu
Sumbawanga
KALEMIE
LILONGWE
BLANTYRE
Healthcare Facility
Map data © OpenStreetMap (openstreetmap.org) and contributors, CC-BY-SA (creativecommons.org) © CARTO

Tanzania

Located on the coast of East Africa, the United Republic of Tanzania is home to 58.6 million people representing more than 120 local indigenous groups. Formerly two separate nations, Tanganyika and Zanzibar unified in 1964 to become modern-day Tanzania, where English and Swahili are the country's official languages. Most of Tanzania's diverse population can be found living in the rural part of the country, while approximately 34 percent are in urban centers. The country's incredible natural features include Mount Kilimanjaro, diverse wildlife, and several UNESCO World Heritage Sites. Tanzania's rich history dates back 1.75 million years, with Olduvai Gorge being the site of some of the oldest known human ancestor remains.

Since its formation, the country has seen improvements in its economic conditions and political stability. Tanzania still faces a variety of development challenges such as poor infrastructure, low education levels, and disparities in population health. Additionally, there exist significant social and economic inequities between urban and rural populations regarding access to opportunity and basic services, such as access to clean water.

The Tanzanian government is both the major provider and financier of health services in the country. The national Tanzanian health system supports local village-based health centers, while larger, more advanced hospitals are located in urban areas. Health indicators such as life expectancy and under-five and under-one mortality rates have improved over time, but challenges to health in the region persist. Diseases among the top causes of death in Tanzania include neonatal disorders, lower respiratory infections, HIV/AIDS, tuberculosis, malaria, diarrheal diseases, and protein-energy malnutrition. Increasingly, non-communicable diseases such as congenital defects, stroke, ischemic heart diseases, and cirrhosis have increased over time to also contribute substantially as top causes of death in Tanzania. To address major health challenges in the country, national health policies have focused on preventive medicine and health.

58.6M
Population

$1,122
GDP Per Capita

65 years
Life Expectancy
↑ Improving

1.4
Doctors/100k
Physician Density

70
Beds/100k
Hospital Bed Density

524
Deaths/100k
Maternal Mortality

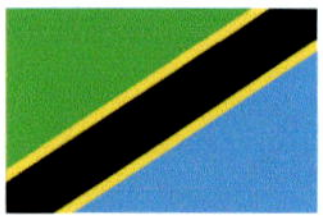

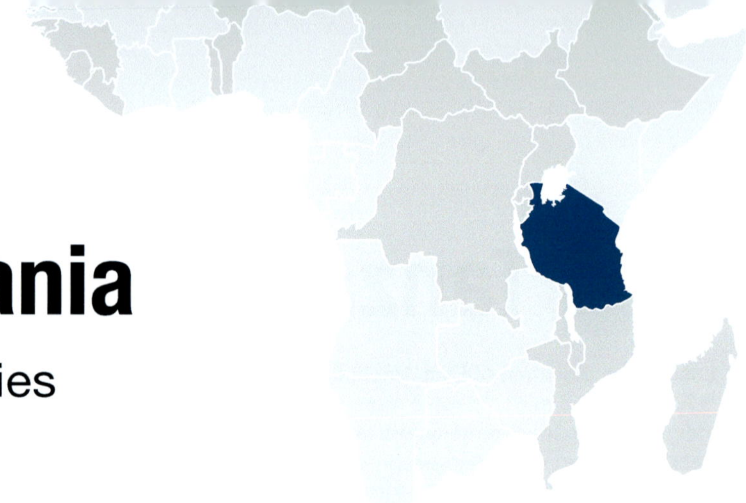

Tanzania

Healthcare Facilities

Aga Khan Hospital, Dar es Salaam
Seaview Road, Dar es Salaam, Coastal Zone, Tanzania
🌐 https://vfapp.org/8aac

AICC Hospital
Nyerere Road, Arusha, Arusha, Tanzania
🌐 https://vfapp.org/f8fe

AL Ijumaa Hospital
Lumumba, Mwanza, Mwanza, Tanzania
🌐 https://vfapp.org/9f78

Amana Referral Hospital
Dar es Salaam, Tanzania
🌐 https://vfapp.org/46dc

Arusha Hospital
T5, Kwa Idd, Arusha, Tanzania
🌐 https://vfapp.org/bbee

Arusha Lutheran Medical Centre
Wachaga Street, Arusha, Arusha, Tanzania
🌐 https://vfapp.org/b763

Bagamoyo District Hospital
Bagamoyo Road, Bagamoyo, Pwani, Tanzania
🌐 https://vfapp.org/6ec3

Bahama Hospital
Balewa Road, Mwanza, Mwanza, Tanzania
🌐 https://vfapp.org/7537

Bariadi Hospital
Bariadi, Shinyanga Region, Tanzania
🌐 https://vfapp.org/8315

Besha Hospital
Tanga, Tanzania
🌐 https://vfapp.org/a845

Biharamulo Designated District Hospital
Biharamulo Road, Biharamulo, Kagera, Tanzania
🌐 https://vfapp.org/255c

Bochi Hospital Limited
Dar es Salaam, Tanzania
🌐 https://vfapp.org/8ad9

Bombo Hospital
Bombo Road, Tanga, Tanzania
🌐 https://vfapp.org/73d4

Bombo Regional Referral Hospital
Makongoro Road, Tanga, Tanzania
🌐 https://vfapp.org/851b

Bugando Medical Center
Mwanza, Tanzania
🌐 https://vfapp.org/7b67

Buguruni Hospital
Mnyamani Road, Dar es Salaam, Coastal Zone, Tanzania
🌐 https://vfapp.org/a91b

Bukombe
Rwanda Road, Bukombe, Geita, Tanzania
🌐 https://vfapp.org/728d

Bukombe District Hospital
Bukombe, Tanzania
🌐 https://vfapp.org/8ffe

Bukumbi Hospital
T4, Kigongo, Mwanza, Tanzania
🌐 https://vfapp.org/99fe

Bulongwa Lutheran Hospital
Church Road, Iniho, Njombe, Tanzania
🌐 https://vfapp.org/61c9

Bunda DDH Hospital
T4, Balili, Mara, Tanzania
🌐 https://vfapp.org/ab3c

Busekwa
Bujora Minor Road, Bujora, Mwanza, Tanzania
🌐 https://vfapp.org/f86d

Butiama Hospital
R193, Butiama, Mara, Tanzania
🌐 https://vfapp.org/5422

Cardinal Rugambwa Hospital
R759, Dar es Salaam, Coastal Zone, Tanzania
🌐 https://vfapp.org/3685

Catholic Mission Hospital
Usokami, Iringa, Tanzania
🌐 https://vfapp.org/ef88

CCBRT Hospital
Ali Bin Said Road, Dar es Salaam, Coastal Zone, Tanzania
🌐 https://vfapp.org/82ee

CF Hospital
Station Road, Mwanza, Mwanza, Tanzania
https://vfapp.org/f3f2

Chake Chake Hospital
Tibirinzi Street, Chake Chake, Kusini Pemba, Tanzania
https://vfapp.org/8e19

Chambala
Kinampanda, Shinyanga, Tanzania
https://vfapp.org/37b5

Chikunja
R853, Naipanga, Masasi, Tanzania
https://vfapp.org/8efe

Children's Ward
Sengerema, Tanzania
https://vfapp.org/7875

Chimala Mission Hospital
S.L.P. 724, Mbeya, Tanzania
https://vfapp.org/5abe

Chingulungulu
Masasi, Tanzania
https://vfapp.org/8f4d

Chingungwe
Tandahimba, Tanzania
https://vfapp.org/bbd9

Chipuputa
T42, Mangaka, Masasi, Tanzania
https://vfapp.org/a437

Chisegu
T6, Masasi, Masasi, Tanzania
https://vfapp.org/42e4

Chiwonga
R875, Kitangari, Mtwara, Tanzania
https://vfapp.org/86ed

Consolata Hospital Ikonda
Ikonda, Njombe, Tanzania
https://vfapp.org/ad22

Coptic Hospital
T17, Musoma, Mara, Tanzania
https://vfapp.org/9921

Dareda Mission Hospital
Seloto, Manyara, Tanzania
https://vfapp.org/b175

Dodoma Hospital
Dodoma, Tanzania
https://vfapp.org/7331

Dr. Atiman Kristu Mfalme Hospital
T9, Sumbawanga, Rukwa, Tanzania
https://vfapp.org/dccf

Dr. Jakaya M. Kikwete District Hospital
Kishapu, Tanzania
https://vfapp.org/8221

Edward Michaud Hospital
Dar es Salaam, Tanzania
https://vfapp.org/8457

Ekenywa Hospital
Usimulizi Street, Dar es Salaam, Coastal Zone, Tanzania
https://vfapp.org/9c67

Emergency Hospital
Senga Road, Dar es Salaam, Coastal Zone, Tanzania
https://vfapp.org/c7cb

First Health Hospital
Rindi Lane, Moshi, Kilimanjaro, Tanzania
https://vfapp.org/6df2

First Hospital
R151, Nyamizeze, Mwanza, Tanzania
https://vfapp.org/963e

Frelimo District Hospital
R622, Ndiuka, Iringa, Tanzania
https://vfapp.org/39e5

Geita Hospital
T4, Nyanza, Geita, Tanzania
https://vfapp.org/4322

Gonja Lutheran Hospital
Mkomazi-Ndungu Road, Maore, Kilimanjaro, Tanzania
https://vfapp.org/44b3

Hai District Hospital
Hai, Tanzania
https://vfapp.org/ce7b

Haydom Lutheran Hospital
Mbulu, Tanzania
https://vfapp.org/c897

Heri Adventist Hospital
Buhigwe, Tanzania
https://vfapp.org/74ff

Hospital ya Wahind
NKOMO, Mwanza, Mwanza, Tanzania
https://vfapp.org/5c99

Hospitali Teule ya Wilaya Nkansi
Namanyere, Tanzania
https://vfapp.org/ef72

Hospitali ya Masista
Tanzania to Zambia road, Mafinga, Iringa, Tanzania
https://vfapp.org/3447

Hospitali ya Mkoa Mbeya
Regional Hospital Road, Mbeya, Mbeya, Tanzania
https://vfapp.org/8bfe

Hospitali ya Wilaya
T28, Kyela, Mbeya, Tanzania
https://vfapp.org/4cc3

Hospitali ya Wilaya ya Nachingwea
R857, Nachingwea, Lindi, Tanzania
https://vfapp.org/f738

Huruma District Hospital
T21, Mkuu, Kilimanjaro, Tanzania
https://vfapp.org/3ebd

Iambi Lutheran Hospital
Mkalama, Tanzania
https://vfapp.org/2c8d

Idende
Makete, Tanzania
https://vfapp.org/defd

Idunda
Njombe, Tanzania
https://vfapp.org/594f

Igodivaha
Wanging'Ombe, Tanzania
https://vfapp.org/7a4c

Igogwe Hospital
T10, Kiwira, Mbeya, Tanzania
https://vfapp.org/3423

Igumbilo
Igumbilo, Njombe, Tanzania
https://vfapp.org/ffa5

Igunga Hospital
T3, Igunga, Tabora, Tanzania
https://vfapp.org/4ac2

Igwachanya Hospital
R646, Igwachanya, Njombe, Tanzania
https://vfapp.org/7347

Ihanga
Iwawa, Njombe, Tanzania
https://vfapp.org/6c96

Ilembula Lutheran Hospital
T1, Wanging'ombe, Njombe, Tanzania
https://vfapp.org/5d3c

Ilininda
Ilininda, Njombe, Tanzania
https://vfapp.org/da4a

Ilula Mission Hospital
Iringa Road, Kimamba, Iringa, Tanzania
https://vfapp.org/2534

Ilungu
Ludilu, Njombe, Tanzania
https://vfapp.org/b661

Imalilo
Wanging'Ombe, Tanzania
https://vfapp.org/ac64

Imecc
A104, Iringa, Tanzania
https://vfapp.org/e431

IMTU Hospital
Dar es Salaam, Coastal Zone, Tanzania
https://vfapp.org/9343

Iniho
Church Road, Iniho, Njombe, Tanzania
https://vfapp.org/6f34

International Eye Hospital
New Bagamoyo Road, Dar es Salaam, Coastal Zone, Tanzania
https://vfapp.org/f58c

Ipamba Hospital
Tanzania to Zambia Road, Mafinga, Iringa, Tanzania
https://vfapp.org/ccff

Ipelele
Ipelele, Mbeya, Tanzania
https://vfapp.org/1bd8

Iringa
Sokoni Street, Ndiuka, Iringa, Tanzania
https://vfapp.org/b3ec

Isapulano
Makete, Tanzania
https://vfapp.org/3175

Iseresere Hospital
Nyamongo Road, Busawe Village, Mara, Tanzania
https://vfapp.org/4bbe

Isingilo Hospital
R101, Rugasha, Kagera, Tanzania
https://vfapp.org/1566

Isoko Hospital
R599, Ndembo, Mbeya, Tanzania
https://vfapp.org/c5eb

Itete Lutheran Hospital
R600, Mbambo, Mbeya, Tanzania
https://vfapp.org/2b53

Ithna-Asheri Hospital
Mt. Karakana, Arusha, Arusha, Tanzania
https://vfapp.org/c686

Itumba Hospital
Ileje, Mbeya, Tanzania
https://vfapp.org/1376

Jaffery Charitable Medical Services
Ghala Road, Moshi, Tanzania
https://vfapp.org/b9dd

Kagera Regional Hospital
Uganda Road, Bukoba, Kagera, Tanzania
https://vfapp.org/4813

Kagera Sugar Hospital
Missenyi, Tanzania
https://vfapp.org/8ed6

Kagondo Hospital
T4, Muhutwe, Kagera, Tanzania
https://vfapp.org/ec88

Kahama Hospital
Ngaya Road, Kahama, Shinyanga, Tanzania
https://vfapp.org/3722

Kairuki University
Hubert Kairuki Street, Dar es Salaam, Coastal Zone, Tanzania
https://vfapp.org/9e16

Kamanga
T4, Mwanza, Mwanza, Tanzania
https://vfapp.org/22c3

Karatu Lutheran Hospital
B144, Karatu, Arusha, Tanzania
https://vfapp.org/68be

Kasulu District Hospital
R326, Kisodji, Kigoma, Tanzania
https://vfapp.org/8c97

Katavi Regional Referral Hospital
216 Two Way, Mpanda, Katavi, Tanzania
https://vfapp.org/c5e2

Kibena Regional Hospital
T6, Ilunda, Njombe, Tanzania
https://vfapp.org/cb3f

Kibondo
T9, Kibondo, Kigoma, Tanzania
https://vfapp.org/99d9

Kibosho Hospital
Kibosho Road, Kibosho, Kilimanjaro, Tanzania
https://vfapp.org/c79e

Kigoma Baptist Hospital
Katubuka, Kigoma, Tanzania
https://vfapp.org/5a64

Kilimanjaro Christian Medical Centre at Moshi
Moshi, Tanzania
https://vfapp.org/c42e

Kilimanjaro Christian Medical Centre at Same
Same, Tanzania
https://vfapp.org/2d69

Kilindi Cdh
Kilindi, Tanzania
https://vfapp.org/c3b3

Kilosa District Hospital
Kilosa, Tanzania
https://vfapp.org/c6f6

Kimamba Hospital
Gairo, Tanzania
https://vfapp.org/bd46

Kinondoni Hospital
Mahakamani Road, Dar es Salaam, Coastal Zone, Tanzania
https://vfapp.org/92f8

Kinyonga Hospital
Kilwa-Nangurukuru Road, Kilwa Masoko, Lindi, Tanzania
https://vfapp.org/4d2f

Kipatimu Mission Hospital
Kipatimu – Utete Road, Kipatimu, Lindi, Tanzania
https://vfapp.org/8ddc

Kisarawe Hospital
Kisarawe, Tanzania
https://vfapp.org/882f

Kitete Regional Hospital
T8, Tabora, Tabora, Tanzania
https://vfapp.org/38d5

Kiungani Street Hospital
Kiungani Street, Dar es Salaam, Tanzania
https://vfapp.org/f682

Kiwanja Mpaka
Independece Avenue, Mbeya, Mbeya, Tanzania
https://vfapp.org/89a9

KMKM Hospital
Malawi Road, Zanzibar City مدينة زنجبار, Unguja Mjini Magharibi, Tanzania
https://vfapp.org/9a29

KOICA Mbagala Rangi Tatu Hospital
Hospitali Street, Dar es Salaam, Coastal Zone, Tanzania
https://vfapp.org/49e6

Kolandoto Hospital
T8, Ibadakuli, Shinyanga, Tanzania
https://vfapp.org/d94e

Kondoa Hospital
R462, Kondoa, Dodoma, Tanzania
https://vfapp.org/8e78

Kowak Regional Hospital
Kowaki, Tanzania
https://vfapp.org/bd3c

Kusini Hospital
Kusini, Tanzania
https://vfapp.org/ee26

Kyela District Hospital
Kyela, Tanzania
https://vfapp.org/538a

Lancet Hospital
Barabara ya Vumbi Dawasco, Dar es Salaam, Coastal Zone, Tanzania
https://vfapp.org/88bd

Ligula Hospital
T6, Mtwara, Mtwara, Tanzania
https://vfapp.org/cb1b

Likawage Hospital
Likawage, Lindi, Tanzania
https://vfapp.org/7b5e

Litembo Hospital
Litembo, Ruvuma, Tanzania
https://vfapp.org/e364

Liuli Hospital
Liuli, Ruvuma, Tanzania
https://vfapp.org/e869

Lubaga
Old Shinyanga Road, Lubaga Farm, Shinyanga, Tanzania
https://vfapp.org/a2e9

Ludewa District Hospital
T31, Ludewa, Njombe, Tanzania
https://vfapp.org/665a

Lugala Hospital
R675, Malinyi, Morogoro, Tanzania
https://vfapp.org/8fb4

Lugulu
T36, Lugulu kijiji, Simiyu, Tanzania
https://vfapp.org/989b

Lumumba Hospital
Zanzibar, Tanzania
https://vfapp.org/c2ac

Lushoto Hospital
Lushoto, Tanzania
https://vfapp.org/2a54

Lutindi Mental Hospital
Korogwe, Tanzania
https://vfapp.org/65a3

Machame Hospital
Nkwarungo Road, Machame, Kilimanjaro, Tanzania
https://vfapp.org/db9d

Mafiga Hospital
Barabara ya Chamwino, Morogoro, Morogoro, Tanzania
https://vfapp.org/be67

Mafinga District Hospital
Tanzania to Zambia Road, Mafinga, Iringa, Tanzania
https://vfapp.org/18b8

Magomeni Hospital
Minaki Road, Dar es Salaam, Coastal Zone, Tanzania
https://vfapp.org/9779

Magu Hospital
Magu Circle, Isandula, Mwanza, Tanzania
https://vfapp.org/971f

Makambako Hospital
Makambako, Tanzania
https://vfapp.org/5f73

Makandana Hospital
T10, Katumba, Mbeya, Tanzania
https://vfapp.org/8138

Makiungu Hospital
Mungaa, Singida, Tanzania
https://vfapp.org/b825

Makole Hospital
Hospital Road, Dodoma, Dodoma, Tanzania
https://vfapp.org/3789

Malya
R160, Mwandu, Simiyu, Tanzania
https://vfapp.org/fda1

Mama Ngoma Health Service
12 Kilwa Street, Dar es Salaam, Coastal Zone, Tanzania
https://vfapp.org/6885

Manyara Regional Referral Hospital
T14, Singu, Manyara, Tanzania
https://vfapp.org/e445

Marangu Hospital
T21, Marangu, Kilimanjaro, Tanzania
https://vfapp.org/d6a8

Masoko Hospital
Kilwa-Nangurukuru Road, Kilwa Masoko, Lindi, Tanzania
https://vfapp.org/826c

Massana Hospital
Peace Street, Dar es Salaam, Coastal Zone, Tanzania
https://vfapp.org/d448

Maswa District Hospital
T36, Zanzui, Simiyu, Tanzania
https://vfapp.org/acaa

Matema Lutheran Hospital
Matema Road, Matema, Mbeya, Tanzania
https://vfapp.org/3eed

Maweni Hospital
Burega Street, Lutale, Kigoma, Tanzania
https://vfapp.org/f17e

Mawenzi Hospital
Maendeleo Street, Dar es Salaam, Coastal Zone, Tanzania
https://vfapp.org/debb

Mawimbini Medical Centre
Kaskazini A, Tanzania
https://vfapp.org/bedf

Mbalizi Hospital
A104, Mbeya, Tanzania
https://vfapp.org/be9d

Mbesa Mission Hospital
Tunduru, Tanzania
https://vfapp.org/263f

Mbeya Consultant Hospital
Chunya Street, Mbeya, Mbeya, Tanzania
https://vfapp.org/926f

Mbeya Hospital
Mbeya, Tanzania
https://vfapp.org/bf59

Mbeya Referral Hospital
Independece Avenue, Mbeya, Mbeya, Tanzania
https://vfapp.org/9d5f

Mbinga District Hospital
T12, Mbinga, Ruvuma, Tanzania
https://vfapp.org/6912

Mbozi Mission Hospital
Mlowo, Mbeya, Tanzania
https://vfapp.org/69bb

Mbulu Hospital
Mbulu, Tanzania
https://vfapp.org/b17b

Meatu Hospital
T37, Mwanhuzi, Simiyu, Tanzania
https://vfapp.org/9e8e

Meru Hospital
T2, Tengeru, Arusha, Tanzania
https://vfapp.org/ff46

Mirembe Hospital
T5, Dodoma, Dodoma, Tanzania
https://vfapp.org/3e47

Misungwi Hospital
T8, Iteja, Mwanza, Tanzania
https://vfapp.org/9ce2

Mkomaindo District Hospital
Tunduru Road, Mlasi, Masasi, Tanzania
https://vfapp.org/9438

Mkula Hospital
T36, Mkula, Simiyu, Tanzania
https://vfapp.org/b51d

Mnazi Mmoja Hospital Dar es Salaam
Bibi Titi Mohamed Road, Dar es Salaam, Coastal Zone, Tanzania
https://vfapp.org/4ab8

Mnazi Mmoja Hospital Zanzibar
Zanzibar, Tanzania
https://vfapp.org/fb78

Mnero Hospital
R853, Nachingwea, Lindi, Tanzania
https://vfapp.org/f87e

Moravian Leprosy Hospital
T8, Sikonge, Tabora, Tanzania
https://vfapp.org/931e

Morogoro Hospital
Morogoro, Tanzania
https://vfapp.org/376f

Morogoro Regional Hospital
Old Dar es Salaam Road, Morogoro, Morogoro, Tanzania
🌐 https://vfapp.org/1a4b

Mount Meru Regional Hospital
Barabara ya Afrika Mashariki, Arusha, Arusha, Tanzania
🌐 https://vfapp.org/5eef

Moyo Hospital
Kinondoni Shamba Road, Dar es Salaam, Coastal Zone, Tanzania
🌐 https://vfapp.org/a72a

Moyo Safi Wa Maria Health Care
Msewe Street, Dar es Salaam, Coastal Zone, Tanzania
🌐 https://vfapp.org/f8a3

Mpwapwa District Hospital
Road to Kibakwe, Mpwapwa, Dodoma, Tanzania
🌐 https://vfapp.org/65c5

Mrara Hospital
Gorowa Road, Babati, Manyara, Tanzania
🌐 https://vfapp.org/8961

Mugana Designated District Hospital
Kantare, Kagera, Tanzania
🌐 https://vfapp.org/bd29

Muheza Ddh
T13, Muheza, Tanga, Tanzania
🌐 https://vfapp.org/f943

Muhimbili National Hospital
Dar es Salaam, Tanzania
🌐 https://vfapp.org/7f95

Murangi
R186, Lyasembe, Mara, Tanzania
🌐 https://vfapp.org/bd49

Mvumi Mission Hospital
Dodoma, Tanzania
🌐 https://vfapp.org/f2e1

Mwadui Hospital
T8, Maganzo, Shinyanga, Tanzania
🌐 https://vfapp.org/d975

Mwananchi Hospital
Temple Street, Mwanza, Mwanza, Tanzania
🌐 https://vfapp.org/95da

Mwananyamala Hospital
Minazini Street, Dar es Salaam, Coastal Zone, Tanzania
🌐 https://vfapp.org/a477

Mwanekeyi
Mwanekeyi, Mwanza, Tanzania
🌐 https://vfapp.org/2482

Mwembeladu Hospital
Zanzibar, Tanzania
🌐 https://vfapp.org/ab4c

Mzinga Hospital
Morogoro, Tanzania
🌐 https://vfapp.org/5ef8

Ndolage Hospital
R109, Ndolage, Kagera, Tanzania
🌐 https://vfapp.org/6add

Ngoyoni Hospital
Lower Road, Shimbi Mashariki, Kilimanjaro, Tanzania
🌐 https://vfapp.org/fdb7

Ngudu Hospital
R159, Ngudu, Mwanza, Tanzania
🌐 https://vfapp.org/68dd

Ngulyati H/C
R365, Ngulyati, Simiyu, Tanzania
🌐 https://vfapp.org/bd4a

Nguruka Hospital
Urundin Road, Nguruka, Kigoma, Tanzania
🌐 https://vfapp.org/e556

Nkinga Hospital
R390, Nkinga, Tabora, Tanzania
🌐 https://vfapp.org/7c8a

Nkoaranga Hospital
T2, Tengeru, Arusha, Tanzania
🌐 https://vfapp.org/47ad

Nkwenda
R101, Kagenyi, Kagera, Tanzania
🌐 https://vfapp.org/9b5e

Nshambya Hospital
Kashozi Road, Bukoba, Kagera, Tanzania
🌐 https://vfapp.org/b755

Nyakahanga Designated District Hospital
T38, Bisheshe, Kagera, Tanzania
🌐 https://vfapp.org/2729

Nyalwanzaja
R161, Buyagu, Geita, Tanzania
🌐 https://vfapp.org/c518

Nyamagana Hospital
T4, Mwanza, Mwanza, Tanzania
🌐 https://vfapp.org/a466

Nyamiaga Hospital
Ngara-Rusumo Road, Murukulazo, Kagera, Tanzania
🌐 https://vfapp.org/95b2

Nzega Government Hospital
R393, Bukooba, Shinyanga, Tanzania
🌐 https://vfapp.org/64b2

Ocean Road Hospital
Luthuli Street, Dar es Salaam, Coastal Zone, Tanzania
🌐 https://vfapp.org/f37f

Oltrument Hospital
TPRI Road, Ngaramtoni, Arusha, Tanzania
🌐 https://vfapp.org/3ac3

Omubweya Bukoba Rural in Tanzania
Kibirizi, Kagera, Tanzania
🌐 https://vfapp.org/6788

Pasua Hospital
Mill Road, Moshi, Kilimanjaro, Tanzania
🌐 https://vfapp.org/daef

Police Hospital
Mchinga Road, Lindi, Lindi, Tanzania
🌐 https://vfapp.org/2415

Puge Hospital
R390, Puge, Tabora, Tanzania
🌐 https://vfapp.org/86bf

Puma Mission Hospital
T3, Mkiwa village, Singida, Tanzania
🌐 https://vfapp.org/cc64

Queen of Universe Hospital
T3, Mkiwa village, Singida, Tanzania
🌐 https://vfapp.org/b157

Red Cross Hospital
Balewa Road, Mwanza, Tanzania
🌐 https://vfapp.org/6cdf

Regency Hospital
Allykhan Road, Dar es Salaam, Coastal Zone, Tanzania
🌐 https://vfapp.org/877f

Ruvuma Regional Hospital
Sokoine Road, Songea, Ruvuma, Tanzania
🌐 https://vfapp.org/2dd8

Sabasaba Hospital
Kingo Street, Morogoro, Morogoro, Tanzania
🌐 https://vfapp.org/49f4

Saidia Watoto
Makongoro Road, Medical Research, Mwanza, Tanzania
🌐 https://vfapp.org/7467

Salaaman Hospital
Kiongi Road, Dar es Salaam, Coastal Zone, Tanzania
🌐 https://vfapp.org/52e9

Sali Hospital
Yacht Club Road, Dar es Salaam, Coastal Zone, Tanzania
🌐 https://vfapp.org/8789

Sanitas Hospital
168 Mwai Kibaki Rd, Dar es Salaam, Tanzania
🌐 https://vfapp.org/df73

Sekou-Toure Hospital
Machemba Street, Isamilo Kaskazini, Mwanza, Tanzania
🌐 https://vfapp.org/23b1

Selian Lutheran Hospital Ngaramtoni
T2, Arusha, Arusha, Tanzania
🌐 https://vfapp.org/db74

Sengerema District Hospital
R149, Mission, Mwanza, Tanzania
🌐 https://vfapp.org/ffcb

Sengerema Hospital
Sengerema, Tanzania
🌐 https://vfapp.org/2657

Serengeti International Hospital
Serengeti, Tanzania
🌐 https://vfapp.org/8637

Shinyanga Government Hospital
Old Shinyanga Road, Shinyanga, Shinyanga, Tanzania
🌐 https://vfapp.org/7862

Shree Hindu Hospital
Pandit Street, Arusha, Arusha, Tanzania
🌐 https://vfapp.org/89bb

Shree Hindu Mandal Hospital
Wurzburg Road, Mwanza, Mwanza, Tanzania
🌐 https://vfapp.org/fcac

Siha Hospital
R262, Engarenairobi, Kilimanjaro, Tanzania
🌐 https://vfapp.org/59b1

Sikonge District Hospital
T8, Sikonge, Tabora, Tanzania
🌐 https://vfapp.org/d5da

Singida Regional Hospital
T14, Singida, Singida, Tanzania
🌐 https://vfapp.org/9db5

Sinza Hospital
Palestina Hospital Road, Dar es Salaam, Coastal Zone, Tanzania
🌐 https://vfapp.org/dafe

Sokoine Hospital
Mtanda Street, Lindi, Lindi, Tanzania
🌐 https://vfapp.org/fa5a

Somanda District Hospital
Bariadi, Shinyanga Region, Tanzania
🌐 https://vfapp.org/8ae3

Songwe
T1, Ivugula, Mbeya, Tanzania
🌐 https://vfapp.org/ed3f

St. Benedict Hospital
Dar es Salaam, Tanzania
🌐 https://vfapp.org/4645

St. Carolus
Singida, Tanzania
🌐 https://vfapp.org/feae

St. Gemma Hospital
T5, Dodoma, Dodoma, Tanzania
🌐 https://vfapp.org/a7ea

St. Anna Mission Hospital
T8, Tabora, Tabora, Tanzania
🌐 https://vfapp.org/524e

St. Anne's Hospital
Nyasa, Tanzania
🌐 https://vfapp.org/5746

St. Benedict Hospital
St. Benedict Road, Dar es Salaam, Coastal Zone, Tanzania
🌐 https://vfapp.org/2ed2

St. Benedict's Hospital
Masasi, Tanzania
🌐 https://vfapp.org/2bb5

St. Elizabeth Hospital
Kigoma Street, Arusha, Arusha, Tanzania
🌐 https://vfapp.org/132e

St. John's Hospital
Lugarawa, Njombe, Tanzania
🌐 https://vfapp.org/d6b2

St. Joseph Hospital
Mailimoja Road, Soweto, Kilimanjaro, Tanzania
🌐 https://vfapp.org/79b6

St. Otto Hospital
T4, Kikomakoma, Kagera, Tanzania
https://vfapp.org/4f31

St. Walburgs Hospital
Nyangao, Tanzania
https://vfapp.org/23a6

Sumbawanga Regional Hospital
Sokoine Street, Sumbawanga, Rukwa, Tanzania
https://vfapp.org/5ad8

Sumve DDH Hospital
R160, Koromije, Mwanza, Tanzania
https://vfapp.org/e5fc

Sumve District Designated Hospital
Kwimba, Tanzania
https://vfapp.org/375c

Swaya
Halengo Road, Mbeya, Mbeya, Tanzania
https://vfapp.org/d4c6

Tandale Hospital
Sokoni Road, Dar es Salaam, Coastal Zone, Tanzania
https://vfapp.org/6617

Tanzania Charitable Hospital
Zimbili Road, Dar es Salaam, Coastal Zone, Tanzania
https://vfapp.org/21da

Tanzania Occupational Health Service
Dar es Salaam, Tanzania
https://vfapp.org/5151

Tarime District Hospital
R194, Tarime, Mara, Tanzania
https://vfapp.org/f1b6

Temeke District Referral Hospital
Temeke Road, Dar es Salaam, Coastal Zone, Tanzania
https://vfapp.org/7a27

Teule
T13, Muheza, Tanga, Tanzania
https://vfapp.org/1462

The Aga Khan University Hospital
Seth Benjamin Street, Arusha, Arusha, Tanzania
https://vfapp.org/4219

TMJ Hospital
Old Bagamoyo Road, Dar es Salaam, Coastal Zone, Tanzania
https://vfapp.org/c971

TPC Hospital
Newvillage Road, Arusha Chini, Manyara, Tanzania
https://vfapp.org/9831

Tumaini Hospital
Magore Street, Dar es Salaam, Tanzania
https://vfapp.org/f1cf

Uhuru Hospital
Rufiji, Tanzania
https://vfapp.org/29db

Ukerewe Hospital
R141, Bukongo, Mwanza, Tanzania
https://vfapp.org/f885

Urambo Hospital
T18, Urambo, Tabora, Tanzania
https://vfapp.org/65e9

Usalama Hospital
Senga Road, Dar es Salaam, Coastal Zone, Tanzania
https://vfapp.org/fd46

Usangi Hospital
Usangi, Kilimanjaro, Tanzania
https://vfapp.org/2575

Uvinza Hospital
Uvinza, Tanzania
https://vfapp.org/9868

Uyole Hospital
3344 T10, Uyole, Mbeya, Tanzania
https://vfapp.org/24c3

Vingunguti Hospital
Mzambarauni Street, Dar es Salaam, Coastal Zone, Tanzania
https://vfapp.org/69c2

Vwawa District Hospital
Vwawa, Tanzania
https://vfapp.org/1e6b

Wasso Hospital
Wasso, Arusha, Tanzania
https://vfapp.org/83d4

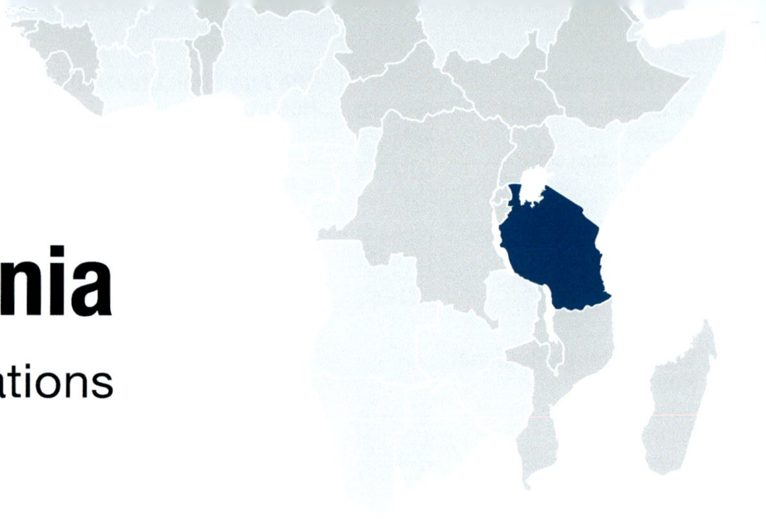

Tanzania

Nonprofit Organizations

A Broader View Volunteers
Provides developing countries around the world with significant volunteer programs that both aid the neediest communities and forge a lasting bond between those volunteering and those they have helped.

Dent-OMFS, ER Med, Infect Dis, MF Med
📞 +1 215-780-1845
🌐 https://vfapp.org/3bec

Abt Associates
Seeks to improve the quality of life and economic well-being of people worldwide, while striving to meet and exceed the highest professional standards.

General, Logist-Op, MF Med, OB-GYN, Peds
📞 +1 212-779-7700
🌐 https://vfapp.org/cec2

Ace Africa
Aims to enable children and their communities to participate in and take responsibility for their own health, well-being, and development.

Infect Dis, Logist-Op, Nutr, Peds
📞 +44 20 7933 2994
🌐 https://vfapp.org/df7f

Action Against Hunger
Aims to end life-threatening hunger for good through treating and preventing malnutrition across more than forty-five countries.

📞 +1 212-967-7800
🌐 https://vfapp.org/2dbc

Addis Clinic, The
Utilizes telemedicine to care for people living in medically underserved areas, connects volunteer physicians with global health challenges, and provides support to local partner organizations and frontline health workers.

General, Infect Dis
📞 +1 339-225-9886
🌐 https://vfapp.org/f82f

Advance Family Planning
Aims to achieve global expansion and access to quality contraceptive information, services, and supplies through financial investment and political commitment.

General, MF Med, Pub Health
📞 +1 410-502-8715
🌐 https://vfapp.org/7478

Africa CDC
Aims to strengthen the capacity and capability of Africa's public health institutions as well as partnerships to detect and respond quickly and effectively to disease threats and outbreaks, based on data-driven interventions and programs.

Infect Dis, Logist-Op, Pub Health
📞 +251 11 551 7700
🌐 https://vfapp.org/339c

Africa Indoor Residual Spraying Project (AIRS)
Aims to protect millions of people in Africa from malaria by spraying insecticide on the walls, ceilings, and other indoor resting places of mosquitoes that transmit malaria.

Infect Dis
📞 +1 301-347-5000
🌐 https://vfapp.org/9bd1

African Christian Hospitals
Aims to provide excellent healthcare services to all in Nigeria, Ghana, and Tanzania, and equips and empowers African healthcare workers through medical scholarships and investments in hospitals.

General, Surg
📞 +1 501-268-9511
🌐 https://vfapp.org/5ff9

African Field Epidemiology Network (AFENET)
Strengthens field epidemiology and public health laboratory capacity to contribute effectively to addressing epidemics and other major public health problems in Africa.

All-Immu, Infect Dis, Path, Pub Health
🌐 https://vfapp.org/df2e

Africa Inland Mission International
Seeks to establish churches and community development programs including health care projects, based in Christian ministry.

Anesth, Dent-OMFS, ER Med, General, MF Med, Medicine, OB-GYN, OB-GYN, Ophth-Opt, Ped Surg, Peds, Rehab
🌐 https://vfapp.org/f2f6

Aid Africa's Children
Aims to empower impoverished African children and communities with healthcare, food, clean water, educational, and entrepreneurial opportunities.

ER Med, General, Infect Dis, Nutr, OB-GYN,

Palliative, Peds, Pub Health
+1 708-269-1139
https://vfapp.org/5e2e

Aloha Medical Mission
Bringing hope and changing the lives of the people served overseas and in Hawai'i.
Anesth, Crit-Care, Dent-OMFS, ENT, ER Med, General, Medicine, OB-GYN, Ophth-Opt, Ortho, Ped Surg, Peds, Plast, Surg, Urol
+1 808-847-3400
https://vfapp.org/72ac

Alshifa Ltd.
Seeks to provide end-stage renal disease with dialysis services at minimum cost, with free services for the low-income community.
Dent-OMFS, Derm, ENT, General, Heme-Onc, Heme-Onc, Nephro, Path, Peds
+255 22 227 7646
https://vfapp.org/3f97

American Academy of Pediatrics
Seeks to attain optimal physical, mental, and social health and well-being for all infants, children, adolescents, and young adults.
Anesth, Crit-Care, Neonat, Ped Surg
+1 800-433-9016
https://vfapp.org/9633

American Heart Association (AHA)
Fights heart disease and stroke, striving to save and improve lives.
CV Med, Crit-Care, General, Heme-Onc, Medicine, Peds
+1 212-878-5900
https://vfapp.org/4747

American International Health Alliance (AIHA)
Strengthens health systems and workforce capacity worldwide through locally-driven, peer-to-peer institutional partnerships.
CV Med, ER Med, Infect Dis, Medicine, OB-GYN
+1 202-789-1136
https://vfapp.org/69fd

American Stroke Association
Works to prevent, treat, and beat stroke by funding innovative research, fighting for stronger public health policies, and providing lifesaving tools and information.
CV Med, Crit-Care, Heme-Onc, Medicine, Neuro, Pub Health, Pulm-Critic, Vasc Surg
+1 800-242-8721
https://vfapp.org/746f

Americares
Saves lives and improves health for people affected by poverty or disaster and responds with life-changing medicine, medical supplies, and health programs including domestic and global medical clinics.
All-Immu, ER Med, General, Infect Dis, MF Med, Nutr
+1 203-658-9500
https://vfapp.org/e567

Amref Health Africa
Serves millions of people across thirty-five countries in Sub-Saharan Africa, strengthening health systems, and training African health workers to respond to the continent's most critical health issues.
All-Immu, General, Infect Dis, Logist-Op, MF Med, OB-GYN, Path, Pub Health, Surg
+254 20 6993000
https://vfapp.org/6985

Amsterdam Institute for Global Health and Development (AIGHD)
Provides sustainable solutions to major health problems across our planet by forging synergies between disciplines, healthcare delivery, research, and education.
Infect Dis
+31 20 210 3960
https://vfapp.org/d73d

AO Alliance
Builds solutions to lessen the burden of injuries in low- and middle-income countries, while enhancing the care of the injured to reduce human suffering, disability, and poverty.
Ortho, Surg
https://vfapp.org/8cd5

Arms Around Africa Foundation
Supports children, empowers women, and helps young people to overcome poverty through talent promotion, education, good health, life skills development, entrepreneurship, and enhanced access to other resources for social and economic development.
General, Infect Dis, OB-GYN, Peds
+256 200 900277
https://vfapp.org/ad98

Assist International
Designs and implements humanitarian programs that build capacity, develop opportunities, and save lives around the world.
Infect Dis, Ped Surg, Peds
+1 831-438-4582
https://vfapp.org/9a3b

Avinta Care
Offers quality healthcare while providing a full suite of services from diagnosis to treatment, specializing in fertility and dermatology.
Derm, MF Med, OB-GYN, Path
https://vfapp.org/52a6

Baylor College of Medicine: Global Surgery
Trains leaders in academic global surgery and remains dedicated to advancements in the arenas of patient care, biomedical research, and medical education.
ENT, Infect Dis, OB-GYN, Ortho, Ped Surg, Plast, Pub Health, Radiol, Surg, Urol
+1 713-798-6078
https://vfapp.org/21f5

Baylor International Pediatric AIDS Initiative (BIPAI) at Texas Children's Hospital
Provides high-quality, high-impact, highly ethical pediatric and family-centered healthcare, health professional training, and clinical research focused on HIV/AIDS, tuberculosis, malaria, malnutrition, and other conditions impacting the health of children worldwide.
Infect Dis, Medicine, OB-GYN, Peds, Pub Health, Surg
+1 832-822-1038
https://vfapp.org/e6ba

BFIRST – British Foundation for International Reconstructive Surgery & Training
Supports projects across the developing world to train surgeons in their local environment to effectively manage devastating injuries.
Anesth, Plast, Surg
+44 20 7831 5161
https://vfapp.org/ad4f

Boston Children's Hospital: Global Health Program
Helps solve pediatric global health care challenges by transferring expertise through long-term partnerships with scalable impact, while working in the field to strengthen healthcare systems, advocate, research and provide care delivery or education as a way of sustainably improving the health of children worldwide.
Anesth, CV Med, Crit-Care, ER Med, Heme-Onc, Infect Dis, Medicine, Nutr, Palliative, Ped Surg, Peds
+1 617-919-6438
https://vfapp.org/f9f8

BRAC USA
Seeks to empower people and communities in situations of poverty, illiteracy, disease, and social injustice. Interventions aim to achieve large-scale, positive changes through economic and social programs that enable everyone to realize their potential.
ER Med, General, Infect Dis, Logist-Op, MF Med, OB-GYN
+1 212-808-5615
https://vfapp.org/9d9e

Bridge of Life
Aims to strengthen healthcare globally through sustainable programs that prevent and treat chronic disease.
Logist-Op, Nephro, OB-GYN, Peds, Surg
+1 888-374-8185
https://vfapp.org/5b68

Bridge2Aid
Provides access to simple, safe, emergency dental treatment.
Dent-OMFS
+44 1453 546776
https://vfapp.org/e682

Bridge2Aid Australia
Seeks to provide access to simple, safe, emergency dental treatment for all.
Anesth, Dent-OMFS
+255 754 033 003
https://vfapp.org/a899

Burn Care International
Seeks to improve the lives of burn survivors around the world through effective rehabilitation.
Derm, Nutr, Psych, Surg
+1 843-662-6717
https://vfapp.org/78d1

Canada-Africa Community Health Alliance
Sends Canadian volunteer teams on two- to three-week missions to African communities to work hand-in-hand with local partners.
General, Infect Dis, MF Med, OB-GYN, Peds, Surg
+1 613-234-9992
https://vfapp.org/4c94

Canadian Foundation for Women's Health
Seeks to advance the health of women in Canada and around the world through research, education, and advocacy in obstetrics and gynecology.
MF Med, OB-GYN
+1 613-730-4192
https://vfapp.org/f41e

Canadian Network for International Surgery, The
Aims to improve maternal health, increase safety, and build local capacity in low-income countries by creating and providing surgical and midwifery courses, training domestically, and transferring skills.
Logist-Op, Surg
+1 877-217-8856
https://vfapp.org/86ff

CardioStart International
Provides free heart surgery and associated medical care to children and adults living in underserved regions of the world, irrespective of political or religious affiliation, through the collective skills of healthcare experts.
Anesth, CT Surg, CV Med, Crit-Care, Pub Health, Pulm-Critic
+1 813-304-2163
https://vfapp.org/85ef

CARE
Works around the globe to save lives, defeat poverty, and achieve social justice.
ER Med, General
+1 800-422-7385
https://vfapp.org/7232

Care for Africa
Seeks to empower communities with sustainable access to healthcare through its Rural School Health Clinic. Works with counterparts in Tanzania Tarime region to share resources and knowledge and build capacity.
ER Med, General, Infect Dis, Ortho, Ped Surg, Peds, Rehab, Surg
+61 408 994 883
https://vfapp.org/bd21

Carter Center, The
Seeks to prevent and resolve conflicts, enhance freedom and democracy, and improve health, while remaining committed to human rights and the alleviation of human suffering.
Infect Dis, MF Med, Ophth-Opt
+1 800-550-3560
https://vfapp.org/6556

Catholic World Mission
Works to rebuild communities worldwide by helping to alleviate poverty and empower underserved areas, while spreading the message of the Catholic Church.
ER Med, General, Nutr, Peds
+1 770-828-4966
https://vfapp.org/7b5f

Center for Private Sector Health Initiatives
Aims to improve the health and well-being of people in developing countries by facilitating partnerships between the public and private sectors.
Infect Dis, Nutr, Peds
+1 202-884-8334
https://vfapp.org/b198

Chain of Hope
Provides lifesaving heart operations for children around the world and supports the development of cardiac services in numerous developing and war-torn countries.
Anesth, CT Surg, CV Med, Crit-Care, Ped Surg, Peds, Pulm-Critic, Surg
+44 20 7351 1978
https://vfapp.org/1b1b

Challenge Initiative, The
Seeks to rapidly and sustainably scale up proven reproductive health solutions among the urban poor.
MF Med, OB-GYN, Peds
+1 410-502-8715
https://vfapp.org/2f77

CharityVision International
Focuses on restoring curable sight impairment worldwide by empowering local physicians and creating sustainable solutions.
Logist-Op, Ophth-Opt, Surg
+1 435-200-4910
https://vfapp.org/6231

Child Family Health International (CFHI)
Connect students with local health professionals and community leaders transforming perspectives about self, global health, and healing.
General, Infect Dis, OB-GYN, Ophth-Opt, Palliative, Peds
+1 415-957-9000
https://vfapp.org/729e

Children Without Worms
Enhances the health and development of children by reducing intestinal worm infections.
Infect Dis, Pub Health
+1 404-371-0466
https://vfapp.org/6bee

Christian Aid Ministries
Strives to be a trustworthy and efficient channel for Amish, Mennonite, and other conservative Anabaptist groups and individuals to minister to physical and spiritual needs around the world.
CT Surg, ER Med, Logist-Op, Ortho, Pub Health
+1 330-893-2428
https://vfapp.org/7b33

Christian Blind Mission (CBM)
Aims to improve the quality of life of persons with disabilities in the poorest countries, addressing poverty as a cause, and a consequence, of disability, and working in partnership to create a society for all.
ENT, General, Infect Dis, OB-GYN, Ophth-Opt, Ortho, Peds, Psych, Rehab, Surg
+49 6251 131131
https://vfapp.org/3824

Christian Connections for International Health (CCIH)
Promotes global health and wholeness from a Christian perspective.
All-Immu, General, Infect Dis, MF Med, Neonat, OB-GYN, Psych
+1 703-923-8960
https://vfapp.org/fa5d

Circle of Health International (COHI)
Aligns with local, community-based organizations led and powered by women to help respond to the needs of the women and children that they serve. Helps with the provision of professional volunteers, capacity training, and procurement of requested and appropriate supplies and equipment. Raises funds for the organizations to provide the services required.
ER Med, Logist-Op, MF Med, Neonat, OB-GYN, Psych
+1 512-210-7710
https://vfapp.org/8b63

Cleft Africa
Strives to provide underserved Africans with cleft lips and palates with access to the best possible treatment for their condition, so that they can live a life free of the health problems caused by cleft.
Anesth, Dent-OMFS, Ped Surg, Surg
https://vfapp.org/8298

Clinton Health Access Initiative (CHAI)
Aims to save lives and reduce the burden of disease in low- and middle-income countries. Works with partners to strengthen the capabilities of governments and the private sector to create and sustain high-quality health systems.
General, Heme-Onc, Infect Dis, Logist-Op, MF Med, Medicine, Neonat, Nutr, OB-GYN, Path, Peds, Rad-Onc
+1 617-774-0110
https://vfapp.org/9ed7

Comprehensive Community Based Rehabilitation in Tanzania (CCBRT)
Aims to become a healthcare social enterprise serving the community and the most vulnerable with accessible, specialized services and development programs.
General, MF Med, Neonat, OB-GYN
+255 699 990 001
https://vfapp.org/be24

Core Group
Aims to improve and expand community health practices for underserved populations, especially women and children, through collaborative action and learning.
General, Infect Dis, MF Med, Medicine, OB-GYN, Peds, Pub Health
+1 202-380-3400
https://vfapp.org/9de3

Creighton University School of Medicine: Global Surgery Fellowship
Aims to significantly impact the absence of acute surgical care in developing countries by providing free surgery to underserved patients and surgical training for developing country trainees.
Anesth, Ped Surg, Surg
+1 402-250-6196
https://vfapp.org/777f

Cura for the World
Seeks to heal, nourish, and embrace the neglected by building medical clinics in remote communities in dire need of medical care.
ER Med, General, Peds
https://vfapp.org/c55f

CURE
Operates charitable hospitals and programs in underserved countries worldwide where patients receive surgical treatment, based in Christian ministry.

Anesth, Neurosurg, Ortho, Ped Surg, Peds, Rehab, Surg

+1 616-512-3105

https://vfapp.org/aa16

CureCervicalCancer
Focuses on the early detection and prevention of cervical cancer around the globe for the women who need it most.

Heme-Onc, OB-GYN

+1 310-601-3002

https://vfapp.org/ace1

D-tree Digital Global Health
Demonstrates and advocates for the potential of digital technology to transform health systems and improve health and wellbeing for all.

Logist-Op, MF Med, OB-GYN, Peds, Pub Health

+1 978-238-9122

https://vfapp.org/1f79

Direct Relief
Improves the health and lives of people affected by poverty or emergency situations by mobilizing and providing essential medical resources needed for their care.

ER Med, Logist-Op

+1 805-964-4767

https://vfapp.org/58e5

Doctors with Africa (CUAMM)
Advocates for the universal right to health and promotes the values of international solidarity, justice, and peace. Works to protect and improve the well-being and health of vulnerable communities in Africa with a long-term development perspective.

ER Med, Infect Dis, MF Med, Neonat, OB-GYN, Peds

https://vfapp.org/d2fb

Doctors Without Borders/Médecins Sans Frontières (MSF)
Responds to emergencies and provides lifesaving medical care where needed most, including during disasters, conflicts, and epidemics.

Anesth, Crit-Care, ER Med, General, Infect Dis, Nutr, OB-GYN, Ped Surg, Peds, Psych, Pub Health, Surg

+1 212-679-6800

https://vfapp.org/f363

Dodoma Christian Medical Centre Trust (DCMCT)
Works to bring health and hope to the people of central Tanzania and beyond.

CV Med, Crit-Care, Dent-OMFS, General, Infect Dis, OB-GYN, Path, Peds, Radiol, Surg

+255 26 232 1051

https://vfapp.org/f9cc

Dodoma Tanzania Health Development
Aims to ensure high-quality, compassionate, Tanzanian-led healthcare for the people of Central Tanzania by developing the capacity and sustainability of Dodoma Christian Medical Center.

Anesth, Crit-Care, Dent-OMFS, General, Infect Dis, MF Med, Medicine, OB-GYN, Ophth-Opt, Path, Ped Surg, Peds, Radiol, Rehab, Surg

+1 763-432-6589

https://vfapp.org/c33a

Dream Sant'Egidio
Seeks to counter HIV/AIDS in Africa by eliminating the transmission of HIV from mother to child, with a focus on women because of the importance of their role in the community.

Infect Dis, MF Med, Neonat, OB-GYN, Path, Peds

+39 06 899 2225

https://vfapp.org/f466

Drugs for Neglected Diseases Initiative
Develops lifesaving medicines for people with neglected diseases around the world, having developed eight treatments for five deadly diseases and saving millions of lives since 2003.

Infect Dis, Pub Health

+41 22 906 92 30

https://vfapp.org/969c

Duke University: Global Health Institute
Sparks innovation in global health research and education, and brings together knowledge and resources to address the most important global health issues of our time.

All-Immu, Infect Dis, MF Med, OB-GYN, Pub Health

+1 919-681-7760

https://vfapp.org/c4cd

East Africa Children's Healthcare Foundation
Provides healthcare insurance for children in order to treat disease more quickly, thereby opening up more opportunities for them to further their education and become successful adults in the Tanzanian community.

Peds

https://vfapp.org/ff32

Elizabeth Glaser Pediatric AIDS Foundation
Seeks to end global pediatric HIV/AIDS through prevention and treatment programs, research, and advocacy.

Infect Dis, Nutr, OB-GYN, Peds

+1 888-499-4673

https://vfapp.org/d6ec

Elton John Aids Foundation
Seeks to address and overcome the stigma, discrimination, and neglect that prevents ending AIDS by funding local experts to challenge discrimination, prevent infections, and provide treatment.

Infect Dis, Pub Health

+1 212-219-0670

https://vfapp.org/9d31

Empower Tanzania
Works in partnership with Tanzanians to develop models that sustainably improve the quality of life and resilience of rural areas through health improvements, education, and economic empowerment.

General, Infect Dis, MF Med, OB-GYN, Palliative

https://vfapp.org/ba24

Enabel
As the development agency of the Belgian federal government, charged with implementing Belgium's international development policy, carries out public service assignments in Belgium and abroad pursuant to the 2030 Agenda for Sustainable Development.

General, Infect Dis, Logist-Op, MF Med, OB-GYN, Peds, Pub Health
+32 2 505 37 00
https://vfapp.org/5af7

END Fund, The
Aims to control and eliminate the most prevalent neglected diseases among the world's poorest and most vulnerable people.
Infect Dis
+1 646-690-9775
https://vfapp.org/2614

EngenderHealth
Works to implement high-quality, gender-equitable programs that advance sexual and reproductive health and rights.
General, MF Med, OB-GYN, Peds
+1 202-902-2000
https://vfapp.org/1cb2

Episcopal Relief & Development
Provides relief in times of disaster and promotes sustainable development by identifying and addressing the root causes of suffering.
Infect Dis, MF Med, Neonat, Nutr, Peds
+1 855-312-4325
https://vfapp.org/7cfa

eRanger
Provides sustainable solutions to transportation and medical provision such as ambulances and mobile clinics in developing countries.
ER Med, General, Logist-Op
+27 40 654 3207
https://vfapp.org/4c18

Evidence Project, The
Improves family-planning policies, programs, and practices through the strategic generation, translation, and use of evidence.
General, MF Med
+1 202-237-9400
https://vfapp.org/f9e7

Eye Care Foundation
Helps prevent and cure avoidable blindness and visual impairment in low-income countries.
Ophth-Opt, Surg
+31 20 647 3879
https://vfapp.org/c8f9

Fertility Education & Medical Management (FEMM)
Aims to make knowledge-based reproductive health accessible to all women and enables them to be informed partners in the choice and delivery of their medical care and services.
MF Med, OB-GYN
https://vfapp.org/e8b2

Fistula Foundation
Aims to engage the support of people worldwide who are eager to see the day when no woman suffers from obstetric fistula. Raises and directs funds to doctors and hospitals providing life-transforming surgery to women in need.
OB-GYN
+1 408-249-9596
https://vfapp.org/e958

Forever Projects
Aims to empower women and their families with self-sustainability and build a brighter future for themselves.
Nutr
+255 756 977 339
https://vfapp.org/5ea5

Foundation for African Medicine & Education (FAME)
Improves access and advances patient-centered care for under-resourced communities in rural Tanzania.
General, Infect Dis, Logist-Op, MF Med, OB-GYN, Peds, Surg
+1 530-229-1071
https://vfapp.org/cb82

Foundation For International Education In Neurological Surgery (FIENS), The
Provides hands-on training and education to neurosurgeons around the world.
Neuro, Neurosurg, Surg
https://vfapp.org/bab8

Fracarita International
Provides support and services in the fields of mental healthcare, care for people with a disability, and education.
Psych, Rehab
https://vfapp.org/8d3c

Friends of UNFPA
Promotes the health, dignity, and rights of women and girls around the world by supporting the lifesaving work of UNFPA, the United Nations reproductive health and rights agency, through education, advocacy, and fundraising.
MF Med, OB-GYN
+1 646-649-9100
https://vfapp.org/2a3a

Gift of Life International
Provides lifesaving cardiac treatment to children in developing countries while developing sustainable pediatric cardiac programs by implementing screening, surgical, and training missions.
Anesth, CT Surg, CV Med, Crit-Care, Ped Surg, Peds, Pulm-Critic
+1 855-734-3278
https://vfapp.org/f2f9

Global Alliance to Prevent Prematurity and Stillbirth (GAPPS)
Seeks to improve birth outcomes worldwide by reducing the burden of premature birth and stillbirth.
All-Immu, Infect Dis, MF Med, Neonat, Neonat, OB-GYN
+1 206-413-7954
https://vfapp.org/3f74

Global Eye Mission
Strives to bring hope and healing to the lives of those living in underserved regions of the world by providing high-quality eye care to help the blind see, and improving the quality of life for individuals and entire communities.
Ophth-Opt, Surg
+1 952-484-9710
https://vfapp.org/197e

Global Eye Project
Empowers local communities by building locally managed, sustainable eye clinics through education initiatives and volunteer-run professional training services.
Anesth, Ophth-Opt, Surg
https://vfapp.org/cdba

Global Ministries – The United Methodist Church
As the worldwide mission and development agency of The United Methodist Church, Global Ministries works with more than 300 hospitals and clinics around the world through its Global Health Unit.
Anesth, CT Surg, CV Med, Crit-Care, Dent-OMFS, Derm, ER Med, GI, General, Infect Dis, Logist-Op, MF Med, Medicine, Neonat, Nephro, Nutr, OB-GYN, Ophth-Opt, Ortho, Palliative, Peds, Pod, Psych, Pub Health, Rehab, Rheum, Surg, Urol
+1 800-862-4246
https://vfapp.org/1723

Global Oncology (GO)
Brings the best in cancer care to underserved patients around the world and collaborates across geographic, professional, and academic borders to improve cancer care, research, and education.
Heme-Onc, Path, Rad-Onc
https://vfapp.org/fcb8

Global Surgical Access Foundation
Partners with underserved communities to provide competent, safe, and sustainable surgical care.
Anesth, Surg
+1 786-223-5046
https://vfapp.org/ea5f

Global Telehealth Network (GTN)
Provides telehealth services with dedicated physician volunteers for people located in medically underserved areas, including low- and medium-resource countries, refugee camps, conflict zones, and disaster areas, as well as in the U.S.
ER Med, General, Path, Peds, Psych, Radiol, Surg
+1 415-847-1239
https://vfapp.org/4345

Grassroot Soccer
Leverages the power of soccer to educate, inspire, and mobilize at risk youth in developing countries to overcome their greatest health challenges, live healthier more productive lives, and be agents for change in their communities.
Infect Dis
+1 603-277-9685
https://vfapp.org/3521

Harvard Global Health Institute
Devoted to improving global health and pioneering the next generation of global health research, education, policy, and practice, with an evidence-based, innovative, integrative and collaborative approach, harnessing the unique breadth of excellence within Harvard.
General, Infect Dis, Logist-Op
+1 617-384-5431
https://vfapp.org/5867

Healing Little Hearts
Sends specialist medical teams to perform free lifesaving heart surgery on babies and children in developing parts of the world.
Anesth, CT Surg, CV Med, Ped Surg, Peds, Surg
+44 116 271 1479
https://vfapp.org/ffc1

Healing the Children Northeast
Helps underserved children around the world secure the medical care they need to lead more fulfilling lives.
Anesth, Dent-OMFS, ENT, General, Medicine, Ophth-Opt, Ped Surg, Peds, Plast
+1 860-355-1828
https://vfapp.org/16ba

Health Equity Initiative
Aims to build and sustain a global community that engages across sectors and disciplines to advance health equity.
Pub Health
https://vfapp.org/e2e2

Health Improvement Project Zanzibar
Works with the government and communities of Zanzibar toward the goal of achieving universal health coverage, while managing two hospitals, training local staff, and running a progressive mental health program.
ER Med, General, Logist-Op, Medicine, Neonat, Nutr, OB-GYN, Peds, Psych, Surg
https://vfapp.org/33ad

Health Tanzania
Seeks to improve the health and education of underserved Tanzanians, with the help of its partners. Inspired by the Christian faith, it works to provide out-patient and in-patient care, community health and prevention programs, and primary education.
All-Immu, Anesth, General, Infect Dis, MF Med, OB-GYN, Peds, Psych, Pub Health
https://vfapp.org/8141

Health Volunteers Overseas (HVO)
Improves the availability and quality of healthcare through the education, training, and professional development of the health workforce in resource-scarce countries.
All-Immu, Anesth, CV Med, Dent-OMFS, Derm, ENT, ER Med, Endo, GI, Heme-Onc, Infect Dis, Medicine, Medicine, Nephro, Neuro, OB-GYN, Ophth-Opt, Ortho, Peds, Plast, Psych, Pulm-Critic, Rehab, Rheum, Surg
+1 202-296-0928
https://vfapp.org/42b2

Health[e] Foundation
Supports health professionals and community workers in the world's most vulnerable societies to ensure quality health for everyone in need by providing digital education and information, using e-learning and m-health.
Logist-Op
https://vfapp.org/b73b

Healthy Child Uganda
Supports medical training and clinical care and initiates a community-cased education project targeting child health.
Logist-Op, Peds
+1 403-210-6161
https://vfapp.org/ebc5

Healthy Developments
Provides Germany-supported health and social protection programs around the globe in a collaborative knowledge management process.
All-Immu, General, Infect Dis, Logist-Op, MF Med
https://vfapp.org/dc31

Heart to Heart International
Strengthens communities through improving health access, providing humanitarian development, and administering crisis relief worldwide. Engages volunteers, collaborates with partners, and deploys resources to achieve this mission.
Anesth, ER Med, General, Logist-Op, Medicine, Path, Path, Peds, Psych, Pub Health, Surg
+1 913-764-5200
https://vfapp.org/aacb

Heineman Medical Outreach
Provides medical and educational assistance globally to promote sustainable healthcare and enhanced living standards in underserved communities through the International Medical Outreach (IMO) program, a collaborative partnership between Heineman Medical Outreach and Atrium Health.
Anesth, CT Surg, CV Med, ER Med, General, Heme-Onc, Logist-Op, Medicine, Neonat, OB-GYN, Ped Surg, Peds, Surg, Vasc Surg
+1 704-374-0505
https://vfapp.org/389b

Helen Keller International
Seeks to eliminate preventable vision loss, malnutrition, and diseases of poverty.
Infect Dis, Nutr, OB-GYN, Ophth-Opt, Peds
+1 212-532-0544
https://vfapp.org/b654

HelpAge International
Works to ensure that people everywhere understand how much older people contribute to society and that they must enjoy their right to healthcare, social services, economic, and physical security.
General, Geri, Infect Dis, Medicine, Pub Health
+44 20 7148 7623
https://vfapp.org/5d91

Hope and Healing International
Gives hope and healing to children and families trapped by poverty and disability.
General, Nutr, Ophth-Opt, Peds, Rehab
+1 905-640-6464
https://vfapp.org/c638

Humanity First
Provides aid and assistance to those in need, offering sustainable development solutions to society while providing and empowering local communities with the resources to help themselves.
ER Med, General, MF Med, Ophth-Opt
+44 20 8417 0082
https://vfapp.org/13cc

ICAP at Columbia University
Serves as global leader in supporting the scale-up of multidisciplinary HIV/AIDS prevention, care, and treatment programs based on a family-focused approach.
General, Infect Dis, MF Med, Medicine, OB-GYN, Pub Health
+1 212-342-0505
https://vfapp.org/a8ef

IMA World Health
Works to build healthier communities by collaborating with key partners to serve vulnerable people with a focus on health, healing, and well-being for all.
Infect Dis, MF Med, Nutr, OB-GYN, Pub Health
+1 202-888-6200
https://vfapp.org/8316

IMPACT Foundation
Works to prevent and alleviate needless disability by restoring sight, mobility, and hearing.
ENT, MF Med, OB-GYN, Ophth-Opt, Ortho, Peds, Surg
+44 1444 457080
https://vfapp.org/ba28

International Agency for the Prevention of Blindness (IAPB), The
Leads international efforts in blindness-prevention activities, works toward a world where no one is needlessly visually impaired, and ensures that everyone has access to the best possible standard of eye health.
Infect Dis, Ophth-Opt, Pub Health
https://vfapp.org/87a2

International Campaign for Women's Right to Safe Abortion
Works to build an international network and campaign that brings together organizations with an interest in promoting and providing safe abortion to create a shared platform for advocacy, debate, and dialogue and the sharing of skills and experience.
OB-GYN, Pub Health, Surg
https://vfapp.org/f341

International Children's Heart Fund
Aims to promote the international growth and quality of cardiac surgery, particularly in children and young adults.
CT Surg, Ped Surg
https://vfapp.org/33fb

International Council of Ophthalmology
Works with ophthalmologic societies and others to enhance ophthalmic education and improve access to the highest quality eye care in order to preserve and restore vision for the people of the world.
Ophth-Opt
https://vfapp.org/ffd2

International Eye Foundation (IEF)
Eliminates preventable and treatable blindness by making quality sustainable eye care services accessible and affordable worldwide.
Infect Dis, Logist-Op, Ophth-Opt
+1 240-290-0263
https://vfapp.org/e839

International Federation of Gynecology and Obstetrics (FIGO)
Implements global projects on specific women's health issues.
MF Med, Medicine, Neonat, OB-GYN, Surg, Urol

📞 +44 20 7928 1166
🌐 https://vfapp.org/c4b4

International Federation of Red Cross and Red Crescent Societies (IFRC)
Coordinates and directs international assistance following natural and man-made disasters in nonconflict situations through the world's largest humanitarian and development network. Provides disaster-preparedness programs, healthcare activities, and promotes humanitarian values.
ER Med, General, Infect Dis, Nutr
📞 +1 212-338-0161
🌐 https://vfapp.org/b4ee

International Health Partners – U.S. Inc.
Seeks to improve healthcare for the people of Tanzania by integrating medical knowledge, techniques, and best practices within the East African culture.
Derm, General, Infect Dis, MF Med, Medicine, Path, Peds
📞 +1 870-404-4491
🌐 https://vfapp.org/d4dd

International Hope Missions
Improves local standards of care by enabling complex procedures for women and children and mentoring local medical teams.
General, MF Med, OB-GYN
📞 +1 929-344-9093
🌐 https://vfapp.org/c5c7

International Medical and Surgical Aid (IMSA)
Aims to save lives and alleviate suffering through education, healthcare, surgical camps, and quality medical programs.
Anesth, General, Ped Surg, Surg
📞 +44 7598 088806
🌐 https://vfapp.org/2561

International Medical Relief
Provides sustainable education, training, medical and dental care, and disaster relief and response in vulnerable communities worldwide.
Dent-OMFS, General, Infect Dis, Medicine, OB-GYN
📞 +1 970-635-0110
🌐 https://vfapp.org/b3ed

International Organization for Migration (IOM) – The UN Migration Agency
Promotes evidence-informed policies and holistic, preventive, and curative health programs that are beneficial, accessible, and equitable for vulnerable migrants.
General, Infect Dis, OB-GYN
📞 +27 12 342 2789
🌐 https://vfapp.org/621a

International Pediatric Nephrology Association (IPNA)
Leads the global efforts to successfully address the care for all children with kidney disease through advocacy, education, and training.
Medicine, Nephro, Peds
🌐 https://vfapp.org/b59d

International Planned Parenthood Federation (IPPF)
Leads a locally owned, globally connected civil society movement that provides and enables services and champions sexual and reproductive health and rights for all, especially the underserved.
Infect Dis, MF Med, OB-GYN
📞 +44 20 7939 8200
🌐 https://vfapp.org/dc97

International Rescue Committee (IRC)
Responds to the world's worst humanitarian crises and helps people whose lives and livelihoods are shattered by conflict and disaster to survive, recover, and gain control of their future.
ER Med, General, Infect Dis, MF Med, Peds
📞 +1 212-551-3000
🌐 https://vfapp.org/5d24

International Smile Power
Partners with people to improve and sustain dental health and build bridges of friendship around the world.
Dent-OMFS
🌐 https://vfapp.org/ba69

International Trachoma Initiative (iTi)
Works toward a world free from trachoma, a preventable cause of blindness, and provides comprehensive support to national ministries of health and governmental and nongovernmental organizations to implement a comprehensive approach to fight trachoma.
Infect Dis, Ophth-Opt
📞 +1 404-371-0466
🌐 https://vfapp.org/3278

International Union Against Tuberculosis and Lung Disease
Develops, implements, and assesses anti-tuberculosis, lung health, and noncommunicable disease programs.
Infect Dis, Pub Health, Pulm-Critic
📞 +33 1 44 32 03 60
🌐 https://vfapp.org/3e82

IntraHealth International
Improves the performance of health workers and strengthens the systems in which they work.
CV Med, Endo, General, Infect Dis, MF Med, Neonat, Nutr, OB-GYN
📞 +1 919-313-3554
🌐 https://vfapp.org/ddc8

IVUmed
Aims to make quality urological care available worldwide by providing medical and surgical education for physicians and nurses and treatment for thousands of children and adults.
Anesth, OB-GYN, Ped Surg, Surg, Urol
📞 +1 801-524-0201
🌐 https://vfapp.org/e619

Jakaya Kikwete Cardiac Institute
Provides high-quality affordable cardiovascular care for patients and facilitates sustainable delivery of tertiary cardiovascular care services, while providing specialized and super-specialized postgraduate courses in the field of cardiovascular medicine.
Anesth, CV Med, Crit-Care, Surg
📞 +255 22 215 2392
🌐 https://vfapp.org/bb41

Jesus Harvesters Ministries
Reaches communities through medical clinics, dental care, veterinarian outreach, pastor training, and community service, based in Christian ministry.
Dent-OMFS, General, Infect Dis
https://vfapp.org/8a23

Jhpiego
Creates and delivers transformative healthcare solutions that save lives in partnership with national governments, health experts, and local communities.
General, Infect Dis, OB-GYN, Surg
+1 410-537-1800
https://vfapp.org/45b8

John Snow, Inc. (JSI)
Aims to improve the health and well-being of underserved and vulnerable people and communities throughout the world.
General, Infect Dis, Logist-Op, MF Med, OB-GYN, Peds, Psych, Pub Health
+1 617-482-9485
https://vfapp.org/ba78

Johns Hopkins Center for Communication Programs
Believes in the power of communication to save lives, by empowering people to adopt healthy behaviors for themselves, their families, and their communities.
General, Infect Dis, Logist-Op, OB-GYN, Pub Health
+1 410-659-6300
https://vfapp.org/1bf9

Johns Hopkins Center for Global Health
Facilitates and focuses the extensive expertise and resources of the Johns Hopkins institutions together with global collaborators to effectively address and ameliorate the world's most pressing health issues.
General, Genetics, Logist-Op, MF Med, Peds, Psych, Pub Health, Pulm-Critic
+1 410-502-9872
https://vfapp.org/54ce

Joint United Nations Programme on HIV/AIDS (UNAIDS)
Aims to place people living with HIV and people affected by the virus at the decision-making table and at the center of designing, delivering, and monitoring the AIDS response.
Infect Dis
+41 22 791 36 66
https://vfapp.org/464a

Kagondo St. Joseph Hospital Foundation
Improves the accessibility of services for orthopedic care, treatment of trauma, skin grafting, birth defect correction, and artificial limbs, and supplies orthopedic implants and other necessary equipment for people in Tanzania.
Endo, Ortho, Ped Surg, Peds, Surg
https://vfapp.org/2848

Kaya Responsible Travel
Promotes sustainable social, environmental, and economic development, empowers communities, and cultivates educated, compassionate global citizens through responsible travel.
All-Immu, Crit-Care, Dent-OMFS, ER Med, General, Geri, Infect Dis, MF Med, Medicine, Nutr, OB-GYN, Peds, Psych, Pub Health, Rehab
+1 413-517-0266
https://vfapp.org/b2cf

Kids Care Everywhere
Seeks to empower physicians in under-resourced environments with multimedia, state-of-the-art medical software, and to inspire young professionals to become future global healthcare leaders.
Logist-Op, Ped Surg, Peds
https://vfapp.org/bc23

KidzCare Tanzania
Provides underprivileged children and orphans with education, nutrition, and medical programs.
Dent-OMFS, Nutr, Ortho, Ped Surg, Peds
https://vfapp.org/5a57

Kilimanjaro Christian Medical Centre
Excels in quality service, training, and research, providing accessible and quality healthcare services as key referral hospital.
Dent-OMFS, ENT, ER Med, Endo, General, General, Heme-Onc, Medicine, Medicine, OB-GYN, Ophth-Opt, Ortho, Path, Peds, Psych, Radiol, Rehab, Urol
+255 27 275 4377
https://vfapp.org/bbc5

Kletjian Foundation
Works toward a world in which all people have access to safe, sustainable, and high-quality medical care, building collaborative networks and supporting entrepreneurial leaders that promote global health equity.
CT Surg, ENT, General, Ortho, Surg
https://vfapp.org/12c2

Kupona Foundation
Works to prevent disability and maternal and neonatal mortality and morbidity, and to provide equitable access to affordable, quality medical rehabilitative services.
MF Med, Neonat, OB-GYN, Rehab
+1 518-595-9007
https://vfapp.org/4198

Lay Volunteers International Association (LVIA)
Fosters local and global change to help overcome extreme poverty, reinforce equitable and sustainable development, and enhance dialogue between Italian and African communities.
ER Med, Logist-Op, MF Med, Neonat, Nutr, OB-GYN, Peds
+39 0171 696975
https://vfapp.org/ecd4

Leprosy Mission: Northern Ireland, The
Leads the fight against leprosy by supporting people living with leprosy today and serving future generations by working to end the transmission of the disease.
General, Infect Dis
+44 28 9262 9500
https://vfapp.org/e265

Life for a Child
Supports the provision of the best possible health care, given local circumstances, to all children and youth with diabetes in less-resourced countries, through the strengthening of existing diabetes services.
Endo, Medicine, Peds
https://vfapp.org/d712

Life Support Foundation
Aims to prevent deaths due to acute, life-threatening conditions in low-income countries through improving the access to, and quality of, basic lifesaving interventions.
Anesth, Crit-Care, ER Med, OB-GYN, Peds
https://vfapp.org/799e

Lifebox
Seeks to provide safer surgery and anesthesia in low-resource countries by investing in tools, training, and partnerships for safe surgery.
Anesth, Crit-Care, Surg
+44 20 3286 0402
https://vfapp.org/2d4d

Light for the World
Contributes to a world in which persons with disabilities fully exercise their rights and assists persons with disabilities living in poverty.
Ophth-Opt, Rehab
+43 1 8101300
https://vfapp.org/3ff6

Lions Clubs International
Empowers volunteers to serve their communities, meet humanitarian needs, encourage peace, and promote international understanding through Lions clubs.
Heme-Onc, Medicine, Nutr, Ophth-Opt
+1 630-571-5466
https://vfapp.org/7b12

London School of Hygiene & Tropical Medicine: International Centre for Eye Health
Works to improve eye health and eliminate avoidable visual impairment and blindness with a focus on low-income populations.
Logist-Op, Ophth-Opt, Pub Health
+44 20 7958 8316
https://vfapp.org/6f5f

Maasai Women Development Organization (MWEDO)
Aims to empower Maasai women economically and socially through improved access to education, health services, and economic opportunities.
General, Infect Dis, MF Med, Nutr, OB-GYN, Peds, Surg
+255 27 254 4290
https://vfapp.org/2a9a

Madaktari Africa
Aims to advance medical expertise and care in Sub-Saharan Africa through the training and education of local medical personnel.
CT Surg, CV Med, ER Med, Nephro, Neurosurg
+1 434-942-9016
https://vfapp.org/7856

Management Sciences for Health (MSH)
Works with countries and communities to save lives and improve the health of the world's poorest and most vulnerable people by building strong, resilient, sustainable health systems.
Infect Dis, Logist-Op, Pub Health
+1 617-250-9500
https://vfapp.org/6aa2

MAP International
Provides medicines and health supplies to those in need around the world so they might experience life to the fullest.
Logist-Op
+1 800-225-8550
https://vfapp.org/deed

Marie Stopes International
Provides the contraception and safe abortion services that enable women all over the world to choose their own futures.
Infect Dis, MF Med, Neonat, OB-GYN, Pub Health
+44 20 7636 6200
https://vfapp.org/9525

Maternity Foundation
Works to ensure safer childbirth for women and newborns everywhere through innovative mobile health solutions such as the Safe Delivery App, a mobile training tool for skilled birth attendants.
MF Med, OB-GYN, Pub Health
https://vfapp.org/ff4f

Maternity Worldwide
Works with communities and partners to identify and develop appropriate and effective ways to reduce maternal and newborn mortality and morbidity, facilitate communities to access quality skilled maternity care, and support the provision of quality skilled care.
MF Med, OB-GYN
+44 1273 234033
https://vfapp.org/822b

McGill University Health Centre: Centre for Global Surgery
Works to reduce the impact of injury by advancing surgical care through research and education in resource-limited settings.
ER Med, Logist-Op, Ped Surg, Surg
+1 514-934-1934
https://vfapp.org/7246

MCW Global
Works to address communities' pressing needs by empowering current leaders and readying leaders of tomorrow.
Dent-OMFS
+1 212-453-5811
https://vfapp.org/1547

Médecins du Monde/Doctors of the World
Provides care, bears witness, and supports social change worldwide with innovative medical programs and evidence-based advocacy initiatives.
ER Med, General, Infect Dis, MF Med, Neonat, OB-GYN, Peds, Pub Health
+33 1 44 92 15 15
https://vfapp.org/a43d

Medical Missions for Children (MMFC)
Provides quality surgical and dental services to poor and underprivileged children and young adults in various countries throughout the world, as well as facilitates the transfer of education, knowledge, and recent innovations to the local medical communities.
Dent-OMFS, ENT, Endo, Ortho, Ped Surg, Peds, Plast
+1 508-697-5821
https://vfapp.org/1631

Medical Missions for Global Health
Seeks to reduce health disparities by providing surgical, medical, and health care services and education to underserved communities and developing communities throughout Africa, the Caribbean, Central and South America, and the U.S.

Dent-OMFS, General, Surg

+1 212-951-1431

https://vfapp.org/cf52

Medical Missions Outreach
Visits developing countries to provide quality, ethical healthcare and outreach to those in need, based in Christian ministry.

Dent-OMFS, Ophth-Opt, Ortho, Surg

+1 410-391-7000

https://vfapp.org/1197

Medical Relief International
Exists to provide dental, medical, humanitarian aid, and other services deemed necessary for the benefit of people in need.

Dent-OMFS, General

+1 206-819-2551

https://vfapp.org/192b

Medical Teams International
Seeks to restore health as the first step to restoring hope, working to bring basic but lifesaving medical care to those in need.

Dent-OMFS, ER Med, General, MF Med, Pub Health

+1 503-624-1000

https://vfapp.org/8d1c

MEDLIFE Movement
Partners with low-income communities in Latin America and Africa to improve access to medicine, education, and community development projects.

Dent-OMFS, General, Peds, Pub Health

+1 844-633-5433

https://vfapp.org/de87

MedSend
Funds qualified healthcare professionals to serve the physical and spiritual needs of people around the world, enabling healthcare providers to work where they have been called.

General

+1 203-891-8223

https://vfapp.org/661c

MedShare
Aims to improve the quality of life of people, communities, and the planet by sourcing and directly delivering surplus medical supplies and equipment to communities in need around the world.

Logist-Op

+1 770-323-5858

https://vfapp.org/c8bc

Mending Kids
Provides free, lifesaving surgical care to sick children worldwide by deploying volunteer medical teams and teaching communities to become medically self-sustaining by educating local medical staff.

Anesth, CT Surg, ENT, Ortho, Ortho, Ped Surg, Plast, Surg

+1 818-843-6363

https://vfapp.org/4d61

MHS-Massana Hospital
Promotes the health and well-being of the local population in Mbezi Beach Area and from all over Dar es Salaam city and Tanzania at large.

Endo, General, MF Med, Medicine, OB-GYN, Ophth-Opt, Peds, Radiol

+255 22 262 7177

https://vfapp.org/8df5

Midwife Vision
Promotes maternal and child health through education, global community participation, and the provision of resources for the nursing and midwifery force.

MF Med, Neonat, OB-GYN

https://vfapp.org/21d7

Miga Solutions Foundation
Improves global healthcare through the donations of medical equipment to underserved communities in the U.S. and around the world.

Logist-Op

+1 763-225-8418

https://vfapp.org/2bf2

Millen Magese Foundation
Empowers women and girls in Tanzania to promote gender equality through access to education and reproductive health, by building schools, securing education supplies, and providing access to health services.

MF Med, OB-GYN

https://vfapp.org/3eae

MiracleFeet
Brings low-cost treatment to every child on the planet born with clubfoot, a leading cause of physical disability.

Ortho, Peds, Rehab

+1 919-240-5572

https://vfapp.org/bda8

Mission: Restore
Trains medical professionals abroad in complex reconstructive surgery in order to create a sustainable infrastructure where long-term relationships are forged and permanent change is made.

Plast, Surg

+1 855-777-1350

https://vfapp.org/3f5f

Missions for Humanity
Provides medical, dental, and humanitarian aid to those in the world's neediest communities, serving with utmost respect for the preservation of human dignity and rooted in the teachings of the Catholic faith.

Dent-OMFS, General, Ophth-Opt

+1 508-672-7996

https://vfapp.org/5bca

mothers2mothers (m2m)
Employs and trains local women living with HIV as community health workers called Mentor Mothers to support women, children, and adolescents with vital medical services, education, and support.

Infect Dis, MF Med, OB-GYN, Peds, Pub Health

+27 21 466 9160

https://vfapp.org/6557

MSD for Mothers
Designs scalable solutions that help end preventable maternal deaths.
MF Med, OB-GYN, Pub Health
https://vfapp.org/9f99

Mufindi Orphans
Provides educational opportunities and health access for vulnerable children and families in Tanzania.
General, Infect Dis, Nutr, Peds
+1 785-550-7565
https://vfapp.org/976e

NEST 360
Works to ensure that hospitals in Africa can deliver lifesaving care for small and sick newborns, by developing and distributing high-quality technologies and services.
MF Med, Neonat, Peds, Pub Health
+1 713-348-4174
https://vfapp.org/cea9

Okoa Project, The
Designs motorcycle ambulances, creates jobs, and saves lives one ride at a time.
ER Med, Logist-Op
https://vfapp.org/1f6c

Olmoti Clinic/Our One Community
Provides comprehensive medical care and transformative education as a foundation for a sustainable Maasai community.
General, Infect Dis, MF Med, OB-GYN, Ophth-Opt, Surg
+1 650-862-7800
https://vfapp.org/911e

OneSight
Brings eye exams and glasses to the people who lack access to vision care.
Ophth-Opt
+1 888-935-4589
https://vfapp.org/3ecc

Open Heart International
Provides surgical interventions and best practices to the most disadvantaged communities on the planet.
CT Surg, MF Med, OB-GYN, Ophth-Opt, Plast, Surg
+61 2 9487 9295
https://vfapp.org/dab2

Operation Fistula
Exists to end obstetric fistula by building models of care that serve every woman, everywhere.
MF Med, OB-GYN, Surg
+1 512-687-3479
https://vfapp.org/ce8e

Operation International
Offers medical aid to adults and children suffering from lack of quality healthcare in impoverished countries.
Dent-OMFS, ER Med, Heme-Onc, OB-GYN, Ophth-Opt, Ortho, Ped Surg, Plast, Surg
+1 631-287-6202
https://vfapp.org/b52a

Operation Walk
Provides the gift of mobility through life-changing joint replacement surgeries at no cost for those in need in the U.S. and globally.
Anesth, Ortho, Rehab, Surg
+1 310-493-8073
https://vfapp.org/bafe

Options
Believes in a world where women and children can access the high-quality health services they need, without financial burden.
Logist-Op, MF Med, Neonat, OB-GYN
+44 20 7430 1900
https://vfapp.org/3a48

OPTIVEST Foundation
Funds strategic opportunities that are holistic and collaborative, inspired by the Christian faith.
General, Nutr
https://vfapp.org/f1e6

Optometry Giving Sight
Delivers eye exams and low or no-cost glasses, provides training for local eye care professionals, and establishes optometry schools, vision centers and optical labs.
Ophth-Opt
+1 303-526-0430
https://vfapp.org/33ea

Orbis International
Works to prevent and treat blindness through hands-on training and improved access to quality eye care.
Anesth, Ophth-Opt, Surg
+1 646-674-5500
https://vfapp.org/f2b2

Oxford University Global Surgery Group (OUGSG)
Aims to contribute to the provision of high-quality surgical care globally, particularly in low- and middle-income countries (LMICs) while bringing together students, researchers, and clinicians with an interest in global surgery, anaesthesia, and obstetrics and gynecology.
Anesth, MF Med, OB-GYN, Ortho, Surg
+44 1865 737543
https://vfapp.org/c624

Pact
Works on the ground to improve the lives of those who are challenged by poverty and marginalization, striving for a world where all people are heard, capable, and vibrant.
Infect Dis, Logist-Op, MF Med, Pub Health
+1 202-466-5666
https://vfapp.org/9a6c

Pan African Thoracic Society (PATS)
Aims to promote lung health in Africa, the continent most afflicted by morbidity and death from respiratory diseases, by promoting education, research, advocacy, optimal care, and the development of African capacity to address respiratory challenges in the continent.
CV Med, Crit-Care, Pulm-Critic
https://vfapp.org/5457

Pan-African Academy of Christian Surgeons (PAACS)
Exists to train and support African surgeons to provide excellent, compassionate care to those most in need, inspired by the Christian faith.
Anesth, CT Surg, Neurosurg, OB-GYN, Ortho,

Ped Surg, Plast, Surg
+1 847-571-9926
https://vfapp.org/85ba

Partners for Development (PfD)
Works to improve quality of life for vulnerable people in underserved communities through local and international partnerships.
Infect Dis, MF Med, Neonat, Peds
+1 301-608-0426
https://vfapp.org/d2f6

Partners for World Health
Sorts, evaluates, repackages, and prepares supplies and equipment for distribution to individuals, communities, and healthcare facilities in need, both locally and internationally.
ER Med, General, Logist-Op
+1 207-774-5555
https://vfapp.org/982e

PATH
Advances health equity through innovation and partnerships so people, communities, and economies can thrive.
All-Immu, CV Med, Endo, Heme-Onc, Infect Dis, MF Med, Neonat, Nutr, OB-GYN, Path, Peds, Pulm-Critic
+1 202-822-0033
https://vfapp.org/b4db

Pathfinder International
Champions sexual and reproductive health and rights worldwide, mobilizing communities most in need to break through barriers and forge paths to a healthier future.
OB-GYN
+1 617-924-7200
https://vfapp.org/a7b3

Pediatric Health Initiative
Supports the spread of quality pediatric care and its development and progress in low- and middle-income countries.
ER Med, Infect Dis, Neonat, Palliative, Ped Surg, Peds
https://vfapp.org/614b

Pepal
Brings together NGOs, global corporations, and the public sector to co-create solutions to big social issues, creating immediate and scalable solutions and developing leaders who are capable of driving change in their communities.
Heme-Onc, Infect Dis, Pub Health
https://vfapp.org/6dc5

Phil Simon Clinic: Tanzania Project
Provides medical, surgical, and psychosocial support in Tanzania.
General, Infect Dis
+1 626-397-5480
https://vfapp.org/8a68

PINCC Preventing Cervical Cancer
Seeks to prevent female-specific diseases in developing countries by utilizing low-cost and low-technology methods to create sustainable programs through patient education, medical personnel training, and facility outfitting.
OB-GYN
+1 830-708-6009
https://vfapp.org/9666

Plaster House, The
Provides low-cost surgical rehabilitation to Tanzanian children living with treatable congenital and traumatic disabilities.
Dent-OMFS, Logist-Op, Ortho, Ped Surg, Plast, Pub Health, Rehab
+255 685 838 215
https://vfapp.org/7ab9

Project Concern International (PCI)
Drives innovation from the ground up to enhance health, end hunger, overcome hardship, and advance women and girls—resulting in meaningful and measurable change in people's lives.
Infect Dis, MF Med, Nutr, OB-GYN, Peds
+1 858-279-9690
https://vfapp.org/5ed7

Project SOAR
Conducts HIV operations research around the world to identify practical solutions to improve HIV prevention, care, and treatment services.
ER Med, General, MF Med, OB-GYN, Psych
+1 202-237-9400
https://vfapp.org/1a77

Provision Charitable Foundation
Improves the lives of Tanzanian people suffering from epilepsy and seizures through education, healthcare, and opportunities.
Dent-OMFS, MF Med, Neonat, Neuro
https://vfapp.org/af24

PSI – Population Services International
Dedicates efforts to improving the health of people in the developing world by focusing on challenges such as a lack of family planning, HIV/AIDS, barriers to maternal health, and the greatest threats to children under the age of 5, including malaria, diarrhea, pneumonia, and malnutrition.
Infect Dis, MF Med, OB-GYN, Peds
+1 202-785-0072
https://vfapp.org/ffe3

RAD-AID International
Improves and optimizes access to medical imaging and radiology in low-resource regions of the world.
Rad-Onc, Radiol
https://vfapp.org/537f

REACH Shirati
Works in partnership with local communities in rural Tanzania to enhance education, improve healthcare, and promote community development.
General, Infect Dis, OB-GYN, Peds, Pub Health, Surg
+1 510-273-9044
https://vfapp.org/a3ff

Reconstructing Women International
Treats patients in their local communities through groups of international volunteers made up of female plastic surgeons using local medical facilities, in cooperation with local medical professionals.
Anesth, Plast, Rehab, Surg
https://vfapp.org/924a

RestoringVision
Empowers lives by restoring vision for millions of people in need.
Ophth-Opt
📞 +1 209-980-7323
🌐 https://vfapp.org/e121

ReSurge International
Provides reconstructive surgical care and builds surgical capacity in developing countries.
Anesth, Dent-OMFS, Ped Surg, Plast, Surg
📞 +1 408-737-8743
🌐 https://vfapp.org/9937

RHD Action
Seeks to reduce the burden of rheumatic heart disease in vulnerable populations throughout the world.
CV Med, Medicine, Pub Health
🌐 https://vfapp.org/f5d9

Rockefeller Foundation, The
Works to promote the well-being of humanity.
Logist-Op, Nutr, Pub Health
📞 +1 212-869-8500
🌐 https://vfapp.org/5424

Rotary International
Provides service to others, improves lives, and advances world understanding, goodwill, and peace through its fellowship of business, professional, and community leaders.
ER Med, General, Infect Dis, MF Med, OB-GYN
🌐 https://vfapp.org/8fb5

Rotaplast International
Helps children and families worldwide by eliminating the burden of cleft lip and/or palate, burn scarring, and other deformities by sending medical teams to provide free reconstructive surgery, ancillary treatment, and training.
Anesth, Dent-OMFS, ENT, Ped Surg, Plast, Surg
📞 +1 415-252-1111
🌐 https://vfapp.org/78b3

ROW Foundation
Works to improve the quality of training for healthcare providers, and the diagnosis and treatment available to people with epilepsy and associated psychiatric disorders in under-resourced areas of the world.
Neuro, Psych
📞 +1 630-791-0247
🌐 https://vfapp.org/25eb

Safe Anaesthesia Worldwide
Provides anesthesia to those in need in low-income countries to enable lifesaving surgery.
Anesth, Plast
📞 +44 7527 506969
🌐 https://vfapp.org/134a

Salvation Army International, The
Seeks to meet human needs through services in education, healthcare, community support, emergency response, and ministry development, inspired by the Christian faith.
Dent-OMFS, Derm, ER Med, Infect Dis, MF Med, Medicine, Nutr, OB-GYN, Ophth-Opt, Palliative, Psych, Rehab, Surg
📞 +44 20 7332 0101
🌐 https://vfapp.org/8eb3

Sanofi Espoir Foundation
Contributes to reducing health inequalities among populations that need it most by applying a socially responsible approach focused on fighting childhood cancers in low-income countries, improving maternal and newborn health, and improving access to care.
ER Med, OB-GYN, Peds
📞 +33 1 53 77 91 38
🌐 https://vfapp.org/943b

Save A Child's Heart
Provides lifesaving cardiac treatment to children in developing countries, and trains healthcare professionals from these countries to deliver quality care in their communities.
CT Surg, CV Med, Crit-Care, Ped Surg, Peds
📞 +1 240-223-3940
🌐 https://vfapp.org/1bef

Save the Children
Gives children around the world a healthy start in life, the opportunity to learn, and protection from harm.
All-Immu, Crit-Care, ER Med, General, Infect Dis, MF Med, Medicine, Neonat, OB-GYN, Peds, Psych, Pub Health
📞 +1 800-728-3843
🌐 https://vfapp.org/2e73

SEE International
Provides sustainable medical, surgical, and educational services through volunteer ophthalmic surgeons, with the objectives of restoring sight and preventing blindness to disadvantaged individuals worldwide.
Ophth-Opt, Surg
📞 +1 805-963-3303
🌐 https://vfapp.org/6e1b

SEVA
Delivers vital eye care services to the world's most vulnerable, including women, children, and Indigenous peoples.
Ophth-Opt, Surg
📞 +1 510-845-7382
🌐 https://vfapp.org/1e87

Shirati Health, Education, and Development (SHED) Foundation
Provides healthcare, education, and development services to underserved communities in Tanzania.
General, Heme-Onc, Infect Dis, OB-GYN, Ped Surg, Peds
📞 +255 621 045 742
🌐 https://vfapp.org/1e1b

Sightsavers
Prevents avoidable blindness in some of the poorest parts of the world by treating debilitating eye diseases.
Infect Dis, Ophth-Opt, Surg
📞 +1 800-707-9746
🌐 https://vfapp.org/aa52

SIGN Fracture Care International
Builds orthopedic capacity around the world and provides the injured poor access to fracture surgery by donating orthopedic education and implant systems to surgeons in developing countries.
Ortho, Rehab, Surg
📞 +1 509-371-1107
🌐 https://vfapp.org/123d

Simavi
Strives for a world in which all women and girls are socially and economically empowered and pursue their rights to live a healthy life, free from discrimination, coercion, and violence.
MF Med, OB-GYN
+31 88 313 1500
https://vfapp.org/b57b

Smile Train
Seeks to give every child with a cleft the opportunity for a healthy, productive life by providing free cleft repair surgery and comprehensive cleft care in their own communities.
Dent-OMFS, ENT, Plast
+1 800-932-9541
https://vfapp.org/f21d

SOS Children's Villages International
Supports children through alternative care and family strengthening.
ER Med, Peds
+43 1 36824570
https://vfapp.org/aca1

St. Benedict Ndanda Referral Hospital
Provides quality healthcare services to all patients, irrespective of faith and socio-economic status.
Dent-OMFS, ER Med, Endo, Nephro, OB-GYN, Ophth-Opt, Peds, Radiol, Rehab, Surg
+255 786 353 135
https://vfapp.org/4656

Sustainable Kidney Care Foundation (SKCF)
Works to provide treatment for kidney injury where none exists, and aims to reduce mortality from treatable acute kidney injury (AKI).
Infect Dis, Medicine, Nephro
https://vfapp.org/1926

Swiss Tropical and Public Health Institute
Contributes to the improvement of the health of populations internationally, nationally, and locally through excellence in research, education, and services.
Infect Dis, Pub Health
+41 61 284 81 11
https://vfapp.org/2ee4

Tanzanian Cardiac Hospital Foundation, Inc. (TCHF)
Seeks to build and sustain a Catholic cardiac hospital in Tanzania and provide cardiac services to the Tanzanian community.
CT Surg, CV Med, Crit-Care, General, MF Med, Surg
+1 772-359-9085
https://vfapp.org/3f3c

Task Force for Global Health, The
Consists of programs and focus areas that cover a range of global health issues including neglected tropical diseases, infectious diseases, vaccines, field epidemiology, public health informatics, health workforce development, and global health ethics.
Infect Dis, Logist-Op, Medicine, Ophth-Opt, Peds
+1 404-371-0466
https://vfapp.org/714c

Tearfund
Responds to crisis and partners with local churches to bring restoration to those living in poverty, inspired by the Christian faith.
ER Med, Logist-Op
+44 20 3906 3906
https://vfapp.org/f6cf

Texas Children's Global Health
Addresses healthcare needs in resource-limited settings locally and globally by improving maternal and child health through the implementation of innovative, sustainable, in-country programs to train health professionals and build functional healthcare infrastructure.
Anesth, ER Med, Heme-Onc, Infect Dis, MF Med, Nutr, OB-GYN, Peds, Pub Health, Surg
+1 832-824-1141
https://vfapp.org/4a1d

THET Partnerships for Global Health
Trains and educates health workers in Africa and Asia, working in partnership with organizations and volunteers from across the UK.
General
+44 20 7290 3891
https://vfapp.org/f937

Third World Eye Care Society (TWECS)
Collects old, unused eyeglasses and distributes them in conjunction with eye exams given by properly trained individuals.
Logist-Op, Ophth-Opt
+1 604-874-2733
https://vfapp.org/8618

Total Health Africa
Aims to increase the capacity of local healthcare providers to deliver quality healthcare to underserved communities through training and providing resources.
General, Infect Dis, OB-GYN, Peds
+1 515-758-0445
https://vfapp.org/9f62

Touch Foundation
Seeks to save lives and relieve human suffering by strengthening healthcare in Sub-Saharan Africa, providing better access to care and improving the quality of local health systems.
General, MF Med, Neonat, OB-GYN
+1 646-779-2414
https://vfapp.org/fdbb

U.S. President's Malaria Initiative (PMI)
Supports low-income countries to help control and eliminate malaria through cost-effective, lifesaving malaria interventions.
Infect Dis, MF Med, OB-GYN
+1 202-712-0000
https://vfapp.org/dc8b

Umoja
Provides education and welfare support to the most vulnerable children and young people in Tanzania, empowering them to develop the knowledge and skills needed to create positive change for themselves and the wider community.
General, Peds, Psych
+255 783 009 332
https://vfapp.org/c978

Union for International Cancer Control (UICC)
Unites and supports the cancer community to reduce the

global cancer burden, promote greater equity, and ensure that cancer control continues to be a priority in the world health and development agenda.

Heme-Oc, Pub Health

+41 22 809 18 11

https://vfapp.org/88b1

United Methodist Volunteers in Mission (UMVIM)

Engages in short-term missions each year in ministries as varied as disaster response, community development, pastor training, microenterprise, agriculture, Vacation Bible School, building repair and construction, and medical/dental services.

Dent-OMFS, ER Med, General

https://vfapp.org/1ee6

United Nations Children's Fund (UNICEF)

Works in over 190 countries and territories to save children's lives, to defend their rights, and to help them fulfill their potential, from early childhood through adolescence.

All-Immu, Infect Dis, MF Med, Neonat, Nutr, OB-GYN, Ped Surg, Peds, Pub Health

https://vfapp.org/42d7

United Nations Development Programme (UNDP)

Helps countries achieve the simultaneous eradication of extreme poverty and significant reduction of inequalities and exclusion using a sustainable human development approach.

Infect Dis, Logist-Op, Pub Health

https://vfapp.org/935c

United Nations High Commissioner for Refugees (UNHCR)

Safeguards the rights and well-being of people who have been forced to flee, ensuring that everybody has the right to seek asylum and find safe refuge in another country, with the goal of seeking lasting solutions.

General, MF Med, Medicine, OB-GYN, Peds, Psych, Pub Health

https://vfapp.org/6636

United Nations Population Fund (UNFPA)

Supports reproductive healthcare for women and youth in more than 150 countries, focusing on delivering a world where every pregnancy is wanted, every childbirth is safe, and every young person's potential is fulfilled.

Infect Dis, MF Med, Neonat, OB-GYN, Peds, Pub Health

+1 212-963-6008

https://vfapp.org/c969

United States President's Emergency Plan for AIDS Relief (PEPFAR)

The U.S. global HIV/AIDS response works to prevent new HIV infections and accelerate progress to control the global epidemic in more than 50 countries, by partnering with governments to support sustainable, integrated, and country-led responses to HIV/AIDS.

Infect Dis, Pub Health

https://vfapp.org/a57c

University of California, Berkeley: Bixby Center for Population, Health & Sustainability

Aims to help manage population growth, improve maternal health, and address the unmet need for family planning within a human rights framework.

OB-GYN

+1 510-642-6915

https://vfapp.org/ff2b

University of California San Francisco: Institute for Global Health Sciences

Dedicates its efforts to improving health and reducing the burden of disease in the world's most vulnerable populations by integrating expertise in the health, social, and biological sciences to train global health leaders and develop solutions to the most pressing health challenges.

Infect Dis, OB-GYN, Pub Health

+1 415-476-5494

https://vfapp.org/6587

University of Chicago: Center for Global Health

Collaborates with communities locally and globally to democratize education, increase service learning opportunities, and advance sustainable solutions to improve health and well-being while reducing global health inequities.

Genetics, MF Med, Peds, Pub Health

+1 773-702-5959

https://vfapp.org/4f8f

University of Colorado: Global Emergency Care Initiative

Strives to sustainably improve emergency care outcomes in low- and middle-income communities worldwide by linking cutting-edge academics with excellent on-the-ground implementation.

ER Med

https://vfapp.org/417a

University of New Mexico School of Medicine: Project Echo

Seeks to improve health outcomes worldwide through the use of a technology called telementoring, a guided-practice model in which the participating clinician retains responsibility for managing the patient.

General, Infect Dis, MF Med, OB-GYN, Path, Peds

+1 505-750-3246

https://vfapp.org/6c9a

University of Virginia: Anesthesiology Department Global Health Initiatives

Educates and trains physicians, to help people achieve healthy productive lives, and advances knowledge in the medical sciences.

Anesth, Pub Health

+1 434-924-2283

https://vfapp.org/1b8b

University of Washington: Department of Global Health

Improves health for all through research, education, training, and service, addresses the causes of disease and health inequities at multiple levels, and collaborates with partners to develop and sustain locally-led, quality health systems, programs and policies.

Infect Dis, Logist-Op, Pub Health

+1 206-616-1159

https://vfapp.org/f543

University of Washington: The International Training and Education Center for Health (I-TECH)

Works with local partners to develop skilled healthcare workers and strong national health systems in resource-limited countries.

Infect Dis, Pub Health
📞 +1 206-744-8493
🌐 https://vfapp.org/642f

USAID: Maternal and Child Survival Program
Works to prevent child and maternal deaths.
Infect Dis, MF Med, Neonat, OB-GYN, Peds
🌐 https://vfapp.org/6fcf

USAID: A2Z The Micronutrient and Child Blindness Project
Aims to increase the use of key micronutrient and blindness interventions to improve child and maternal health.
MF Med, Neonat, Nutr, Ophth-Opt, Surg
📞 +1 202-884-8785
🌐 https://vfapp.org/c5f1

USAID: Deliver Project
Builds a global supply chain to deliver lifesaving health products to people in order to enable countries to provide family planning, protect against malaria, and limit the spread of pandemic threats.
Infect Dis, Logist-Op, MF Med
📞 +1 202-712-0000
🌐 https://vfapp.org/374e

USAID: EQUIP Health
Exists as an effective, efficient response mechanism to achieving global HIV epidemic control by delivering the right intervention at the right place and in the right way.
Infect Dis
📞 +27 11 276 8850
🌐 https://vfapp.org/d76a

USAID: Health Finance and Governance Project
Uses research to implement strategies to help countries develop robust governance systems, increase their domestic resources for health, manage those resources more effectively, and make wise purchasing decisions.
Logist-Op
📞 +1 202-712-0000
🌐 https://vfapp.org/8652

USAID: Health Policy Initiative
Provides field-level programming in health policy development and implementation.
General, Infect Dis, MF Med, OB-GYN, Peds
🌐 https://vfapp.org/8f84

USAID: Human Resources for Health 2030 (HRH2030)
Helps low- and middle-income countries develop the health workforce needed to prevent maternal and child deaths, support the goals of Family Planning 2020, control the HIV/AIDS epidemic, and protect communities from infectious diseases.
Logist-Op
📞 +1 202-955-3300
🌐 https://vfapp.org/9ea8

USAID: Leadership, Management and Governance Project
Improves leadership, management, and governance practices to strengthen health systems and improve health for all, including vulnerable populations worldwide.
Logist-Op
🌐 https://vfapp.org/d35e

USAID: Maternal and Child Health Integrated Program
Works to improve the health of women and their families, including programs for maternal, newborn, and child health, immunization, family planning, nutrition, malaria, and HIV/AIDS.
All-Immu, General, Infect Dis, MF Med
📞 +1 202-835-3136
🌐 https://vfapp.org/4415

Vision Care
Restores sight and helps patients get regular treatment at short-term eye camps and long-term base clinics by having doctors, missionaries, volunteers, and sponsors work together.
Ophth-Opt
📞 +1 212-769-3056
🌐 https://vfapp.org/9d7c

Vision Health International
Brings high-quality eye care to underserved communities around the world.
Ophth-Opt
📞 +1 970-462-7279
🌐 https://vfapp.org/e97f

Vision Outreach International
Advocates for helping the blind in underserved regions of the world and empowers the poor through sight restoration.
Ophth-Opt
📞 +1 269-428-3300
🌐 https://vfapp.org/9721

Vital Strategies
Helps governments strengthen their public health systems to contend with the most important and difficult health challenges, while accelerating progress on the world's most pressing health problems.
CV Med, Infect Dis, Peds
📞 +1 212-500-5720
🌐 https://vfapp.org/fe25

Vitamin Angels
Helps at-risk populations in need—specifically pregnant women, new mothers, and children under age five—to gain access to life-changing vitamins and minerals.
General, Nutr
📞 +1 805-564-8400
🌐 https://vfapp.org/7da1

Voices for a Malaria-Free Future
Seeks to expand national movements of private and public sector leaders to mobilize political and popular support for malaria control.
Infect Dis, Path
🌐 https://vfapp.org/4213

Voluntary Service Overseas (VSO)
Works with health workers, communities, and governments to improve health services and rights for women, babies, youth, people with disabilities, and prisoners.
General, MF Med, OB-GYN
📞 +44 20 8780 7500
🌐 https://vfapp.org/213d

VOSH (Volunteer Optometric Services to Humanity) International
Facilitates the provision and the sustainability of vision care

worldwide for people who can neither afford nor obtain such care.

Ophth-Opt

https://vfapp.org/a149

Wajamama Wellness Center

Empowers women, children, and communities in Zanzibar through health promotion and disease prevention.

General, OB-GYN, Peds

+255 758 648 885

https://vfapp.org/5349

Watsi

Uses technology to make healthcare a reality for those who might not otherwise be able to afford it.

Pub Health, Surg

+1 256-792-8747

https://vfapp.org/41a3

Weill Cornell Medicine: Center for Global Health

Collaborates with international partners to improve the health of people in resource-poor countries through research, training, and service.

General, Infect Dis, OB-GYN

+1 646-962-8140

https://vfapp.org/1813

WellShare International

Partners with diverse communities to promote health and well-being, to achieve equitable healthcare and resources where all individuals are able to live healthy and fulfilling lives.

Geri, MF Med, Nutr, Pulm-Critic

+1 612-871-3759

https://vfapp.org/2e9c

White Ribbon Alliance, The

Leads a movement for reproductive, maternal, and newborn health and accelerates progress by putting citizens at the center of global, national, and local health efforts.

MF Med, OB-GYN

+1 202-204-0324

https://vfapp.org/496b

Women Orthopaedist Global Outreach (WOGO)

Provides free, life-altering orthopedic surgery that eliminates debilitating arthritis and restores disabled joints so that women can reclaim their ability to care for themselves, their families, and their communities.

Anesth, Ortho, Rehab, Surg

+1 844-588-9646

https://vfapp.org/6386

Women's Refugee Commission

Seeks to improve lives by protecting the rights of women, children, and youth displaced by conflict and crisis through researching their needs, identifying solutions, and advocating for programs and policies to strengthen their resilience.

General, MF Med, Neonat, OB-GYN, Peds, Psych

+1 212-551-3115

https://vfapp.org/3d8f

World Blind Union (WBU)

Represents those experiencing blindness, speaking to governments and international bodies on issues concerning visual impairments.

Ophth-Opt

https://vfapp.org/2bd3

World Health Organization, The (WHO)

The United Nations' agency for health provides leadership on global health matters, shapes the health research agenda, setting norms and standards, articulates evidence-based policy options, provides technical support and monitoring to countries, and assesses health trends.

ER Med, General, Infect Dis, Logist-Op, MF Med, OB-GYN, Peds, Psych, Pub Health

+41 22 791 21 11

https://vfapp.org/c476

World Heart Federation

Leads the global fight against heart disease and stroke, with a focus on low- and middle-income countries.

CV Med, Crit-Care, Heme-Onc, Medicine, Peds

+41 22 807 03 20

https://vfapp.org/ea51

World Medical Relief

Facilitates the distribution of surplus medical resources where they are needed.

Logist-Op

+1 313-866-5333

https://vfapp.org/72dc

World Vision International

Works with vulnerable communities around the world to overcome poverty and injustice with child-focused programs.

ER Med, General, Infect Dis, MF Med, Nutr, OB-GYN, Peds

+1 626-303-8811

https://vfapp.org/2642

Worldwide Healing Hands

Works to improve the quality of healthcare for women and children in the most underserved areas of the world and to stop the preventable deaths of mothers.

General, MF Med, Neonat, OB-GYN

+1 707-279-8733

https://vfapp.org/b331

YORGHAS Foundation

Supports mothers, pregnant women, infants, people with disabilities, and those suffering from humanitarian crises, poverty, or social inequalities, with particular emphasis on women's and children's rights.

MF Med, Neonat

+48 501 844 438

https://vfapp.org/9e44

Zanzibar Outreach Program

Aims to improve the community's access to healthcare, clean water, and education.

Dent-OMFS, ENT, General, Geri, OB-GYN, Ophth-Opt, Ortho, Pub Health, Surg

+255 773 047 979

https://vfapp.org/7e96

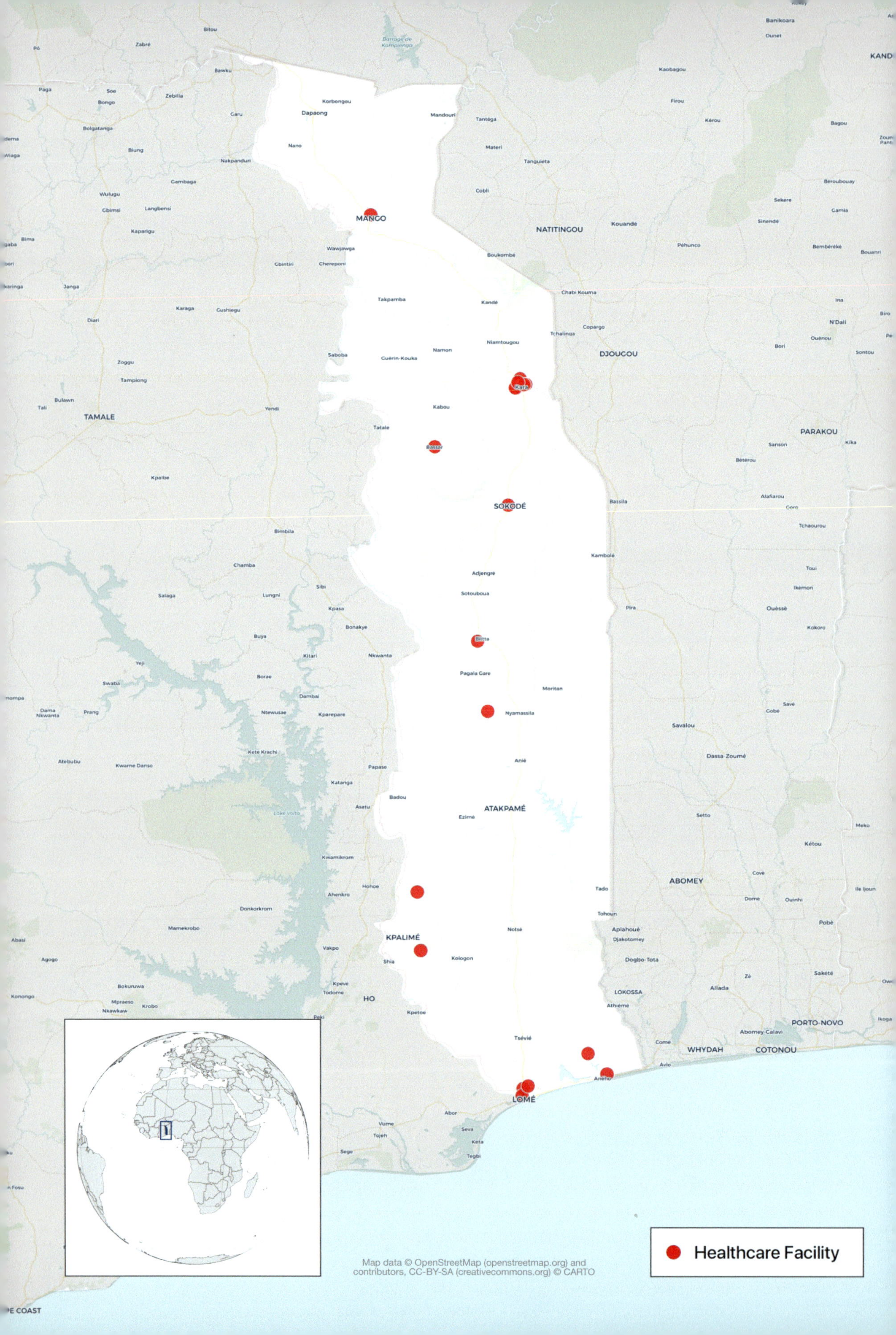
Dapaong
Korbongou
Mandouri
Nano
MANGO
NATITINGOU
Wawjawga
Chereponi
Takpamba
Kandé
Niamtougou
Saboba
Guérin-Kouka
Namon
DJOUGOU
Kara
Kabou
TAMALE
Tatale
Bassar
PARAKOU
SOKODÉ
Bassila
Bimbila
Kambolé
Adjengré
Sotouboua
Blitta
Pagala Gare
Nyamassila
Anié
Badou
ATAKPAMÉ
Ezimé
ABOMEY
Tado
Notsé
KPALIMÉ
Kologon
HO
Kpetoe
Tsévié
LOMÉ
Aného
WHYDAH
COTONOU
PORTO-NOVO
Map data © OpenStreetMap (openstreetmap.org) and contributors, CC-BY-SA (creativecommons.org) © CARTO
Healthcare Facility

Togo

Sandwiched between Ghana and Benin in West Africa, the Togolese Republic (Togo) is one of the smallest countries on the continent. It boasts a rapidly increasing population of 8.6 million people representing at least 37 different ethnic groups. While many people speak one of the four major Togolese languages, French is the official language of the country. Togo boasts a wide array of natural landscapes, including beaches, forests, hills, and savannas.

Since gaining independence in 1960—after control by German, French, and British governments—Togo has struggled to maintain consistent economic and political stability and suffers from occasional demonstrations, strikes, and marches. And while poverty has decreased by several percentage points over the past two decades, it is still widespread, especially in rural areas, where about 70 percent of households live below the poverty line. Togo's economy is based mainly on agriculture, with nearly 60 percent of the workforce employed in the subsistence and commercial farming of crops such as coffee, cocoa, cotton, yams, cassava, corn, beans, rice, millet, and sorghum. Togo is also a mining nation with large quantities of phosphate.

Life expectancy in Togo has increased significantly, from age 53 to 61, between 2000 and 2018. Similarly, under-five mortality rates decreased from 144 to 67 deaths per 1,000 live births. While these are overall improvements, the population is still vulnerable to poor health. Currently, leading causes of death in Togo include diseases such as diarrheal diseases, malaria, neonatal disorders, lower respiratory infections, HIV/AIDS, and tuberculosis. However, non-communicable diseases have also increased substantially in recent years, and top causes of death now include ischemic heart disease, stroke, and cirrhosis. Trauma and mortality from road injuries is also significant.

8.6M
Population

$676
GDP Per Capita

61 years
Life Expectancy
↑ Improving

7.7
Doctors/100k
Physician Density

70
Beds/100k
Hospital Bed Density

396
Deaths/100k
Maternal Mortality

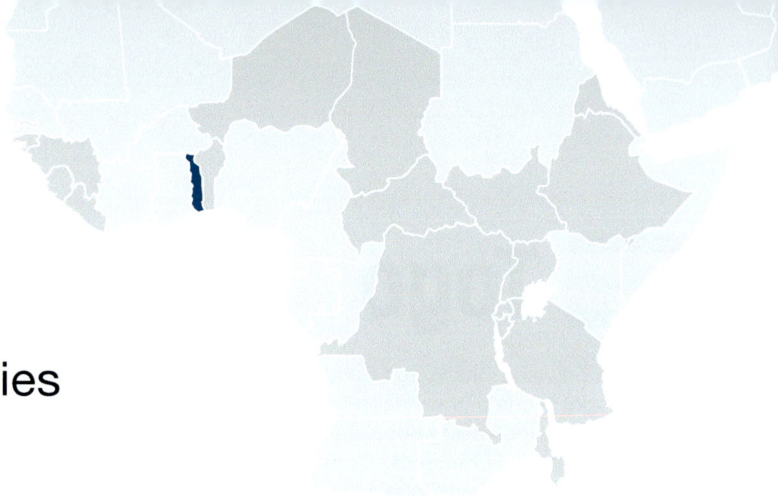

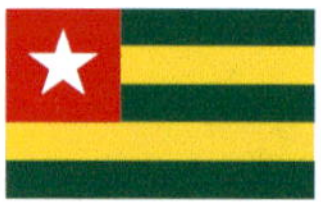

Togo

Healthcare Facilities

Aneho Psychiatric Hospital
N36, Aného, Région Maritime, Togo
https://vfapp.org/d4cd

Association Espoir Pour Demain (AED)
Rue Wakada, Kara, Région de la Kara, Togo
https://vfapp.org/f998

CHP Bassar
N17, Bassar, Région de la Kara, Togo
https://vfapp.org/cf66

CHR de Sokodé
Sokodé – Bassar, Sokodé, Région Centrale, Togo
https://vfapp.org/66c6

CHU du Campus
N1, Lomé, Togo
https://vfapp.org/9198

CHU Kara
Kara, Togo
https://vfapp.org/d1df

CHU Tokoin
Avenue de la Victoire, Lomé, Togo
https://vfapp.org/ee4c

Croix-Rouge at Kara
Avenue Maman N'Danida, Kara, Région de la Kara, Togo
https://vfapp.org/c2d7

Hospital of Hope
Lomé – Ouagadougou, Mango, Région des Savanes, Togo
https://vfapp.org/5ba1

Hôpital Baptiste Biblique
Tsiko, Togo
https://vfapp.org/9668

Hôpital Bethesda
Kloto, Togo
https://vfapp.org/7414

Hôpital Bon Sécours de Kegué
Route de la Nouvelle Présidence, Lomé, Togo
https://vfapp.org/873e

Hôpital de Blitta
Lomé – Cinkassé, Blitta, Région Centrale, Togo
https://vfapp.org/3f84

Hôpital de Sotouboua
Sotouboua, Togo
https://vfapp.org/56de

Hôpital Mère et Enfants SOS
Avenue Maman N'Danida, Kara, Région de la Kara, Togo
https://vfapp.org/8fe7

Hôpital Préfectoral de Vogan
Route Lomé – Vogan, Vogan, Région Maritime, Togo
https://vfapp.org/fed4

USP
Rue Wakada, Kara, Région de la Kara, Togo
https://vfapp.org/f4b5

USP de Lama-Kpédah
Rue Bakali, Poudè, Région de la Kara, Togo
https://vfapp.org/2611

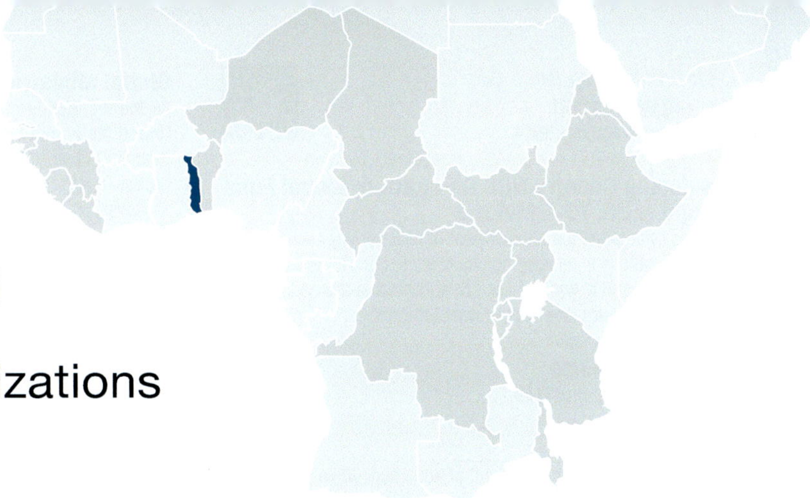

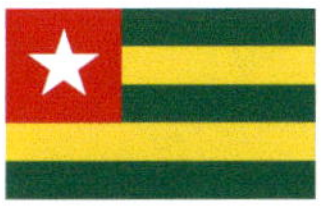

Togo

Nonprofit Organizations

Advance Family Planning
Aims to achieve global expansion and access to quality contraceptive information, services, and supplies through financial investment and political commitment.

General, MF Med, Pub Health

📞 +1 410-502-8715

🌐 **https://vfapp.org/7478**

African Health Now
Promotes and provides information and access to sustainable primary healthcare to women, children, and families living across Sub-Saharan Africa.

Dent-OMFS, Endo, General, Infect Dis, MF Med, OB-GYN

🌐 **https://vfapp.org/c766**

Against Malaria Foundation
Helps protect people from malaria. Funds anti-malaria nets, specifically long-lasting insecticidal nets (LLINs), and works with distribution partners to ensure they are used. Tracks and reports on net use and malaria case data.

Infect Dis

📞 +44 20 7371 8735

🌐 **https://vfapp.org/337d**

AO Alliance
Builds solutions to lessen the burden of injuries in low- and middle-income countries, while enhancing the care of the injured to reduce human suffering, disability, and poverty.

Ortho, Surg

🌐 **https://vfapp.org/8cd5**

Assist Africa
Believes that through education, entrepreneurial support, and access to healthcare, the quality of life for many people can be improved dramatically and that sustainable economic growth and overall well-being can be fostered by focusing on these three cornerstones.

Dent-OMFS, General, Surg

🌐 **https://vfapp.org/37fd**

Beta Humanitarian Help
Provides plastic surgery in underserved areas of the world.

Anesth, Plast

📞 +49 228 909075778

🌐 **https://vfapp.org/7221**

BroadReach
Collaborates with governments, multinational health organizations, donors, and private sector companies to affect healthcare reform and solve the world's biggest health challenges.

Logist-Op

📞 +27 21 514 8300

🌐 **https://vfapp.org/7812**

CARE
Works around the globe to save lives, defeat poverty, and achieve social justice.

ER Med, General

📞 +1 800-422-7385

🌐 **https://vfapp.org/7232**

Carter Center, The
Seeks to prevent and resolve conflicts, enhance freedom and democracy, and improve health, while remaining committed to human rights and the alleviation of human suffering.

Infect Dis, MF Med, Ophth-Opt

📞 +1 800-550-3560

🌐 **https://vfapp.org/6556**

Center for Strategic and International Studies (CSIS) Commission on Strengthening America's Health Security
Brings together a distinguished and diverse group of high-level opinion leaders bridging security and health, with the core aim to chart a bold vision for the future of U.S. leadership in global health.

ER Med, Infect Dis, MF Med, Pub Health

📞 +1 202-887-0200

🌐 **https://vfapp.org/6d7f**

Chain of Hope (La Chaîne de l'Espoir)
Helps underprivileged children around the world by providing them with access to healthcare.

Anesth, CT Surg, Crit-Care, ER Med, Neurosurg, Ortho, Ped Surg, Surg, Vasc Surg

📞 +33 1 44 12 66 66

🌐 **https://vfapp.org/e871**

Christian Blind Mission (CBM)
Aims to improve the quality of life of persons with disabilities in the poorest countries, addressing poverty as a cause, and a consequence, of disability, and working in partnership to create a society for all.

ENT, General, Infect Dis, OB-GYN, Ophth-Opt,

Ortho, Peds, Psych, Rehab, Surg
+49 6251 131131
https://vfapp.org/3824

Developing Country NGO Delegation: Global Fund to Fight AIDS, TB & Malaria
Works to strengthen the engagement of civil society actors and organizations in developing countries to contribute toward achieving a world in which AIDS, TB, and Malaria are no longer global, public health, and human rights threats.
Infect Dis, Pub Health
+254 20 2515790
https://vfapp.org/3149

Dianova
Works in prevention and treatment of addiction, while promoting social progress in international forums.
Psych, Pub Health
+34 936 36 57 30
https://vfapp.org/1998

Direct Relief
Improves the health and lives of people affected by poverty or emergency situations by mobilizing and providing essential medical resources needed for their care.
ER Med, Logist-Op
+1 805-964-4767
https://vfapp.org/58e5

Duke University: Global Health Institute
Sparks innovation in global health research and education, and brings together knowledge and resources to address the most important global health issues of our time.
All-Immu, Infect Dis, MF Med, OB-GYN, Pub Health
+1 919-681-7760
https://vfapp.org/c4cd

EngenderHealth
Works to implement high-quality, gender-equitable programs that advance sexual and reproductive health and rights.
General, MF Med, OB-GYN, Peds
+1 202-902-2000
https://vfapp.org/1cb2

eRanger
Provides sustainable solutions to transportation and medical provision such as ambulances and mobile clinics in developing countries.
ER Med, General, Logist-Op
+27 40 654 3207
https://vfapp.org/4c18

Fondation Follereau
Promotes the quality of life of the most vulnerable African communities. Alongside trusted partners, the foundation supports local initiatives in healthcare and education.
General, Infect Dis, OB-GYN
+352 44 66 06 34
https://vfapp.org/bcc7

Global Clubfoot Initiative (GCI)
Promotes and resources the treatment of children with clubfoot in developing countries using the Ponseti technique.
Ortho, Ped Surg
https://vfapp.org/f229

Global Ministries – The United Methodist Church
As the worldwide mission and development agency of The United Methodist Church, Global Ministries works with more than 300 hospitals and clinics around the world through its Global Health Unit.
Anesth, CT Surg, CV Med, Crit-Care, Dent-OMFS, Derm, ER Med, GI, General, Infect Dis, Logist-Op, MF Med, Medicine, Neonat, Nephro, Nutr, OB-GYN, Ophth-Opt, Ortho, Palliative, Peds, Pod, Psych, Pub Health, Rehab, Rheum, Surg, Urol
+1 800-862-4246
https://vfapp.org/1723

Global Oncology (GO)
Brings the best in cancer care to underserved patients around the world and collaborates across geographic, professional, and academic borders to improve cancer care, research, and education.
Heme-Onc, Path, Rad-Onc
https://vfapp.org/fcb8

Grassroot Soccer
Leverages the power of soccer to educate, inspire, and mobilize at risk youth in developing countries to overcome their greatest health challenges, live healthier more productive lives, and be agents for change in their communities.
Infect Dis
+1 603-277-9685
https://vfapp.org/3521

Health & Development International (HDI)
Aims to prevent obstetric fistula and deaths from obstructed labor, preventing postpartum hemorrhage, and eradicating Guinea worm disease and lymphatic filariasis in Africa and elsewhere. Goal is to advance world public health, human dignity, and socioeconomics.
Infect Dis, OB-GYN
+1 858-245-2410
https://vfapp.org/25cd

Healthy Developments
Provides Germany-supported health and social protection programs around the globe in a collaborative knowledge management process.
All-Immu, General, Infect Dis, Logist-Op, MF Med
https://vfapp.org/dc31

Heart to Heart International
Strengthens communities through improving health access, providing humanitarian development, and administering crisis relief worldwide. Engages volunteers, collaborates with partners, and deploys resources to achieve this mission.
Anesth, ER Med, General, Logist-Op, Medicine, Path, Path, Peds, Psych, Pub Health, Surg
+1 913-764-5200
https://vfapp.org/aacb

HelpMeSee
Trains local cataract specialists in Manual Small Incision Cataract Surgery (MSICS) in significant numbers, to meet the increasing demand for surgical services in the communities most impacted by cataract blindness.
Anesth, Ophth-Opt, Surg
+1 844-435-7638
https://vfapp.org/973c

Hope Walks
Frees children, families, and communities from the burden of clubfoot, inspired by the Christian faith.
Ortho, Ped Surg, Peds, Rehab
+1 717-502-4400
https://vfapp.org/f6d4

Hospital of Hope
Works to meet patients' physical, emotional, and spiritual needs and offers an outpatient clinic with 11 consultation rooms including OB, surgery, and medicine.
Dent-OMFS, General, Infect Dis, Neonat, OB-GYN, Peds, Radiol, Surg
https://vfapp.org/c623

Humanity & Inclusion
Works alongside people with disabilities and vulnerable populations, taking action and bearing witness in order to respond to their essential needs, improve their living conditions and health, and promote respect for their dignity and fundamental rights.
General, Infect Dis, MF Med, Medicine, Ortho, Peds, Psych, Pub Health, Rehab
+1 301-891-2138
https://vfapp.org/16b7

Humanity First
Provides aid and assistance to those in need, offering sustainable development solutions to society while providing and empowering local communities with the resources to help themselves.
ER Med, General, MF Med, Ophth-Opt
+44 20 8417 0082
https://vfapp.org/13cc

International Agency for the Prevention of Blindness (IAPB), The
Leads international efforts in blindness-prevention activities, works toward a world where no one is needlessly visually impaired, and ensures that everyone has access to the best possible standard of eye health.
Infect Dis, Ophth-Opt, Pub Health
https://vfapp.org/87a2

International Council of Ophthalmology
Works with ophthalmologic societies and others to enhance ophthalmic education and improve access to the highest quality eye care in order to preserve and restore vision for the people of the world.
Ophth-Opt
https://vfapp.org/ffd2

International Federation of Red Cross and Red Crescent Societies (IFRC)
Coordinates and directs international assistance following natural and man-made disasters in nonconflict situations through the world's largest humanitarian and development network. Provides disaster-preparedness programs, healthcare activities, and promotes humanitarian values.
ER Med, General, Infect Dis, Nutr
+1 212-338-0161
https://vfapp.org/b4ee

International Medical Relief
Provides sustainable education, training, medical and dental care, and disaster relief and response in vulnerable communities worldwide.
Dent-OMFS, General, Infect Dis, Medicine, OB-GYN
+1 970-635-0110
https://vfapp.org/b3ed

International Organization for Migration (IOM) – The UN Migration Agency
Promotes evidence-informed policies and holistic, preventive, and curative health programs that are beneficial, accessible, and equitable for vulnerable migrants.
General, Infect Dis, OB-GYN
+27 12 342 2789
https://vfapp.org/621a

International Planned Parenthood Federation (IPPF)
Leads a locally owned, globally connected civil society movement that provides and enables services and champions sexual and reproductive health and rights for all, especially the underserved.
Infect Dis, MF Med, OB-GYN
+44 20 7939 8200
https://vfapp.org/dc97

IntraHealth International
Improves the performance of health workers and strengthens the systems in which they work.
CV Med, Endo, General, Infect Dis, MF Med, Neonat, Nutr, OB-GYN
+1 919-313-3554
https://vfapp.org/ddc8

Ipas
Focuses efforts on women and girls who want contraception or abortion, and builds programs around their needs and how best to support them.
OB-GYN
https://vfapp.org/8e39

Jhpiego
Creates and delivers transformative healthcare solutions that save lives in partnership with national governments, health experts, and local communities.
General, Infect Dis, OB-GYN, Surg
+1 410-537-1800
https://vfapp.org/45b8

Johns Hopkins Center for Communication Programs
Believes in the power of communication to save lives, by empowering people to adopt healthy behaviors for themselves, their families, and their communities.
General, Infect Dis, Logist-Op, OB-GYN, Pub Health
+1 410-659-6300
https://vfapp.org/1bf9

Joint United Nations Programme on HIV/AIDS (UNAIDS)
Aims to place people living with HIV and people affected by the virus at the decision-making table and at the center of designing, delivering, and monitoring the AIDS response.
Infect Dis
+41 22 791 36 66
https://vfapp.org/464a

Life for a Child
Supports the provision of the best possible health care, given local circumstances, to all children and youth with diabetes in less-

resourced countries, through the strengthening of existing diabetes services.

Endo, Medicine, Peds

https://vfapp.org/d712

Light in the World Development Foundation

Enhances the dignity and quality of life in underserved areas of Africa by ensuring access to clean water, quality education, and affordable healthcare.

General, Infect Dis, MF Med

+1 539-777-2984

https://vfapp.org/e1d6

Lions Clubs International

Empowers volunteers to serve their communities, meet humanitarian needs, encourage peace, and promote international understanding through Lions clubs.

Heme-Onc, Medicine, Nutr, Ophth-Opt

+1 630-571-5466

https://vfapp.org/7b12

Management Sciences for Health (MSH)

Works with countries and communities to save lives and improve the health of the world's poorest and most vulnerable people by building strong, resilient, sustainable health systems.

Infect Dis, Logist-Op, Pub Health

+1 617-250-9500

https://vfapp.org/6aa2

MAP International

Provides medicines and health supplies to those in need around the world so they might experience life to the fullest.

Logist-Op

+1 800-225-8550

https://vfapp.org/deed

Maternity Foundation

Works to ensure safer childbirth for women and newborns everywhere through innovative mobile health solutions such as the Safe Delivery App, a mobile training tool for skilled birth attendants.

MF Med, OB-GYN, Pub Health

https://vfapp.org/ff4f

Médecins du Monde/Doctors of the World

Provides care, bears witness, and supports social change worldwide with innovative medical programs and evidence-based advocacy initiatives.

ER Med, General, Infect Dis, MF Med, Neonat, OB-GYN, Peds, Pub Health

+33 1 44 92 15 15

https://vfapp.org/a43d

MedSend

Funds qualified healthcare professionals to serve the physical and spiritual needs of people around the world, enabling healthcare providers to work where they have been called.

General

+1 203-891-8223

https://vfapp.org/661c

MedShare

Aims to improve the quality of life of people, communities, and the planet by sourcing and directly delivering surplus medical supplies and equipment to communities in need around the world.

Logist-Op

+1 770-323-5858

https://vfapp.org/c8bc

Mercy Ships

Operates hospital ships staffed by volunteers to bring hope, healing, and healthcare to underserved communities worldwide.

Anesth, Dent-OMFS, Logist-Op, Neonat, OB-GYN, Ophth-Opt, Ortho, Palliative, Plast, Psych, Surg

+1 903-939-7000

https://vfapp.org/2e99

Mérieux Foundation

Committed to fighting infectious diseases that affect developing countries by capacity building, particularly in clinical laboratories, and focusing on diagnosis.

Logist-Op, Path

+33 4 72 40 79 79

https://vfapp.org/a23a

Pathfinder International

Champions sexual and reproductive health and rights worldwide, mobilizing communities most in need to break through barriers and forge paths to a healthier future.

OB-GYN

+1 617-924-7200

https://vfapp.org/a7b3

Philips Foundation

Aims to reduce healthcare inequality by providing access to quality healthcare for disadvantaged communities.

CV Med, OB-GYN, Ped Surg, Peds, Surg, Urol

https://vfapp.org/bacb

RestoringVision

Empowers lives by restoring vision for millions of people in need.

Ophth-Opt

+1 209-980-7323

https://vfapp.org/e121

Rockefeller Foundation, The

Works to promote the well-being of humanity.

Logist-Op, Nutr, Pub Health

+1 212-869-8500

https://vfapp.org/5424

Rotary Action Group for Family Health & AIDS Prevention (RFHA)

Works to save and improve the lives of children and families who lack access to preventive healthcare and education.

Dent-OMFS, Infect Dis, OB-GYN, Ophth-Opt, Peds

+27 83 456 3923

https://vfapp.org/6563

Rotary International

Provides service to others, improves lives, and advances world understanding, goodwill, and peace through its fellowship of business, professional, and community leaders.

ER Med, General, Infect Dis, MF Med, OB-GYN

https://vfapp.org/8fb5

Rotaplast International

Helps children and families worldwide by eliminating the burden of cleft lip and/or palate, burn scarring, and other deformities by sending medical teams to provide free reconstructive surgery, ancillary treatment, and training.

Anesth, Dent-OMFS, ENT, Ped Surg, Plast, Surg

+1 415-252-1111

https://vfapp.org/78b3

Salvation Army International, The

Seeks to meet human needs through services in education, healthcare, community support, emergency response, and ministry development, inspired by the Christian faith.

Dent-OMFS, Derm, ER Med, Infect Dis, MF Med, Medicine, Nutr, OB-GYN, Ophth-Opt, Palliative, Psych, Rehab, Surg

+44 20 7332 0101

https://vfapp.org/8eb3

Samaritan's Purse International Disaster Relief

Provides spiritual and physical aid to hurting people around the world, such as victims of war, poverty, natural disasters, disease, and famine, based in Christian ministry.

Anesth, CT Surg, Crit-Care, Dent-OMFS, Derm, ENT, ER Med, Endo, GI, General, Heme-Onc, Infect Dis, MF Med, Neonat, Nephro, Neuro, Neurosurg, Nutr, OB-GYN, Ophth-Opt, Ortho, Path, Ped Surg, Peds, Plast, Psych, Pulm-Critic, Radiol, Rehab, Rheum, Surg, Urol, Vasc Surg

+1 800-528-1980

https://vfapp.org/87e3

Sanofi Espoir Foundation

Contributes to reducing health inequalities among populations that need it most by applying a socially responsible approach focused on fighting childhood cancers in low-income countries, improving maternal and newborn health, and improving access to care.

ER Med, OB-GYN, Peds

+33 1 53 77 91 38

https://vfapp.org/943b

Santé Diabète

Addresses the lack of access to care for people with diabetes in Africa with the mission to save lives through disease prevention and management and improving quality of life through care delivery.

Endo, Medicine, Vasc Surg

+33 6 24 51 82 69

https://vfapp.org/7652

Save A Child's Heart

Provides lifesaving cardiac treatment to children in developing countries, and trains healthcare professionals from these countries to deliver quality care in their communities.

CT Surg, CV Med, Crit-Care, Ped Surg, Peds

+1 240-223-3940

https://vfapp.org/1bef

SEE International

Provides sustainable medical, surgical, and educational services through volunteer ophthalmic surgeons, with the objectives of restoring sight and preventing blindness to disadvantaged individuals worldwide.

Ophth-Opt, Surg

+1 805-963-3303

https://vfapp.org/6e1b

Sightsavers

Prevents avoidable blindness in some of the poorest parts of the world by treating debilitating eye diseases.

Infect Dis, Ophth-Opt, Surg

+1 800-707-9746

https://vfapp.org/aa52

SIGN Fracture Care International

Builds orthopedic capacity around the world and provides the injured poor access to fracture surgery by donating orthopedic education and implant systems to surgeons in developing countries.

Ortho, Rehab, Surg

+1 509-371-1107

https://vfapp.org/123d

Smile Train

Seeks to give every child with a cleft the opportunity for a healthy, productive life by providing free cleft repair surgery and comprehensive cleft care in their own communities.

Dent-OMFS, ENT, Plast

+1 800-932-9541

https://vfapp.org/f21d

Swiss Tropical and Public Health Institute

Contributes to the improvement of the health of populations internationally, nationally, and locally through excellence in research, education, and services.

Infect Dis, Pub Health

+41 61 284 81 11

https://vfapp.org/2ee4

Task Force for Global Health, The

Consists of programs and focus areas that cover a range of global health issues including neglected tropical diseases, infectious diseases, vaccines, field epidemiology, public health informatics, health workforce development, and global health ethics.

Infect Dis, Logist-Op, Medicine, Ophth-Opt, Peds

+1 404-371-0466

https://vfapp.org/714c

Terre Des Hommes

Works to improve the conditions of the most vulnerable children worldwide by improving the health of children under the age of 3, protecting migrant children, providing humanitarian aid to children and their families in times of crisis, and preventing child exploitation.

ER Med, MF Med, Neonat, OB-GYN, Ped Surg, Peds

+41 58 611 06 66

https://vfapp.org/2689

Turing Foundation

Aims to contribute toward a better world and a better society by focusing on efforts such as health, art, education, and nature.

Infect Dis

+31 20 520 0010

https://vfapp.org/6bcc

Union for International Cancer Control (UICC)

Unites and supports the cancer community to reduce the global cancer burden, promote greater equity, and ensure that cancer control continues to be a priority in the world health and development agenda.

Heme-Onc, Pub Health

+41 22 809 18 11

https://vfapp.org/88b1

United Nations Development Programme (UNDP)
Helps countries achieve the simultaneous eradication of extreme poverty and significant reduction of inequalities and exclusion using a sustainable human development approach.
Infect Dis, Logist-Op, Pub Health
🌐 https://vfapp.org/935c

United Nations High Commissioner for Refugees (UNHCR)
Safeguards the rights and well-being of people who have been forced to flee, ensuring that everybody has the right to seek asylum and find safe refuge in another country, with the goal of seeking lasting solutions.
General, MF Med, Medicine, OB-GYN, Peds, Psych, Pub Health
🌐 https://vfapp.org/6636

United Nations Population Fund (UNFPA)
Supports reproductive healthcare for women and youth in more than 150 countries, focusing on delivering a world where every pregnancy is wanted, every childbirth is safe, and every young person's potential is fulfilled.
Infect Dis, MF Med, Neonat, OB-GYN, Peds, Pub Health
📞 +1 212-963-6008
🌐 https://vfapp.org/c969

United Surgeons for Children (USFC)
Pursues greater health and opportunity for children in the most neglected pockets of the world, with a specific focus and expertise in surgery.
Anesth, CT Surg, Neonat, Neurosurg, OB-GYN, Peds, Radiol, Surg
🌐 https://vfapp.org/3b4c

USAID: African Strategies for Health
Identifies and advocates for best practices, enhancing technical capacity of African regional institutions and engaging African stakeholders to address health issues in a sustainable manner.
All-Immu, Infect Dis, OB-GYN, Peds
🌐 https://vfapp.org/c272

USAID: Human Resources for Health 2030 (HRH2030)
Helps low- and middle-income countries develop the health workforce needed to prevent maternal and child deaths, support the goals of Family Planning 2020, control the HIV/AIDS epidemic, and protect communities from infectious diseases.
Logist-Op
📞 +1 202-955-3300
🌐 https://vfapp.org/9ea8

Vision Outreach International
Advocates for helping the blind in underserved regions of the world and empowers the poor through sight restoration.
Ophth-Opt
📞 +1 269-428-3300
🌐 https://vfapp.org/9721

Vitamin Angels
Helps at-risk populations in need—specifically pregnant women, new mothers, and children under age five—to gain access to life-changing vitamins and minerals.
General, Nutr
📞 +1 805-564-8400
🌐 https://vfapp.org/7da1

World Blind Union (WBU)
Represents those experiencing blindness, speaking to governments and international bodies on issues concerning visual impairments.
Ophth-Opt
🌐 https://vfapp.org/2bd3

World Health Organization, The (WHO)
The United Nations' agency for health provides leadership on global health matters, shapes the health research agenda, setting norms and standards, articulates evidence-based policy options, provides technical support and monitoring to countries, and assesses health trends.
ER Med, General, Infect Dis, Logist-Op, MF Med, OB-GYN, Peds, Psych, Pub Health
📞 +41 22 791 21 11
🌐 https://vfapp.org/c476

World Medical Relief
Facilitates the distribution of surplus medical resources where they are needed.
Logist-Op
📞 +1 313-866-5333
🌐 https://vfapp.org/72dc

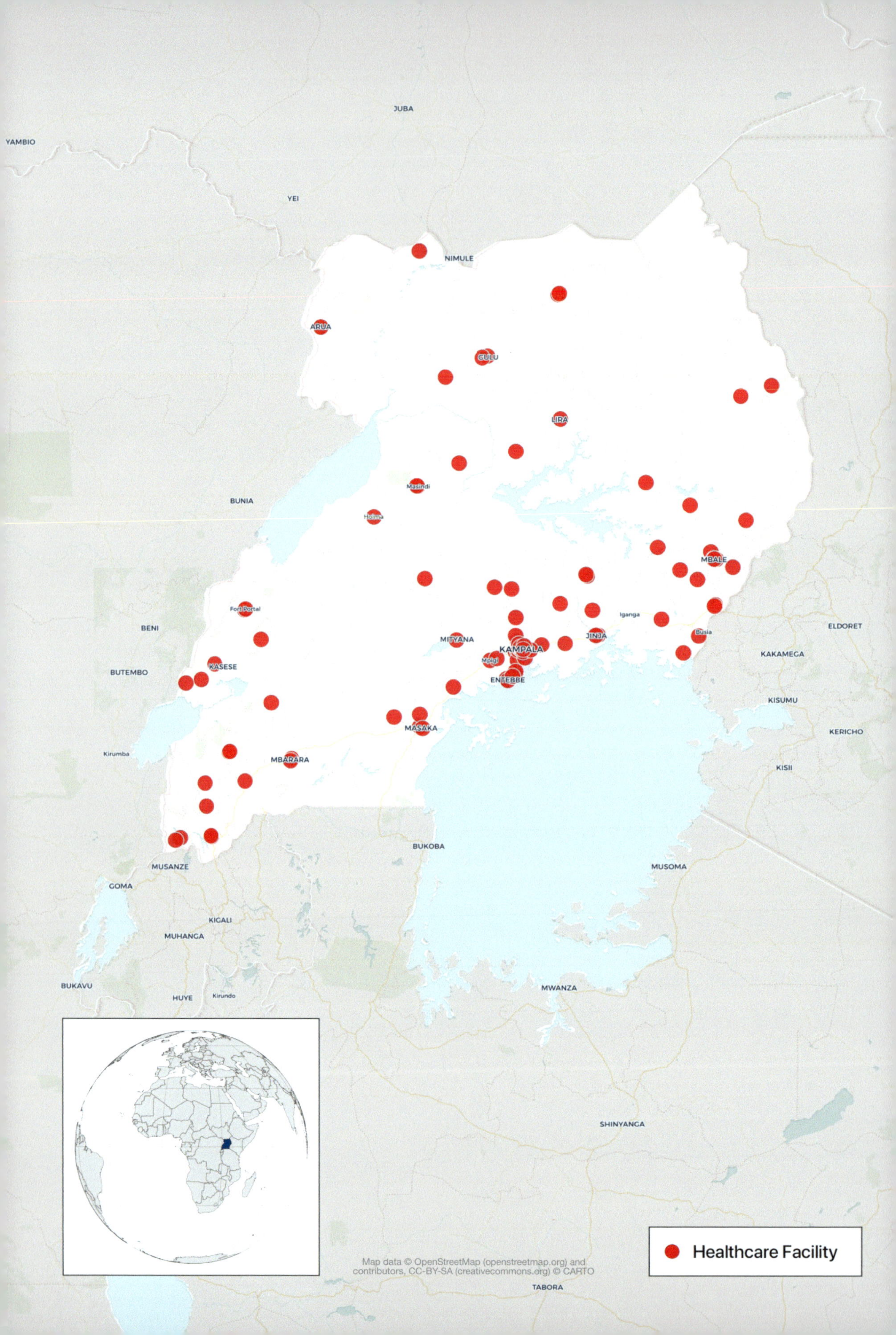
JUBA
YAMBIO
YEI
NIMULE
ARUA
GULU
LIRA
Masindi
Hoima
BUNIA
MBALE
Fort Portal
BENI
Iganga
ELDORET
MITYANA
JINJA
Busia
KAMPALA
KAKAMEGA
KASESE
Mpigi
BUTEMBO
ENTEBBE
KISUMU
MASAKA
KERICHO
Kirumba
MBARARA
KISII
BUKOBA
MUSANZE
MUSOMA
GOMA
KIGALI
MUHANGA
BUKAVU
MWANZA
HUYE
Kirundo
SHINYANGA
Healthcare Facility
Map data © OpenStreetMap (openstreetmap.org) and contributors, CC-BY-SA (creativecommons.org) © CARTO
TABORA

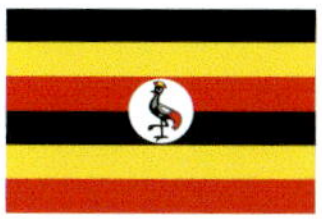

Uganda

The Republic of Uganda, landlocked in East-Central Africa, has a large and burgeoning population of about 43.3 million people. The population density of Uganda is high relative to other African countries, and many people live in the capital city of Kampala, in the central and southern regions, and along the shorelines of Lake Albert and Lake Victoria. English is the official language, with Swahili also widely spoken. This scenic nation is known for Lake Victoria, the largest lake in Africa.

After the country won its independence from Britain in 1962, Uganda experienced a period of political instability and violence, but things have improved significantly since the 1980s. Poverty was reduced by half between 1992 and 2013, mainly due to the growth and development of the agriculture sector, which now employs as much as 70 percent of Ugandans. The country's population is one of the youngest and most rapidly increasing in the world. This is fueled by a high fertility rate—5.8 children per woman. However, Uganda faces specific challenges when it comes to its economy, education, livelihood, and especially health.

Uganda has some of the highest maternal mortality rates in the world, and one-third of children under five are stunted due to malnutrition. However, the Ugandan government has significantly improved the country's health infrastructure, supplies, and training. The result: A decrease in the under-one mortality rate—from about 95 deaths per 1,000 live births down to 42 per 1,000 live births between 1990 and 2017—and an overall improvement in life expectancy. While overall improvements have been made to health, diseases such as neonatal disorders, malaria, HIV/AIDS, lower respiratory infections, tuberculosis, stroke, diarrheal diseases, ischemic heart disease, congenital defects, and meningitis cause the most death in the country. Notably, sexually transmitted infections are also a top cause of death in Uganda, and have increased over time.

43.3M
Population

$777
GDP Per Capita

63 years
Life Expectancy
↑ Improving

16.8
Doctors/100k
Physician Density

50
Beds/100k
Hospital Bed Density

375
Deaths/100k
Maternal Mortality

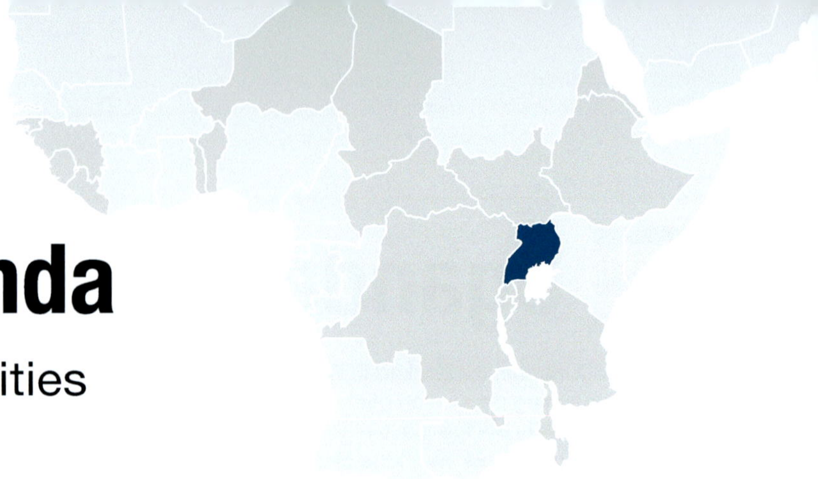

Uganda

Healthcare Facilities

Anaka Hospital
Anaka, Nwoya, Uganda
https://vfapp.org/3f66

Apac General Hospital
Olelpek Road, Apac, Apac, Uganda
https://vfapp.org/bb13

Arua Regional Referral Hospital
Hospital Road, River Oli, Arua, Uganda
https://vfapp.org/69fe

Baylor
Kampala, Uganda
https://vfapp.org/c763

Bishop Caesar Asili Hospital
Gulu – Kampala Road, Luweero, Uganda
https://vfapp.org/befb

Bombo Military Hospital
Gulu – Kampala Road, Bombo, Luweero, Uganda
https://vfapp.org/5218

Bududa Hospital
Bududa Ring, Namaitsu, Bududa, Uganda
https://vfapp.org/b5f2

Bugiri Main Hospital
Bugiri, Uganda
https://vfapp.org/9abc

Buhinga Fort Portal Regional Referral Hospital
Mugurusi Road, Fort Portal, Kabarole, Uganda
https://vfapp.org/6256

Butabika Hospital
Butabika Road, Kampala, Central Region, Uganda
https://vfapp.org/be9e

Buwenge Hospital
Jinja Kamuli Road, Kasambira, Kamuli, Uganda
https://vfapp.org/d1a2

Bwera Hospital
Kaserengethe II, Kasese, Uganda
https://vfapp.org/e5af

Bwindi Community Hospital
Kanungu, Uganda
https://vfapp.org/831f

China-Uganda Friendship Hospital
Shoprite Road, Kampala, Central Region, Uganda
https://vfapp.org/e6f6

CoRSU Hospital
Kawuku, Entebbe Road, Uganda
https://vfapp.org/47f6

Cure Childrens Hospital at Uganda
Mbale, Uganda
https://vfapp.org/9dae

Dabani Hospital
B1, Bumulimba, Busia, Uganda
https://vfapp.org/9393

Eggwonero Life Saving Hospital
Kawempe I 2482, Kampala, Central Region, Uganda
https://vfapp.org/d647

Entebbe Hospital
Kampala Road, Entebbe, Wakiso, Uganda
https://vfapp.org/b383

Gulu Hospital
Awere Road, Gulu, Uganda
https://vfapp.org/2c91

Hoima Regional Referral Hospital
Main Street, Hoima, Uganda
https://vfapp.org/66e2

Hope and Faith
Kibuye Natete Road, Kampala, Central Region, Uganda
https://vfapp.org/f3db

International Hospital Kampala
4686 St. Barnabas Road, Kampala, Central Region, Uganda
https://vfapp.org/6a87

Ishaka Adventist Hospital
Nungamo – Katunguru Road, Kashenyi, Bushenyi, Uganda
https://vfapp.org/dfd5

Islamic Hospital
Gulu – Kampala Road,
Matugga, Wakiso, Uganda
https://vfapp.org/3b2b

Itojo Hospital
Itojo, Uganda
https://vfapp.org/3d37

Jinja Hospital
Naranbhai Road, Jinja, Uganda
https://vfapp.org/4e48

Jinja Main Hospital
Nile Avenue, Jinja, Uganda
https://vfapp.org/28e3

Kabale Regional Hospital
Corryndon Road, Kabale,
Kabale, Uganda
https://vfapp.org/fbd2

Kabarole Hospital
Fort Portal – Kasese Road,
Kasusu, Kabarole, Uganda
https://vfapp.org/d7e8

Kadic Hospital
Kiira Road, Kampala, Central
Region, Uganda
https://vfapp.org/3e9a

Kagando Hospital
Kagando, Kasese, Uganda
https://vfapp.org/f8ff

Kampala Hospital
Plot 6C Makindu Close,
Kampala, Central Region,
Uganda
https://vfapp.org/3271

Kampala Medical Chambers Hospital
Buganda, Kampala, Uganda
https://vfapp.org/9b36

Kamu Medical Centre
Wakoli, Jinja, Uganda
https://vfapp.org/6941

Kamuli General Hospital
Kamuli, Uganda
https://vfapp.org/b14d

Kamuli Mission Hospital
Gabula Road, Kamuli, Kamuli,
Uganda
https://vfapp.org/23b5

Kapchorwa Hospital
Mbale-Sironko-Kapchorwa
Highway, Kapchorwa,
Kapchorwa, Uganda
https://vfapp.org/e2ab

Katabi UPDAF Hospital
Katabi, Uganda
https://vfapp.org/5626

Katimba Parish Hospital
Kabingo Road, Katimba,
Sembabule, Uganda
https://vfapp.org/8495

Kawolo Hospital
Jinja – Kampala Road,
Najjembe, Buikwe, Uganda
https://vfapp.org/dada

Kayunga Hospital
Busaana Road, Kaazi, Kayunga,
Uganda
https://vfapp.org/ce34

Kiboga Hospital
Hoima – Kampala Road,
Munsambya, Kyankwanzi,
Uganda
https://vfapp.org/d435

Kibuli Muslim Hospital
Prince Badru Kakungulu Road,
Kampala, Central Region,
Uganda
https://vfapp.org/1358

Kilembe Hospital
Kilembe Road, Chanjojo,
Kasese, Uganda
https://vfapp.org/6e57

Kiruddu General Referral Hospital
Salaama Road, Kampala,
Central Region, Uganda
https://vfapp.org/38c1

Kiryandongo Hospital
Gulu – Kampala Road,
Kigumba, Kiryandongo, Uganda
https://vfapp.org/dc13

Kisiizi Hospital
Rukungiri, Uganda
https://vfapp.org/4ef6

Kisoro Hospital
Kisoro – Bunagana Road,
Bunagana Trading Centre,
Kisoro, Uganda
https://vfapp.org/299f

Kisubi Hospital
Road to White House Sister's
Residence, Kisubi, Wakiso,
Uganda
https://vfapp.org/c524

Kitara Medical Center
Hoima Road, Masindi, Uganda
https://vfapp.org/9796

Kitgum Hospital
Gulu-Kitgum Road, Acholibur,
Pader, Uganda
https://vfapp.org/732a

Kitovu General Hospital
Senyange Road, Masaka,
Masaka, Uganda
https://vfapp.org/f272

KIU Teaching Hospital
Kabirisi Road, Ishaka,
Bushenyi, Uganda
https://vfapp.org/fcc1

Kiwoko Hospital
Kiwoko Road, Kiwoko,
Nakaseke, Uganda
https://vfapp.org/d72a

Kololo Hospital Kampala
16 Kawalya Kaggwa Close,
Kampala, Central Region, Uganda
https://vfapp.org/e412

Kumi Hospital
Ongino Road, Kumi, Uganda
https://vfapp.org/96fa

Lira Regional Referral Hospital
Plot 9/19, 21-41 Ngetta Road
Police Rd, Lira, Uganda
https://vfapp.org/c5fa

Makerere University Hospital
Kagugube Semuliki Walk,
Kampala, Central Region,
Uganda
https://vfapp.org/edb7

Masaka Referral Hospital
Alex Ssebowa Road, Masaka, Masaka, Uganda
https://vfapp.org/ad2e

Masindi District Hospital
Kijunjubwa Road, Masindi, Uganda
https://vfapp.org/1bce

Mayanja Memorial Hospital
Mbarara, Uganda
https://vfapp.org/562d

Mbale General Hospital
Lira – Mbale Road, Mbale, Uganda
https://vfapp.org/c5b6

Mbale Regional Referral Hospital
Lira – Mbale Road, Mbale, Uganda
https://vfapp.org/645e

Mbarara District Regional Referral Hospital
Hospital Road, Mbarara, Mbarara, Uganda
https://vfapp.org/22cc

Medik Hospital
Bombo Road, Kampala, Central Region, Uganda
https://vfapp.org/a336

Mengo Hospital
Catherdral Hill Road, Kampala, Central Region, Uganda
https://vfapp.org/8ff1

MGH
Ggaba Road, Kampala, Central Region, Uganda
https://vfapp.org/c391

Middle East Hospital & Diagnostic Centre
Spring Road, Kampala, Uganda
https://vfapp.org/51b2

Mildmay Uganda
Entebbe Road, Lubowa, Wakiso, Uganda
https://vfapp.org/586e

Mityana Hospital
Fort Portal – Kampala Road, Zigoti, Mityana, Uganda
https://vfapp.org/7977

Moroto Regional Referral Hospital
Moroto Highway and Mainstreet, Moroto, Uganda
https://vfapp.org/895d

Moyo Hospital
Okudi Road, Moyo, Moyo, Uganda
https://vfapp.org/efcd

Mpigi Hospital
Mpigi Kabasanda Road, Mpigi, Uganda
https://vfapp.org/cb33

MRC/UVRI & LSHTM Uganda Research Unit
Nakiwogo Road, Entebbe, Uganda
https://vfapp.org/8362

Mt Elgon Hospital
Cathedral Avenue, Mbale, Uganda
https://vfapp.org/4125

Mukesh Madhvani Children's Hospital
Clive Road, Jinja, Uganda
https://vfapp.org/9fc7

Mukono Church of Uganda Hospital
Jinja – Kampala Road, Mukono, Mukono, Uganda
https://vfapp.org/4146

Mulago National Referral Hospital
Upper Mulago Hill Road, Kampala, Central Region, Uganda
https://vfapp.org/83da

Mundindi
Busia, Busia, Uganda
https://vfapp.org/3ab9

Mutolere Hospital
Mutolere Road, Mutolere, Kisoro, Uganda
https://vfapp.org/c652

Nakasero Hospital
Nakasero Hill, Kampala, Uganda
https://vfapp.org/5f4d

Nansanga Hospital
Nansanga, Uganda
https://vfapp.org/3355

Nile International Hospital
Kyabazinga Road, Jinja, Uganda
https://vfapp.org/7495

Nkozi Hospital
Nkozi, Mpigi, Uganda
https://vfapp.org/68bb

Norvik Hospital
Bombo Road, Kampala, Central Region, Uganda
https://vfapp.org/16b2

Nyakibale Hospital
Kambuga – Ntungamo, Rukungiri, Uganda
https://vfapp.org/944a

Pallisa Hospital
Kanyumu Road, Pallisa, Uganda
https://vfapp.org/c97b

Paragon Hospital
6A/7A Luthuli Avenue, Kampala, Central Region, Uganda
https://vfapp.org/ed72

Rubaga Hospital
Muteesa Road, Kampala, Central Region, Uganda
https://vfapp.org/47e2

Rugarama Hospital
Rugarama Road, Rugarama, Kabale, Uganda
https://vfapp.org/b3c1

Rushere Community Hospital
Rushere, Kiruhura District, Western Region, Uganda
https://vfapp.org/b619

Ruth Gaylord Hospital Maganjo
Bombo Road, Kampala, Central Region, Uganda
https://vfapp.org/78fe

Saint Catherine's Hospital
Buganda, Kampala, Uganda
https://vfapp.org/fac1

Salem Hospital
Nakaloke-Kabwangasi, Nakaloke, Mbale, Uganda
https://vfapp.org/36be

Soroti Regional Referral Hospital
A104, Opuyo, Soroti, Uganda
https://vfapp.org/3bb4

St. Joseph's Hospital
Gulu-Kitgum Road, Acholibur, Pader, Uganda
https://vfapp.org/c4fc

St. Monica Katende HC III
Kampala – Masaka Road, Katende, Mpigi, Uganda
https://vfapp.org/dbd1

St. Anthony's Hospital
Busia Road, Tororo, Uganda
https://vfapp.org/adc9

St. Francis Hospital Nsambya
Nsambya Road, Kampala, Central Region, Uganda
https://vfapp.org/afae

St. Kizito Hospital
Matany, Napak, Uganda
https://vfapp.org/7275

St. Mary's Hospital Lacor
Nimule – Gulu Road, Aciak, Amuru, Uganda
https://vfapp.org/e14f

Taso
Italy Road, Mbale, Uganda
https://vfapp.org/9a39

The Spontaneous Healing Center
Mbale-Nkokonjeru, Mbale, Uganda
https://vfapp.org/9916

Tororo Hospital
Station Road, Railway Village, Tororo, Uganda
https://vfapp.org/9e69

Uganda Cancer Institute
Upper Mulago Hill Road, Kampala, Uganda
https://vfapp.org/c41a

Uganda Children's Hospital
Jinja – Mbale Road, Mbale, Uganda
https://vfapp.org/d3b3

Uganda Martyrs Ibanda
Ibanda, Uganda
https://vfapp.org/37e4

Uganda Red Cross
Maluku, Mbale, Uganda
https://vfapp.org/a212

Victoria Hospital
Kiira Road, Kampala, Central Region, Uganda
https://vfapp.org/e281

Villa Maria Hospital
Weaver Bird Road, Masaka, Uganda
https://vfapp.org/fc59

Whisper's Magical Children's Hospital
32 Madhvani Road, Jinja, Uganda
https://vfapp.org/25b3

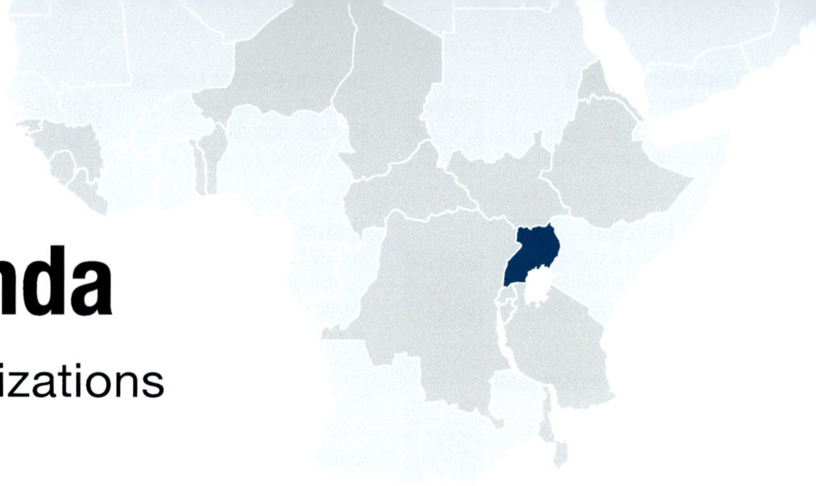

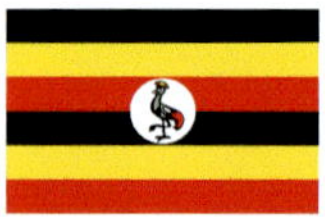

Uganda

Nonprofit Organizations

100X Development Foundation
Empowers children and families for a more hopeful and productive future through the support and care of orphaned children, education and job training for those in need, help for vulnerable youth to escape trafficking, and healthy nutrition and medical care for mothers to enable a safe birth.

ER Med, Infect Dis, OB-GYN, Peds, Psych

📞 +1 334-387-1178

🌐 https://vfapp.org/b629

1789 Fund, The
Promotes gender equality worldwide through investment in the economic empowerment of women and the health of mothers and newborns.

MF Med, Neonat, OB-GYN

📞 +1 215-439-3256

🌐 https://vfapp.org/7145

A Broader View Volunteers
Provides developing countries around the world with significant volunteer programs that both aid the neediest communities and forge a lasting bond between those volunteering and those they have helped.

Dent-OMFS, ER Med, Infect Dis, MF Med

📞 +1 215-780-1845

🌐 https://vfapp.org/3bec

A Reason to Smile (ARTS)
Empowers communities without access to dental professionals to achieve and maintain a higher level of oral health by providing hygiene education, direct treatment, and dental supplies.

Dent-OMFS

🌐 https://vfapp.org/3bae

A Stitch in Time
Seeks to address socially crippling but readily treatable conditions, such as genital prolapse in women who lack access, by providing technically advanced pelvic reconstructive surgery free of charge to restore women's bodies in geographically or access remote areas of the world.

Anesth, OB-GYN

📞 +1 516-528-4757

🌐 https://vfapp.org/6474

Abalon Trust
Provides ophthalmic eye services in developing countries.

Ophth-Opt

📞 +44 20 3778 0743

🌐 https://vfapp.org/d7ed

Abt Associates
Seeks to improve the quality of life and economic well-being of people worldwide, while striving to meet and exceed the highest professional standards.

General, Logist-Op, MF Med, OB-GYN, Peds

📞 +1 212-779-7700

🌐 https://vfapp.org/cec2

Accomplish Children's Trust
Provides education and medical care to children with disabilities. Also addresses the financial implications of caring for a child with disabilities by helping families to earn an income.

Neuro, Peds, Rehab

🌐 https://vfapp.org/de84

Action Against Hunger
Aims to end life-threatening hunger for good through treating and preventing malnutrition across more than forty-five countries.

📞 +1 212-967-7800

🌐 https://vfapp.org/2dbc

Adara Group
Seeks to bridge the world of business with the people in extreme poverty, and to support vulnerable communities with health, education, and other essential services.

General, MF Med, Neonat, OB-GYN, Ped Surg, Peds

📞 +1 425-967-5115

🌐 https://vfapp.org/c8b4

Advance Family Planning
Aims to achieve global expansion and access to quality contraceptive information, services, and supplies through financial investment and political commitment.

General, MF Med, Pub Health

📞 +1 410-502-8715

🌐 https://vfapp.org/7478

Africa CDC
Aims to strengthen the capacity and capability of Africa's public health institutions as well as partnerships to detect and respond quickly and effectively to disease threats and outbreaks, based on data-driven interventions and programs.

Infect Dis, Logist-Op, Pub Health
+251 11 551 7700
https://vfapp.org/339c

Africa Humanitarian Action (AHA)
Responds to crises, conflicts, and disasters in Africa, while informing and advising the international community, governments, civil society, and the private sector on humanitarian issues of concern to Africa. Supports institutional and organizational development efforts.
General, Infect Dis, MF Med, Nutr, OB-GYN
+251 11 660 4800
https://vfapp.org/3ca2

African Community Center for Social Sustainability (ACCESS)
Works with vulnerable people in resource-limited settings by providing medical care, education, and economic empowerment to create long-lasting change that is owned by entire communities.
General, Infect Dis, MF Med, Neonat, Peds
+256 783 095856
https://vfapp.org/f9cf

African Field Epidemiology Network (AFENET)
Strengthens field epidemiology and public health laboratory capacity to contribute effectively to addressing epidemics and other major public health problems in Africa.
All-Immu, Infect Dis, Path, Pub Health
https://vfapp.org/df2e

Africa Inland Mission International
Seeks to establish churches and community development programs including health care projects, based in Christian ministry.
Anesth, Dent-OMFS, ER Med, General, MF Med, Medicine, OB-GYN, OB-GYN, Ophth-Opt, Ped Surg, Peds, Rehab
https://vfapp.org/f2f6

Against Malaria Foundation
Helps protect people from malaria. Funds anti-malaria nets, specifically long-lasting insecticidal nets (LLINs), and works with distribution partners to ensure they are used. Tracks and reports on net use and malaria case data.
Infect Dis
+44 20 7371 8735
https://vfapp.org/337d

AIDS Healthcare Foundation
Provides cutting-edge HIV/AIDS medical care and advocacy to over one million people in forty-three countries.
Infect Dis
+1 323-860-5200
https://vfapp.org/b27c

AIDS Information Centre – Uganda
Provides sustainable, collaborative, and Integrated HIV and AIDS and other related health services in Uganda.
Infect Dis, Logist-Op, Pub Health
+256 41 4231528
https://vfapp.org/672f

AISPO
Implements international initiatives in the healthcare sector and remains involved in a variety of projects to combat poverty, social injustice, and disease in the world.
All-Immu, ER Med, GI, General, Infect Dis, Logist-Op, MF Med, Neonat, OB-GYN, Peds, Psych, Pub Health, Radiol
+39 02 2643 4481
https://vfapp.org/c9e6

ALIGHT
Works closely with refugees, trafficked persons, economic migrants, and other displaced persons to co-design solutions that help them build full and fulfilling lives by providing healthcare, clean water, shelter protection, and economic opportunity.
ER Med, General, Infect Dis, MF Med, Neonat, Peds
+1 800-875-7060
https://vfapp.org/5993

American Academy of Pediatrics
Seeks to attain optimal physical, mental, and social health and well-being for all infants, children, adolescents, and young adults.
Anesth, Crit-Care, Neonat, Ped Surg
+1 800-433-9016
https://vfapp.org/9633

American Foundation for Children with AIDS
Provides critical comprehensive services to infected and affected HIV-positive children and their caregivers.
Infect Dis, Nutr, Pub Health
+1 888-683-8323
https://vfapp.org/6258

American International Health Alliance (AIHA)
Strengthens health systems and workforce capacity worldwide through locally-driven, peer-to-peer institutional partnerships.
CV Med, ER Med, Infect Dis, Medicine, OB-GYN
+1 202-789-1136
https://vfapp.org/69fd

Americares
Saves lives and improves health for people affected by poverty or disaster and responds with life-changing medicine, medical supplies, and health programs including domestic and global medical clinics.
All-Immu, ER Med, General, Infect Dis, MF Med, Nutr
+1 203-658-9500
https://vfapp.org/e567

Amref Health Africa
Serves millions of people across thirty-five countries in Sub-Saharan Africa, strengthening health systems, and training African health workers to respond to the continent's most critical health issues.
All-Immu, General, Infect Dis, Logist-Op, MF Med, OB-GYN, Path, Pub Health, Surg
+254 20 6993000
https://vfapp.org/6985

Amsterdam Institute for Global Health and Development (AIGHD)
Provides sustainable solutions to major health problems across our planet by forging synergies between disciplines, healthcare delivery, research, and education.
Infect Dis
+31 20 210 3960
https://vfapp.org/d73d

AO Alliance
Builds solutions to lessen the burden of injuries in low- and middle-income countries, while enhancing the care of the injured to reduce human suffering, disability, and poverty.
Ortho, Surg
https://vfapp.org/8cd5

Arms Around Africa Foundation
Supports children, empowers women, and helps young people to overcome poverty through talent promotion, education, good health, life skills development, entrepreneurship, and enhanced access to other resources for social and economic development.
General, Infect Dis, OB-GYN, Peds
+256 200 900277
https://vfapp.org/ad98

Assist International
Designs and implements humanitarian programs that build capacity, develop opportunities, and save lives around the world.
Infect Dis, Ped Surg, Peds
+1 831-438-4582
https://vfapp.org/9a3b

AYINET – African Youth Initiative Network
Mobilizes and empowers youth and communities in promoting a healthy, peaceful, and just society.
Infect Dis, Psych, Pub Health, Rehab, Surg
+256 789 622661
https://vfapp.org/9bac

Baylor College of Medicine: Global Surgery
Trains leaders in academic global surgery and remains dedicated to advancements in the arenas of patient care, biomedical research, and medical education.
ENT, Infect Dis, OB-GYN, Ortho, Ped Surg, Plast, Pub Health, Radiol, Surg, Urol
+1 713-798-6078
https://vfapp.org/21f5

Baylor International Pediatric AIDS Initiative (BIPAI) at Texas Children's Hospital
Provides high-quality, high-impact, highly ethical pediatric and family-centered healthcare, health professional training, and clinical research focused on HIV/AIDS, tuberculosis, malaria, malnutrition, and other conditions impacting the health of children worldwide.
Infect Dis, Medicine, OB-GYN, Peds, Pub Health, Surg
+1 832-822-1038
https://vfapp.org/e6ba

Bega Kwa Bega Uganda
Enables communities in Uganda to support their orphans and vulnerable children so they may live in their own homes and on land with their basic needs ensured—and through education gain the knowledge and skills needed to become self-sufficient.
General, Infect Dis, Nutr, OB-GYN, Peds, Pub Health
+44 20 8743 0655
https://vfapp.org/a373

Benjamin H. Josephson, MD Fund
Provides healthcare professionals with the financial resources necessary to deliver medical services for those in need throughout the world.
General, OB-GYN
+1 908-522-2853
https://vfapp.org/6acc

Beta Humanitarian Help
Provides plastic surgery in underserved areas of the world.
Anesth, Plast
+49 228 909075778
https://vfapp.org/7221

BethanyKids
Transforms the lives of African children with surgical conditions and disabilities through pediatric surgery, rehabilitation, public education, spiritual ministry, and training health professionals.
Neurosurg, Nutr, Ortho, Ped Surg, Peds, Rehab, Surg
https://vfapp.org/db4e

Bill & Melinda Gates Foundation
Focuses on global issues, from poverty to health, to education, offering the opportunity to dramatically improve the quality of life for billions of people, by building partnerships that bring together resources, expertise, and vision to identify issues, find answers, and drive change.
All-Immu, General, Infect Dis, MF Med, Neonat, OB-GYN, Pub Health
https://vfapp.org/7cf2

Birth With Dignity
Seeks to educate, support, and equip nurses and midwives of Uganda to improve care for patients and families with high-risk perinatal needs with the goal of decreasing maternal and neonatal deaths, as well as caring for families with perinatal loss.
MF Med
https://vfapp.org/7696

Blessing Foundation, The
Mobilizes resources that promote education, create employment, and enhance healthy living for the underserved and disadvantaged population in Africa.
General, Infect Dis, MF Med, Ophth-Opt
+1 412-260-9008
https://vfapp.org/89af

Boston Children's Hospital: Global Health Program
Helps solve pediatric global health care challenges by transferring expertise through long-term partnerships with scalable impact, while working in the field to strengthen healthcare systems, advocate, research and provide care delivery or education as a way of sustainably improving the health of children worldwide.
Anesth, CV Med, Crit-Care, ER Med, Heme-Onc, Infect Dis, Medicine, Nutr, Palliative, Ped Surg, Peds
+1 617-919-6438
https://vfapp.org/f9f8

BRAC USA
Seeks to empower people and communities in situations of poverty, illiteracy, disease, and social injustice. Interventions aim to achieve large-scale, positive changes through economic and social programs that enable everyone to realize their potential.
ER Med, General, Infect Dis, Logist-Op, MF Med, OB-GYN
+1 212-808-5615
https://vfapp.org/9d9e

Braveheart
Aims to inspire hope and improve the quality of life for people coping with illness, the loss of a loved one, or emotional trauma through ongoing peer-to-peer support.
Dent-OMFS, Infect Dis, Nutr, Peds, Pod
https://vfapp.org/8aeb

Brick by Brick
Creates partnerships to improve education, health, and economic opportunity in East Africa.
Neonat, OB-GYN, Peds
+256 200 902073
https://vfapp.org/71c3

Bridge to Health Medical and Dental
Seeks to provide health care to those who need it most based on a philosophy of partnership, education, and community development. Strives to bring solutions to global health issues in underserved communities through clinical outreach and medical and dental training.
Dent-OMFS, General, Infect Dis, MF Med, OB-GYN, Ophth-Opt, Ortho, Pub Health, Radiol
https://vfapp.org/bb2c

Brigham and Women's Center for Surgery and Public Health
Advances the science of surgical care delivery by studying effectiveness, quality, equity, and value at the population level, and develops surgeon-scientists committed to excellence in these areas.
Anesth, ER Med, Infect Dis, Pub Health, Surg
+1 617-525-7300
https://vfapp.org/5d64

Brigham and Women's Hospital Global Health Hub
Cares for patients in underserved settings, provides education to staff who work in those areas to create sustainable change, and conducts research designed to improve health in such settings.
General, Infect Dis
https://vfapp.org/a8a3

Bright Eyes Uganda
Cares for the underserved populations of Uganda, specifically children, by improving the infrastructure of rural villages, and providing clean water, nutritional food, accessible health care, and quality education.
General, Infect Dis, Nutr, Peds
+1 904-249-3374
https://vfapp.org/146e

BroadReach
Collaborates with governments, multinational health organizations, donors, and private sector companies to affect healthcare reform and solve the world's biggest health challenges.
Logist-Op
+27 21 514 8300
https://vfapp.org/7812

Bulamu Healthcare
Strives to improve the well-being of rural Ugandans by providing affordable access to primary healthcare and related services.
Dent-OMFS, General, Infect Dis, OB-GYN, Ophth-Opt, Ped Surg, Peds
+1 650-799-7296
https://vfapp.org/df64

Canada-Africa Community Health Alliance
Sends Canadian volunteer teams on two- to three-week missions to African communities to work hand-in-hand with local partners.
General, Infect Dis, MF Med, OB-GYN, Peds, Surg
+1 613-234-9992
https://vfapp.org/4c94

Canadian Network for International Surgery, The
Aims to improve maternal health, increase safety, and build local capacity in low-income countries by creating and providing surgical and midwifery courses, training domestically, and transferring skills.
Logist-Op, Surg
+1 877-217-8856
https://vfapp.org/86ff

CardioStart International
Provides free heart surgery and associated medical care to children and adults living in underserved regions of the world, irrespective of political or religious affiliation, through the collective skills of healthcare experts.
Anesth, CT Surg, CV Med, Crit-Care, Pub Health, Pulm-Critic
+1 813-304-2163
https://vfapp.org/85ef

CARE
Works around the globe to save lives, defeat poverty, and achieve social justice.
ER Med, General
+1 800-422-7385
https://vfapp.org/7232

Care Old Age & Child Foundation
Works toward empowering orphans and vulnerable children under the direct care of elderly-headed households in the Ssese Islands of Uganda by providing healthcare services and economic education and support.
General, General, Geri, Infect Dis, Palliative, Peds
+256 788 549682
https://vfapp.org/8d36

Carter Center, The
Seeks to prevent and resolve conflicts, enhance freedom and democracy, and improve health, while remaining committed to human rights and the alleviation of human suffering.
Infect Dis, MF Med, Ophth-Opt
+1 800-550-3560
https://vfapp.org/6556

Catholic Organization for Relief & Development Aid (CORDAID)
Provides humanitarian assistance and creates opportunities to improve security, healthcare, education, and inclusive economic growth in fragile and conflict-affected areas.
ER Med, Infect Dis, MF Med, OB-GYN, Peds, Psych
+31 70 313 6300
https://vfapp.org/8ae5

Catholic World Mission
Works to rebuild communities worldwide by helping to alleviate poverty and empower underserved areas, while spreading the message of the Catholic Church.
ER Med, General, Nutr, Peds
+1 770-828-4966
https://vfapp.org/7b5f

Chain of Hope
Provides lifesaving heart operations for children around the world and supports the development of cardiac services in numerous developing and war-torn countries.
Anesth, CT Surg, CV Med, Crit-Care, Ped Surg, Peds, Pulm-Critic, Surg
+44 20 7351 1978
https://vfapp.org/1b1b

Challenge Initiative, The
Seeks to rapidly and sustainably scale up proven reproductive health solutions among the urban poor.
MF Med, OB-GYN, Peds
+1 410-502-8715
https://vfapp.org/2f77

Cherish Uganda
Focuses on helping Ugandan children with HIV/AIDS by providing healing, hope, and a future.
General, Infect Dis, Logist-Op, MF Med, Peds, Pub Health
+1 512-803-9430
https://vfapp.org/232c

Child Care and Youth Empowerment Foundation
Improves the well-being of vulnerable children and youth through education, socio-economic interventions, nutrition, WASH, and primary healthcare.
General, Nutr, OB-GYN, Peds
+256 701 148054
https://vfapp.org/bd62

Child Family Health International (CFHI)
Connect students with local health professionals and community leaders transforming perspectives about self, global health, and healing.
General, Infect Dis, OB-GYN, Ophth-Opt, Palliative, Peds
+1 415-957-9000
https://vfapp.org/729e

ChildFund Australia
Works to reduce poverty for children in many of the world's most disadvantaged communities.
ER Med, General, Peds
+1 800023600
https://vfapp.org/13df

Children & Charity International
Puts people first by providing education, leadership, and nutrition programs along with mentoring and healthcare support services to children, youth, and families.
Nutr, Peds
+1 202-234-0488
https://vfapp.org/6538

Children Care Uganda (CCU)
Provides vulnerable children, disabled children, poor single young mothers, and jobless youths with hope for a brighter future, encouragement, and support in any medical or educational issue in their daily lives.
General, Infect Dis, Peds
+256 787 558691
https://vfapp.org/a3f8

Children of the Nations
Provides holistic, Christ-centered care for orphaned children, enabling them to create positive and lasting change in their nations.
Anesth, Dent-OMFS, General, Surg
+1 360-698-7227
https://vfapp.org/cc52

Children of Uganda (UK)
Provides educational, vocational, and welfare support, as well as infrastructure programs to enhance the health and well-being of children and village communities in Uganda.
General, Peds
+44 778696532
https://vfapp.org/c341

Christian Aid Ministries
Strives to be a trustworthy and efficient channel for Amish, Mennonite, and other conservative Anabaptist groups and individuals to minister to physical and spiritual needs around the world.
CT Surg, ER Med, Logist-Op, Ortho, Pub Health
+1 330-893-2428
https://vfapp.org/7b33

Christian Blind Mission (CBM)
Aims to improve the quality of life of persons with disabilities in the poorest countries, addressing poverty as a cause, and a consequence, of disability, and working in partnership to create a society for all.
ENT, General, Infect Dis, OB-GYN, Ophth-Opt, Ortho, Peds, Psych, Rehab, Surg
+49 6251 131131
https://vfapp.org/3824

Christian Connections for International Health (CCIH)
Promotes global health and wholeness from a Christian perspective.
All-Immu, General, Infect Dis, MF Med, Neonat, OB-GYN, Psych
+1 703-923-8960
https://vfapp.org/fa5d

Christian Health Service Corps
Brings Christian doctors, health professionals, and health educators who are committed to serving the poor to places that have little or no access to healthcare.
Anesth, Dent-OMFS, General, Medicine, Peds, Surg
+1 903-962-4000
https://vfapp.org/da57

Cleft Africa
Strives to provide underserved Africans with cleft lips and palates with access to the best possible treatment for their condition, so that they can live a life free of the health problems caused by cleft.
Anesth, Dent-OMFS, Ped Surg, Surg
https://vfapp.org/8298

Clinton Health Access Initiative (CHAI)
Aims to save lives and reduce the burden of disease in low- and middle-income countries. Works with partners to strengthen the capabilities of governments and the private sector to create and sustain high-quality health systems.
General, Heme-Onc, Infect Dis, Logist-Op, MF Med, Medicine, Neonat, Nutr, OB-GYN, Path, Peds, Rad-Onc
+1 617-774-0110
https://vfapp.org/9ed7

Columbia University: Global Mental Health Programs
Pioneers research initiatives, promotes mental health, and aims to reduce the burden of mental illness worldwide.
Psych
+1 646-774-5308
https://vfapp.org/c5cd

Comitato Collaborazione Medica (CCM)
Supports development processes that safeguard and promote the right to health with a global approach, working on health needs and influencing socio-economic factors, identifying poverty as the main cause for the lack of health.
All-Immu, General, Infect Dis, MF Med, OB-GYN
+39 011 660 2793
https://vfapp.org/4272

Confident Children Out of Conflict
Provides vulnerable children with a safe space to sleep, eat, learn, and play to help them develop into young adults, fulfilling their potential, and supports households to develop a protective environment for safe reintegration of these children into communities.
All-Immu, General, Peds, Psych
+211 955 065 445
https://vfapp.org/daf7

Core Group
Aims to improve and expand community health practices for underserved populations, especially women and children, through collaborative action and learning.
General, Infect Dis, MF Med, Medicine, OB-GYN, Peds, Pub Health
+1 202-380-3400
https://vfapp.org/9de3

Cura for the World
Seeks to heal, nourish, and embrace the neglected by building medical clinics in remote communities in dire need of medical care.
ER Med, General, Peds
https://vfapp.org/c55f

CURE
Operates charitable hospitals and programs in underserved countries worldwide where patients receive surgical treatment, based in Christian ministry.
Anesth, Neurosurg, Ortho, Ped Surg, Peds, Rehab, Surg
+1 616-512-3105
https://vfapp.org/aa16

Dentaid
Seeks to treat, equip, train, and educate people in need of dental care.
Dent-OMFS
+44 1794 324249
https://vfapp.org/a183

Dental Hope for Children
Seeks to provide dental services to children in underserved areas, based in Christian ministry.
Dent-OMFS
https://vfapp.org/1426

Direct Relief
Improves the health and lives of people affected by poverty or emergency situations by mobilizing and providing essential medical resources needed for their care.
ER Med, Logist-Op
+1 805-964-4767
https://vfapp.org/58e5

Direct Relief of Poverty & Sickness Foundation (DROPS)
Volunteer led organization that utilizes all donations toward direct relief of poverty and illness through initiatives in healthcare education, improving healthcare systems and providing essential medical help to children and aged people in need.
Dent-OMFS, General, Ophth-Opt
+49 171 3637659
https://vfapp.org/af95

Doctors with Africa (CUAMM)
Advocates for the universal right to health and promotes the values of international solidarity, justice, and peace. Works to protect and improve the well-being and health of vulnerable communities in Africa with a long-term development perspective.
ER Med, Infect Dis, MF Med, Neonat, OB-GYN, Peds
https://vfapp.org/d2fb

Doctors Without Borders/Médecins Sans Frontières (MSF)
Responds to emergencies and provides lifesaving medical care where needed most, including during disasters, conflicts, and epidemics.
Anesth, Crit-Care, ER Med, General, Infect Dis, Nutr, OB-GYN, Ped Surg, Peds, Psych, Pub Health, Surg
+1 212-679-6800
https://vfapp.org/f363

Double Cure Medical Centre Kalagala – MPIGI
Extends quality affordable medical care closer to the rural areas in the mid-region of Uganda (including the four counties of Gomba, Butambala, Busiro, and Mawokota) and provides quality medical care to all, including free community outreach care twice a month.
Dent-OMFS, General, Infect Dis, OB-GYN
+256 774 228399
https://vfapp.org/9cec

Drugs for Neglected Diseases Initiative
Develops lifesaving medicines for people with neglected diseases around the world, having developed eight treatments for five deadly diseases and saving millions of lives since 2003.
Infect Dis, Pub Health
+41 22 906 92 30
https://vfapp.org/969c

Duke Health Global Neurosurgery and Neurology
Promotes health in low- and middle-income countries through a multi-faceted, evidence-based, and collaborative approach to improve patient access to care and health outcomes, strengthen health systems, and inform policy.
Anesth, Neuro, Neurosurg
https://vfapp.org/d9d4

Duke University School of Medicine: Global Pediatric Surgery
Engages in active partnerships in Guatemala and Uganda that include capacity building, research, and service initiatives to

address global surgical needs.
Anesth, Heme-Onc, Logist-Op, Ped Surg, Peds
☎ +1 919-681-3445
🌐 https://vfapp.org/2d75

Duke University: Global Health Institute
Sparks innovation in global health research and education, and brings together knowledge and resources to address the most important global health issues of our time.
All-Immu, Infect Dis, MF Med, OB-GYN, Pub Health
☎ +1 919-681-7760
🌐 https://vfapp.org/c4cd

Elizabeth Glaser Pediatric AIDS Foundation
Seeks to end global pediatric HIV/AIDS through prevention and treatment programs, research, and advocacy.
Infect Dis, Nutr, OB-GYN, Peds
☎ +1 888-499-4673
🌐 https://vfapp.org/d6ec

Elton John Aids Foundation
Seeks to address and overcome the stigma, discrimination, and neglect that prevents ending AIDS by funding local experts to challenge discrimination, prevent infections, and provide treatment.
Infect Dis, Pub Health
☎ +1 212-219-0670
🌐 https://vfapp.org/9d31

EMERGENCY
Provides free, high-quality healthcare to victims of war, poverty, and landmines. Also builds hospitals and trains local staff, while pursuing human-rights-based medicine.
ER Med, Neonat, OB-GYN, Ophth-Opt, Ped Surg
☎ +39 02 881881
🌐 https://vfapp.org/c361

Empower Through Health
Aims to improve healthcare access to the world's most vulnerable by providing direct evidence-based medical care, helping build local healthcare capacity, and addressing root causes of poor health outcomes, with the full participation of communities.
GI, General, Infect Dis, OB-GYN, Path, Peds, Pub Health, Radiol
🌐 https://vfapp.org/68ff

Enabel
As the development agency of the Belgian federal government, charged with implementing Belgium's international development policy, carries out public service assignments in Belgium and abroad pursuant to the 2030 Agenda for Sustainable Development.
General, Infect Dis, Logist-Op, MF Med, OB-GYN, Peds, Pub Health
☎ +32 2 505 37 00
🌐 https://vfapp.org/5af7

EngenderHealth
Works to implement high-quality, gender-equitable programs that advance sexual and reproductive health and rights.
General, MF Med, OB-GYN, Peds
☎ +1 202-902-2000
🌐 https://vfapp.org/1cb2

Engeye
Empowers the people of Ddegeya Village in rural Uganda by supporting healthcare, education, and community development initiatives.
General, MF Med, Neonat, OB-GYN, Peds
☎ +51 82 270579
🌐 https://vfapp.org/6b8d

eRanger
Provides sustainable solutions to transportation and medical provision such as ambulances and mobile clinics in developing countries.
ER Med, General, Logist-Op
☎ +27 40 654 3207
🌐 https://vfapp.org/4c18

Evidence Action
Aims to be a world leader in scaling evidence-based and cost-effective programs to reduce the burden of poverty.
General, Infect Dis
☎ +1 202-888-9886
🌐 https://vfapp.org/94b6

Evidence Project, The
Improves family-planning policies, programs, and practices through the strategic generation, translation, and use of evidence.
General, MF Med
☎ +1 202-237-9400
🌐 https://vfapp.org/f9e7

Eye Health Uganda
Provides and supports quality eye healthcare services to mitigate preventable blindness as a means to empower individuals and communities.
Ophth-Opt
☎ +256 789 642152
🌐 https://vfapp.org/8cfc

Fertility Education & Medical Management (FEMM)
Aims to make knowledge-based reproductive health accessible to all women and enables them to be informed partners in the choice and delivery of their medical care and services.
MF Med, OB-GYN
🌐 https://vfapp.org/e8b2

Finn Church Aid
Supports people in the most vulnerable situations within fragile and disaster-affected regions in three thematic priority areas: right to peace, livelihood, and education.
ER Med, Psych, Pub Health
☎ +358 20 7871201
🌐 https://vfapp.org/9623

USAID: Fistula Care Plus
A fistula repair and prevention project from USAID that builds on, enhances, and expands the work undertaken by the previous Fistula Care project (2007–2013), with attention to new areas of focus so that obstetric fistula can become a rare event for future generations.
MF Med, OB-GYN, Surg
☎ +1 202-902-2000
🌐 https://vfapp.org/a7cd

Fistula Foundation
Aims to engage the support of people worldwide who are eager to see the day when no woman suffers from obstetric fistula. Raises and directs funds to doctors and hospitals providing life-

transforming surgery to women in need.

OB-GYN

☏ +1 408-249-9596

🌐 https://vfapp.org/e958

Fondation d'Harcourt

Promotes national and international projects and partnerships in the fields of mental health and psychosocial support; provides grants to organizations with specific expertise in mental health or psychosocial support to implement projects, and provides direct services.

Psych, Pub Health

☏ +41 22 716 00 23

🌐 https://vfapp.org/4a8a

Fondazione Corti Onlus

Provides medical screening for children with congenital heart defects and helps establish pediatric cardiac care wherever there is need, inspired by the Christian faith.

All-Immu, Anesth, General, Infect Dis, Ortho, Peds, Surg

☏ +39 02 805 4728

🌐 https://vfapp.org/4a3b

Foundation for International Medical Relief of Children (FIMRC)

Provides access to healthcare for low-resource and medically underserved families around the world.

General, Infect Dis, Peds, Pub Health

☏ +1 888-211-8575

🌐 https://vfapp.org/78b9

Friends of East Africa Foundation

Provides high-quality, comprehensive, and affordable medical services to all who need them by funding the Ruth Gaylord Hospital Maganjo in Kampala, Uganda.

Dent-OMFS, Infect Dis, MF Med, Neonat, OB-GYN, Ophth-Opt, Peds, Surg

☏ +1 651-962-8520

🌐 https://vfapp.org/9315

Gift of Life International

Provides lifesaving cardiac treatment to children in developing countries while developing sustainable pediatric cardiac programs by implementing screening, surgical, and training missions.

Anesth, CT Surg, CV Med, Crit-Care, Ped Surg, Peds, Pulm-Critic

☏ +1 855-734-3278

🌐 https://vfapp.org/f2f9

Global Alliance to Prevent Prematurity and Stillbirth (GAPPS)

Seeks to improve birth outcomes worldwide by reducing the burden of premature birth and stillbirth.

All-Immu, Infect Dis, MF Med, Neonat, Neonat, OB-GYN

☏ +1 206-413-7954

🌐 https://vfapp.org/3f74

Global Emergency Care

Aims to make lifesaving medical care available to all by training non-physician clinicians in emergency medicine to increase the availability of highly trained providers in areas where there are none.

ER Med, General, Radiol

🌐 https://vfapp.org/1fad

Global Force for Healing

Works to end preventable maternal and newborn deaths by supporting the scaling of effective grassroots. community-led, culturally respectful care and education in underserved areas around the globe using the midwifery model of care.

Neonat, OB-GYN

🌐 https://vfapp.org/deb2

Global Health Corps

Mobilizes a diverse community of leaders to build the movement for global health equity, working toward a world where every person lives a healthy life.

ER Med, General, Pub Health

🌐 https://vfapp.org/31c6

Global Health Network

Promotes, protects, and preserves the health of all Ugandans through good leadership, public-private partnerships, innovation, and concerted action in primary healthcare and reproductive health.

General, Infect Dis, MF Med, OB-GYN, Peds

🌐 https://vfapp.org/f84c

Global Medical and Surgical Teams

Provides cleft lip and palate surgery for patients in underserved areas by providing surgical care free of charge to children with cleft lip and palate deformities. Works through medical and surgical missions, education, training, technology, and donor relationships to provide specialized medical and surgical care.

Anesth, Dent-OMFS, ENT, Ped Surg, Plast, Surg

🌐 https://vfapp.org/6d3e

Global Ministries – The United Methodist Church

As the worldwide mission and development agency of The United Methodist Church, Global Ministries works with more than 300 hospitals and clinics around the world through its Global Health Unit.

Anesth, CT Surg, CV Med, Crit-Care, Dent-OMFS, Derm, ER Med, GI, General, Infect Dis, Logist-Op, MF Med, Medicine, Neonat, Nephro, Nutr, OB-GYN, Ophth-Opt, Ortho, Palliative, Peds, Pod, Psych, Pub Health, Rehab, Rheum, Surg, Urol

☏ +1 800-862-4246

🌐 https://vfapp.org/1723

Global Oncology (GO)

Brings the best in cancer care to underserved patients around the world and collaborates across geographic, professional, and academic borders to improve cancer care, research, and education.

Heme-Onc, Path, Rad-Onc

🌐 https://vfapp.org/fcb8

Global Strategies

Empowers communities in the most neglected areas of the world to improve the lives of women and children through healthcare.

MF Med, Neonat, OB-GYN, Peds

☏ +1 415-451-1814

🌐 https://vfapp.org/ef92

Global Telehealth Network (GTN)

Provides telehealth services with dedicated physician volunteers for people located in medically underserved areas, including low- and medium-resource countries, refugee camps, conflict zones, and disaster areas, as well as in the U.S.

ER Med, General, Path, Peds, Psych, Radiol, Surg
+1 415-847-1239
https://vfapp.org/4345

GOAL
Works with the most vulnerable communities to help them respond to and recover from humanitarian crises, and to assist them in building transcendent solutions to mitigate poverty and vulnerability.
ER Med, General, Pub Health
+353 1 280 9779
https://vfapp.org/bbea

Grassroot Soccer
Leverages the power of soccer to educate, inspire, and mobilize at risk youth in developing countries to overcome their greatest health challenges, live healthier more productive lives, and be agents for change in their communities.
Infect Dis
+1 603-277-9685
https://vfapp.org/3521

Harvard Global Health Institute
Devoted to improving global health and pioneering the next generation of global health research, education, policy, and practice, with an evidence-based, innovative, integrative and collaborative approach, harnessing the unique breadth of excellence within Harvard.
General, Infect Dis, Logist-Op
+1 617-384-5431
https://vfapp.org/5867

Head and Neck Outreach
Seeks to improve healthcare in developing countries through sustainable education, research, and surgical programs. Aims to develop sustainable healthcare programs to improve head and neck care.
Anesth, ENT, Surg
+1 574-870-1639
https://vfapp.org/f7b1

Healing Kadi Foundation
Works with the people of South Sudan and Uganda to provide sustainable high-quality healthcare, education for local healthcare providers, and psychological and spiritual counseling.
All-Immu, Dent-OMFS, General, Infect Dis, MF Med, Neonat, OB-GYN, Peds, Psych
+1 951-315-7070
https://vfapp.org/a7f1

Healing the Children
Helps underserved children around the world secure the medical care they need to lead more fulfilling lives.
Anesth, Dent-OMFS, ENT, General, Medicine, Ophth-Opt, Ped Surg, Peds, Plast, Surg
+1 509-327-4281
https://vfapp.org/d4ee

Health Equity Initiative
Aims to build and sustain a global community that engages across sectors and disciplines to advance health equity.
Pub Health
https://vfapp.org/e2e2

Health Poverty Action
Works in partnership with people around the world who are pursuing change in their own communities to demand health justice and challenge power imbalances.
ER Med, General, Infect Dis, Psych, Pub Health
+44 20 7840 3777
https://vfapp.org/ee58

Health Volunteers Overseas (HVO)
Improves the availability and quality of healthcare through the education, training, and professional development of the health workforce in resource-scarce countries.
All-Immu, Anesth, CV Med, Dent-OMFS, Derm, ENT, ER Med, Endo, GI, Heme-Onc, Infect Dis, Medicine, Medicine, Nephro, Neuro, OB-GYN, Ophth-Opt, Ortho, Peds, Plast, Psych, Pulm-Critic, Rehab, Rheum, Surg
+1 202-296-0928
https://vfapp.org/42b2

Health[e] Foundation
Supports health professionals and community workers in the world's most vulnerable societies to ensure quality health for everyone in need by providing digital education and information, using e-learning and m-health.
Logist-Op
https://vfapp.org/b73b

HealthRight International
Leverages global resources to address local health challenges and create sustainable solutions that empower marginalized communities to live healthy lives.
General, Infect Dis, MF Med, OB-GYN, Psych, Pub Health
+1 212-226-9890
https://vfapp.org/129d

Healthy Child Uganda
Supports medical training and clinical care and initiates a community-cased education project targeting child health.
Logist-Op, Peds
+1 403-210-6161
https://vfapp.org/ebc5

Heart Healers International
Brings lifesaving heart diagnostics and treatments to children in Africa with the goal that no child with a treatable heart will be left behind. Works alongside the local medical teams in caring for patients, conducting ongoing research, and providing education, including telemedicine.
Anesth, CT Surg, CV Med, Infect Dis, Logist-Op, Ped Surg, Peds
https://vfapp.org/f34a

Heart to Heart International
Strengthens communities through improving health access, providing humanitarian development, and administering crisis relief worldwide. Engages volunteers, collaborates with partners, and deploys resources to achieve this mission.
Anesth, ER Med, General, Logist-Op, Medicine, Path, Path, Peds, Psych, Pub Health, Surg
+1 913-764-5200
https://vfapp.org/aacb

Heineman Medical Outreach
Provides medical and educational assistance globally to promote sustainable healthcare and enhanced living standards in underserved communities through the International Medical

Outreach (IMO) program, a collaborative partnership between Heineman Medical Outreach and Atrium Health.

Anesth, CT Surg, CV Med, ER Med, General, Heme-Onc, Logist-Op, Medicine, Neonat, OB-GYN, Ped Surg, Peds, Surg, Vasc Surg

📞 +1 704-374-0505

🌐 https://vfapp.org/389b

HelpAge International

Works to ensure that people everywhere understand how much older people contribute to society and that they must enjoy their right to healthcare, social services, economic, and physical security.

General, Geri, Infect Dis, Medicine, Pub Health

📞 +44 20 7148 7623

🌐 https://vfapp.org/5d91

Helping Hands Medical Missions

Delivers compassionate healthcare by hosting medical missions and treating patients in underserved communities around the world, based in Christian ministry.

Anesth, Dent-OMFS, ER Med, General, OB-GYN, Ophth-Opt, Surg

📞 +1 972-253-1800

🌐 https://vfapp.org/8efd

Holy Innocents Children's Hospital Uganda

Works to bring better health to all children of Mbarara, Uganda, and its surrounding villages through better medical care and prevention.

Ped Surg, Peds

🌐 https://vfapp.org/4964

Hope and Healing International

Gives hope and healing to children and families trapped by poverty and disability.

General, Nutr, Ophth-Opt, Peds, Rehab

📞 +1 905-640-6464

🌐 https://vfapp.org/c638

Hope Health Action

Facilitates sustainable, lifesaving health, and disability care for the world's most vulnerable, without any discrimination.

ER Med, MF Med, Neonat, Nutr, OB-GYN, Peds, Rehab

📞 +44 20 8462 5256

🌐 https://vfapp.org/86f7

Hope Line Organisation

Builds schools to provide free basic education to young children, supports women's community development, and provides healthcare outreach in Buikwe District in Central Uganda.

Dent-OMFS, General, Infect Dis, Peds

📞 +256 782 295902

🌐 https://vfapp.org/5426

Hope Smiles

Develops and empowers healthcare leaders to restore hope and transform lives by mobilizing and equipping sustainable dental teams in unreached communities.

Dent-OMFS, Pub Health, Surg

📞 +1 615-324-3904

🌐 https://vfapp.org/8a76

Humanity & Inclusion

Works alongside people with disabilities and vulnerable populations, taking action and bearing witness in order to respond to their essential needs, improve their living conditions and health, and promote respect for their dignity and fundamental rights.

General, Infect Dis, MF Med, Medicine, Ortho, Peds, Psych, Pub Health, Rehab

📞 +1 301-891-2138

🌐 https://vfapp.org/16b7

Humanity First

Provides aid and assistance to those in need, offering sustainable development solutions to society while providing and empowering local communities with the resources to help themselves.

ER Med, General, MF Med, Ophth-Opt

📞 +44 20 8417 0082

🌐 https://vfapp.org/13cc

Hunger Project, The

Aims to end hunger and poverty by pioneering sustainable, grassroots, women-centered strategies and advocating for their widespread adoption in countries throughout the world.

Infect Dis, Nutr, OB-GYN, Pub Health

📞 +1 212-251-9100

🌐 https://vfapp.org/3a49

ICAP at Columbia University

Serves as global leader in supporting the scale-up of multidisciplinary HIV/AIDS prevention, care, and treatment programs based on a family-focused approach.

General, Infect Dis, MF Med, Medicine, OB-GYN, Pub Health

📞 +1 212-342-0505

🌐 https://vfapp.org/a8ef

IMA World Health

Works to build healthier communities by collaborating with key partners to serve vulnerable people with a focus on health, healing, and well-being for all.

Infect Dis, MF Med, Nutr, OB-GYN, Pub Health

📞 +1 202-888-6200

🌐 https://vfapp.org/8316

Imaging the World

Develops sustainable models for ultrasound imaging in the world's lowest resource settings and uses a technology-enabled solution to improve healthcare access, integrating lifesaving ultrasound and training programs in rural communities.

Logist-Op, OB-GYN, Radiol

🌐 https://vfapp.org/59e4

Infectious Diseases Institute: College of Health Sciences, Makerere University

Works to strengthen health systems in Africa, with a strong emphasis on infectious diseases, through research and capacity development.

General, Infect Dis, Logist-Op, Pub Health

📞 +256 31 2211422

🌐 https://vfapp.org/9fc3

Interface Uganda

Aims to provide essential reconstructive surgery and to equip and train local specialists in Uganda and the surrounding areas.

Anesth, Dent-OMFS, Ped Surg, Plast, Surg

📞 +44 1392 860732

🌐 https://vfapp.org/837b

International Agency for the Prevention of Blindness (IAPB), The
Leads international efforts in blindness-prevention activities, works toward a world where no one is needlessly visually impaired, and ensures that everyone has access to the best possible standard of eye health.
Infect Dis, Ophth-Opt, Pub Health
https://vfapp.org/87a2

International Campaign for Women's Right to Safe Abortion
Works to build an international network and campaign that brings together organizations with an interest in promoting and providing safe abortion to create a shared platform for advocacy, debate, and dialogue and the sharing of skills and experience.
OB-GYN, Pub Health, Surg
https://vfapp.org/f341

International Children's Heart Fund
Aims to promote the international growth and quality of cardiac surgery, particularly in children and young adults.
CT Surg, Ped Surg
https://vfapp.org/33fb

International Federation of Gynecology and Obstetrics (FIGO)
Implements global projects on specific women's health issues.
MF Med, Medicine, Neonat, OB-GYN, Surg, Urol
+44 20 7928 1166
https://vfapp.org/c4b4

International Federation of Red Cross and Red Crescent Societies (IFRC)
Coordinates and directs international assistance following natural and man-made disasters in nonconflict situations through the world's largest humanitarian and development network. Provides disaster-preparedness programs, healthcare activities, and promotes humanitarian values.
ER Med, General, Infect Dis, Nutr
+1 212-338-0161
https://vfapp.org/b4ee

International Learning Movement (ILM UK)
Supports some of the world's poorest people in developing countries with core projects in education, safe drinking water, and healthcare.
General, Ophth-Opt
+44 1254 265451
https://vfapp.org/b974

International Medical Professionals Initiative Inc.
Works to improve healthcare in developing nations.
General, Nutr
+1 954-862-2235
https://vfapp.org/514a

International Medical Relief
Provides sustainable education, training, medical and dental care, and disaster relief and response in vulnerable communities worldwide.
Dent-OMFS, General, Infect Dis, Medicine, OB-GYN
+1 970-635-0110
https://vfapp.org/b3ed

International Organization for Migration (IOM) – The UN Migration Agency
Promotes evidence-informed policies and holistic, preventive, and curative health programs that are beneficial, accessible, and equitable for vulnerable migrants.
General, Infect Dis, OB-GYN
+27 12 342 2789
https://vfapp.org/621a

International Outreach Program of St. Joseph's Health System
Works to save lives in developing countries by training doctors through partnerships with universities, medical schools, and teaching hospitals in countries that need more doctors.
Logist-Op
+1 905-522-1155
https://vfapp.org/a751

International Pediatric Nephrology Association (IPNA)
Leads the global efforts to successfully address the care for all children with kidney disease through advocacy, education, and training.
Medicine, Nephro, Peds
https://vfapp.org/b59d

International Planned Parenthood Federation (IPPF)
Leads a locally owned, globally connected civil society movement that provides and enables services and champions sexual and reproductive health and rights for all, especially the underserved.
Infect Dis, MF Med, OB-GYN
+44 20 7939 8200
https://vfapp.org/dc97

International Rescue Committee (IRC)
Responds to the world's worst humanitarian crises and helps people whose lives and livelihoods are shattered by conflict and disaster to survive, recover, and gain control of their future.
ER Med, General, Infect Dis, MF Med, Peds
+1 212-551-3000
https://vfapp.org/5d24

International Smile Power
Partners with people to improve and sustain dental health and build bridges of friendship around the world.
Dent-OMFS
https://vfapp.org/ba69

International Trachoma Initiative (iTi)
Works toward a world free from trachoma, a preventable cause of blindness, and provides comprehensive support to national ministries of health and governmental and nongovernmental organizations to implement a comprehensive approach to fight trachoma.
Infect Dis, Ophth-Opt
+1 404-371-0466
https://vfapp.org/3278

International Union Against Tuberculosis and Lung Disease
Develops, implements, and assesses anti-tuberculosis, lung health, and noncommunicable disease programs.
Infect Dis, Pub Health, Pulm-Critic
+33 1 44 32 03 60
https://vfapp.org/3e82

InterSurgeon
Fosters collaborative partnerships in the field of global surgery that will advance clinical care, teaching, training, research, and the provision and maintenance of medical equipment.

ENT, Neurosurg, Ortho, Ped Surg, Plast, Surg, Urol

🌐 **https://vfapp.org/6f8a**

IntraHealth International
Improves the performance of health workers and strengthens the systems in which they work.

CV Med, Endo, General, Infect Dis, MF Med, Neonat, Nutr, OB-GYN

📞 **+1 919-313-3554**

🌐 **https://vfapp.org/ddc8**

Ipas
Focuses efforts on women and girls who want contraception or abortion, and builds programs around their needs and how best to support them.

OB-GYN

🌐 **https://vfapp.org/8e39**

Iris Global
Serves the poor, the destitute, the lost, and the forgotten by providing adoration, outreach, family, education, relief, development, healing, and the arts.

General, Infect Dis, Nutr, Pub Health

📞 **+1 530-255-2077**

🌐 **https://vfapp.org/37f8**

Islamic Medical Association of North America
Fosters health promotion, disease prevention, and health maintenance in communities around the world through direct patient care and health programs.

Anesth, Dent-OMFS, ER Med, General, Logist-Op, Ophth-Opt, Peds, Plast, Surg

📞 **+1 630-932-0000**

🌐 **https://vfapp.org/a157**

Island Mission Uganda
Aims to improve the lives of people living with HIV/AIDS, especially children, and integrates primary healthcare services in the remote island communities of Lake Victoria.

Infect Dis, Peds

📞 **+256 755 365130**

🌐 **https://vfapp.org/a778**

IsraAID
Supports people affected by humanitarian crisis and partners with local communities around the world to provide urgent aid, assist recovery, and reduce the risk of future disasters.

ER Med, Infect Dis, Psych, Rehab

📞 **+972 3-947-7766**

🌐 **https://vfapp.org/de96**

IVUmed
Aims to make quality urological care available worldwide by providing medical and surgical education for physicians and nurses and treatment for thousands of children and adults.

Anesth, OB-GYN, Ped Surg, Surg, Urol

📞 **+1 801-524-0201**

🌐 **https://vfapp.org/e619**

Jesus Harvesters Ministries
Reaches communities through medical clinics, dental care, veterinarian outreach, pastor training, and community service, based in Christian ministry.

Dent-OMFS, General, Infect Dis

🌐 **https://vfapp.org/8a23**

Jhpiego
Creates and delivers transformative healthcare solutions that save lives in partnership with national governments, health experts, and local communities.

General, Infect Dis, OB-GYN, Surg

📞 **+1 410-537-1800**

🌐 **https://vfapp.org/45b8**

John Snow, Inc. (JSI)
Aims to improve the health and well-being of underserved and vulnerable people and communities throughout the world.

General, Infect Dis, Logist-Op, MF Med, OB-GYN, Peds, Psych, Pub Health

📞 **+1 617-482-9485**

🌐 **https://vfapp.org/ba78**

Johns Hopkins Center for Communication Programs
Believes in the power of communication to save lives, by empowering people to adopt healthy behaviors for themselves, their families, and their communities.

General, Infect Dis, Logist-Op, OB-GYN, Pub Health

📞 **+1 410-659-6300**

🌐 **https://vfapp.org/1bf9**

Johns Hopkins Center for Global Health
Facilitates and focuses the extensive expertise and resources of the Johns Hopkins institutions together with global collaborators to effectively address and ameliorate the world's most pressing health issues.

General, Genetics, Logist-Op, MF Med, Peds, Psych, Pub Health, Pulm-Critic

📞 **+1 410-502-9872**

🌐 **https://vfapp.org/54ce**

Joint Aid Management (JAM)
Provides food security, nutrition, water, and sanitation to vulnerable communities in Africa in dignified and sustainable ways.

ER Med, Nutr

📞 **+27 11 548 3900**

🌐 **https://vfapp.org/dcac**

Joint United Nations Programme on HIV/AIDS (UNAIDS)
Aims to place people living with HIV and people affected by the virus at the decision-making table and at the center of designing, delivering, and monitoring the AIDS response.

Infect Dis

📞 **+41 22 791 36 66**

🌐 **https://vfapp.org/464a**

Kagando Rural Development Center (KARUDEC)
Provides integrated community programs and holistic care through Kagando Hospital, microfinance projects, farms, community outreach for palliative care, mental health, water supply, and entrepreneurship programs.

Crit-Care, Dent-OMFS, Ophth-Opt, Path, Psych, Radiol, Rehab

📞 **+256 70011028**

🌐 **https://vfapp.org/997d**

Kajo Keji Health Training Institute (KKHTI)
Addresses the severe shortage of medical personnel in South Sudan by training quality healthcare workers.
General, Infect Dis, MF Med
+211 954 338 623
https://vfapp.org/ff59

Kamuli Friends
Organizes support to Kamuli Mission Hospital in the form of building projects, medical equipment, and international volunteers in response to the needs of the hospital.
General, Medicine, OB-GYN, Peds, Surg
https://vfapp.org/1e99

Karin Community Initiatives Uganda (KCIU)
Seeks to transform lives and heal communities by providing quality healthcare services, inspired by the Christian faith.
General, Infect Dis, MF Med, OB-GYN, Peds
+256 793 852129
https://vfapp.org/31ed

Katalemwa Cheshire Home
Provides holistic rehabilitation services, such as quality medical care, social economic support, and orthopedic appliances to children and young persons with disabilities.
Ortho, Peds, Rehab
+256 41 4590739
https://vfapp.org/1edd

Kaya Responsible Travel
Promotes sustainable social, environmental, and economic development, empowers communities, and cultivates educated, compassionate global citizens through responsible travel.
All-Immu, Crit-Care, Dent-OMFS, ER Med, General, Geri, Infect Dis, MF Med, Medicine, Nutr, OB-GYN, Peds, Psych, Pub Health, Rehab
+1 413-517-0266
https://vfapp.org/b2cf

Kimbra Foundation
Provides opportunity to African children in need.
General, Nutr, Peds
+1 561-784-7852
https://vfapp.org/f11d

Kletjian Foundation
Works toward a world in which all people have access to safe, sustainable, and high-quality medical care, building collaborative networks and supporting entrepreneurial leaders that promote global health equity.
CT Surg, ENT, General, Ortho, Surg
https://vfapp.org/12c2

Kumi Hospital Uganda
Provides holistic, preventive, curative, and rehabilitative services, based in Christian ministry.
All-Immu, General, Infect Dis, OB-GYN, Ortho, Peds, Surg
+256 776 221443
https://vfapp.org/4942

Last Mile Health
Links community health workers with frontline health workers—nurses, doctors, and midwives at community clinics—and supports them to bring lifesaving services to the doorsteps of people living far from care.
General, Logist-Op, OB-GYN, Pub Health
+1 617-880-6163
https://vfapp.org/37da

Life for a Child
Supports the provision of the best possible health care, given local circumstances, to all children and youth with diabetes in less-resourced countries, through the strengthening of existing diabetes services.
Endo, Medicine, Peds
https://vfapp.org/d712

LifeNet International
Transforms African healthcare by equipping and empowering existing local health centers to provide quality, sustainable, and lifesaving care to patients.
General, Infect Dis, MF Med, Neonat, OB-GYN, Pub Health
+1 407-630-9518
https://vfapp.org/e5d2

Light for the World
Contributes to a world in which persons with disabilities fully exercise their rights and assists persons with disabilities living in poverty.
Ophth-Opt, Rehab
+43 1 8101300
https://vfapp.org/3ff6

Lions Clubs International
Empowers volunteers to serve their communities, meet humanitarian needs, encourage peace, and promote international understanding through Lions clubs.
Heme-Onc, Medicine, Nutr, Ophth-Opt
+1 630-571-5466
https://vfapp.org/7b12

Living Goods
Leverages a powerful combination of catalytic technology, high-impact training, and quality treatments that empower government community health workers (CHWs) to deliver quality care to their neighbors' doorsteps.
Infect Dis, Logist-Op, MF Med
+1 202-792-7833
https://vfapp.org/d6d2

London School of Hygiene & Tropical Medicine
Seeks to improve health and health equity in the UK and worldwide, working in partnership to achieve excellence in public and global health research, education and translation of knowledge into policy and practice.
Infect Dis, Pub Health
+44 20 7636 8636
https://vfapp.org/349a

London School of Hygiene & Tropical Medicine: Health in Humanitarian Crises Centre
Advances health and health equity in crisis-affected countries through research, education, and translation of knowledge into policy and practice.
ER Med, Infect Dis, Pub Health
+44 20 7636 8636
https://vfapp.org/96ad

Love One International
Ensures the children of Uganda receive the emergency healthcare and rehabilitative services they need.

General, Infect Dis, Peds
https://vfapp.org/ef2e

Lámha Suas

Aims to improve the lives of young women in Uganda by supporting the education and healthcare of girls.
General, Nutr, OB-GYN, Rehab
https://vfapp.org/a489

Management Sciences for Health (MSH)

Works with countries and communities to save lives and improve the health of the world's poorest and most vulnerable people by building strong, resilient, sustainable health systems.
Infect Dis, Logist-Op, Pub Health
+1 617-250-9500
https://vfapp.org/6aa2

MAP International

Provides medicines and health supplies to those in need around the world so they might experience life to the fullest.
Logist-Op
+1 800-225-8550
https://vfapp.org/deed

Maranatha Health

Works to improve health outcomes, empower the poor, and make positive, lasting change in Uganda by collaborating with local communities in rural Western Uganda, namely Kamwenge and Kabarole Districts, to improve health, inspired by the Christian faith.
Anesth, ENT, Infect Dis, Neonat, Nutr, OB-GYN, Ophth-Opt, Ped Surg, Peds, Radiol, Surg
+61 414 440 498
https://vfapp.org/c4a9

Marie Stopes International

Provides the contraception and safe abortion services that enable women all over the world to choose their own futures.
Infect Dis, MF Med, Neonat, OB-GYN, Pub Health
+44 20 7636 6200
https://vfapp.org/9525

Mary Mission Incorporated

Restores hope and dignity in a peaceful and safe environment by providing for the needs of the poor and vulnerable with education, food, clothing, healthcare, and shelter.
General
+1 701-530-9310
https://vfapp.org/3ec5

Massachusetts General Hospital Global Surgery Initiative

Aims to improve surgical education and access to advanced surgical care in resource-limited settings around the world by performing surgical operations as visitors, training local surgeons, and sharing medical technology through international partnerships across disciplines.
Anesth, Crit-Care, ER Med, Heme-Onc, Peds, Surg
+1 617-724-4093
https://vfapp.org/31b1

Maternity Worldwide

Works with communities and partners to identify and develop appropriate and effective ways to reduce maternal and newborn mortality and morbidity, facilitate communities to access quality skilled maternity care, and support the provision of quality skilled care.
MF Med, OB-GYN
+44 1273 234033
https://vfapp.org/822b

Maverick Collective

Aims to build a global community of strategic philanthropists and informed advocates who use their intellectual and financial resources to create change.
Infect Dis, MF Med, OB-GYN
+1 202-785-0072
https://vfapp.org/ea49

McGill University Health Centre: Centre for Global Surgery

Works to reduce the impact of injury by advancing surgical care through research and education in resource-limited settings.
ER Med, Logist-Op, Ped Surg, Surg
+1 514-934-1934
https://vfapp.org/7246

Medical Missions Foundation

Provides surgical and medical care in underserved communities throughout the world and hopes to positively impact the lives of children and their families.
Anesth, Ped Surg, Surg
+1 913-338-0343
https://vfapp.org/f385

Medical Teams International

Seeks to restore health as the first step to restoring hope, working to bring basic but lifesaving medical care to those in need.
Dent-OMFS, ER Med, General, MF Med, Pub Health
+1 503-624-1000
https://vfapp.org/8d1c

MedShare

Aims to improve the quality of life of people, communities, and the planet by sourcing and directly delivering surplus medical supplies and equipment to communities in need around the world.
Logist-Op
+1 770-323-5858
https://vfapp.org/c8bc

MENTOR Initiative

Saves lives in emergencies through tropical disease control, and helps people recover from crisis with dignity, working side by side with communities, health workers, and health authorities to leave a lasting impact.
ER Med, Infect Dis
+44 1444 412171
https://vfapp.org/3bd5

Merck for Mothers

Hopes to create a world where no woman has to die giving life by collaborating with partners to improve the health and well-being of women during pregnancy, childbirth, and the postpartum period.
MF Med, OB-GYN
https://vfapp.org/5b51

Mercy Ships
Operates hospital ships staffed by volunteers to bring hope, healing, and healthcare to underserved communities worldwide.
Anesth, Dent-OMFS, Logist-Op, Neonat, OB-GYN, Ophth-Opt, Ortho, Palliative, Plast, Psych, Surg
+1 903-939-7000
https://vfapp.org/2e99

MicroResearch: Africa/Asia
Seeks to improve health outcomes in Africa by training, mentoring, and supporting local multidisciplinary health professional researchers.
Infect Dis, Nutr, OB-GYN, Psych
https://vfapp.org/13e7

Mildmay
Transforms and empowers lives through the delivery of quality health services, treatment, and care in the UK and Africa.
Infect Dis, MF Med, Neuro, Psych
+44 20 7613 6300
https://vfapp.org/3fd8

MiracleFeet
Brings low-cost treatment to every child on the planet born with clubfoot, a leading cause of physical disability.
Ortho, Peds, Rehab
+1 919-240-5572
https://vfapp.org/bda8

Mission Bambini
Helps to support children living in poverty, sickness, and without education, giving them the opportunity and hope of a better life.
CT Surg, CV Med, Crit-Care, ER Med, Ped Surg, Peds
+39 02 210 0241
https://vfapp.org/dc1a

Mission to Heal
Aims to heal underserved people and train local practitioners in the most remote areas of the world through global healthcare missions.
Anesth, Infect Dis, OB-GYN, Surg
https://vfapp.org/4718

Mission Vision
Seeks to decrease blindness and other eye-related disabilities, as well as to increase academic performance and general quality of life.
Ophth-Opt
+1 724-553-3114
https://vfapp.org/83d8

More Than Medicine
Provides ENT head/neck care while supporting local doctors to grow the quality of medicine abroad.
Anesth, ENT, Heme-Onc, Surg
+1 501-268-9511
https://vfapp.org/c4e8

Mothers and Children Support International
Provides education and health services in rural Uganda, focusing on orphans, mothers, and children.
General, Infect Dis, Pub Health
+1 484-908-1614
https://vfapp.org/fd5f

mothers2mothers (m2m)
Employs and trains local women living with HIV as community health workers called Mentor Mothers to support women, children, and adolescents with vital medical services, education, and support.
Infect Dis, MF Med, OB-GYN, Peds, Pub Health
+27 21 466 9160
https://vfapp.org/6557

MPACT for Mankind
Transforms communities by improving health outcomes, enhancing knowledge, and providing hope while promoting sustainable growth.
ER Med, General
+1 469-998-1381
https://vfapp.org/1c61

MSD for Mothers
Designs scalable solutions that help end preventable maternal deaths.
MF Med, OB-GYN, Pub Health
https://vfapp.org/9f99

Multi-Agency International Training and Support (MAITS)
Improves the lives of some of the world's poorest people living with disabilities through better access to quality health and education services and support.
Neuro, Psych, Rehab
+44 20 7258 8443
https://vfapp.org/9dcd

NCD Alliance
Unites and strengthens civil society to stimulate collaborative advocacy, action, and accountability for NCD (noncommunicable disease) prevention and control.
All-Immu, CV Med, General, Heme-Onc, Medicine, Peds, Psych
+41 22 809 18 11
https://vfapp.org/abdd

NuVasive Spine Foundation (NSF)
Partners with leading spine surgeons, nonprofits, and in-country medical professionals/facilities to bring life-changing spine surgery to under-resourced communities around the world.
Logist-Op, Ortho, Ped Surg, Rehab, Surg
+1 800-455-1476
https://vfapp.org/6ccc

Omni Med
Promotes health volunteerism and provides innovative, cooperative, and sustainable programs with measurable impact.
ER Med, Endo, Medicine, Neuro, OB-GYN, Ophth-Opt, Ortho, Palliative, Peds, Vasc Surg
+1 617-332-9614
https://vfapp.org/2969

OneWorld Health
Provides quality, affordable healthcare to communities in need and empowers communities to achieve long-term improvements in health and quality of life.
Dent-OMFS, General, Infect Dis, Ortho, Peds,

Rehab, Surg
+1 843-203-3280
https://vfapp.org/71d7

Operation Fistula
Exists to end obstetric fistula by building models of care that serve every woman, everywhere.
MF Med, OB-GYN, Surg
+1 512-687-3479
https://vfapp.org/ce8e

Operation Healthy Africa
Organizes and participates in medical missions, disease treatment and prevention, vision and hearing care, and other medical services around the world, while also providing medical equipment and other supplies in the areas where it operates.
Dent-OMFS, General, Infect Dis, Logist-Op, MF Med, OB-GYN, Ophth-Opt, Surg
+1 310-534-5483
https://vfapp.org/c99b

Operation Hernia
Provides high-quality surgery at minimal costs to patients that otherwise would not receive it.
Anesth, Ortho, Surg
https://vfapp.org/6e9a

Operation International
Offers medical aid to adults and children suffering from lack of quality healthcare in impoverished countries.
Dent-OMFS, ER Med, Heme-Onc, OB-GYN, Ophth-Opt, Ortho, Ped Surg, Plast, Surg
+1 631-287-6202
https://vfapp.org/b52a

Options
Believes in a world where women and children can access the high-quality health services they need, without financial burden.
Logist-Op, MF Med, Neonat, OB-GYN
+44 20 7430 1900
https://vfapp.org/3a48

Optometry Giving Sight
Delivers eye exams and low or no-cost glasses, provides training for local eye care professionals, and establishes optometry schools, vision centers and optical labs.
Ophth-Opt
+1 303-526-0430
https://vfapp.org/33ea

Orbis International
Works to prevent and treat blindness through hands-on training and improved access to quality eye care.
Anesth, Ophth-Opt, Surg
+1 646-674-5500
https://vfapp.org/f2b2

Ostomates Uganda
Brings attention to the suffering of ostomates, lobbies for support, provides education opportunities, and provides psycho-social support for the ostomates and their families.
GI, Psych
+256 783 005064
https://vfapp.org/ad24

Oxford University Global Surgery Group (OUGSG)
Aims to contribute to the provision of high-quality surgical care globally, particularly in low- and middle-income countries (LMICs) while bringing together students, researchers, and clinicians with an interest in global surgery, anaesthesia, and obstetrics and gynecology.
Anesth, MF Med, OB-GYN, Ortho, Surg
+44 1865 737543
https://vfapp.org/c624

Pact
Works on the ground to improve the lives of those who are challenged by poverty and marginalization, striving for a world where all people are heard, capable, and vibrant.
Infect Dis, Logist-Op, MF Med, Pub Health
+1 202-466-5666
https://vfapp.org/9a6c

Partners for World Health
Sorts, evaluates, repackages, and prepares supplies and equipment for distribution to individuals, communities, and healthcare facilities in need, both locally and internationally.
ER Med, General, Logist-Op
+1 207-774-5555
https://vfapp.org/982e

PATH
Advances health equity through innovation and partnerships so people, communities, and economies can thrive.
All-Immu, CV Med, Endo, Heme-Onc, Infect Dis, MF Med, Neonat, Nutr, OB-GYN, Path, Peds, Pulm-Critic
+1 202-822-0033
https://vfapp.org/b4db

Pathfinder International
Champions sexual and reproductive health and rights worldwide, mobilizing communities most in need to break through barriers and forge paths to a healthier future.
OB-GYN
+1 617-924-7200
https://vfapp.org/a7b3

Pediatric Health Initiative
Supports the spread of quality pediatric care and its development and progress in low- and middle-income countries.
ER Med, Infect Dis, Neonat, Palliative, Ped Surg, Peds
https://vfapp.org/614b

Pepal
Brings together NGOs, global corporations, and the public sector to co-create solutions to big social issues, creating immediate and scalable solutions and developing leaders who are capable of driving change in their communities.
Heme-Onc, Infect Dis, Pub Health
https://vfapp.org/6dc5

Perspective for Children
Supports HIV/AIDS affected and disabled children and adolescents in Uganda.
General, Infect Dis, MF Med, OB-GYN
+43 676 9356521
https://vfapp.org/efd6

Physicians Across Continents
Provides high-quality medical care to people affected by crises and disasters.
CV Med, Dent-OMFS, Heme-Onc, MF Med, Nephro, Nephro, OB-GYN, Ped Surg, Plast, Surg
+44 20 7993 6900
https://vfapp.org/fe5d

Poole Africa Link
Provides a link of training for doctors, nurses, midwives, and student nurses between Poole Hospital NHS Foundation Trust and Wau Hospital in South Sudan.
Logist-Op, OB-GYN
+44 1202 448182
https://vfapp.org/1f6f

Programme for Nutrition and Eye Care (PRONEC)
Champions access to affordable eye care, nutrition education, and services, including HIV/AIDS education, among the rural poor in Uganda.
General, Infect Dis, Nutr, Ophth-Opt
+256 753 150492
https://vfapp.org/ac8b

Project Concern International (PCI)
Drives innovation from the ground up to enhance health, end hunger, overcome hardship, and advance women and girls—resulting in meaningful and measurable change in people's lives.
Infect Dis, MF Med, Nutr, OB-GYN, Peds
+1 858-279-9690
https://vfapp.org/5ed7

Project SOAR
Conducts HIV operations research around the world to identify practical solutions to improve HIV prevention, care, and treatment services.
ER Med, General, MF Med, OB-GYN, Psych
+1 202-237-9400
https://vfapp.org/1a77

Project Turquoise
Raises awareness and supports the needs of displaced families and provides humanitarian support locally and abroad.
Dent-OMFS, ER Med
https://vfapp.org/88bf

RAD-AID International
Improves and optimizes access to medical imaging and radiology in low-resource regions of the world.
Rad-Onc, Radiol
https://vfapp.org/537f

Rakai Health Sciences Program
Conducts innovative and relevant health research in infectious diseases, communicable and non-communicable diseases, and reproductive health, and provides health-related services in order to improve public health and inform policy.
GI, Infect Dis, Neuro, Path, Pub Health
+256 200 900384
https://vfapp.org/ee73

Rays of Hope Hospice Jinja
Provides palliative care and improves the quality of life for all people with life-limiting illnesses and their families in the Busoga Region and neighboring districts.
+256 771 619991
https://vfapp.org/9816

Real Medicine Foundation (RMF)
Provides humanitarian support to people living in disaster and poverty-stricken areas, focusing on the person as a whole by providing medical/physical, emotional, economic, and social support.
ER Med, General, Infect Dis, Nutr, Peds, Psych
+44 20 8638 0637
https://vfapp.org/d45a

Rescue Hope
Connects medical professionals with opportunities to serve around the world and bring physical and spiritual healing to nations abroad.
ER Med, General
+1 936-537-1959
https://vfapp.org/1428

RestoringVision
Empowers lives by restoring vision for millions of people in need.
Ophth-Opt
+1 209-980-7323
https://vfapp.org/e121

RHD Action
Seeks to reduce the burden of rheumatic heart disease in vulnerable populations throughout the world.
CV Med, Medicine, Pub Health
https://vfapp.org/f5d9

Rockefeller Foundation, The
Works to promote the well-being of humanity.
Logist-Op, Nutr, Pub Health
+1 212-869-8500
https://vfapp.org/5424

Rose Charities International
Aims to support communities to improve quality of life and reduce the effects of poverty through innovative, self-sustaining projects and partnerships.
ENT, ER Med, General, Infect Dis, Neonat, OB-GYN, Ophth-Opt, Ped Surg, Peds, Rehab, Urol
+1 604-733-0442
https://vfapp.org/53df

Rotary Action Group for Family Health & AIDS Prevention (RFHA)
Works to save and improve the lives of children and families who lack access to preventive healthcare and education.
Dent-OMFS, Infect Dis, OB-GYN, Ophth-Opt, Peds
+27 83 456 3923
https://vfapp.org/6563

Rotary International
Provides service to others, improves lives, and advances world understanding, goodwill, and peace through its fellowship of business, professional, and community leaders.
ER Med, General, Infect Dis, MF Med, OB-GYN
https://vfapp.org/8fb5

ROW Foundation
Works to improve the quality of training for healthcare providers, and the diagnosis and treatment available to people with epilepsy and associated psychiatric disorders in under-resourced areas of the world.

Neuro, Psych

☎ +1 630-791-0247

🌐 https://vfapp.org/25eb

Rural Health Care Foundation Uganda
Works to make a difference in local communities by providing basic healthcare and programs supporting people with HIV/AIDS, access to clean, safe water, education on sustainable hygiene and sanitation practices, and treating opportunistic infections.

General, Infect Dis, Nutr, OB-GYN, Peds, Urol

☎ +256 758 446912

🌐 https://vfapp.org/d65d

Ruth Gaylord Hospital Maganjo
Provides self-sustaining, affordable, and equitable community-based healthcare services through a dedicated and professional workforce.

Crit-Care, Infect Dis, OB-GYN, Ophth-Opt

☎ +256 701 791373

🌐 https://vfapp.org/2d7e

Safe Anaesthesia Worldwide
Provides anesthesia to those in need in low-income countries to enable lifesaving surgery.

Anesth, Plast

☎ +44 7527 506969

🌐 https://vfapp.org/134a

Safe Places Uganda Foundation
Works to improve the mental health and well-being of the people in Uganda and seeks to build an inclusive society that values mental health, respects the rights of persons with mental illnesses, and is free of any related stigma.

General, Peds, Psych

☎ +256 782 740522

🌐 https://vfapp.org/b3fc

Salvation Army International, The
Seeks to meet human needs through services in education, healthcare, community support, emergency response, and ministry development, inspired by the Christian faith.

Dent-OMFS, Derm, ER Med, Infect Dis, MF Med, Medicine, Nutr, OB-GYN, Ophth-Opt, Palliative, Psych, Rehab, Surg

☎ +44 20 7332 0101

🌐 https://vfapp.org/8eb3

Samaritan's Purse International Disaster Relief
Provides spiritual and physical aid to hurting people around the world, such as victims of war, poverty, natural disasters, disease, and famine, based in Christian ministry.

Anesth, CT Surg, Crit-Care, Dent-OMFS, Derm, ENT, ER Med, Endo, GI, General, Heme-Onc, Infect Dis, MF Med, Neonat, Nephro, Neuro, Neurosurg, Nutr, OB-GYN, Ophth-Opt, Ortho, Path, Ped Surg, Peds, Plast, Psych, Pulm-Critic, Radiol, Rehab, Rheum, Surg, Urol, Vasc Surg

☎ +1 800-528-1980

🌐 https://vfapp.org/87e3

Sanofi Espoir Foundation
Contributes to reducing health inequalities among populations that need it most by applying a socially responsible approach focused on fighting childhood cancers in low-income countries, improving maternal and newborn health, and improving access to care.

ER Med, OB-GYN, Peds

☎ +33 1 53 77 91 38

🌐 https://vfapp.org/943b

Save A Child's Heart
Provides lifesaving cardiac treatment to children in developing countries, and trains healthcare professionals from these countries to deliver quality care in their communities.

CT Surg, CV Med, Crit-Care, Ped Surg, Peds

☎ +1 240-223-3940

🌐 https://vfapp.org/1bef

Save the Children
Gives children around the world a healthy start in life, the opportunity to learn, and protection from harm.

All-Immu, Crit-Care, ER Med, General, Infect Dis, MF Med, Medicine, Neonat, OB-GYN, Peds, Psych, Pub Health

☎ +1 800-728-3843

🌐 https://vfapp.org/2e73

Save the Mothers
Promotes maternal health in developing countries through education, public awareness, and advocacy.

General, MF Med, Neonat, OB-GYN, Peds

☎ +1 905-928-7283

🌐 https://vfapp.org/498f

Saving Mothers
Seeks to eradicate preventable maternal deaths and birth-related complications in low-resource settings.

MF Med, Neonat, OB-GYN, Surg

🌐 https://vfapp.org/ed94

SEE International
Provides sustainable medical, surgical, and educational services through volunteer ophthalmic surgeons, with the objectives of restoring sight and preventing blindness to disadvantaged individuals worldwide.

Ophth-Opt, Surg

☎ +1 805-963-3303

🌐 https://vfapp.org/6e1b

Seed Global Health
Focuses on human resources for health capacity building at the individual, institutional, and national level through sustained collaborative engagement with partners.

Logist-Op

☎ +1 617-366-1650

🌐 https://vfapp.org/d12e

Senior Citizens Agecare Foundation Uganda (SCACFU)
Fights isolation, loneliness, neglect, abuse, and poverty to ensure senior citizens live self-fulfilled lives by encouraging active aging and that they retire gracefully with dignity.

Geri

☎ +1 617-230-8326

🌐 https://vfapp.org/1c4c

SEVA
Delivers vital eye care services to the world's most vulnerable, including women, children, and Indigenous peoples.
Ophth-Opt, Surg
+1 510-845-7382
https://vfapp.org/1e87

Share Uganda
Focuses on providing quality and sustainable health services, supporting the education of local healthcare professionals, and developing collaborative solutions to local healthcare challenges.
General, Infect Dis, Neonat, OB-GYN, Pub Health
https://vfapp.org/c6e6

Shines Children's Foundation
Aims to protect the rights of children and provide them access to education, healthcare, and shelter.
General, Infect Dis, Nutr, Pub Health
+256 754 546113
https://vfapp.org/da64

Sightsavers
Prevents avoidable blindness in some of the poorest parts of the world by treating debilitating eye diseases.
Infect Dis, Ophth-Opt, Surg
+1 800-707-9746
https://vfapp.org/aa52

SIGN Fracture Care International
Builds orthopedic capacity around the world and provides the injured poor access to fracture surgery by donating orthopedic education and implant systems to surgeons in developing countries.
Ortho, Rehab, Surg
+1 509-371-1107
https://vfapp.org/123d

Simavi
Strives for a world in which all women and girls are socially and economically empowered and pursue their rights to live a healthy life, free from discrimination, coercion, and violence.
MF Med, OB-GYN
+31 88 313 1500
https://vfapp.org/b57b

Smile Train
Seeks to give every child with a cleft the opportunity for a healthy, productive life by providing free cleft repair surgery and comprehensive cleft care in their own communities.
Dent-OMFS, ENT, Plast
+1 800-932-9541
https://vfapp.org/f21d

Soft Power Health
Provides primary healthcare, health education and prevention, and health-promoting activities for people in need.
General, Infect Dis, MF Med, Nutr, Pub Health
+1 914-282-7354
https://vfapp.org/e587

SOS Children's Villages International
Supports children through alternative care and family strengthening.
ER Med, Peds
+43 1 36824570
https://vfapp.org/aca1

Sovereign Wings of Hope Ministries (SWOH)
Renders medical, spiritual, and humanitarian services to enrich communities in Uganda.
Palliative
+1 713-503-8011
https://vfapp.org/937d

St. Francis Hospital Nsambya
Provides sustainable quality healthcare, training, and research, while supporting economically disadvantaged communities.
Dent-OMFS, Heme-Onc, Medicine, Neonat, Path, Peds, Radiol, Surg
+256 41 4267012
https://vfapp.org/d9f8

St. Mary's Hospital Lacor
Provides healthcare to those in need and helps to fight disease and poverty.
Anesth, ER Med, General, Infect Dis, MF Med, OB-GYN, Peds, Surg
+256 790 915167
https://vfapp.org/ecc1

Stanford Global Health Neurosurgery Initiative
Shares knowledge and expertise in areas where neurosurgeons are few and access to neurosurgical treatment is lacking, sending nurses, residents, and surgeons to different parts of the world to provide clinical care and conduct research.
Anesth, Neuro, Neurosurg, Ortho, Rehab, Surg
+1 650-721-6736
https://vfapp.org/f4d4

Sustainable Cardiovascular Health Equity Development Alliance
Fights cardiovascular disease in underserved populations globally via education, training, and increasing interventional capacity.
CV Med, Pub Health, Radiol
+1 608-338-3357
https://vfapp.org/799c

Sustainable Kidney Care Foundation (SKCF)
Works to provide treatment for kidney injury where none exists, and aims to reduce mortality from treatable acute kidney injury (AKI).
Infect Dis, Medicine, Nephro
https://vfapp.org/1926

Sustainable Medical Missions
Trains and supports Indigenous healthcare and faith leaders in underdeveloped communities to treat neglected tropical diseases (NTDs) and other endemic conditions affecting the poorest community members by pairing faith-based solutions with best practices.
Infect Dis, Pub Health
+1 513-543-2896
https://vfapp.org/9165

Swedish Organization for Global Health
Aims to improve the quality and accessibility of healthcare and health promotion through local and international partnerships.
Logist-Op, OB-GYN, Pub Health
https://vfapp.org/a5b1

Swiss Tropical and Public Health Institute
Contributes to the improvement of the health of populations

internationally, nationally, and locally through excellence in research, education, and services.

Infect Dis, Pub Health

+41 61 284 81 11

https://vfapp.org/2ee4

Task Force for Global Health, The

Consists of programs and focus areas that cover a range of global health issues including neglected tropical diseases, infectious diseases, vaccines, field epidemiology, public health informatics, health workforce development, and global health ethics.

Infect Dis, Logist-Op, Medicine, Ophth-Opt, Peds

+1 404-371-0466

https://vfapp.org/714c

Team Canada Healing Hands

Provides and develops interdisciplinary rehabilitation treatment, education, and training in areas of need.

ENT, Neuro, Psych, Rehab

+1 506-363-3836

https://vfapp.org/2eaf

Tearfund

Responds to crisis and partners with local churches to bring restoration to those living in poverty, inspired by the Christian faith.

ER Med, Logist-Op

+44 20 3906 3906

https://vfapp.org/f6cf

Teasdale-Corti Foundation/St. Mary's Hospital Lacor

Guarantees affordable medical services, especially to those most in need, and ensures the continuity of healthcare, training, and growth of Lacor Hospital in Uganda.

CV Med, Crit-Care, General, Infect Dis, MF Med, OB-GYN, Ped Surg, Peds

+1 514-253-1737

https://vfapp.org/f1da

Terrewode Women's Fund

Supports quality surgical treatment and social reintegration to thousands of Ugandan women suffering from obstetric fistula.

MF Med, OB-GYN, Surg

https://vfapp.org/1d12

Texas Children's Global Health

Addresses healthcare needs in resource-limited settings locally and globally by improving maternal and child health through the implementation of innovative, sustainable, in-country programs to train health professionals and build functional healthcare infrastructure.

Anesth, ER Med, Heme-Onc, Infect Dis, MF Med, Nutr, OB-GYN, Peds, Pub Health, Surg

+1 832-824-1141

https://vfapp.org/4a1d

THET Partnerships for Global Health

Trains and educates health workers in Africa and Asia, working in partnership with organizations and volunteers from across the UK.

General

+44 20 7290 3891

https://vfapp.org/f937

Think Humanity

Saves lives and provides hope for refugees and underdeveloped communities in Africa by improving provisions for healthcare, clean water, education and socio-economic development.

General, Infect Dis, Peds

+1 970-667-9335

https://vfapp.org/e537

U.S. President's Malaria Initiative (PMI)

Supports low-income countries to help control and eliminate malaria through cost-effective, lifesaving malaria interventions.

Infect Dis, MF Med, OB-GYN

+1 202-712-0000

https://vfapp.org/dc8b

Uganda Child Cancer Foundation

Supports children and young persons with cancer in Uganda through direct support, advocacy, and awareness about cancer.

Heme-Onc, Ped Surg, Peds

+256 39 2834441

https://vfapp.org/ea73

Uganda Kidney Foundation

Works in the prevention and management of kidney disease through awareness, education, and research.

Nephro

+256 772 442700

https://vfapp.org/5848

Uganda Rural Fund

Empowers orphans, underprivileged youth, and women to fight poverty in Uganda's rural communities through the creation of educational and sustainable development opportunities.

General, Infect Dis, Pub Health

+1 763-291-1102

https://vfapp.org/6657

Uganda Spine Surgery Mission

Provides the best possible spine care to Ugandan patients afflicted by infectious, degenerative, traumatic, and congenital spinal ailments.

Ortho, Surg

https://vfapp.org/b413

Uganda Village Project

Facilitates community health and well-being in rural Uganda through improved access, education, and prevention.

General, Infect Dis, MF Med, OB-GYN, Surg

+1 860-748-5358

https://vfapp.org/76ac

Union for International Cancer Control (UICC)

Unites and supports the cancer community to reduce the global cancer burden, promote greater equity, and ensure that cancer control continues to be a priority in the world health and development agenda.

Heme-Onc, Pub Health

+41 22 809 18 11

https://vfapp.org/88b1

United Methodist Volunteers in Mission (UMVIM)

Engages in short-term missions each year in ministries as varied as disaster response, community development, pastor training, microenterprise, agriculture, Vacation Bible School, building repair and construction, and medical/dental services.

Dent-OMFS, ER Med, General

https://vfapp.org/1ee6

United Nations Children's Fund (UNICEF)

Works in over 190 countries and territories to save children's lives, to defend their rights, and to help them fulfill their potential, from early childhood through adolescence.

All-Immu, Infect Dis, MF Med, Neonat, Nutr, OB-GYN, Ped Surg, Peds, Pub Health

https://vfapp.org/42d7

United Nations Development Programme (UNDP)

Helps countries achieve the simultaneous eradication of extreme poverty and significant reduction of inequalities and exclusion using a sustainable human development approach.

Infect Dis, Logist-Op, Pub Health

https://vfapp.org/935c

United Nations High Commissioner for Refugees (UNHCR)

Safeguards the rights and well-being of people who have been forced to flee, ensuring that everybody has the right to seek asylum and find safe refuge in another country, with the goal of seeking lasting solutions.

General, MF Med, Medicine, OB-GYN, Peds, Psych, Pub Health

https://vfapp.org/6636

United Nations Population Fund (UNFPA)

Supports reproductive healthcare for women and youth in more than 150 countries, focusing on delivering a world where every pregnancy is wanted, every childbirth is safe, and every young person's potential is fulfilled.

Infect Dis, MF Med, Neonat, OB-GYN, Peds, Pub Health

+1 212-963-6008

https://vfapp.org/c969

United States Agency for International Development (USAID)

Promotes and demonstrates democratic values abroad and advances a free, peaceful, and prosperous world. Leads the U.S. government's international development and disaster assistance through partnerships and investments that save lives.

ER Med, Infect Dis, MF Med, OB-GYN, Peds

+1 202-712-0000

https://vfapp.org/9a99

United States President's Emergency Plan for AIDS Relief (PEPFAR)

The U.S. global HIV/AIDS response works to prevent new HIV infections and accelerate progress to control the global epidemic in more than 50 countries, by partnering with governments to support sustainable, integrated, and country-led responses to HIV/AIDS.

Infect Dis, Pub Health

https://vfapp.org/a57c

United Way

Aims to improve lives by mobilizing the caring power of communities around the world to advance the common good by fighting for the health, education, and financial stability of every person.

General, Infect Dis, Pub Health

+1 703-836-7112

https://vfapp.org/c812

University of California, San Francisco: Center for Global Surgery and Health Equity

Leads and supports academic global surgery, while strengthening surgical-care systems in low-resource settings through research and education.

Anesth, OB-GYN, Surg

+1 415-206-4352

https://vfapp.org/564f

University of California Los Angeles: David Geffen School of Medicine Global Health Program

Catalyzes opportunities to improve health globally by engaging in multi-disciplinary and innovative education programs, research initiatives, and bilateral partnerships that provide opportunities for trainees, faculty, and staff to contribute to sustainable health initiatives and to address health inequities facing the world today.

All-Immu, Infect Dis, Logist-Op, MF Med, Medicine, Neonat, OB-GYN, Ortho, Ped Surg, Peds, Radiol

+1 310-312-0531

https://vfapp.org/f1a4

University of California San Francisco: Institute for Global Health Sciences

Dedicates its efforts to improving health and reducing the burden of disease in the world's most vulnerable populations by integrating expertise in the health, social, and biological sciences to train global health leaders and develop solutions to the most pressing health challenges.

Infect Dis, OB-GYN, Pub Health

+1 415-476-5494

https://vfapp.org/6587

University of Colorado: Global Emergency Care Initiative

Strives to sustainably improve emergency care outcomes in low- and middle-income communities worldwide by linking cutting-edge academics with excellent on-the-ground implementation.

ER Med

https://vfapp.org/417a

University of Michigan Medical School Global REACH

Aims to facilitate health research, education, and collaboration among Michigan Medicine learners and faculty with our global partners to reduce health disparities for the benefit of communities worldwide.

ENT, General, Ophth-Opt, Peds, Psych, Pub Health, Urol

+1 734-615-5692

https://vfapp.org/5f19

University of Minnesota: Global Surgery & Disparities Program

Works to understand and improve surgical, anesthesia, and OBGYN care in underserved areas through partnerships with local providers, while training the next generation of academic global surgery leaders.

All-Immu, Dent-OMFS, ER Med, Heme-Onc, MF Med, Neurosurg, OB-GYN, Ophth-Opt, Path, Ped Surg, Plast, Surg, Urol

+1 612-626-1999

https://vfapp.org/e59a

University of New Mexico School of Medicine: Project Echo
Seeks to improve health outcomes worldwide through the use of a technology called telementoring, a guided-practice model in which the participating clinician retains responsibility for managing the patient.

General, Infect Dis, MF Med, OB-GYN, Path, Peds
+1 505-750-3246
https://vfapp.org/6c9a

University of Virginia: Anesthesiology Department Global Health Initiatives
Educates and trains physicians, to help people achieve healthy productive lives, and advances knowledge in the medical sciences.

Anesth, Pub Health
+1 434-924-2283
https://vfapp.org/1b8b

University of Washington: Department of Global Health
Improves health for all through research, education, training, and service, addresses the causes of disease and health inequities at multiple levels, and collaborates with partners to develop and sustain locally-led, quality health systems, programs and policies.

Infect Dis, Logist-Op, Pub Health
+1 206-616-1159
https://vfapp.org/f543

USAID: Maternal and Child Survival Program
Works to prevent child and maternal deaths.

Infect Dis, MF Med, Neonat, OB-GYN, Peds
https://vfapp.org/6fcf

USAID: A2Z The Micronutrient and Child Blindness Project
Aims to increase the use of key micronutrient and blindness interventions to improve child and maternal health.

MF Med, Neonat, Nutr, Ophth-Opt, Surg
+1 202-884-8785
https://vfapp.org/c5f1

USAID: EQUIP Health
Exists as an effective, efficient response mechanism to achieving global HIV epidemic control by delivering the right intervention at the right place and in the right way.

Infect Dis
+27 11 276 8850
https://vfapp.org/d76a

USAID: Human Resources for Health 2030 (HRH2030)
Helps low- and middle-income countries develop the health workforce needed to prevent maternal and child deaths, support the goals of Family Planning 2020, control the HIV/AIDS epidemic, and protect communities from infectious diseases.

Logist-Op
+1 202-955-3300
https://vfapp.org/9ea8

USAID: Leadership, Management and Governance Project
Improves leadership, management, and governance practices to strengthen health systems and improve health for all, including vulnerable populations worldwide.

Logist-Op
https://vfapp.org/d35e

USAID: Maternal and Child Health Integrated Program
Works to improve the health of women and their families, including programs for maternal, newborn, and child health, immunization, family planning, nutrition, malaria, and HIV/AIDS.

All-Immu, General, Infect Dis, MF Med
+1 202-835-3136
https://vfapp.org/4415

Vision Care
Restores sight and helps patients get regular treatment at short-term eye camps and long-term base clinics by having doctors, missionaries, volunteers, and sponsors work together.

Ophth-Opt
+1 212-769-3056
https://vfapp.org/9d7c

Vision for the Poor
Reduces human suffering and improves quality of life through the recovery of sight by building sustainable eye hospitals in developing countries, empowering local eye specialists, funding essential ophthalmic infrastructure, and partnering with like-minded agencies.

Ophth-Opt
+1 814-823-4486
https://vfapp.org/528e

Vital Strategies
Helps governments strengthen their public health systems to contend with the most important and difficult health challenges, while accelerating progress on the world's most pressing health problems.

CV Med, Infect Dis, Peds
+1 212-500-5720
https://vfapp.org/fe25

Vitamin Angels
Helps at-risk populations in need—specifically pregnant women, new mothers, and children under age five—to gain access to life-changing vitamins and minerals.

General, Nutr
+1 805-564-8400
https://vfapp.org/7da1

Voices for a Malaria-Free Future
Seeks to expand national movements of private and public sector leaders to mobilize political and popular support for malaria control.

Infect Dis, Path
https://vfapp.org/4213

Voluntary Service Overseas (VSO)
Works with health workers, communities, and governments to improve health services and rights for women, babies, youth, people with disabilities, and prisoners.

General, MF Med, OB-GYN
+44 20 8780 7500
https://vfapp.org/213d

Volunteering in Uganda
Constructs volunteer programs with purpose and focus on community development, education, healthcare, and childcare.

General, Peds
+256 39 2003218
https://vfapp.org/8414

VOSH (Volunteer Optometric Services to Humanity) International
Facilitates the provision and the sustainability of vision care worldwide for people who can neither afford nor obtain such care.
Ophth-Opt
https://vfapp.org/a149

Watsi
Uses technology to make healthcare a reality for those who might not otherwise be able to afford it.
Pub Health, Surg
+1 256-792-8747
https://vfapp.org/41a3

Waves of Health, The
Supports the primary healthcare needs of underserved communities and educates others about the medical challenges in the developing world.
ER Med, Infect Dis, Medicine
+1 973-771-6902
https://vfapp.org/63ff

WellShare International
Partners with diverse communities to promote health and well-being, to achieve equitable healthcare and resources where all individuals are able to live healthy and fulfilling lives.
Geri, MF Med, Nutr, Pulm-Critic
+1 612-871-3759
https://vfapp.org/2e9c

White Ribbon Alliance, The
Leads a movement for reproductive, maternal, and newborn health and accelerates progress by putting citizens at the center of global, national, and local health efforts.
MF Med, OB-GYN
+1 202-204-0324
https://vfapp.org/496b

Willing and Abel
Seeks to provide connections between children in developing nations and specialist centers, helping with visas, passports, transportation, and finances.
Anesth, Dent-OMFS, Ped Surg
https://vfapp.org/9dc7

Women and Children First
Pioneers approaches that support communities to solve problems themselves.
MF Med, Neonat, OB-GYN, Peds
+44 20 7700 6309
https://vfapp.org/cdc9

Women's Refugee Commission
Seeks to improve lives by protecting the rights of women, children, and youth displaced by conflict and crisis through researching their needs, identifying solutions, and advocating for programs and policies to strengthen their resilience.
General, MF Med, Neonat, OB-GYN, Peds, Psych
+1 212-551-3115
https://vfapp.org/3d8f

World Blind Union (WBU)
Represents those experiencing blindness, speaking to governments and international bodies on issues concerning visual impairments.
Ophth-Opt
https://vfapp.org/2bd3

World Children's Initiative (WCI)
Aims to improve and rebuild the healthcare and educational infrastructure for children in developing areas, both domestically and worldwide.
CV Med, Ped Surg, Surg
+1 408-554-4188
https://vfapp.org/9ca7

World Compassion Fellowship (WCF)
Serves the global poor and persecuted through relief, medical care, development, and training.
CV Med, ER Med, Endo, GI, General, Infect Dis, Medicine, Nutr, OB-GYN, Ortho, Peds, Psych, Pub Health, Rehab
+1 646-535-2344
https://vfapp.org/7b97

World Gospel Mission
Mobilizes volunteers to transform the world through healthcare, education, evangelism, and Christ.
ER Med, General
+1 765-664-7331
https://vfapp.org/efa4

World Health Organization, The (WHO)
The United Nations' agency for health provides leadership on global health matters, shapes the health research agenda, setting norms and standards, articulates evidence-based policy options, provides technical support and monitoring to countries, and assesses health trends.
ER Med, General, Infect Dis, Logist-Op, MF Med, OB-GYN, Peds, Psych, Pub Health
+41 22 791 21 11
https://vfapp.org/c476

World Medical Relief
Facilitates the distribution of surplus medical resources where they are needed.
Logist-Op
+1 313-866-5333
https://vfapp.org/72dc

World Vision International
Works with vulnerable communities around the world to overcome poverty and injustice with child-focused programs.
ER Med, General, Infect Dis, MF Med, Nutr, OB-GYN, Peds
+1 626-303-8811
https://vfapp.org/2642

Worldwide Fistula Fund
Protects and restores the health and dignity of the world's most vulnerable women by preventing and treating devastating childbirth injuries.
OB-GYN
+1 847-592-2438
https://vfapp.org/8813

Worldwide Healing Hands
Works to improve the quality of healthcare for women and children in the most underserved areas of the world and to stop the preventable deaths of mothers.

General, MF Med, Neonat, OB-GYN
+1 707-279-8733
https://vfapp.org/b331

Yale School of Medicine: Global Surgery Division

Addresses the rising worldwide surgical disease burden in low-resource settings both domestically and internationally by mobilizing a community of surgical leaders to engage in international partnerships, implement quality improvement and training protocols.

ER Med, Infect Dis, Medicine, Peds
+1 203-785-2844
https://vfapp.org/2bf7

YORGHAS Foundation

Supports mothers, pregnant women, infants, people with disabilities, and those suffering from humanitarian crises, poverty, or social inequalities, with particular emphasis on women's and children's rights.

MF Med, Neonat
+48 501 844 438
https://vfapp.org/9e44

Sources of Data for Country Introductions

"10 Most Censored Countries." Committee to Protect Journalists. Committee to Protect Journalists. Accessed October 22, 2020. https://cpj.org/reports/2019/09/10-most-censored-eritrea-north-korea-turkmenistan-journalist/#1.

"2014–2016 Ebola Outbreak in West Africa." Centers for Disease Control and Prevention. U.S. Department of Health & Human Services. Accessed October 22, 2020. https://www.cdc.gov/vhf/ebola/history/2014-2016-outbreak/index.html.

Adotevi, Stanislas Spero, et al. Britannica. Encyclopædia Britannica, Inc. Accessed October 23, 2020. https://www.britannica.com/place/Benin.

"Africa: Benin." The World Factbook. Central Intelligence Agency. October 21, 2020. https://www.cia.gov/library/publications/the-world-factbook/geos/bn.html.

"Africa: Burundi." The World Factbook. Central Intelligence Agency. October 21, 2020. https://www.cia.gov/library/publications/the-world-factbook/geos/by.html/.

"Africa: Central African Republic." The World Factbook. Central Intelligence Agency. October 6, 2020. https://www.cia.gov/library/publications/the-world-factbook/geos/ct.html.

"Africa: Chad." The World Factbook. Central Intelligence Agency. October 21, 2020. https://www.cia.gov/library/publications/the-world-factbook/geos/cd.html.

"Africa: Eritrea." The World Factbook. Central Intelligence Agency. October 21, 2020. https://www.cia.gov/library/publications/the-world-factbook/geos/er.html.

"Africa: Gambia, The." The World Factbook. Central Intelligence Agency. October 21, 2020. https://www.cia.gov/library/publications/the-world-factbook/geos/ga.html.

"Africa: Liberia." The World Factbook. Central Intelligence Agency. October 15, 2020. https://www.cia.gov/library/publications/the-world-factbook/geos/li.html.

"Africa: Malawi." The World Factbook. Central Intelligence Agency. October 9, 2020. https://www.cia.gov/library/publications/the-world-factbook/geos/mi.html.

"Africa: Niger." The World Factbook. Central Intelligence Agency. October 16, 2020. https://www.cia.gov/library/publications/the-world-factbook/geos/ng.html.

"Africa: Rwanda." Accessed October 23, 2020. https://www.cia.gov/library/publications/the-world-factbook/geos/print_rw.html.

"Africa: Sierra Leone." The World Factbook. Central Intelligence Agency. October 16, 2020. https://www.cia.gov/library/publications/the-world-factbook/geos/sl.html.

"Africa: Togo." The World Factbook. Central Intelligence Agency. October 16, 2020. https://www.cia.gov/library/publications/the-world-factbook/geos/to.html.

"Africa: Uganda." The World Factbook. Central Intelligence Agency. October 19, 2020. https://www.cia.gov/library/publications/the-world-factbook/geos/ug.html.

"An overview of Tanzania's political history." Oxford Business Group. Oxford Business Group. Accessed October 23, 2020. https://oxfordbusinessgroup.com/overview/clearing-hurdles-country-stable-political-ground.

"Annex 5. Tanzania." Accessed October 23, 2020. https://www.who.int/workforcealliance/knowledge/resources/MLHWCountryCaseStudies_annex5_Tanzania.pdf.

"Benin." IHME (Institute for Health Metrics and Evaluation). University of Washington. Accessed October 23, 2020. http://www.healthdata.org/benin/.

"Benin." Lonely Planet. Lonely Planet. Accessed October 23, 2020. https://www.lonelyplanet.com/benin.

"Benin." Nations Online. Nationsonline.org. Accessed October 23, 2020. https://www.nationsonline.org/oneworld/benin.htm.

"Benin." The World Bank. World Bank Group. Accessed October 23, 2020. https://data.worldbank.org/country/BJ/.

"Benin." World Factbook. February 2020. https://www.cia.gov/library/publications/resources/the-world-factbook/attachments/summaries/BN-summary.pdf.

"Benin – Airports." iExplore. iExplore. Accessed October 23, 2020. https://www.iexplore.com/articles/travel-guides/africa/benin/airports.

"Benin country profile." BBC. BBC. April 29, 2019. https://www.bbc.com/news/world-africa-13037572.

"Benin – History and Culture." iExplore. iExplore. Accessed October 23, 2020. https://www.iexplore.com/articles/travel-guides/africa/benin/history-and-culture.

"Burundi." IHME (Institute for Health Metrics and Evaluation). University of Washington. Accessed November 6, 2020. http://www.healthdata.org/burundi.

"Burundi." World Factbook. June 2020. https://www.cia.gov/library/publications/resources/the-world-factbook/attachments/summaries/BY-summary.pdf.

"Burundi: Control of corruption." TheGlobalEconomy.com. TheGlobalEconomy.com. Accessed October 23, 2020. https://www.theglobaleconomy.com/Burundi/wb_corruption/.

"Burundi: Political stability." TheGlobalEconomy.com. TheGlobalEconomy.com. Accessed October 23, 2020. https://www.theglobaleconomy.com/Burundi/wb_political_stability/.

"Burundi: Poverty ratio." TheGlobalEconomy.com. TheGlobalEconomy.com. Accessed October 23, 2020. https://www.theglobaleconomy.com/Burundi/poverty_ratio/.

Camera, Mohamed, and Yassima Camara. "The healthcare system in Africa: the case of Guinea." *International Journal of Community Medicine and Public Health* 2, no. 4 (January 2015): 685–689. https://www.researchgate.net/publication/283239841_The_healthcare_system_in_Africa_the_case_of_guinea.

"Case Counts." Centers for Disease Control and Prevention. U.S. Department of Health & Human Services. Accessed October 22, 2020. https://www.cdc.gov/vhf/ebola/history/2014-2016-outbreak/case-counts.html.

"CDC in Benin." Centers for Disease Control and Prevention. U.S. Department of Health and Human Services. Accessed October 23, 2020. https://www.cdc.gov/globalhealth/countries/benin/pdf/Benin_Factsheet.pdf.

"Central African Republic." International Crisis Group. International Crisis Group. Accessed October 15, 2020. https://www.crisisgroup.org/africa/central-africa/central-african-republic.

"Central African Republic." IHME (Institute for Health Metrics and Evaluation). University of Washington. Accessed November 6, 2020. http://www.healthdata.org/central-african-republic.

"Central African Republic." World Factbook. August 2020. https://www.cia.gov/library/publications/resources/the-world-factbook/attachments/summaries/CT-summary.pdf.

"Central African Republic." World Health Organization. World Health Organization. Accessed October 15, 2020. https://www.who.int/countries/caf/.

"Central African Republic: Life expectancy." TheGlobalEconomy.com. TheGlobalEconomy.com. Accessed October 15, 2020. https://www.theglobaleconomy.com/Central-African-Republic/Life_expectancy/.

"Chad." Global Health Workforce Alliance. WHO. Accessed October 22, 2020. https://www.who.int/workforcealliance/countries/tcd/en/.

"Chad." IHME (Institute for Health Metrics and Evaluation). University of Washington. Accessed November 6, 2020. http://www.healthdata.org/chad.

"Chad." UNHCR: The UN Refugee Agency. UNHCR: The UN Refugee Agency. Accessed October 22, 2020. https://reporting.unhcr.org/node/2533#_ga=2.96357343.270408414.1571428048-115620519.1571428048.

"Chad." United Nations World Food Programme. World Food Programme. Accessed October 22, 2020. https://www.wfp.org/countries/chad/.

"Chad." World Factbook. August 2020. https://www.cia.gov/library/publications/resources/the-world-factbook/attachments/summaries/CD-summary.pdf.

"Chad country profile." BBC. BBC. May 8, 2018. https://www.bbc.com/news/world-africa-13164686.

"Chad – History and Culture." iExplore. iExplore. Accessed October 22, 2020. https://www.iexplore.com/articles/travel-guides/africa/chad/history-and-culture.

"Chad travel guide." World Travel Guide. Columbus Travel Media Ltd. Accessed October 22, 2020. https://www.worldtravelguide.net/guides/africa/chad/.

Clay, Daniel, et al. "Rwanda." Britannica. Encyclopædia Britannica, Inc. Accessed October 23, 2020. https://www.britannica.com/place/Rwanda.

"Congo, Dem. Rep." The World Bank. World Bank Group. Accessed October 22, 2020. https://data.worldbank.org/country/congo-dem-rep.

"Culture." Embassy of the Republic of Malawi in the United States. Embassy of the Republic of Malawi. Accessed October 22, 2020. http://www.malawiembassy-dc.org/page/culture.

"Democratic Republic of the Congo." World Factbook. April 2020. https://www.cia.gov/library/publications/resources/the-world-factbook/attachments/summaries/CG-summary.pdf.

"Democratic Republic of the Congo." IHME (Institute for Health Metrics and Evaluation). University of Washington. Accessed November 6, 2020. http://www.healthdata.org/democratic-republic-congo.

"Democratic Republic of Congo in Detail: Flights & getting there." Lonely Planet. Lonely Planet. Accessed October 22, 2020. https://www.lonelyplanet.com/democratic-republic-of-congo/narratives/practical-information/transport/getting-there-away.

"Ebola virus disease." World Health Organization. World Health Organization. February 10, 2020. https://www.who.int/news-room/fact-sheets/detail/ebola-virus-disease.

Echenberg, Myron. "Togo." Britannica. Encyclopædia Britannica, Inc. Accessed October 23, 2020. https://www.britannica.com/place/Togo.

Eggers, Ellen Kahan, et al. Britannica. Encyclopædia Britannica, Inc. Accessed October 23, 2020. https://www.britannica.com/place/Burundi.

"Eritrea." Global Health Workforce Alliance. WHO. Accessed October 22, 2020. https://www.who.int/workforcealliance/countries/eri/en/.

"Eritrea." IHME (Institute for Health Metrics and Evaluation). University of Washington. Accessed November 6, 2020. http://www.healthdata.org/eritrea.

"Eritrea." Lonely Planet. Lonely Planet. Accessed October 22, 2020. https://www.lonelyplanet.com/eritrea.

"Eritrea." World Factbook. August 2020. https://www.cia.gov/library/publications/resources/the-world-factbook/attachments/summaries/ER-summary.pdf.

"Eritrea country profile." BBC. BBC. November 15, 2018. https://www.bbc.com/news/world-africa-13349078.

"Eritrea profile - Timeline." BBC. BBC. November 15, 2018. https://www.bbc.com/news/world-africa-13349395.

"Ethiopia." IHME (Institute for Health Metrics and Evaluation). University of Washington. Accessed November 6, 2020. http://www.healthdata.org/ethiopia.

"Ethiopia." World Health Organization. WHO. Accessed October 22, 2020. https://www.who.int/hac/donorinfo/callsformobilisation/eth/en/.

"Field Listing: Population." The World Factbook. Central Intelligence Agency. Accessed October 25, 2020. https://www.cia.gov/library/publications/resources/the-world-factbook/fields/335.html#GA.

Fuglestad, Finn, et al. "Niger." Britannica. Encyclopædia Britannica, Inc. Accessed October 23, 2020. https://www.britannica.com/place/Niger.

Gailey, Harry A., et al. "The Gambia." Britannica. Encyclopædia Britannica, Inc. Accessed October 22, 2020. https://www.britannica.com/place/The-Gambia.

Galli, Rosemary Elizabeth, et al. "Guinea-Bissau." Britannica. Encyclopædia Britannica, Inc. September 9, 2020. https://www.britannica.com/place/Guinea-Bissau.

"Gambia." IHME (Institute for Health Metrics and Evaluation). University of Washington. Accessed October 22, 2020. http://www.healthdata.org/gambia.

"Gambia." United Nations World Food Programme. World Food Programme. Accessed October 22, 2020. https://www.wfp.org/countries/gambia#:~:text=The%20Gambia's%20poverty%20rate%20remains,leading%20a%20food%20security%20emergency.

"Gambia: Political stability." TheGlobalEconomy.com. TheGlobalEconomy.com. Accessed October 22, 2020. https://www.theglobaleconomy.com/Gambia/wb_political_stability/.

"Gambia, The." The World Bank. World Bank Group. Accessed October 22, 2020. https://data.worldbank.org/country/gambia-the.

"Getting Around Benin." World Travel Guide. Columbus Travel Media Ltd. Accessed October 23, 2020. https://www.worldtravelguide.net/guides/africa/benin/getting-around/.

"GDP per capita (current US$)." The World Bank. The World Bank Group. Accessed October 25, 2020. https://data.worldbank.org/indicator/NY.GDP.PCAP.CD.

"Getting Around Burundi." World Travel Guide. Columbus Travel Media Ltd. Accessed October 23, 2020. https://www.worldtravelguide.net/guides/africa/burundi/getting-around/

"Getting Around." Malawi: The Warm Heart of Africa. Malawi Travel Marketing Consortium. Accessed October 22, 2020. https://www.malawitourism.com/getting-around/.

"Getting Around Chad." World Travel Guide. Columbus Travel Media Ltd. Accessed October 22, 2020. https://www.worldtravelguide.net/guides/africa/chad/getting-around/.

"Getting Around Eritrea." World Travel Guide. Columbus Travel Media Ltd. Accessed October 22, 2020. https://www.worldtravelguide.net/guides/africa/eritrea/getting-around/.

"Getting Around Haiti." World Travel Guide. Columbus Travel Media Ltd. Accessed October 22, 2020. https://www.worldtravelguide.net/guides/caribbean/haiti/getting-around/.

"Getting Around Uganda." World Travel Guide. Columbus Travel Media Ltd. Accessed October 23, 2020. https://www.worldtravelguide.net/guides/africa/uganda/getting-around/.

"Getting There." Malawi: The Warm Heart of Africa. Malawi Travel Marketing Consortium. Accessed October 22, 2020. https://www.malawitourism.com/getting-there/.

"Global Health." USAID. USAID. Accessed October 23, 2020. https://www.usaid.gov/burundi/global-health#:~:text=Burundi's%20health%20system%20suffers%20from,health%2C%20and%20strengthen%20health%20systems.

"Global Health – Guinea." Centers for Disease Control and Prevention. U.S. Department of Health & Human Services. June 4, 2019.

"Global Health – Liberia." Centers for Disease Control and Prevention. U.S. Department of Health & Human Services. Accessed October 22, 2020. https://www.cdc.gov/globalhealth/countries/liberia/default.htm.

Grove, Alfred Thomas, et al. "Chad." Britannica. Encyclopædia Britannica, Inc. Accessed October 22, 2020. https://www.britannica.com/place/Chad.

Guerreiro, Cátia Sá, Augusto Paulo Silva, Tomé Cá, and Paulo Ferrinho. "Strategic planning in Guiné-Bissau's health sector: evolution, influences and process." Anais do IHMT. An Inst Hig MedTrop 2017, 16 (Supl. 1): S55–S68. https://research.unl.pt/ws/portalfiles/portal/4168743/Planeamento_estrat_gico_no_setor_da_sa_de.pdf.

"Guinea." IHME (Institute for Health Metrics and Evaluation). University of Washington. Accessed November 6, 2020. http://www.healthdata.org/guinea.

"Guinea." World Health Organization. World Health Organization. Accessed October 22, 2020. https://www.who.int/countries/gin/.

"Guinea-Bissau." IHME (Institute for Health Metrics and Evaluation). University of Washington. Accessed October 22, 2020. http://www.healthdata.org/guinea-bissau.

"Guinea-Bissau." The World Bank. The World Bank Group. Accessed October 22, 2020. https://data.worldbank.org/country/guinea-bissau.

"Guinea History, Language and Culture." World Travel Guide. Columbus Travel Media Ltd. Accessed October 22, 2020. https://www.worldtravelguide.net/guides/africa/guinea/history-language-culture/.

"Guinea: Poverty ratio." TheGlobalEconomy.com. TheGlobalEconomy.com. Accessed October 22, 2020. https://www.theglobaleconomy.com/Guinea/poverty_ratio/.

"Guinea profile – Timeline." BBC. BBC. May 14, 2018. https://www.bbc.com/news/world-africa-13443183.

"Gunneweg@TheHealthFactory." Gunneweg@TheHealthFactory. THE HEALTH FACTORY:

Health System Strengthening & Governance and Decentralised Health Management. Accessed October 23, 2020. https://www.gunneweg-thehealthfactory.nl/.

Habtom, Gebremichael Kibreab. "Designing innovative pro-poor healthcare financing system in sub-Saharan Africa: The case of Eritrea." *Journal of Public Administration and Policy Research* 9, no. 4 (May 18, 2017): 51–67. https://academicjournals.org/journal/JPAPR/article-full-text-pdf/9B68E9D65935.

"Haiti." Health in the Americas. Pan American Health Organization. Accessed October 22, 2020. https://www.paho.org/salud-en-las-americas-2017/?p=4110#:~:text=The%20health%20care%20delivery%20system,specialized%20centers%20provide%20tertiary%20care.

"Haiti." IHME (Institute for Health Metrics and Evaluation). University of Washington. Accessed October 22, 2020. http://www.healthdata.org/haiti.

"Haiti country profile." BBC. BBC. February 11, 2019. https://www.bbc.com/news/world-latin-america-19548810.

"Haiti: Country profile." World Health Organization. World Health Organization. Accessed October 22, 2020. https://www.who.int/hac/crises/hti/background/profile/en/.

Hibbett, Kristen. "Addressing the Barriers to Proper Health Care in Ethiopia." The Borgen Project. The Borgen Project. June 1, 2018. https://borgenproject.org/addressing-the-barriers-to-proper-health-care-in-ethiopia/.

"Hospital beds (per 10 000 population)." World Health Organization. World Health Organization. Accessed October 25, 2020. https://www.who.int/data/gho/data/indicators/indicator-details/GHO/hospital-beds-(per-10-000-population).

"Human Capital Index and Components, 2018." The World Bank. The World Bank Group. October 18, 2018. https://www.worldbank.org/en/data/interactive/2018/10/18/human-capital-index-and-components-2018.

"Human Development Reports." United Nations Development Programme. United Nations Development Programme. Accessed October 22, 2020. http://hdr.undp.org/en/composite/HDI.

Ingham, Kenneth. "Malawi." Encyclopædia Britannica, Inc. Accessed October 22, 2020. https://www.britannica.com/place/Malawi.

Jones, Abeodu Bowen, et al. "Liberia." Encyclopædia Britannica, Inc. Accessed October 22, 2020. https://www.britannica.com/place/Liberia.

Lawless, Robert, et al. "Haiti." Britannica. Encyclopædia Britannica, Inc. Accessed October 22, 2020. https://www.britannica.com/place/Haiti.

"Least Developed Country Category: Niger Profile." United Nations: Department of Economic and Social Affairs. United Nations. 2018. Accessed October 23, 2020. https://www.un.org/development/desa/dpad/least-developed-country-category-niger.html.

"Liberia." IHME (Institute for Health Metrics and Evaluation). University of Washington. Accessed October 6, 2020. http://www.healthdata.org/liberia.

"Liberia." Travel.State.Gov. U.S. Department of State. Accessed October 22, 2020. https://travel.state.gov/content/travel/en/international-travel/International-Travel-Country-Information-Pages/Liberia.html.

"Liberia country profile." BBC. BBC. January 22, 2018. https://www.bbc.com/news/world-africa-13729504.

"Liberia: Life Expectancy." TheGlobalEconomy.com. TheGlobalEconomy.com. Accessed October 22, 2020. https://www.theglobaleconomy.com/Liberia/Life_expectancy/.

"Liberia: Political stability." TheGlobalEconomy.com. TheGlobalEconomy.com. Accessed October 22, 2020. https://www.theglobaleconomy.com/Liberia/wb_political_stability/#:~:text=Liberia%3A%20Political%20stability%20index%20(%2D2.5%20weak%3B%202.5%20strong)&text=For%20comparison%2C%20the%20world%20average,195%20countries%20is%20%2D0.05%20points.&text=The%20index%20is%20an%20average,Political%20Risk%20Services%2C%20among%20others.

"Liberia: Poverty ratio." TheGlobalEconomy.com. TheGlobalEconomy.com. Accessed October 22, 2020. https://www.theglobaleconomy.com/Liberia/poverty_ratio/.

"Liberia profile – Timeline." BBC. BBC. January 22, 2018. https://www.bbc.com/news/world-africa-13732188.

"Life expectancy at birth, total (years)." The World Bank. The World Bank Group. Accessed October 25, 2020. https://data.worldbank.org/indicator/SP.DYN.LE00.IN.

"Life expectancy at birth, total (years) – Rwanda." The World Bank. The World Bank Group. Accessed October 23, 2020. https://data.worldbank.org/indicator/SP.DYN.LE00.IN?locations=RW.

"Life expectancy at birth, total (years) – Togo." The World Bank. The World Bank Group. Accessed October 23, 2020. https://data.worldbank.org/indicator/SP.DYN.LE00.IN?locations=TG.

"Life expectancy at birth, total (years) – Uganda." The World Bank. The World Bank Group. Accessed October 23, 2020. https://data.worldbank.org/indicator/SP.DYN.LE00.IN?locations=UG.

"Life Expectancy of the World Population." Worldometer. Worldometer. Accessed October 22, 2020. https://www.worldometers.info/demographics/life-expectancy/.

Lyons, Maryinez. "Uganda." Britannica. Encyclopædia Britannica, Inc. September 8, 2020. https://www.britannica.com/place/Uganda.

Mackenzie, Lindsay. "WHO warns against potential Ebola spread in DR Congo and beyond." UN News. United Nations. September 11, 2020. https://news.un.org/en/story/2020/09/1072152/.

"Madagascar." IHME (Institute for Health Metrics and Evaluation). University of Washington. Accessed October 22, 2020. http://www.healthdata.org/madagascar.

"Madagascar." The World Bank. The World Bank Group. Accessed October 22, 2020. https://data.worldbank.org/country/madagascar.

"Madagascar country profile." BBC. BBC. November 15, 2019. https://www.bbc.com/news/world-africa-13861843.

"Madagascar: GDP, constant dollars." TheGlobalEconomy.com. TheGlobalEconomy.com. Accessed October 22, 2020. https://www.theglobaleconomy.com/Madagascar/GDP_constant_dollars/.

"Madagascar: Poverty ratio." TheGlobalEconomy.com. TheGlobalEconomy.com. Accessed October 22, 2020. https://www.theglobaleconomy.com/Madagascar/poverty_ratio/.

"Malawi." IHME (Institute for Health Metrics and Evaluation). University of Washington. Accessed October 22, 2020. http://www.healthdata.org/malawi.

"Malawi Government." Malawi Government. Government of the Republic of Malawi. 2013. Accessed October 22, 2020. https://www.malawi.gov.mw/.

"Malawi: Life expectancy." TheGlobalEconomy.com. TheGlobalEconomy.com. Accessed October 22, 2020. https://www.theglobaleconomy.com/Malawi/Life_expectancy/.

"Malawi: Political stability." TheGlobalEconomy.com. TheGlobalEconomy.com. Accessed October 22, 2020. https://www.theglobaleconomy.com/Malawi/wb_political_stability/.

"Malawi: Poverty ratio." TheGlobalEconomy.com. TheGlobalEconomy.com. Accessed October 22, 2020. https://www.theglobaleconomy.com/Malawi/poverty_ratio/.

Markakis, John, et al. "Eritrea." Britannica. Encyclopædia Britannica, Inc. September 12, 2020. https://www.britannica.com/place/Eritrea.

Mascarenhas, Adolfo C., et al. "Tanzania." Britannica. Encyclopædia Britannica, Inc. September 8, 2020. https://www.britannica.com/place/Tanzania.

"Maternal mortality ratio (modeled estimate, per 100,000 live births) – Benin." The World Bank. The World Bank Group. Accessed October 25, 2020. https://data.worldbank.org/indicator/SH.STA.MMRT?locations=BJ.

"Measles – Madagascar." World Health Organization. World Health Organization. January 17, 2019. https://www.who.int/csr/don/17-january-2019-measles-madagascar/en/.

"Medical doctors (per 10 000 population)." World Health Organization. World Health Organization. Accessed October 25, 2020. https://www.who.int/data/gho/data/indicators/indicator-details/GHO/medical-doctors-(per-10-000-population).

"Mozambique." IHME (Institute for Health Metrics and Evaluation). University of Washington. Accessed October 22, 2020. http://www.healthdata.org/mozambique.

"Mozambique." The World Bank. The World Bank Group. Accessed October 22, 2020. https://data.worldbank.org/country/mozambique.

"Mozambique." World Health Organization. World Health Organization. Accessed October 22, 2020. https://www.who.int/countries/moz/areas/health_system/en/index1.html.

"Mozambique: GDP, constant dollars." TheGlobalEconomy.com. TheGlobalEconomy.com. Accessed October 22, 2020. https://www.theglobaleconomy.com/Mozambique/GDP_constant_dollars/.

"Mozambique: Is Cabo Delgado the latest Islamic State outpost?" BBC. BBC. May 4. Accessed October 22, 2020. https://www.bbc.com/news/world-africa-52532741.

Mudge, Lewis. "Central African Republic Events of 2018." Human Rights Watch. Human Rights Watch. 2018. https://www.hrw.org/world-report/2019/country-chapters/central-african-republic#.

"Nepal." IHME (Institute for Health Metrics and Evaluation). University of Washington. Accessed November 6, 2020. http://www.healthdata.org/nepal.

"Niger." IHME (Institute for Health Metrics and Evaluation). University of Washington. Accessed October 23, 2020. http://www.healthdata.org/niger.

"Niger." UNESCO. UNESCO Institute of Statistics. Accessed October 23, 2020. http://uis.unesco.org/en/country/ne.

"Niger country profile." BBC. BBC. February 19, 2018. https://www.bbc.com/news/world-africa-13943662.

"Niger: Nutrition Profile." USAID. USAID. February 2018. Accessed October 23, 2020. https://www.usaid.gov/sites/default/files/documents/1864/Niger-Nutrition-Profile-Mar2018-508.pdf.

"Niger slavery: Background." The Guardian. Guardian News & Media Limited. October 27, 2008. https://www.theguardian.com/world/2008/oct/27/humanrights1.

"Niger 2020 Crime & Safety Report." OSAC. Overseas Security Advisory Council, Bureau of Diplomatic Security, U.S. Department of State. April 16, 2020. https://www.osac.gov/Country/Niger/Content/Detail/Report/bfb3f35d-08e2-4008-ab52-18760b02138a.

Ntembwa, Hyppolite Kalambay and Wim Van Lerberghe. "Improving Health System Efficiency: Democratic Republic of the Congo improving aid coordination in the health sector."

Health Systems Governance & Financing. World Health Organization. 2015. https://apps.who.int/iris/bitstream/handle/10665/186673/WHO_HIS_HGF_CaseStudy_15.4_eng.pdf?sequence=1.

O'Toole, Thomas E. "Guinea." Britannica. Encyclopædia Britannica, Inc. September 9, 2020. https://www.britannica.com/place/Guinea.

Pape, Utz and Arden Finn. "How conflict and economic crises exacerbate poverty in South Sudan." World Bank Blogs. World Bank Group. April 23, 2019. https://blogs.worldbank.org/africacan/how-conflict-and-economic-crises-exacerbate-poverty-in-south-sudan.

Payanzo, Ntsomo, et al. "Democratic Republic of the Congo." Britannica. Encyclopædia Britannica, Inc. Accessed October 22, 2020. https://www.britannica.com/place/Democratic-Republic-of-the-Congo.

"Population, total – Tanzania." The World Bank. The World Bank Group. Accessed October 23, 2020. https://data.worldbank.org/indicator/SP.POP.TOTL?locations=TZ.

Roser, Max, Esteban Ortiz-Ospina, and Hannah Ritchie. "Life Expectancy." Our World in Data. Global Change Data Lab. October 2019. Accessed October 23, 2020. https://ourworldindata.org/life-expectancy#:~:text=The%20inequality%20of%20life%20expectancy,expectancy%20is%2030%20years%20longer.

"Rwanda." IHME (Institute for Health Metrics and Evaluation). University of Washington. Accessed October 23, 2020. http://www.healthdata.org/rwanda.

"Rwanda." PMI: President's Malaria Initiative Fighting Malaria and Saving Lives. U.S. President's Malaria Initiative. 2018. Accessed October 23, 2020. https://www.pmi.gov/docs/default-source/default-document-library/country-profiles/rwanda_profile.pdf?sfvrsn=26.

"Rwanda: Political stability." TheGlobalEconomy.com. TheGlobalEconomy.com. Accessed October 23, 2020. https://www.theglobaleconomy.com/Rwanda/wb_political_stability/.

"Rwanda travel guide." World Travel Guide. Columbus Travel Media Ltd. Accessed October 23, 2020. https://www.worldtravelguide.net/guides/africa/rwanda/.

Sesay, Shekou M. "Sierra Leone." Britannica. Encyclopædia Britannica, Inc. Accessed October 23, 2020. https://www.britannica.com/place/Sierra-Leone.

Sheldon, Kathleen Eddy, et al. "Mozambique." Britannica. Encyclopædia Britannica, Inc. Accessed October 22, 2020. https://www.britannica.com/place/Mozambique.

"Sierra Leone." IHME (Institute for Health Metrics and Evaluation). University of Washington. Accessed October 23, 2020. http://www.healthdata.org/sierra-leone.

"Sierra Leone." World Health Organization. World Health Organization. Accessed October 23, 2020. https://www.who.int/countries/sle/.

"Sierra Leone country profile." BBC. BBC. April 5, 2018. https://www.bbc.com/news/world-africa-14094194.

"Sierra Leone: Economic growth." TheGlobalEconomy.com. TheGlobalEconomy.com. Accessed October 23, 2020. https://www.theglobaleconomy.com/Sierra-Leone/Economic_growth/.

"Sierra Leone: Life expectancy." TheGlobalEconomy.com. TheGlobalEconomy.com. Accessed October 23, 2020. https://www.theglobaleconomy.com/Sierra-Leone/Life_expectancy/.

"South Sudan." Global Health Workforce Alliance. WHO. Accessed October 23, 2020. https://www.who.int/workforcealliance/countries/ssd/en/.

"South Sudan." IHME (Institute for Health Metrics and Evaluation). University of Washington. Accessed October 23, 2020. http://www.healthdata.org/south-sudan.

"South Sudan." World Health Organization. World Health Organization. Accessed October 23, 2020. https://www.who.int/countries/ssd/.

"South Sudan country profile." BBC. BBC. August 6, 2018. https://www.bbc.com/news/world-africa-14069082.

Southall, Aidan William, et al. "Madagascar." Britannica. Encyclopædia Britannica, Inc. September 9, 2020. https://www.britannica.com/place/Madagascar.

Spaulding, Jay L., et al. "South Sudan." Britannica. Encyclopædia Britannica, Inc. Accessed October 23, 2020. https://www.britannica.com/place/South-Sudan.

"Strengthening Maternal and Child Health Service Delivery in Guinea-Bissau." The World Bank. The World Bank. June 13, 2017. 1–13. http://documents1.worldbank.org/curated/pt/753341512739828724/pdf/Concept-Project-Information-Document-Integrated-Safeguards-Data-Sheet.pdf.

"Tajikistan." IHME (Institute for Health Metrics and Evaluation). University of Washington. Accessed November 6, 2020. http://www.healthdata.org/tajikistan.

"Tajikistan profile – Timeline." BBC. BBC. July 31, 2018. https://www.bbc.com/news/world-asia-16201087.

"Tanzania." IHME (Institute for Health Metrics and Evaluation). University of Washington. Accessed November 6, 2020. http://www.healthdata.org/tanzania.

"The 1 largest airports and airlines in Burundi." WorldData.info. WorldData.info. Accessed October 23, 2020. https://www.worlddata.info/africa/burundi/airports.php. "The biggest airports in Liberia." WorldData.info. WorldData.info. Accessed October 22, 2020. https://www.worlddata.info/africa/liberia/airports.php.

"The Gambia." Lonely Planet. Lonely Planet. Accessed October 22, 2020. https://www.lonelyplanet.com/the-gambia.

"The World Bank In Benin." The World Bank. World Bank Group. Accessed October 23, 2020. https://www.worldbank.org/en/country/benin/overview.

"The World Bank In Burundi." The World Bank. World Bank Group. Accessed October 23, 2020. https://www.worldbank.org/en/country/burundi/overview.

"The World Bank in Central African Republic." The World Bank. World Bank Group. Accessed October 15, 2020. https://www.worldbank.org/en/country/centralafricanrepublic/overview.

"The World Bank in Chad." The World Bank. World Bank Group. Accessed October 22, 2020. https://www.worldbank.org/en/country/chad/overview.

"The World Bank in DRC." The World Bank. World Bank Group. Accessed October 22, 2020. https://www.worldbank.org/en/country/drc/overview.

"The World Bank in Eritrea." The World Bank. World Bank Group. Accessed October 22, 2020. https://www.worldbank.org/en/country/eritrea/overview.

"The World Bank in The Gambia." The World Bank. World Bank Group. Accessed October 22, 2020. https://www.worldbank.org/en/country/gambia/overview.

"The World Bank in Guinea. The World Bank. World Bank Group. Accessed October 22, 2020. https://www.worldbank.org/en/country/guinea/overview.

"The World Bank in Guinea-Bissau." The World Bank. World Bank Group. Accessed October 22, 2020. https://www.worldbank.org/en/country/guineabissau/overview.

"The World Bank in Haiti." The World Bank. World Bank Group. Accessed October 22, 2020. https://www.worldbank.org/en/country/haiti/overview.

"The World Bank in Madagascar." The World Bank. World Bank Group. Accessed October

22, 2020. https://www.worldbank.org/en/country/madagascar/overview.

"The World Bank in Malawi." The World Bank. World Bank Group. Accessed October

22, 2020. https://www.worldbank.org/en/country/malawi/overview.

"The World Bank in Mozambique." The World Bank. World Bank Group. Accessed October

22, 2020. https://www.worldbank.org/en/country/mozambique/overview#1.

"The World Bank in Niger." The World Bank. World Bank Group. Accessed October

23, 2020. https://www.worldbank.org/en/country/niger/overview.

"The World Bank in Rwanda." The World Bank. World Bank Group. Accessed October

23, 2020. https://www.worldbank.org/en/country/rwanda/overview.

"The World Bank in Sierra Leone." The World Bank. World Bank Group. Accessed October

23, 2020. https://www.worldbank.org/en/country/sierraleone/overview.

"The World Bank in South Sudan." The World Bank. World Bank Group. Accessed October

23, 2020. https://www.worldbank.org/en/country/southsudan/overview.

"The World Bank in Tajikistan." The World Bank. World Bank Group. Accessed October

23, 2020. https://www.worldbank.org/en/country/tajikistan/overview#1.

"The World Bank in Togo." The World Bank. World Bank Group. Accessed October

23, 2020. https://www.worldbank.org/en/country/togo/overview.

"The World Bank in Uganda." The World Bank. World Bank Group. Accessed October

23, 2020. https://www.worldbank.org/en/country/uganda/overview.

"Togo country profile." BBC. BBC. February 24. Accessed October 23, 2020. https://www.bbc.com/news/world-africa-14106781.

"Togo 2020 Crime & Safety Report." OSAC. Overseas Security Advisory Council, Bureau of

Diplomatic Security, U.S. Department of State. April 9, 2020. https://www.osac.gov/Country/Togo/Content/Detail/Report/1afba1d9-f4a6-414b-b1e1-1867c0edd3f3.

"Togo." IHME (Institute for Health Metrics and Evaluation). University of

Washington. Accessed October 23, 2020. http://www.healthdata.org/togo.

"Travel to Haiti." World Travel Guide. Columbus Travel Media Ltd. Accessed October

22, 2020. https://www.worldtravelguide.net/guides/caribbean/haiti/travel-by/.

"Travel to Mozambique." World Travel Guide. Columbus Travel Media Ltd. Accessed October

22, 2020. https://www.worldtravelguide.net/guides/africa/mozambique/travel-by/.

"Travel to Niger." World Travel Guide. Columbus Travel Media Ltd. Accessed October 23, 2020. https://www.worldtravelguide.net/guides/africa/niger/travel-by/.

"Travel to Uganda." World Travel Guide. Columbus Travel Media Ltd. Accessed October 23, 2020. https://www.worldtravelguide.net/guides/africa/uganda/travel-by/.

"Uganda." IHME (Institute for Health Metrics and Evaluation). University of Washington. Accessed October 23, 2020. http://www.healthdata.org/uganda.

"Uganda country profile." BBC. BBC. May 10, 2018. https://www.bbc.com/news/world-africa-14107906.

"UN list of Least Developed Countries." UNCTAD. United Nations Conference on Trade and Development. Accessed October 15, 2020. https://unctad.org/topic/vulnerable-economies/least-developed-countries/list.

"UNICEF Sierra Leone." UNICEF Sierra Leone. UNICEF. Accessed October 23, 2020. https://www.unicef.org/sierraleone/#:~:text=With%201%2C360%20mothers%20dying%20per,of%20death%20associated%20to%20childbirth.

"United Republic of Tanzania." IHME (Institute for Health Metrics and Evaluation). University of Washington. Accessed October 23, 2020. http://www.healthdata.org/tanzania.

Van Hoogstraten, Jan S.F, et al. "Central African Republic." Britannica. Encyclopædia Britannica, Inc. Accessed October 15, 2020. https://www.britannica.com/place/Central-African-Republic.

"Welcome to Rwanda." Republic of Rwanda. Republic of Rwanda. Accessed October 23, 2020. https://www.gov.rw/.

Index

For Product Safety Concerns and Information please contact our EU representative GPSR@taylorandfrancis.com Taylor & Francis Verlag GmbH, Kaufingerstraße 24, 80331 München, Germany

Batch number: 10777152

Printed by Printforce, the Netherlands